Essentials of Nursing Leadership & Management

Third Edition

Essentials of Nursing Leadership & Management

Third Edition

Patricia Kelly
Professor Emeritus
Purdue University Calumet
School of Nursing
Hammond, Indiana
Consultant
Chicago, Illinois and Fort Myers, Florida

Janice Tazbir
Professor
Purdue University Calumet
School of Nursing
Hammond, Indiana

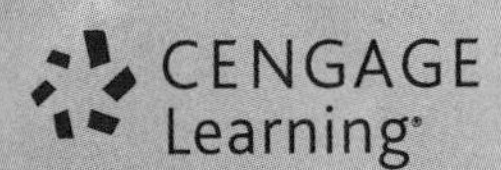

Australia • Brazil • Japan • Korea • Mexico • Singapore • Spain • United Kingdom • United States

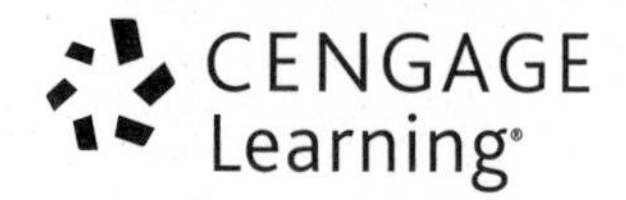

Essentials of Nursing Leadership & Management, Third Edition
Patricia Kelly, Janice Tazbir

Vice President, Careers & Computing: Dave Garza

Publisher, Health Care: Stephen Helba

Director, Development-Careers & Computing: Marah Bellegarde

Executive Editor: Maureen Rosener

Product Development Manager, Careers: Juliet Steiner

Senior Product Manager: Elisabeth Williams

Editorial Assistant: Jennifer Wheaton

Brand Manager: Wendy Mapstone

Market Development Manager: Nancy Bradshaw

Senior Production Director: Wendy A. Troeger

Production Manager: Andrew Crouth

Senior Content Project Manager: Kara A. DiCaterino

Senior Art Director: Jack Pendleton

Cover Image: www.Shutterstock.com

© 2014, 2010, 2004 Delmar, Cengage Learning

ALL RIGHTS RESERVED. No part of this work covered by the copyright herein may be reproduced, transmitted, stored, or used in any form or by any means graphic, electronic, or mechanical, including but not limited to photocopying, recording, scanning, digitizing, taping, Web distribution, information networks, or information storage and retrieval systems, except as permitted under Section 107 or 108 of the 1976 United States Copyright Act, without the prior written permission of the publisher.

For product information and technology assistance, contact us at
Professional & Career Group Customer Support, 1-800-648-7450
For permission to use material from this text or product, submit all requests online at **cengage.com/permissions.**
Further permissions questions can be e-mailed to
permissionrequest@cengage.com

Library of Congress Control Number: 2012953798

ISBN-13: 978-1-133-93558-2

ISBN-10: 1-133-93558-3

Delmar
5 Maxwell Drive
Clifton Park, NY 12065-2919
USA

Cengage Learning products are represented in Canada by Nelson Education, Ltd.

For your lifelong learning solutions, visit **delmar.cengage.com**

Visit our corporate website at **cengage.com**

Notice to the Reader
Publisher does not warrant or guarantee any of the products described herein or perform any independent analysis in connection with any of the product information contained herein. Publisher does not assume, and expressly disclaims, any obligation to obtain and include information other than that provided to it by the manufacturer. The reader is expressly warned to consider and adopt all safety precautions that might be indicated by the activities described herein and to avoid all potential hazards. By following the instructions contained herein, the reader willingly assumes all risks in connection with such instructions. The publisher makes no representations or warranties of any kind, including but not limited to, the warranties of fitness for particular purpose or merchantability, nor are any such representations implied with respect to the material set forth herein, and the publisher takes no responsibility with respect to such material. The publisher shall not be liable for any special, consequential, or exemplary damages resulting, in whole or part, from the readers' use of, or reliance upon, this material.

Printed in the United States of America
1 2 3 4 5 6 7 17 16 15 14 13

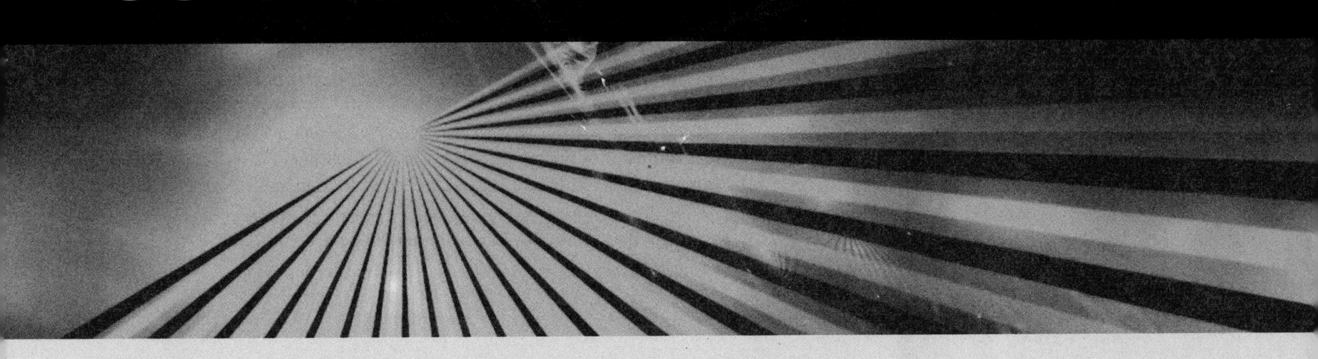

CONTENTS

PREFACE

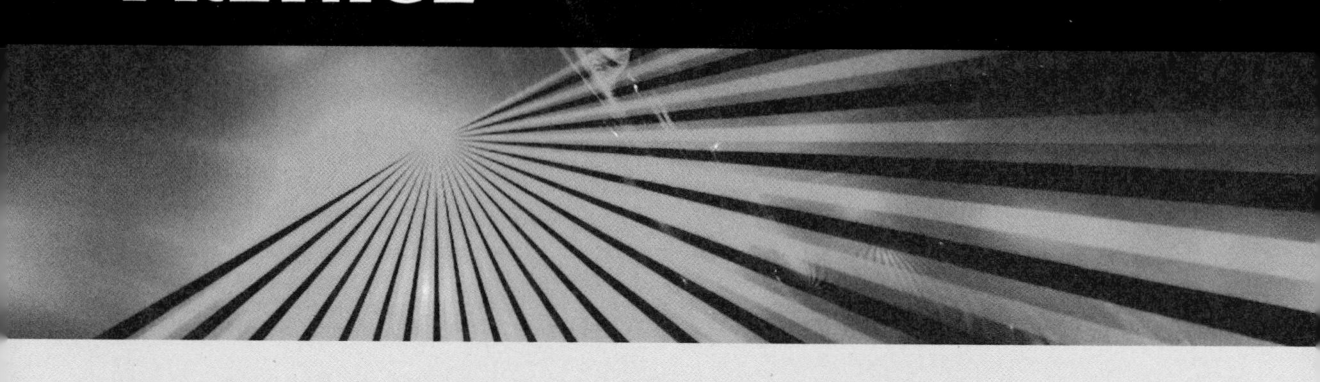

Health care is changing more rapidly than ever. Nurses, as the largest group in the health care workforce, are the champions of many of these changes. The responsibilities and roles of nurses today are expanding and two words, "quality" and "safety," are paramount. The need for patient quality and safety was highlighted in the 1999 Institute of Medicine (IOM) report *To Err is Human: Building a Safer Health System,* where it was noted that at least 44,000 people, and perhaps as many as 98,000 people, die in hospitals each year as a result of medical errors that could have been prevented. Knowing that nurses are vital to the quality and safety of patient care, the Agency for Healthcare Research and Quality, with funding from the Robert Wood Johnson Foundation, published *Patient Safety and Quality: An Evidence-Based Handbook for Nurses* (2008), edited by Ronda G. Hughes, PhD, MHS, RN, to provide all nurses, in whatever environment they care for patients, with evidence-based techniques and interventions to improve patient outcomes. The IOM report *The Future of Nursing: Leading Change, Advancing Health* (2011), recommends that nurses practice to the full extent of their education, improve nursing education, assume nursing leadership positions in health care redesign, and improve data collection for workplace planning and policy making.

In nursing education, the onus is on nurses to prepare future nurses to be able to walk out of the classroom and into health care environments utilizing evidence to provide high-quality, safe health care and to be ready to take leadership roles. A national initiative, Quality and Safety Education for Nurses (QSEN), was funded by the Robert Wood Johnson Foundation. Phases I and II were led by Linda Cronenwett, PhD, FAAN, and Gwen Sherwood, PhD, RN, FAAN. Phase III is led by Mary A. Dolansky, PhD, RN. QSEN pursues strategies to ensure that future nursing graduates develop knowledge, skills, and attitudes (KSAs) in patient-centered care, teamwork and collaboration, evidence-based practice, quality improvement, safety, and informatics. These strategies for nursing students and faculty can be seen at http://www.qsen.org.

Essentials of Nursing Leadership & Management, third edition, is designed to help beginning nurses and nurse leaders to develop knowledge, skills, and attitudes based on evidence, as well as to lead and manage nursing care delivery for patients and future health care redesign. The text prepares beginning nurses and nurse managers and leaders to move into the complex changing health care of today. The text embraces the aforementioned Quality and Safety Education for Nurses text, *Patient Safety and Quality: An Evidence-Based Handbook for Nurses* (2008), and the IOM report *The Future of Nursing: Leading Change, Advancing Health* (2011) as standards from which to draw upon and guide current practice.

The contributors to this edition include nursing faculty and educators, nursing consultants, clinical nurse specialists, nurse lawyers, nurse practitioners, wound and ostomy care nurses, and nurse entrepreneurs. These contributors are from various areas of the United States and Canada, thus allowing them to offer a broad view of nursing leadership and management. Contributors are from California, Florida, Illinois, Indiana, Kentucky, Louisiana, Maine, Maryland, Massachusetts, Minnesota, Missouri, New York, Ohio, Texas, Vermont, Virginia, Washington, Wisconsin, and Winnipeg, Manitoba, Canada.

Each chapter of *Essentials of Nursing Leadership & Management*, third edition, discusses the latest evidence and practice relevant to its specific topic. Various points of view are presented through case studies and interviews with staff nurses, nurse practitioners, nursing administrators, nursing risk managers, nursing faculty, physicians, and patients.

ORGANIZATION

Essentials of Nursing Leadership & Management, third edition, consists of 18 chapters arranged in a conceptual framework (see inside cover of book) that provides beginning nurses with an overview of the nurse's leadership and management responsibilities to the patient, to the health care team, to the health care organization, and to self. The book consists of five units.

- **Unit I** introduces nursing leadership and management and then discusses the health care environment; nursing today; and decision making, critical thinking, technology, and informatics.
- **Unit II** discusses leadership and management of the inter-professional team, including inter-professional teamwork and collaboration; change, innovation, and conflict management; and power and politics.
- **Unit III** discusses leadership and management of patient-centered care, including delegation of patient care; effective staffing; budget concepts for patient care; strategic planning and organizing patient care for quality and safety; and time management and setting patient care priorities.
- **Unit IV** discusses quality improvement of patient outcomes, including quality improvement and evidence-based patient care; legal aspects of health care; ethical aspects of health care; and culture, generational differences, and spirituality.
- **Unit V** discusses leadership and management of self and the future, including NCLEX-RN preparation and your first job; and career planning and achieving balance.

Discussion of timely topics is included throughout the chapters. Examples include: information technology, Health Insurance Portability and Accountability Act (HIPAA, Title II), magnet hospitals, inter-professional teamwork and collaboration, quality and performance improvement, generational differences, balancing personal and professional needs, delegation, ethics, legal aspects, culture and spirituality, decision making, critical thinking, disaster nursing, emotional intelligence, horizontal violence, workforce bullying, and population-based care. The real world of nursing is embraced by presenting a variety of different views.

NEW TO THIS EDITION

The third edition of *Essentials of Nursing Leadership & Management* builds on the strength of the second edition, embraces user feedback, and highlights the complexity of the health care landscape.

Important changes include the following:

- EMPHASIS ON QUALITY AND SAFETY. An enhanced emphasis on quality and safety is threaded throughout all chapters, in reaction to the new QSEN initiative and increased nursing and public awareness of the need for quality and safety.
- MORE CHALLENGING ACTIVITIES. Stronger opening scenarios, Critical Thinking exercises, Case Studies, Review Questions, and Review Activities are included in each chapter for development of key concepts by the entry-level nurse.
- REVISED MATERIAL. All chapters have been revised, updated, and strengthened to reflect the most current information in the field, with an eye to preparing new nurses to competently enter the health care arena.
- MULTIPLE OPPORTUNITIES FOR PRACTICE. NCLEX-style review questions (with answers and rationales available online) have been added in order to provide students

with additional practice opportunities. Expanded NCLEX-style questions now include multiple-response formats.

- CURRENT TRENDS IN THE FIELD. The third edition includes a discussion of timely topics, such as informatics, national safety goals, core measures, sentinel events, high reliability organizations, culture of safety, just culture, and the Quality and Safety Education for Nurses (QSEN) initiative, so that students are adequately prepared for a career in today's health care industry.
- UP-TO-DATE COVERAGE. New information on quality improvement, safety, informatics, team building, evidence-based practice, and patient-centered care has been added throughout the text.
- ONLINE RESOURCES. A new Premium Website offers answers to students for the text's Review Questions and Review Activities.

FEATURES

Several standard chapter features are utilized throughout the text that provide the reader with a consistent format for learning and an assortment of resources for understanding and applying the knowledge presented. Features include the following:

- A health care or nursing quote related to chapter content
- A photo that sets the scene for the chapter
- Objectives that state the chapter's learning goals
- An opening scenario, a mini entry-level nursing case study that relates to the chapter, and two to three critical thinking questions
- Key Concepts, a listing of the primary understandings the reader is to take from the chapter
- Key Terms, a listing of important new terms presented in the chapters
- Review Questions, several NCLEX-style questions at the end of each chapter
- Review Activities, to apply chapter content to entry-level nursing situations
- Exploring the Web activities
- References
- Suggested Readings

Special elements are sprinkled throughout the chapters to enhance learning and encourage critical thinking and application:

- Evidence from the Literature—with synopsis of key findings from nursing and health care literature
- Real World Interviews—with health care leaders and managers, including bedside nursing staff, clinicians, administrators, risk managers, faculty, nursing and medical practitioners, patients, nursing assistive personnel (NAP), and lawyers
- Critical Thinking—exercises related to ethical, legal, cultural, spiritual, delegation, safety, and quality improvement topics of nursing and health care
- Case Studies—to provide the entry-level nurse with a clinical nursing leadership/management situation calling for critical thinking to solve an open-ended problem
- Exploring the Web—notes that guide the reader to the Internet and give Internet addresses for the latest information related to the chapter content
- Review Activities—activities that encourage students to think critically about how to apply chapter content to the workplace and other "real-world" situations, providing reinforcement of key leadership and management skills
- Tables and Figures—these appear throughout the text and provide convenient capsules of information for the student's reference

Learning Package for the Student

The **Premium Website** is available to purchasers of the text and to instructors, and is accessed at **www.CengageBrain.com**. Enter your passcode, found in the front of the book, and the Premium Website will be added to your bookshelf. Here you can access the answers with rationales for the text's Review Questions, and view suggested responses to the text's Review Activities.

ISBN: 978-1-133-93570-4

Teaching Package for the Instructor

The **Instructor Companion Website** is a teaching tool to aid instructors in preparing lessons, creating lectures, and developing quizzes. This website will assist faculty in planning and developing their programs and classes for the most efficient use of time and resources. This resource, complementary for adopters of *Essentials of Nursing Leadership & Management*, third edition, includes:

- Lecture slides in PowerPoint® for each chapter to enhance classroom discussions
- A test bank of several hundred questions, in NCLEX-RN format, with answers and rationales
- Tie to text features: answers with rationales for the text's Review Questions, suggested responses to the text's Review Activities, answers to the text's Case Studies, discussion of the text's chapter-opening scenarios, and suggested responses to the text's Critical Thinking Activities

REFERENCES

Agency for Healthcare Research and Quality (AHRQ). (2008, April). *Patient safety and quality: An evidence-based handbook for nurses.* AHRQ Publication No. 08-0043. Rockville, MD: AHRQ. Retrieved October 1, 2012, from http://www.ahrq.gov/qual/nurseshdbk

Institute of Medicine (IOM). (1999). *To Err is Human: Building a Safer Health System.* Washington, DC: The National Academies Press.

Institute of Medicine (IOM). National Research Council. (2011). *The future of nursing: Leading change, advancing health.* Washington, DC: The National Academies Press.

ACKNOWLEDGMENTS

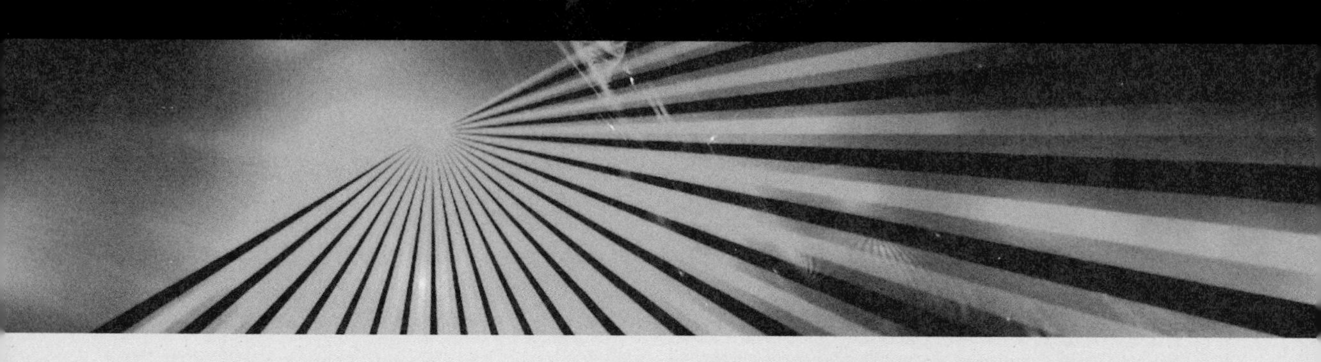

A book such as this requires great effort and the coordination of many people with various areas of expertise. Pat and Janice would like to thank all of the contributors for their time and effort in sharing their knowledge gained through years of experience in both the clinical and academic setting. All of the contributing authors worked within tight time frames to share their expertise. We especially thank Jo Reidy, Mercy Hospital & Medical Center, Chicago, Illinois; Corinne Haviley, Central DuPage Hospital, Cadence Health, Winfield, Illinois; and Dawn Moeller, Advocate Good Shepherd Health Care, Barrington, Illinois, for their help in arranging some of the photographs for the text. Thanks also to Jane Woodruff for her computer support.

We would like to acknowledge and sincerely thank the team who worked to make this book a reality. Beth Williams, Senior Product Manager, and Delia K. Uherec, Associate Acquisitions Editor, at Delmar Cengage Learning; and Mahendran Mani, Project Manager, at Carlisle Publishing Services, India, are great people who worked tirelessly and shared their knowledge, guidance, humor, and attention to help keep us motivated and on track throughout the project.

We also want to thank the reviewers for their time spent critically reviewing the manuscript and providing the valuable comments that have enhanced this text.

Patricia Kelly and Janice Tazbir

Pat adds special thanks to her Dad and Mom, Ed and Jean Kelly; Ron Vana, her special friend; her sisters, Tessie Dybel and Kathy Milch; her Aunt Pat and Uncle Bill Kelly (who convinced Pat to start writing); her Aunt Verna and Uncle Archie Payne; her nieces, Natalie Dybel Bevil, Melissa Milch Arredondo, and Stacey Milch; her nephew, John Milch; her grand nephew, Brock Bevil; her grand niece, Reese Bevil; her nephews-in-law, Tracy Bevil and Peter Arredondo; and her dear friends, Patricia Wojcik, Florence Lebryk, Lee McGuan, Dolores Wynen, and Joan Fox, who have supported Pat throughout the writing of this book and much of her life. Special thanks also go to Pat's wonderful nursing friends, Zenaida Corpuz, Dr. Mary Elaine Koren, Dr. Barbara Mudloff, Dr. Patricia Padjen, Jane McKeon, Kerrie Ellingsen, and especially to Gerri Kane, Janice Klepitch, Sylvia Komyatte, and Julie Martini, as well as Anna Fizer, Judy Ilijanich, Trudy Keilman, Judy Rau, Lillian Rau, and Ivy Schmude, who have supported her throughout the writing of this book and during their fifty years together as nurses. Special thanks to her faculty mentors, Dr. Imogene King, Dr. Joyce Ellis, and Nancy Weber. Pat would also like to thank Janice for her great contributions as coauthor. Janice worked hard within tight deadlines and helped develop this thorough review of *Essentials of Nursing Leadership and Management.*

Patricia Kelly

Janice would like to thank Patricia Kelly for the opportunity to coauthor this text. Her guidance, mentoring, and support are appreciated beyond words. As mentioned, sincerest thanks to the contributors, reviewers, and the Delmar team. A personal thanks to her incredible colleagues at Purdue University Calumet and her entire family for their support through this journey.

Janice Tazbir

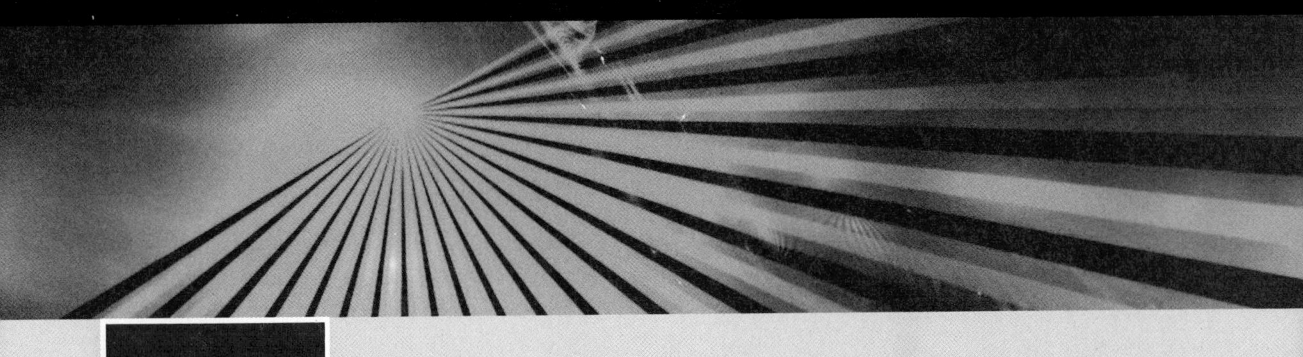

ABOUT THE AUTHORS

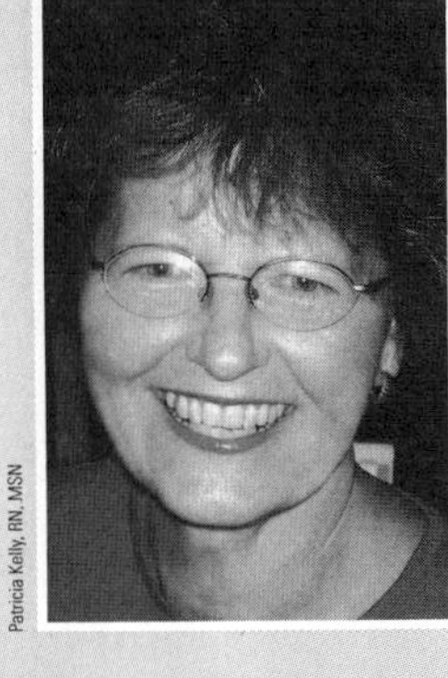

Patricia Kelly, RN, MSN
Professor Emeritus
Purdue University Calumet
School of Nursing
Hammond, Indiana

Patricia Kelly earned a Diploma in Nursing from St. Margaret Hospital School of Nursing, Hammond, Indiana; a Baccalaureate in Nursing from DePaul University in Chicago, Illinois; and a Master's Degree in Nursing from Loyola University in Chicago, Illinois. Pat is Professor Emeritus, Purdue University Calumet, Hammond, Indiana. She has worked as a staff nurse, school nurse, and nurse educator. Pat has traveled extensively in the United States, Canada, and Puerto Rico, teaching conferences for the Joint Commission, Resource Applications, Pediatric Concepts, and Kaplan, Inc. She currently teaches nationwide NCLEX-RN review courses for Evolve Testing & Remediation/Health Education Systems, Inc. (HESI), Houston, Texas.

Pat was Director of Quality Improvement at the University of Chicago Hospitals and Clinics. She has taught at Wesley-Passavant School of Nursing, Chicago State University, and Purdue University Calumet, Hammond, Indiana. Pat has taught fundamentals of nursing, adult nursing, nursing leadership and management, nursing issues, nursing trends, quality improvement, and legal aspects of nursing. Pat is a member of Sigma Theta Tau, the American Nurses Association, and the Emergency Nurses Association. She is listed in *Who's Who in American Nursing, 2000 Notable American Women,* and the *International Who's Who of Professional and Business Women.*

Pat has served on the board of directors of Tri City Mental Health Center, St. Anthony's Home, and the Quality Connection. She is the author of *Nursing Leadership & Management,* currently in its third edition (Delmar Cengage Learning, 2012). This text has also been adapted for Canadian nursing students, i.e., *Nursing Leadership and Management* (Kelly, P. & Crawford, H. (2011). Delmar Cengage Learning). Pat is author of *Essentials of Nursing Leadership and Management* (Delmar Cengage Learning, 2010). She is co-author with Janice Tazbir of *Essentials of*

Nursing Leadership & Management, also in its third edition (Delmar Cengage Learning, 2012). Pat is also coauthor with Maureen Marthaler of *Delegation of Nursing Care* (Delmar Cengage Learning, 2005) and *Nursing Delegation, Setting Priorities, and Making Patient Care Assignments,* second edition (Delmar Cengage Learning, 2011). Pat is currently developing a new text on safety and quality in nursing with Beth Vottero and Carolyn Christie-McAuliffe for Delmar Cengage Learning. Pat contributed a chapter, "Preparing the Undergraduate Student and Faculty to Use Quality Improvement in Practice," to *Improving Quality,* second edition, by Claire Gavin Meisenheimer. Pat also contributed a chapter on obstructive lung disease to *Medical Surgical Nursing,* (Delmar Cengage Learning). Pat has written several articles, including "Chest X-Ray Interpretation" and many articles on quality improvement. She has served as a national disaster volunteer for the American Red Cross and as a volunteer at several church food pantries in Austin, Texas, and Chicago, Illinois. She has gone on health care relief trips to Nicaragua. Throughout most of her career, she has taught nursing at the university level. Pat has been licensed and has worked in many states during her career, including Indiana, Illinois, Wisconsin, Oklahoma, New York, Pennsylvania, and Texas. Pat lives in Chicago most of the year and lives in Florida part of the year. She may be contacted at patkelly777@aol.com.

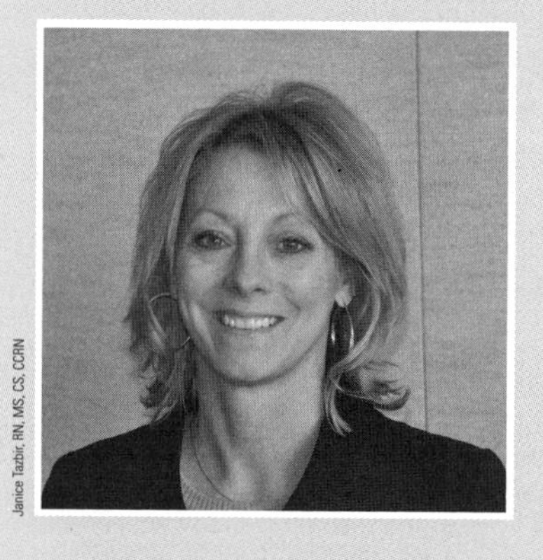

Janice Tazbir, RN, MS, CS, CCRN

Janice Tazbir, RN, MS, CCRN, CS, CNE
Professor of Nursing
Purdue University Calumet
School of Nursing
Hammond, Indiana

Janice Tazbir initially earned an Associate Degree in Science in Nursing at Purdue University Calumet, and then furthered her education earning a Bachelor's Degree, then a Master's Degree as a Clinical Nurse Specialist in Critical Care. Her clinical nursing background is critical care and she has worked there the majority of her career, currently in critical care at the University of Chicago Hospitals. Her teaching career has been at Purdue Calumet since 1997, where she teaches mainly advanced medical surgical nursing, pathophysiology, critical care, capstone in nursing, and NCLEX preparation. Janice attained the status of professor in 2011. She was awarded the Teaching Excellence Award at Purdue University Calumet in 2006; is Quality Matters–certified as a distance-learning educator; is a certified Experiential Educator; and is certified by the Indiana Center for Evidence-Based Practice as a research associate. She became a certified nurse educator (CNE) in 2012.

Janice is a member of many professional organizations including Sigma Theta Tau, the American Association of Critical-Care Nurses, and the American Association of Neuroscience Nurses, to name a few. She is active in service at the university level, sits on the board of governors for the Society of Innovators, and is a peer advisor for a publishing company. She has published numerous refereed articles and book chapters over her career. She has presented locally and nationally, authored the *Clinical Companion to Accompany Contemporary Medical-Surgical Nursing,* now in its second edition (Delmar Cengage Learning, 2011), and has coauthored *The Medical Surgical Atlas* (Delmar Cengage Learning, 2008). Her students are her passion and they are an everyday reminder of the privilege of teaching. She is married to Johnny and they have two beloved daughters, Jade and Joule. They all enjoy traveling together. You may contact her at Tazbir@purduecal.edu.

DEDICATION

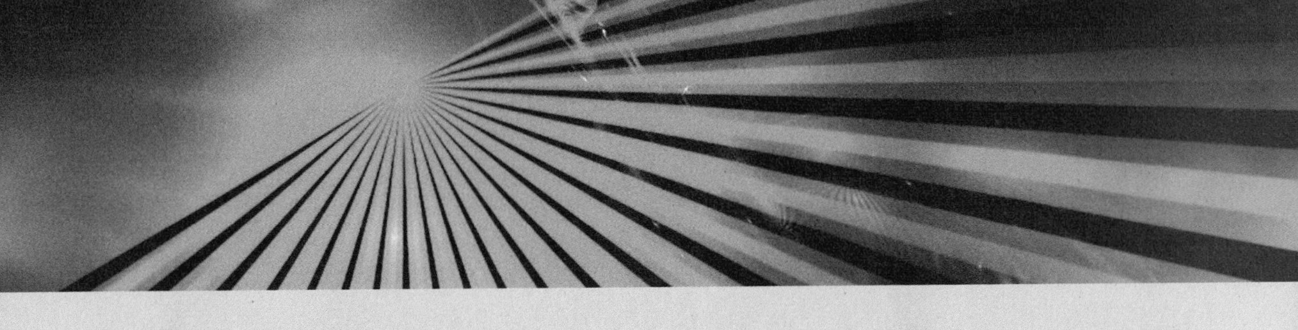

This book is dedicated by Pat to her loving Dad and Mom, Ed and Jean Kelly; to dear Ron Vana; to her super sisters, Tessie Dybel and Kathy Milch; to her dear aunts and uncles, Aunt Verna and Uncle Archie Payne and Aunt Pat and Uncle Bill Kelly; to her nieces, Natalie Dybel Bevil, Melissa Milch Arredondo, and Stacey Milch; to her nephew, John Milch; to her grand-nephew, Brock Bevil, and grand-niece, Reese Bevil; and nephews-in-law, Tracy Bevil and Peter Arredondo.

Janice dedicates this book in loving memory of her parents, Deanna and Bill.

CONTRIBUTORS

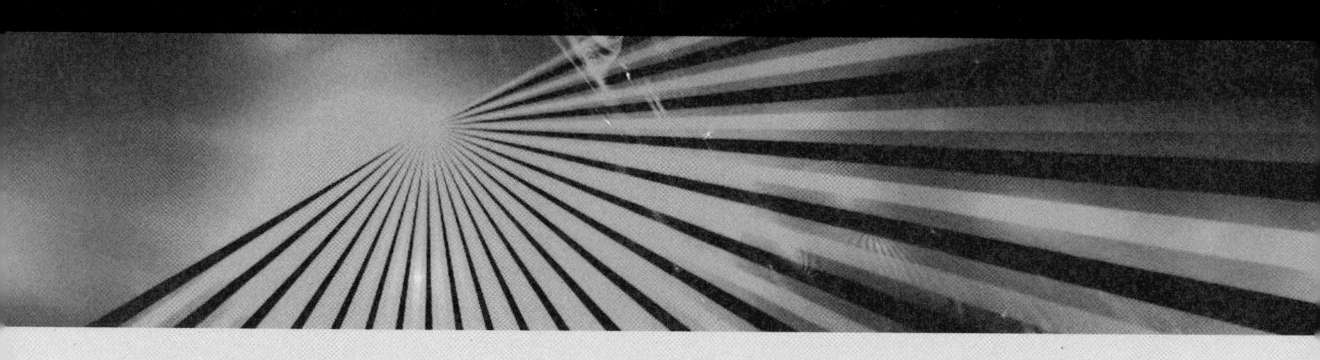

Rinda Alexander, RN, CS, PhD
Professor Emeritus, Nursing
Purdue University Calumet
Hammond, Indiana
and
Professor of Nursing
University of Florida
College of Nursing
Gainesville, Florida
and
Nursing Consultant
Health Care and Administration
Schererville, Indiana

Kim Siarkowski Amer, RN, PhD

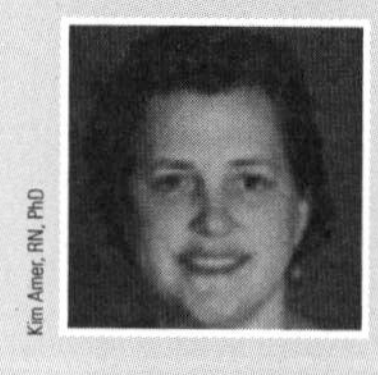
Kim Amer, RN, PhD

Associate Professor
Department of Nursing
DePaul University
Chicago, Illinois

Margaret M. Anderson, RN, CNAA, EdD

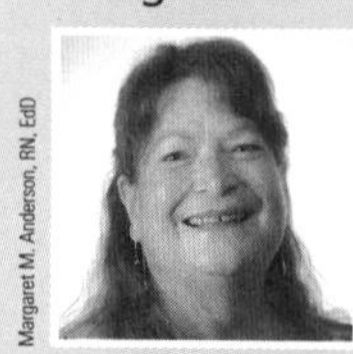
Margaret M. Anderson, RN, EdD

Professor of Nursing and Past Chair
College of Health Professions
Department of Advanced Nursing Studies
Northern Kentucky University
Highland Heights, Kentucky

Ida M. Androwich, RN, BC, FAAN, PhD

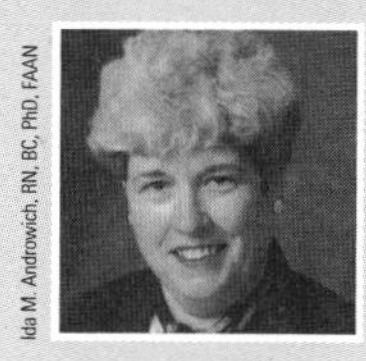
Ida M. Androwich, RN, BC, PhD, FAAN

Professor and Director
Health Systems Management
Niehoff School of Nursing
Loyola University Chicago
Maywood, Illinois

Anne Bernat, RN, MSN, CNAA
Vice President of Patient Care Services (Retired)
Arlington, Virginia

Donna Bowles, RN, MSN, EdD, CNE

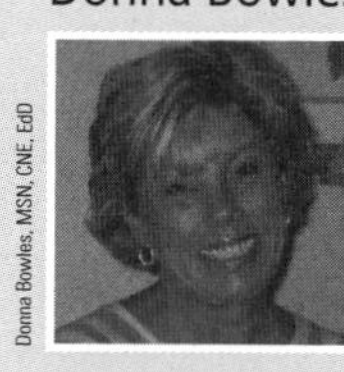
Donna Bowles, MSN, CNE, EdD

Associate Professor
School of Nursing
Indiana University SE
New Albany, Indiana

Nancy Braaten, RN, MS

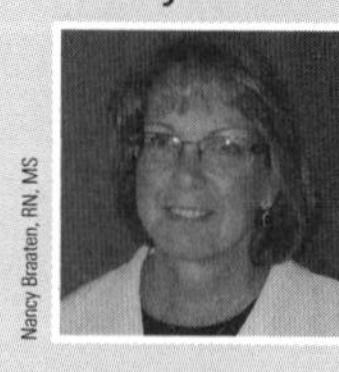
Nancy Braaten, RN, MS

Adult Health Clinical Nurse Specialist
Clinical Analyst, Nursing Information Systems
Northeast Health Acute Care Division
Troy, New York

Kathleen Cain, OSF, JD
Attorney
Franciscan Legal Services
Baton Rouge, Louisiana

Carolyn Christie-McAuliffe, PhD, FNP

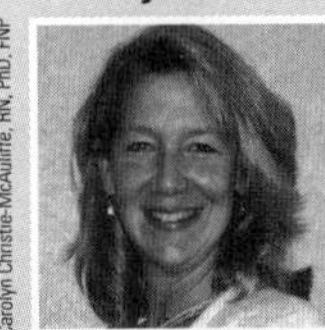
Carolyn Christie-McAuliffe, RN, PhD, FNP

Director of Research
Hematology Oncology Associates of CNY
East Syracuse, New York

Martha Desmond, RN, MS, Post Masters Certificate in Nursing Education

Clinical Nurse Specialist in Critical Care
Northeast Health Acute Care Division
Troy, New York
and
Adjunct Faculty
Excelsior College
Albany, New York

Joan Dorman, RN, MS, CEN

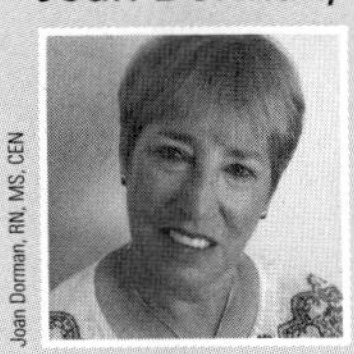
Joan Dorman, RN, MS, CEN

Clinical Associate Professor of Nursing
Purdue University Calumet
Hammond, Indiana

Deborah Erickson, RN, PhD

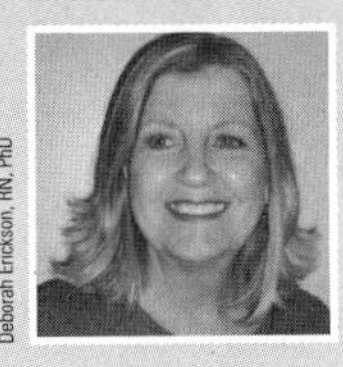
Deborah Erickson, RN, PhD

Assistant Professor
Undergraduate Coordinator
STTI - Epsilon Epsilon Chapter President
Department of Nursing
Bradley University
Peoria, Illinois

Barbara K. Fane, RN, MS, APRN-BC

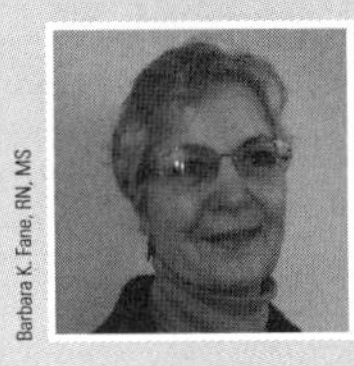
Barbara K. Fane, RN, MS

Clinical Nurse Specialist, Critical Care
Northeast Health Acute Care Division
Troy, New York
and
Adjunct Clinical Faculty
Southern Vermont College
Bennington, Vermont

Mary L. Fisher, RN, CNAA, BC, PhD

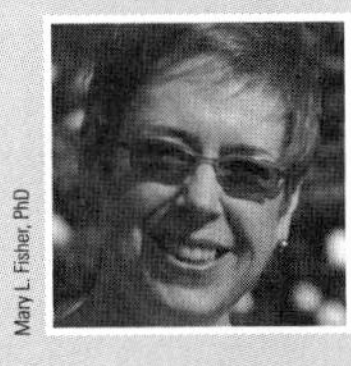
Mary L. Fisher, PhD

Professor and Department Chair
Environments for Health
Indiana University School of Nursing
Indianapolis, Indiana

Charlene C. Gyurko, PhD, RN, CNE

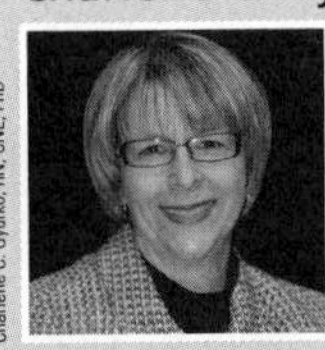
Charlene C. Gyurko, RN, CNE, PhD

Assistant Professor
Purdue University North Central
Department of Nursing
Westville, Indiana

Corinne Haviley, RN, MS, PhD

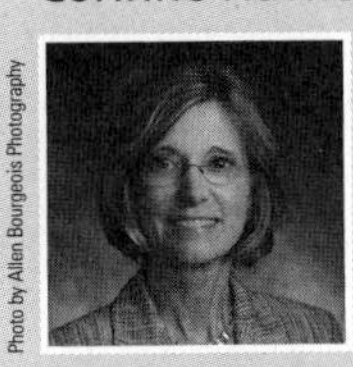
Photo by Allen Bourgeois Photography

Associate Chief Nursing Officer
Outpatient, Emergency and Behavioral Health Services
Central DuPage Hospital
Cadence Health
Winfield, Illinois

Paul Heidenthal, MS

Instructional Designer
Texas Health and Human Services Commission
Austin, Texas

Sara Anne Hook, JD, MLS, MBA

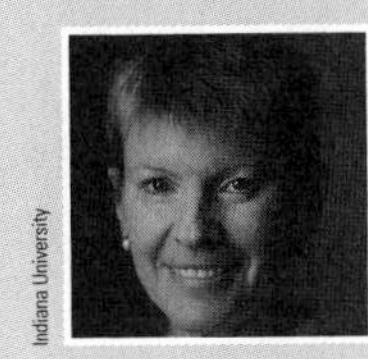
Indiana University

Professor of Informatics
Indiana University
School of Informatics
Indianapolis, Indiana
and
Adjunct Professor of Law
Indiana University School of Law-Indianapolis
Indianapolis, Indiana

Karen Houston, RN, MS

Director of Quality and Continuum of Care
Albany Medical Center
Albany, New York

Ronda G. Hughes, MHS, RN, FAAN, PhD

Associate Professor
Marquette University
Milwaukee, Wisconsin

Mary Anne Jadlos, MS, ACNP-BC, CWOCN

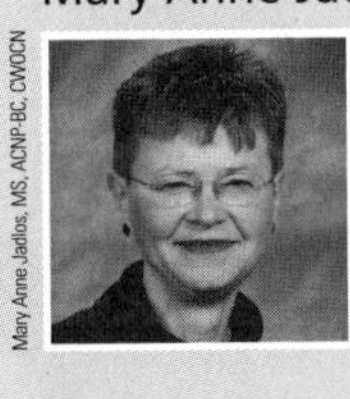
Mary Anne Jadlos, MS, ACNP-BC, CWOCN

Coordinator, Wound, Skin and Ostomy Nursing Service
Northeast Health Acute Care Division
Samaritan Hospital
Troy, New York
and
Albany Memorial Hospital
Albany, New York

Crisamar Javellana-Anunciado, RN, MSN, FNP-BC

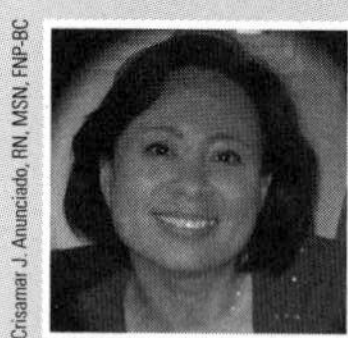
Crisamar J. Anunciado, RN, MSN, FNP-BC

Inpatient Nurse Practitioner
Sharp Chula Vista Medical Center
Chula Vista, California
and
Adjunct Faculty
Southwestern Community College
Associate Degree Nursing Program
Chula Vista, California

Josette Jones, RN, PhD

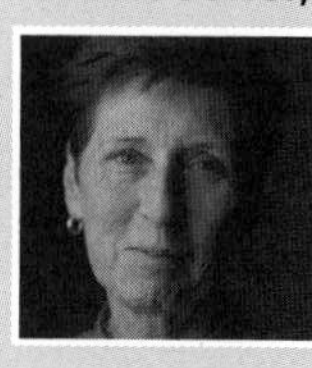
Indiana Board of Trustees (IUPUI)

Assistant Professor
Indiana University
School of Nursing
School of Informatics
Indianapolis, Indiana

Stephen Jones, RN, MS, CPNP ET

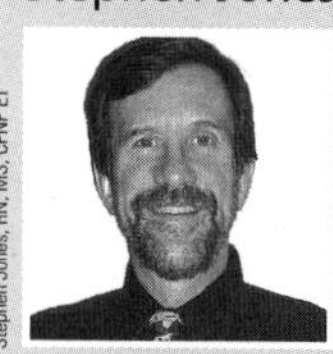
Stephen Jones, RN, MS, CPNP ET

Pediatric Clinical Nurse Specialist/Nurse Practitioner
The Children's Hospital at Albany Medical Center
Albany, New York
and
Founder
Pediatric Concepts
Averill Park, New York

Patricia Kelly, RN, MSN

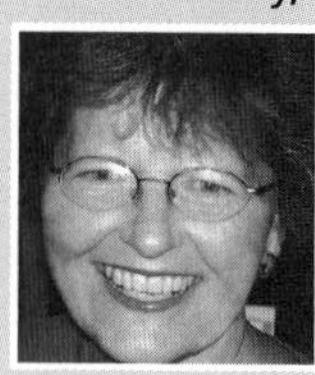
Patricia Kelly, RN, MSN

Professor Emeritus
Purdue University Calumet
School of Nursing
Hammond, Indiana
and
Faculty Evolve Testing and Remediation/Health Education Sytems, Inc. (HESI)
NCLEX-RN Review Courses
Houston, Texas
and
Consultant
Chicago, Illinois
Fort Myers, Florida

Glenda B. Kelman, ACNP-BC, PhD

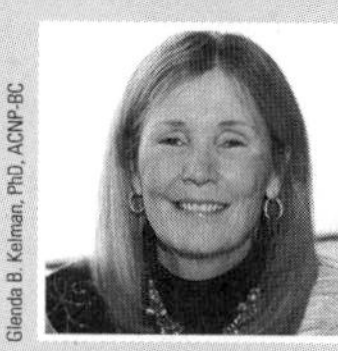
Glenda B. Kelman, PhD, ACNP-BC

Associate Professor and Chair
Nursing Department
The Sage Colleges
Troy, New York
and
Acute Care Nurse Practitioner
Wound, Skin, and Ostomy Nursing Service
Northeast Health Acute Care Division
Samaritan Hospital
Troy, New York
and
Albany Memorial Hospital
Albany, New York

Kathleen Kleefisch, APRN, FNP-BC, DNP

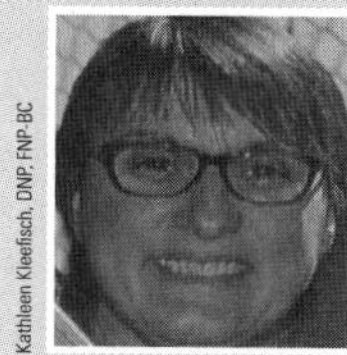
Kathleen Kleefisch, DNP, FNP-BC

Assistant Professor
Purdue University Calumet
School of Nursing
Hammond, Indiana

Mary Elaine Koren, RN, PhD

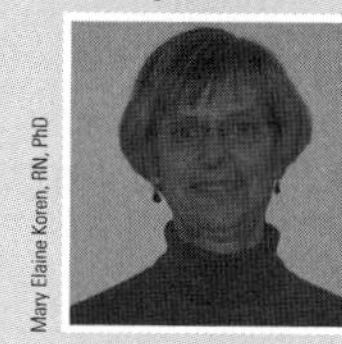
Mary Elaine Koren, RN, PhD

Associate Professor of Nursing
Northern Illinois University
School of Nursing and Health Studies
DeKalb, Illinois

Lyn LaBarre, RN, MS

Patient Care Service Director
Critical Care, Specialty and Emergency Services
Albany Medical Center
Albany, New York

Linda Searle Leach, RN, NEA-BC, PhD

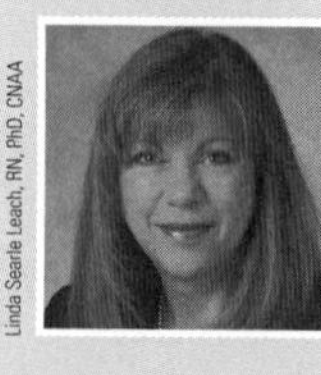
Linda Searle Leach, RN, PhD, CNAA

Assistant Professor
UCLA School of Nursing
Los Angeles, California

Camille B. Little, RN, BSN, MS
Instructional Assistant Professor (Retired)
Mennonite College of Nursing
Illinois State University
Normal, Illinois

Sharon Little-Stoetzel, RN, MS, CNE

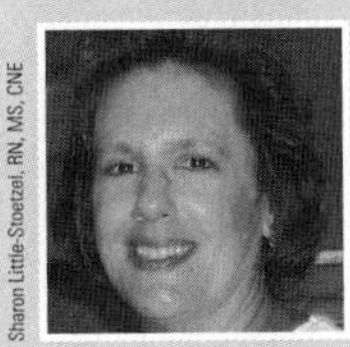
Sharon Little-Stoetzel, RN, MS, CNE

Associate Professor of Nursing
MidAmerica Nazarene University
Independence, Missouri

Miki Magnino-Rabig, RN, PhD
Assistant Professor
University of St. Francis
Joliet, Illinois

Patsy Maloney, RN-BC, NEA-BC, MSN, MA, EdD

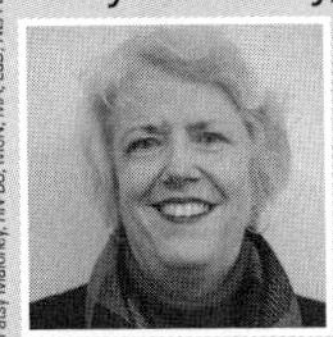
Patsy Maloney, RN-BC, MSN, MA, EdD, NEA-BC

Professor and Director
Continuing Nursing Education
School of Nursing
Pacific Lutheran University
Tacoma, Washington

Richard J. Maloney, BS, MA, MAHRM, EdD

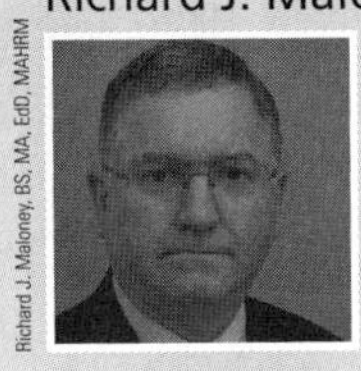
Richard J. Maloney, BS, MA, EdD, MAHRM

Partner
Policy Governance Associates
Tacoma, Washington

Maureen T. Marthaler, RN, MS

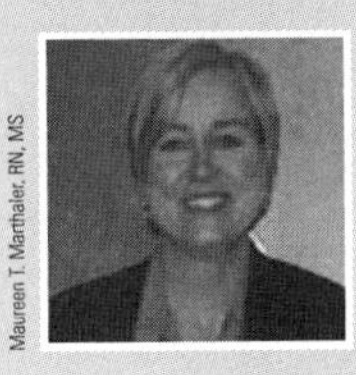
Maureen T. Marthaler, RN, MS

Associate Professor
Purdue University Calumet
School of Nursing
Hammond, Indiana

Judith W. Martin, RN, JD
Attorney
Franciscan Legal Services
Baton Rouge, Louisiana

Edna Harder Mattson, RN, BN, BA(CRS), MDE

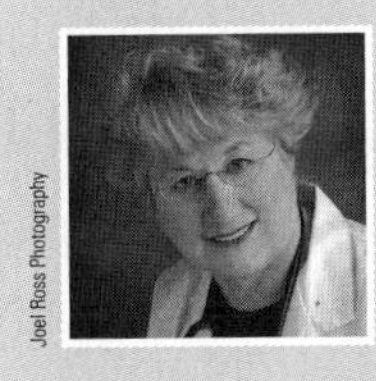
Joel Ross Photography

Doctoral Student in Education
University of Phoenix
and
President
International Nursing Consultation and Tutorial Services
Winnipeg, Manitoba, Canada

Mary McLaughlin, RN, MBA
Assistant Director for Case Management and Social Work
Albany Medical Center
Albany, New York

Kathleen M. McPhaul, RN, MPH, PhD

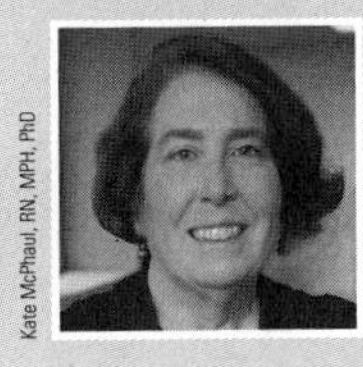
Kate McPhaul, RN, MPH, PhD

Assistant Professor and Specialty Director
Community/Public Health
Department of Family and Community Health
University of Maryland School of Nursing
Baltimore, Maryland

Terry W. Miller, RN, PhD

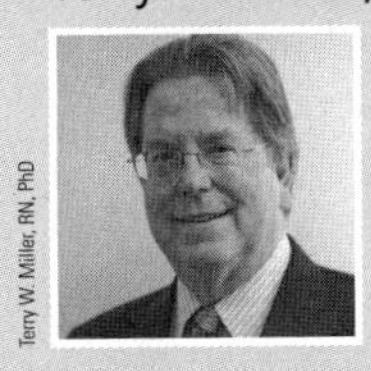
Terry W. Miller, RN, PhD

Dean and Professor
School of Nursing
Pacific Lutheran University
Tacoma, Washington

Peter D. Mills Ph.D., MS.
Director, VA National Center for Patient Safety Field Office
Adjunct Associate Professor of Psychiatry,
Dartmouth Medical School
White River Junction, Vermont

Leslie H. Nicoll, RN, BC, MBA, PhD
President and Owner, Maine Desk, LLC
Portland, Maine

Laura J. Nosek, RN, PhD
Doctor of Nursing Practice Faculty
The Bolton School of Nursing
Case Western Reserve University
Cleveland, Ohio
and
Adjunct Associate Professor of Nursing
Marcella Niehoff School of Nursing
Loyola University Chicago
Chicago, Illinois
and
Course Facilitator
Excelsior College
Albany, New York

Amy Androwich O'Malley, RN, MSN

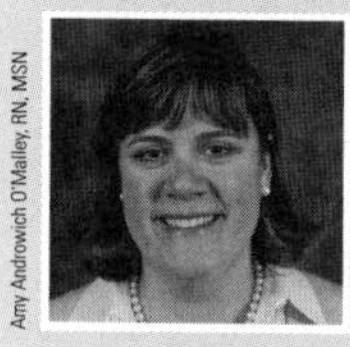
Amy Androwich O'Malley, RN, MSN

Education and Program Manager
Medela, Inc.
McHenry, Illinois

Kristine E. Pfendt, RN, MSN

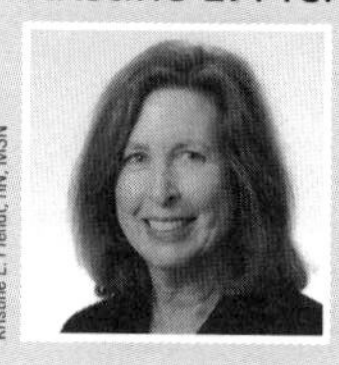
Kristine E. Pfendt, RN, MSN

Associate Professor of Nursing
College of Health Professions
Department of Advanced Nursing Studies
Northern Kentucky University
Highland Heights, Kentucky

Karin Polifko-Harris, RN, CNAA, PhD
Vice President
Organization Development and Research
Naples Community Healthcare System
Naples, Florida

Robyn Pozza-Dollar, JD
Attorney
Cambridge, Massachusetts

Chad S. Priest, RN, MSN, JD

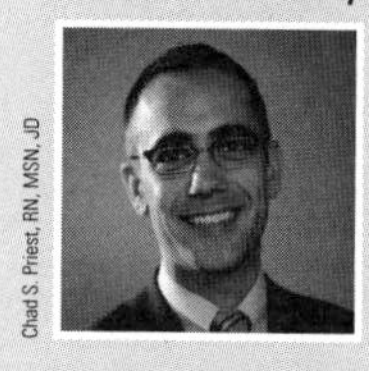
Chad S. Priest, RN, MSN, JD

Chief Executive Officer
MESH, Inc.
Indianapolis, Indiana

Jenny Radsma, RN, PhD
Associate Professor
Division of Nursing
University of Maine at Fort Kent
Fort Kent, Maine

Josephine Reidy, RN, MSN

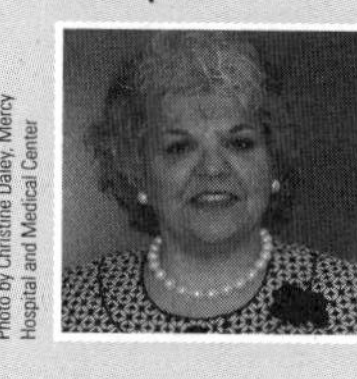
Photo by Christine Daley, Mercy Hospital and Medical Center

Director of the Emergency Department
Mercy Hospital and Medical Center
Chicago, Illinois

Christine Rovinski-Wagner, ARNP, MSN
Accreditation/Performance Improvement Coordinator
Acting System Redesign Coordinator
VA Medical Center
White River Junction, Vermont

Jacklyn L. Ruthman, RN, PhD

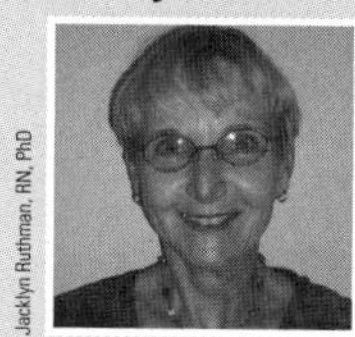
Jacklyn Ruthman, RN, PhD

Associate Professor, Retired
Bradley University
Peoria, Illinois

Patricia M. Schoon, RN, MPH, PHN

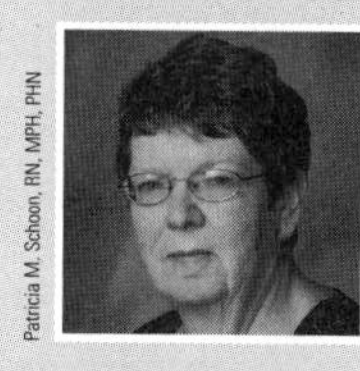
Patricia M. Schoon, RN, MPH, PHN

Adjunct Associate Professor
Graduate and Professional Programs
Saint Mary's University of Minnesota
Minneapolis, Minnesota

Kathleen F. Sellers, RN, PhD

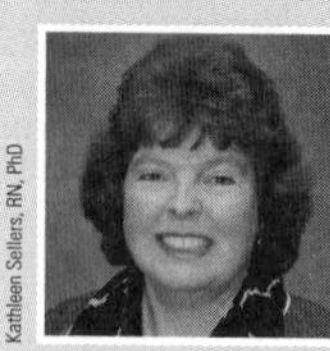
Kathleen Sellers, RN, PhD

Associate Professor
School of Nursing and Health Systems
SUNY Institute of Technology
Utica, New York

Susan Abaffy Shah, MS, ACNP-BC
Division of Cardiology
Albany Medical Center
Albany, New York

Maria R. Shirey, RN, MBA, NEA-BC, FACHE, FAAN, PhD

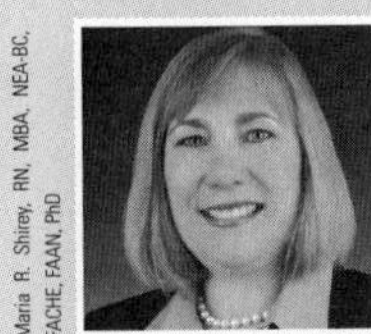
Maria R. Shirey, RN, MBA, NEA-BC, FACHE, FAAN, PhD

Associate Professor
University of Southern Indiana
College of Nursing and Health Professions
Evansville, Indiana

Nancy S. Sisson, RN, MS

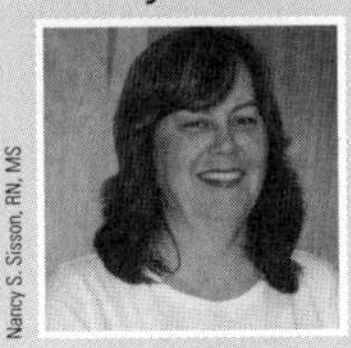
Nancy S. Sisson, RN, MS

Adult Health Clinical Nurse Specialist
Clinical Nurse Specialist—Telemetry
Northeast Health Acute Care Division
Albany, New York

Tanya L. Sleeper, GNP-BC, MSN, MSB

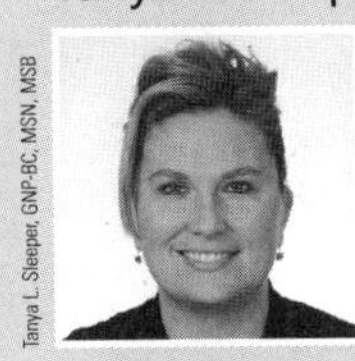
Tanya L. Sleeper, GNP-BC, MSN, MSB

Assistant Professor
Division of Nursing
University of Maine at Fort Kent
Fort Kent, Maine

Erin C. Soucy, RN, MSN

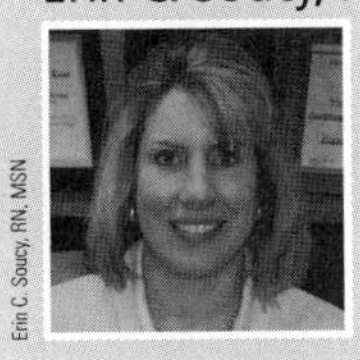
Erin C. Soucy, RN, MSN

Director, Division of Nursing
Assistant Professor of Nursing
University of Maine at Fort Kent
Fort Kent, Maine

Sara Swett, RN, BSN, MSN

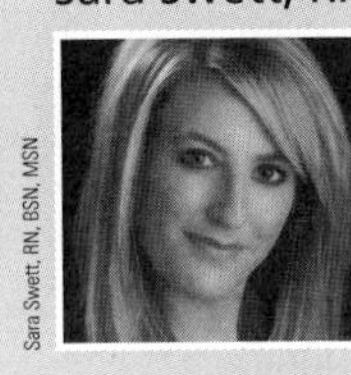
Sara Swett, RN, BSN, MSN

Clinical Instructor
Pacific Lutheran University
School of Nursing
Tacoma, Washington

Janice Tazbir, RN, MS, CCRN, CS, CNE

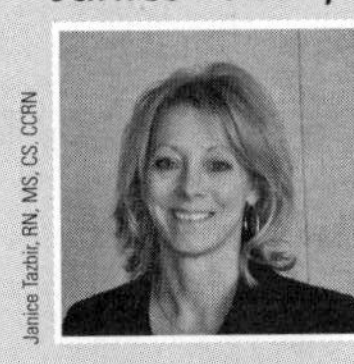
Janice Tazbir, RN, MS, CS, CCRN

Professor of Nursing
Purdue University Calumet
School of Nursing
Hammond, Indiana

Tanya L. Toth, RN, MSN/MBA/HCM, CNOR, CRNFA

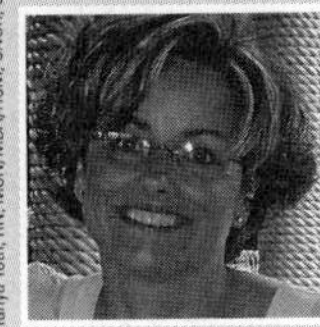
Tanya Toth, RN, MSN/MBA/HCM, CNOR, CRNFA

Lead Academic Coach
Purdue University Calumet
BSN-RN Program
Assistant Director of Nursing Services
LaPorte, Indiana

Beth A. Vottero, PhD, RN, CNE

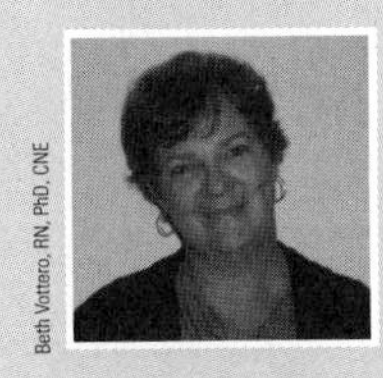
Beth Vottero, RN, PhD, CNE

Assistant Professor of Nursing
Purdue University Calumet
School of Nursing
Hammond, Indiana

Kathryn L. Ward, RN, MS, MA

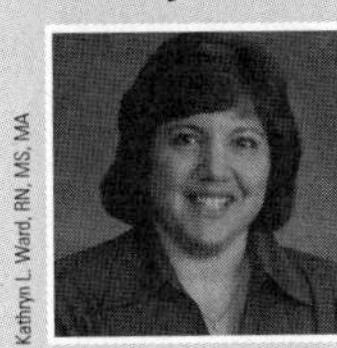
Kathryn L. Ward, RN, MS, MA

Faxton-St. Luke's Healthcare
Utica, New York
and
Clinical Quality Value Analyst
Adjunct Faculty
SUNY Institute of Technology
Utica, New York

Karen Luther Wikoff, RN, PhD

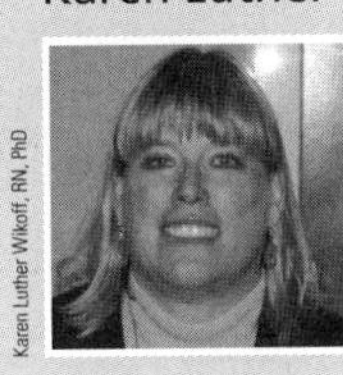
Karen Luther Wikoff, RN, PhD

Assistant Professor
California State University, Stanislaus
Turlock, California

REVIEWERS

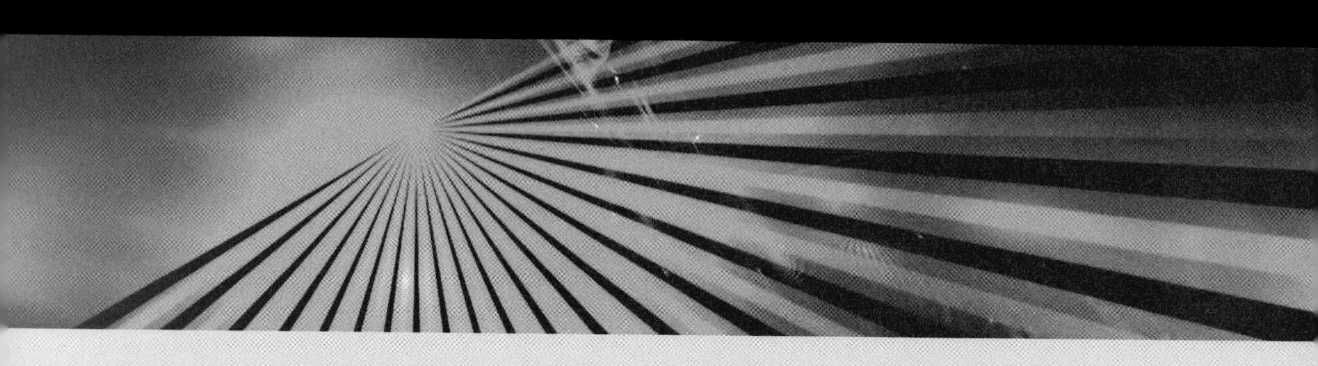

Susan Johnson Garbutt, RN, CNE, CIC, DNP
Adjunct Faculty
Uniformed Services
University of the Health Sciences
Graduate School of Nursing
Bethesda, Maryland

Patricia Kaye Hawley, MEd
Ferris State University
Big Rapids, Michigan

Karla Huntsman, RN, MSN/Ed
Nursing Instructor
AmeriTech College
Draper, Utah

Carolyn McKinney, RN, MSN/Ed, PHN
Professor Emeritus—Nursing
Moorpark College
Moorpark, California
and
Nursing Faculty
California State University
Northridge, California
and
Clinical Nurse Instructor
Oxnard Adult School
Oxnard, California

HOW TO USE THIS BOOK

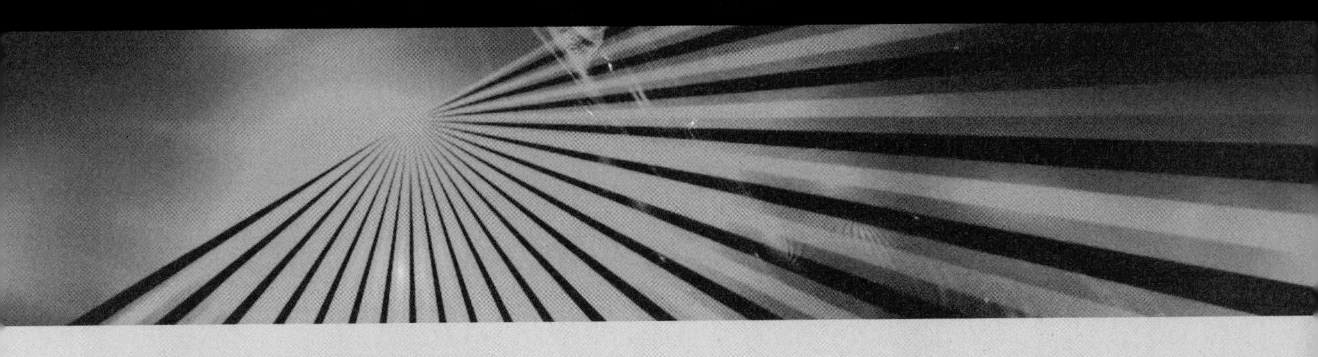

Luck is a matter of preparation meeting opportunity.

—OPRAH WINFREY

QUOTE

A nursing or health care theorist quote gives a professional's perspective regarding the topic at hand; read this quote as you begin each new chapter and see whether your opinion matches or differs, or whether you are in need of further information.

OBJECTIVES

Upon completion of this chapter, the reader should be able to:

1. Discuss preparation for the National Council of State Boards of Nursing Licensure Examination for Registered Nurses (NCLEX-RN).
2. Detail the process of beginning a successful nursing job search.
3. Develop a résumé and cover letter.
4. Identify appropriate preparation for a successful job interview.
5. Discuss potential interview questions and identify acceptable answers.
6. Describe typical components of health care orientation.
7. Discuss elements of performance feedback.

OBJECTIVES

These goals indicate to you the performance-based, measurable objectives that are targeted for mastery upon completion of the chapter.

Mary will be graduating from her nursing education program in two months. She plans to focus her current efforts on preparing to take the NCLEX-RN Licensure Examination. She knows that three important areas of examination preparation are having the knowledge, being adept at testing, and controlling test anxiety.

How should she prepare for the examination?

Where should she focus?

How can she decrease her test anxiety?

OPENING SCENARIO

This mini case study with related critical thinking questions should be read prior to delving into the chapter; it sets the tone for the material to come and helps you identify your knowledge base and perspective.

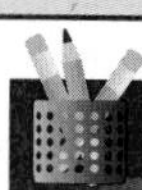

CASE STUDY **16-3**

Sally M. is a 28-year-old RN who has worked on the same critical care unit for five years. During the past three months, the unit has lost four staff who have yet to be replaced, resulting in significant overtime for everyone including Sally. In addition, acuity of the unit has remained high with an unusual number of admissions of young adults as well as deaths. It has been necessary for Sally to work three weekends in a row. She is feeling physically tired but is aware she is feeling emotionally tired as well and is worried she might be depressed.

Could Sally be spiritually distressed? Please discuss.

If this is spiritual distress, what are a few things Sally could do to help herself? What could Sally's manager do to help her as well as her colleagues best attend to their spiritual needs?

CASE STUDY

These short cases with related questions present a beginning, clinical, nursing-management situation calling for judgment, decision making, or analysis in solving an open-ended problem. Familiarize yourself with the types of situations and settings you will later encounter in practice, and challenge yourself to devise solutions that will result in the best outcomes for all parties, within the boundaries of legal and ethical nursing practice.

EVIDENCE FROM THE **LITERATURE**

Citation: Kelley, T. F., Brandon, D. H., & Docherty, S. L. (2011). Electronic nursing documentation as a strategy to improve quality of patient care. *Journal of Nursing Scholarship, 43*, 154–162. doi: 10.1111/j.1547-5069.2011.01397.x

Discussion: This integrative review of the literature examined the relationship between nurses' electronic documentation and the quality of care given to hospitalized patients. Most U.S. hospitals are currently switching from paper-based to electronic documentation, anticipating improved quality. The extent to which nurses' electronic documentation improves the quality of care to hospitalized patients remains unknown because of the lack of effective comparisons with nurses' paper-based documentation.

Implications for Practice: Future research needs to investigate the day-to-day relationship between nurses' electronic documentation and the quality of care provided to patients in the hospital.

EVIDENCE FROM THE LITERATURE

Study these key findings from nursing and health care research, theory, and literature, and ask yourself how they will influence your practice. Do you see ways in which your nursing could be affected by these literature findings and research results? Do you agree with the conclusions drawn by the author?

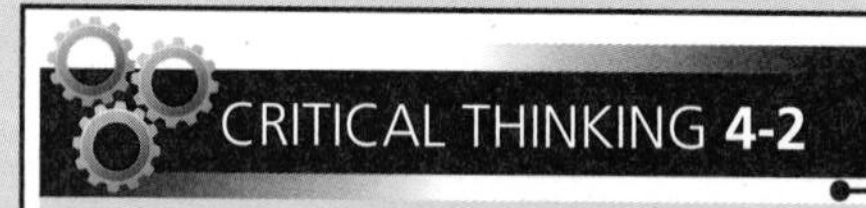

CRITICAL THINKING **4-2**

Visit the American Nurses Credentialing Center at www.nursingworld.org. Click on "careers and credentialing/certification." Choose a specialty in which a nurse can be certified and compare it to the certification in informatics. How are they similar? How are they different?

CRITICAL THINKING

Ethical, cultural, spiritual, legal, delegation, and quality improvement considerations are highlighted in these critical thinking boxes. Before beginning a new chapter, page through and read the Critical Thinking sections and jot down your comments or reactions; then see whether your perspective changes after you complete the chapter.

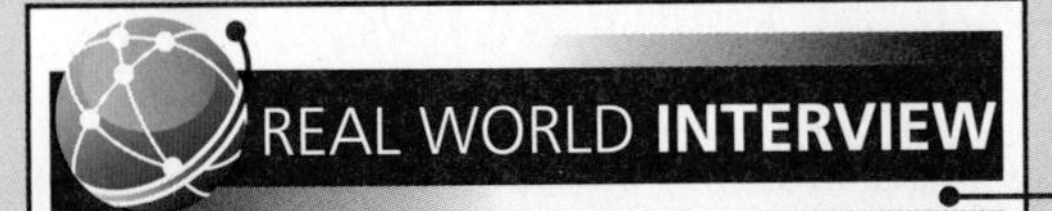

I was in a situation where I just didn't think my patient looked good. I decided to go ahead and start two new IV sites, just in case. The patient arrested two hours later, and we really needed those IV sites. I felt good about my decision.

CHERYL BUNTZ, RN
New Graduate
Independence, Missouri

REAL WORLD INTERVIEWS

Real World Interviews with nurses, doctors, staff, patients, and family members are included. As you read these, ask yourself whether you have ever considered the point of view being represented on the given topic. How would knowing another person's perspective affect the care you deliver?

KEY CONCEPTS

- Ethics is the branch of philosophy that concerns the distinction of right from wrong on the basis of a body of knowledge, not just on the basis of opinions.
- A personal philosophy stems from an individual's beliefs and values. This personal philosophy will influence an individual's philosophy of nursing.
- Values clarification is an important step in helping one understand what is truly important.
- Ethical principles include autonomy and confidentiality, beneficence, nonmaleficence, fidelity, autonomy, respect for others, veracity, and advocacy.
- The Ethical Positioning System is a helpful tool.
- The Patient Care Partnership encourages more effective patient care.
- Organizations have a responsibility to society to practice ethically, with a focus on quality and safety.
- Ethics committees provide guidance for decision making about ethical dilemmas that arise in health care settings.
- The International Council of Nurses' Code of Ethics for Nurses influences patient care.
- Various nursing ethical codes influence patient care.

KEY CONCEPTS

This bulleted list serves as a review and study tool for you as you complete each chapter.

KEY TERMS

autonomy	ethics	philosophy
beneficence	fidelity	trustworthiness
compassion	integrity	values
confidentiality	justice	values clarification
discernment	morality	veracity
ethical dilemma	nonmaleficence	

KEY TERMS

Study this list of key terms prior to reading the chapter, and then again as you complete a chapter to test your true understanding of the terms and concepts covered. Make a study list of terms you need to focus on to thoroughly appreciate the material in the chapter.

REVIEW QUESTIONS

1. A senior nursing student is preparing for the NCLEX-RN exam. The student realizes a variety of formats for questions will be used that include which of the following? Select all that apply.
   A. Fill-in-the-blank calculation
   B. Multiple responses
   C. Case study scenarios
   D. Ordered response
   E. Hot spots
   F. Matching
2. The nursing student is using the ARKO acronym as a strategy for preparing for the NCLEX-RN. The NCLEX-RN question states: "How would the nurse evaluate if the drug enoxaparin (Lovenox) is effective for the postoperative patient?" Using the second step (R), choose the best answer based on the information provided.
   A. What are the adverse effects of the drug?
   B. How long does it take for the drug to become effective?
   C. What is the intended action of the drug?
   D. How will the nurse administer this drug safely?

REVIEW QUESTIONS

These questions will challenge your comprehension of objectives and concepts presented in the chapter and will allow you to demonstrate content mastery, build critical-thinking skills, and achieve integration of the concepts. Multiple-choice and alternate styles of NCLEX-RN questions are included. Answers with rationales can be found on the **Premium Website**.

REVIEW ACTIVITIES

1. Set up a group to study for the NCLEX with several of your friends. Have each member of the group buy an NCLEX review book from a different publisher. Practice answering questions separately for one to two hours daily. Do not mark your answers in the review book. Share your study schedule and your review books with each other to encourage each other and increase your exposure to various authors' test questions.
2. You are graduating in two months from a nursing program. Develop a résumé using the format in this chapter.
3. You are a new nurse who has been asked to interview for a position on the orthopedic floor. Develop a cover letter expressing interest in the position. Make a list of possible interview questions.

REVIEW ACTIVITIES

These thought-provoking activities at the close of a chapter invite you to approach a problem or scenario critically and apply the knowledge you have gained. Suggested responses can be found on the **Premium Website**.

EXPLORING THE WEB

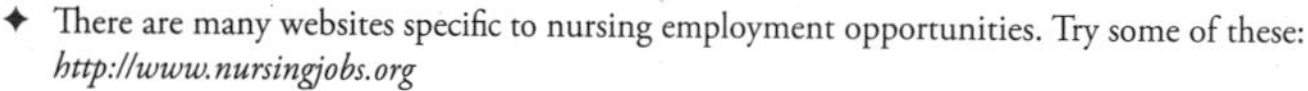

- There are many websites specific to nursing employment opportunities. Try some of these:
  http://www.nursingjobs.org
  http://www.healthecareers.com
  http://www.nurse.com
  http://www.discovernursing.com
  http://www.studentdoc.com/nursing-job-site.html
  http://www.healthcareerweb.com
- Look up several of these nursing sites:
  Association of Pediatric Oncology Nurses: *http://www.apon.org*
  Association of Rehabilitation Nurses: *http://www.rehabnurse.org*
  Association of Women's Health, Obstetric and Neonatal Nurses: *http://www.awhonn.org*
  Trauma Nursing: *http://www.trauma.com*
- Check this site for job opportunities: *http://healthcare.monster.com*
- Check this site:
  National Student Nurses' Association: *http://www.nsna.org*
- Go to: *http://www.learningext.com*

EXPLORING THE WEB

Internet activities encourage you to use your computer to search the Web for additional information on quality and nursing leadership and management.

UNIT I

INTRODUCTION

CHAPTER 1

Nursing Leadership, Management, and Motivation

MAUREEN T. MARTHALER, RN, MS;
LINDA SEARLE LEACH, RN, PHD, CNAA; AND
CHARLENE C. GYURKO, RN, PHD, CNE

Let whoever is in charge keep this simple question in her head (not, how can I always do this right thing myself, but) how can I provide for this right thing to always be done?

– FLORENCE NIGHTINGALE, 1859

OBJECTIVES

Upon completion of this chapter, the reader should be able to:

1. Differentiate between leadership and management.
2. Discuss leadership.
3. Review leadership theories.
4. Discuss management.
5. Review organizational management perspectives.
6. Discuss motivation theories.
7. Discuss Benner's Model of Novice to Expert.

Three nurses have been selected to participate in the hiring of a nurse manager. One of the nurses who works on the unit has applied for the job. Two nurses from nearby hospitals have also applied for the job. The nurses doing the hiring have identified the type of nurse manager they are seeking. The majority of them have determined that a transformational nurse manager would best serve their unit.

What are the pros and cons for the nurse who works on the unit to be hired in this position?

What are the pros and cons for nurses from other hospitals to be hired in this position?

What questions would the hiring nurses ask new applicants for the nurse manager position?

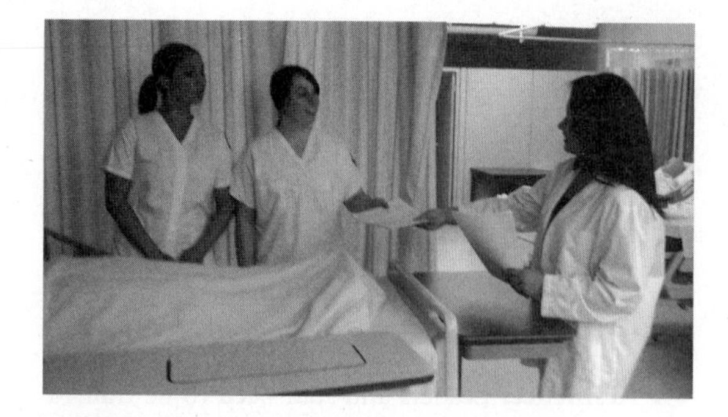

© Cengage Learning 2014

Today more than ever, registered nurses (RNs) have been identified as the much-needed linchpins of health care systems. Historically, nurses have often been considered a cost item versus making a significant contribution to an organization. In 2010, The Robert Wood Johnson Foundation (RWJF) and the Institute of Medicine (IOM) developed an action-oriented blueprint, *The Future of Nursing: Leading Change, Advancing Health* (IOM, 2010). Among the many things they recommended, were that nurses should practice to the full extent of their education and training; nurses should achieve higher levels of education in a system that promotes seamless academic progression; nurses should be full partners, with physicians and other health care professionals, in redesigning health care in the United States; and that effective nursing workforce planning and policy making require a better data collection and information infrastructure.

Nurses make a critical difference every day in leading and managing the care of their patients and patients' families. Nurses often believe those accomplishments are ordinary work, yet those accomplishments often prevent the occurrence of nursing-sensitive indicators. **Nursing-sensitive indicators** reflect the structure, process, and outcomes of nursing care. The structure of nursing care is indicated by the supply of nursing staff, the skill level of the nursing staff, and the education/certification of nursing staff. Process indicators measure aspects of nursing care such as assessment, intervention, and RN job satisfaction. Patient outcomes that are determined to be nursing sensitive are those that improve if there is a greater quantity or quality of nursing care (e.g., pressure ulcers, falls, and intravenous infiltrations) (American Nurses Association, 2012). Nurses make a critical difference whether they are working with an individual patient or managing a patient care unit or an entire nursing department.

Nurses manage and lead patient care in health care organizations that are moving more and more toward becoming high reliability organizations focused on improving patient care. **High reliability organizations** (HROs) create a culture and work processes that radically reduce system failures and effectively respond when failures do occur, thus helping to achieve safety, quality, and efficiency goals. Nurses work to do things right much of the time. But even very infrequent failures in critical work processes can have terrible consequences for a patient. At the core of HROs are five key concepts:

1. **Sensitivity to operations.** The HRO must preserve constant awareness by leaders and staff of the state of the systems and processes that affect patient care is important. This awareness is key to noting risks and preventing them.
2. **Reluctance to simplify.** Simple work processes are good, but simplistic explanations for why things work or fail are risky. Avoiding overly simple explanations of failure (unqualified staff, inadequate training, communication failure, and so on) is essential in order to avoid the true reasons patients are placed at risk.
3. **Preoccupation with failure.** When near-miss errors occur, these are viewed in HROs as evidence of systems that should be improved to

reduce potential harm to patients. Rather than viewing near misses as proof that the system has effective safeguards, near misses are viewed as symptomatic of areas in need of more attention.

4. **Deference to expertise.** If leaders and supervisors are not willing to listen and respond to the insights of staff who know how work processes really work and the risks patients really face, a high reliability organization is not possible.
5. **Resilience.** Leaders and staff need to be trained and prepared to know how to respond when system failures do occur.

This chapter differentiates between leadership and management, identifies theories of leadership, and discusses management. It reviews organizational management perspectives, outlines motivation theories, and discusses Benner's Model of Novice to Expert.

LEADERSHIP AND MANAGEMENT

Leadership and management are different. Hughes, Ginnett, & Curphy (2006) make the following distinctions between managers and leaders:

- Managers administer; leaders innovate
- Managers maintain; leaders develop
- Managers control; leaders inspire
- Managers have a short-term view; leaders have a long-term view
- Managers ask how and when; leaders ask what and why
- Managers initiate; leaders originate
- Managers accept the status quo; leaders challenge it

Not all leaders are managers. Bennis and Nanus (2003) popularized the phrase, "managers are people who do things right; leaders are people who do the right thing." Both roles are crucial in their own way. It is important to avoid thinking that leadership is important and management is insignificant. People need to be managed, as well as inspired and led. Leadership is part of management, not a substitute for it. We need both.

LEADERSHIP

Leadership is a process that occurs between a leader and another individual; between the leader and a group; or between a leader and an organization, a community, or a society; and that influences others, often by inspiring, enlivening, and engaging others to participate in the achievement of goals. Leadership is a subtle art and skill. It is based on inherent qualities of the individual and developed over time, through life events and experiences that range from insignificant to life altering (Comack, 2012). Leadership involves influencing the attitudes, beliefs, behaviors, and feelings of other people (Spector, 2006). The process of leadership involves the leader and the follower in an interaction. This implies that leadership is a reciprocal relationship. Defining leadership as a process helps us to better understand leadership. What this means for nurses as professionals is that they function as leaders when they influence others and make a difference in people's lives. Each nurse has the potential to serve as a leader.

Today's nurse must know how to lead. Effective leadership in health care is paramount. Nurses represent the largest discipline in health care. Nursing and nursing leadership is vital. Leading is also one of four managerial functions, along with planning, organizing and staffing, and controlling. Whereas management is more formal and relies on tools such as planning, budgeting, and controlling, leading involves having a vision and goals for what the organization can become, and then getting the cooperation and teamwork from others to achieve those goals (DuBrin, 2000).

Leadership is introduced early in a nurse's education as part of the nurse's role in providing assistance to others. A student nurse is a leader to patients and their families. Leadership ability grows in the beginning nurse who may demonstrate leadership in working with other staff; for example, the new nurse speaks up about the need for improvement in an element of care delivery. Leadership ability often grows as the nurse becomes more confident and experienced in working with others.

Leadership can be **formal leadership,** as when a person is in a position of authority or in a sanctioned, assigned role within an organization that connotes influence, such as a clinical nurse specialist (Northouse, 2010). **Informal leadership** is when a person demonstrates leadership outside the scope of a formal leadership role, such as a member of a group rather than the head or leader of the group. Staff nurses demonstrate informal leadership when they advocate and speak up for patient needs or when they take action to improve health care.

Leaders and Followers

Leaders and followers are both necessary roles. Leaders need followers in order to lead. Followers need leaders in order to follow. Nurses are alternately leaders and followers when they work with other health care team members to achieve patient care goals, participate in meetings, and so forth. The most valuable followers are skilled, self-directed employees who participate actively in setting the group's direction and invest time and energy in the work of the group, thinking critically and advocating for new ideas (Grossman & Valiga, 2008). Good followers communicate and work well with others, being supportive, yet thoughtful, in their approach to new ideas.

Nurses are leaders. Nurses function as leaders when they influence others toward goal achievement. RNs in staff nurse positions lead nursing practice by setting a direction, aligning people, and motivating and inspiring others toward a vision. Nurses lead other nurses and their community to achieve a collective vision of quality health care. See Table 1-1 for examples of nursing leadership characteristics and role activities.

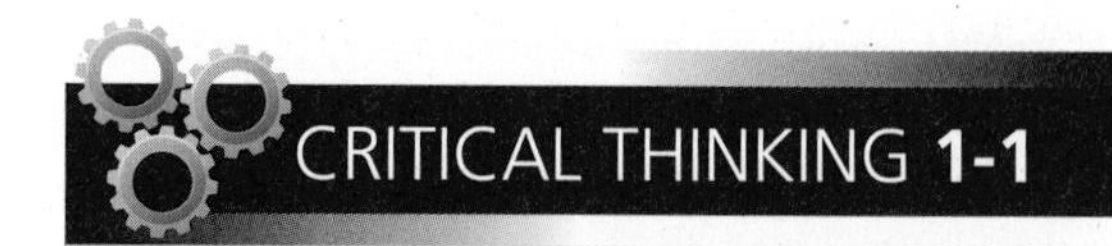

CRITICAL THINKING 1-1

Look for opportunities to gather data about quality clinical performance. What additional quality measures can you monitor in the following areas?

- *Clinical Care:* Number of patients who are triaged within 5 minutes of arrival in the Emergency Department.
- *Utilization:* Number of patients who achieve quality outcomes under normal staffing ratios.
- *Financial:* Number of patients who meet patient care budget goals.
- *Quality:* Number of patients who state they are pleased with their nursing care.

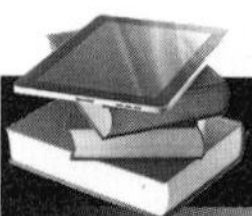

EVIDENCE FROM THE LITERATURE

Citation: Adeniran, R. K., Bhattacharya, A., & Adeniran, A. (2012). Professional excellence and career advancement in nursing: A conceptual framework for clinical leadership development. *Nursing Administration Quarterly, 36*(1), 41–51.

Discussion: One approach for nursing success is standardizing the entry-level education for nurses and developing a uniform professional development and career advancement trajectory with appropriate incentives to encourage participation. A framework to guide and provide scientific evidence of how frontline nurses can be engaged is paramount. A model for professional excellence and career advancement provides a framework that offers a clear path for researchers to examine variables influencing nurses' professional development and career advancement in a systematic manner. This article underscores professional preparedness of a registered nurse as central to leadership development. It also describes the elements that influence nurses' participation in professional development and career advancement under four main categories emphasizing mentorship and self-efficacy as essential variables.

Implications for Practice: The framework presented here highlights the impact of the key factors associated with professional excellence and career advancement among nurses. The framework acknowledges that professional nurses' level of education and professional preparedness make a major contribution toward their ability to engage in career advancement opportunities, drive evidence-based care, and influence decision making, using leadership competencies. Furthermore, the schema presented here identifies the importance of the interactive effect of self-efficacy and mentorship to a nurse's successful engagement in career advancement and leadership.

TABLE 1-1
Nursing Leadership Characteristics and Role Activities

Leadership requires personal mastery.	Nurses demonstrate leadership when they show competence and mastery in the tasks they perform. Nurses are deemed competent by means of a license to practice nursing (NLN, 2010).
Leadership is about values.	Nurses exhibit leadership through their demonstration of cultural values that are embraced through individual belief systems. Nurses display their personal and professional values as they serve others. Values are often entwined with ethical conflicts (Dahnke, 2009). The National League for Nursing (NLN) implements its mission guided by four dynamic and integrated core values that permeate the organization and are reflected in its work: ◆ CARING: promoting health, healing, and hope in response to the human condition ◆ INTEGRITY: respecting the dignity and moral wholeness of every person without conditions or limitation ◆ DIVERSITY: affirming the uniqueness of and differences among persons, ideas, values, and ethnicities ◆ EXCELLENCE: creating and implementing transformative strategies with daring ingenuity (NLN, 2010)
Leadership is about service.	Service learning is a current buzz word in nursing. Service learning links information learned in the classroom or learning environment to the community and can enhance culturally congruent care (Amerson, 2010).
Leadership is about people and relationships.	Nurses demonstrate leadership and play roles in patient outcomes when they build relationships with patients and their significant others (Wong & Cummings, 2007).
Leadership is contextual.	Nurses demonstrate leadership when they adjust their leadership styles, depending on the context that surrounds a particular situation, to achieve nursing goals. A major context evolves around the interrelationships that nurses have with others (Spence Laschinger, Finegan, & Wilk, 2009).
Leadership is about the management of meaning.	Nurses demonstrate leadership when they monitor the meaning of what is being communicated, both verbally and nonverbally, and manage the situation to achieve goals for all involved. The communication must be clear and inspiring (Murphy, 2005).
Leadership is about balancing.	Nurses demonstrate leadership when they multitask and balance all that they do to achieve nursing goals.
Leadership is about continuous learning and improvement.	Nurses demonstrate leadership by continuing to increase and improve their knowledge and expertise. Nightingale argued, ". . . a nurse never stops learning" (Mills, 1964, p. 35).

(Continues)

TABLE 1-1 (Continued)

Leadership is about effective decision making.	Nurses demonstrate leadership when they make effective, evidence-based decisions. Nurses must be autonomous in their decision making and also work with other members of the health care team to assure the best care for their patients (Wong & Cummings, 2007).
Leadership is a political process.	Nurses demonstrate leadership when they participate in nursing organizations and various political processes in their states and nations (Bishop, 2010).
Leadership is about modeling.	Nurses demonstrate leadership when they model learned beliefs and practices as they mentor other nurses.
Leadership is about integrity.	Nurses demonstrate leadership when they consistently model integrity, an expectation of a leader.

Source: Compiled with information from Moore, J. (2004). Leadership: Lessons learned. PowerPoint presentation to Indiana State University PhD Educational Leadership and Foundation Students. Terre Haute, Indiana. Nonpublished PowerPoint presentation.

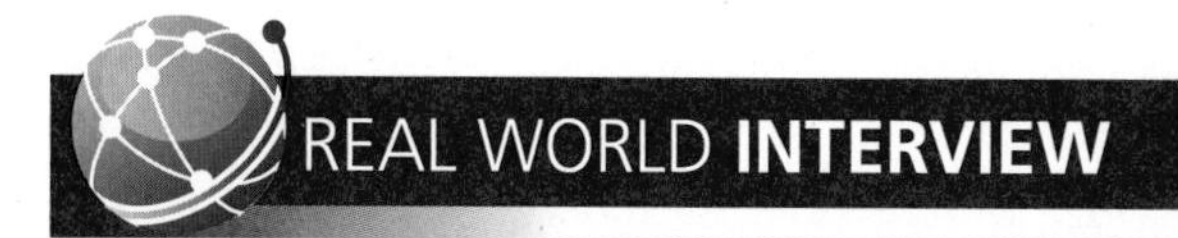

REAL WORLD **INTERVIEW**

It was a Monday. The Emergency Department was very busy as usual. A new patient, a 69-year-old African-American female, was admitted by ambulance following a motor vehicle accident. I went to assess this patient and noted that blood was dripping from a small laceration on her forehead. She was awake, alert, and oriented. She had no pain or nausea. She told me that she was feeling fine, but I noticed that her lips and mouth were pale. I told the charge nurse that I believed that the patient's hemoglobin level was below 5, and I asked her to please tell the physician to come to the room soon to assess the patient. As I believed this patient was not stable, I immediately took the lead and inserted a large-bore intravenous heplock in her vein and collected blood samples for a CBC, BMP, PT, PTT, INR, and type and cross match, just in case. I started a liter of 0.9% normal saline intravenous fluid and connected the patient to the cardiac monitor as well as to the blood pressure, pulse, and pulse oximeter monitors. The patient now began to complain of nausea. At this point, the doctor had not come to see the patient yet. I went and told the doctor to please come to the patient's room and assess her now. I told him that the patient was bleeding and that I believed that her hemoglobin would be reported as below 5. He then came to the room and assessed the patient. He removed the head laceration dressing, which was now soaked in blood. He noted a 1-inch laceration on her forehead that was still bleeding. He sutured the wound and finally ordered the CBC. I asked him if he was sure he only wanted the CBC. He said yes. When the CBC results came back, the patient's hemoglobin was 3.8. I felt good about my assessment and intervention with this patient. The physician then ordered a type and cross match for four units of blood and a CT of the head. After the patient received two units of blood, she was transferred to the ICU.

NIRMALA JOSEPH, RN
Staff Nurse
Houston, Texas

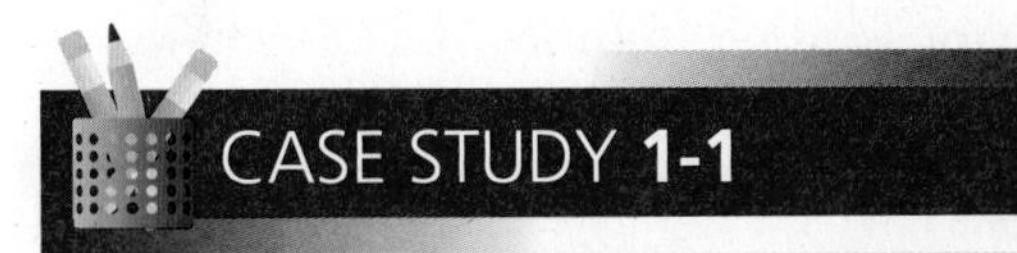

The nurse is caring for five pediatric patients. The nurse assesses one of the children and notes that the child is tachypneic. The child's color is pale, the skin is cool to the touch, and the child is difficult to rouse. The mother is asleep at the bedside but awakes during the commotion of the nurse's intervention. The nurse yells that she needs help. The charge nurse comes in the room, positions the child in a high Fowler's position, and encourages the child to take a deep breath. Several more nurses arrive. The child loses consciousness and a code is called.

What should have been done initially to prevent this patient from deteriorating?

What skill(s) did the charge nurse exhibit that demonstrated leadership?

How can the nurse be more prepared for a situation such as this in the future?

Leadership Characteristics

According to Bennis and Nanus (2003), effective leaders share several personal qualities. The first quality is a vision. Leaders focus on a professional and purposeful vision that provides direction toward the preferred future. The second quality is passion. Passion expressed by the leader involves the ability to inspire and align people toward the promises of life. The third quality is integrity based on knowledge of self, honesty, and maturity that is developed through experience and growth. Another quality associated with leadership is empowerment. Leaders empower others to translate intentions into reality and sustain it. McCall (1998) describes how self-awareness—knowing our strengths and weaknesses—can allow us to use feedback and learn from our mistakes. Daring and curiosity are also basic ingredients of leadership that leaders may use.

In their landmark work, *AACN Standards for Establishing Healthy Work Environments: A Journey to Excellence,* the American Association of Critical-Care Nurses cites authentic leadership as one of their key standards and assert that authentic leadership requires skill in the core competencies of self-knowledge, strategic vision, risk-taking and creativity, interpersonal and communication effectiveness, and inspiration (AACN, 2005).

Certain traits are commonly attributed to leaders. These traits are considered desirable and seem to contribute to the perception of being a leader. They include intelligence, self-confidence, determination, integrity, and sociability (Stodgill, 1948, 1974). Research among 46 hospitals designated as magnet hospitals for their success in attracting and retaining registered nurses emphasized the value of leaders who are visionary and enthusiastic, are supportive and knowledgeable, have high standards and expectations, value education and professional development, demonstrate power and status in the organization, are visible and responsive, communicate openly, and are active in professional associations (McClure & Hinshaw, 2002; Scott, Sochalski, & Aiken, 1999; Kramer, 1990; McClure, Poulin, Sovie, & Wandelt, 1983; Kramer & Schmalenberg, 2005). Research findings from studies of nurses revealed that caring, respectability, trustworthiness, and flexibility were the leader characteristics most valued. In one study, nurse leaders identified managing the dream, mastering change, designing organization structure, learning, and taking initiative as leadership characteristics (Murphy & DeBack, 1991). Research by Kirkpatrick and Locke (1991) concluded that leaders are different from nonleaders across six traits: drive, the desire to lead, honesty and integrity, self-confidence, cognitive ability, and knowledge of the business. Although no set of traits is definitive and reliable in determining who is a leader or who is effective as a leader, many people still rely on personality traits to describe and define leadership characteristics.

Leadership Theories

The major leadership theories can be classified according to the following approaches: behavioral, including autocratic, democratic, and laissez-faire; contingency; and contemporary.

Behavioral Approaches

Leadership studies from the 1930s by Kurt Lewin and colleagues at Iowa State University conveyed information about three leadership styles that are still widely recognized today. The three styles are autocratic, democratic, and laissez-faire leadership (Lewin, 1939; Lewin & Lippitt, 1938; Lewin, Lippitt, & White, 1939).

Autocratic leadership involves centralized decision making, with the leader making decisions and using power to command and control others. The *autocratic* style is used by the leader in situations in which (1) the task or outcome is relatively simple (such as telling the nursing assistive personnel [NAP] to take a temperature); (2) most team members would agree with the decision and provide consensus; and (3) a decision has to be made promptly.

Democratic leadership is participatory, with authority often delegated to others. To be influential, the democratic leader uses expert power and the power base afforded by having close, personal relationships. In the *democratic* style, the leader will ask the opinions of the entire team, but the final decision usually lies with the leader, or there may be mutual decision making by both team members and the leader, with everyone having an equal vote. This process encourages everyone to fully accept the team's conclusion. This style allows all to have the opportunity to provide input and differing perspectives into the decision.

The third style, **laissez-faire leadership**, is passive and permissive, and the leader defers decision making. Lewin (1939) contrasted these styles and concluded that autocratic leaders were associated with high-performing groups, but that close supervision of the group was necessary and feelings of hostility were often present toward the autocratic leader. Democratic leaders engendered positive feelings in their groups; group performance was strong whether or not the democratic leader was present. Low productivity and feelings of frustration in the group were associated with laissez-faire leaders.

Behavioral leadership studies from the University of Michigan and Ohio State University led to the identification of two basic leader behaviors: job-centered and employee-centered behaviors. Effective leadership was described as having a focus on the human needs of subordinates and was called **employee-centered leadership** (Moorhead & Griffin, 2001). **Job-centered leaders** were seen as less effective because of their focus on schedules, costs, and efficiency, resulting in a lack of attention to developing work groups and high-performance goals (Moorhead & Griffin, 2001).

The researchers at Ohio State focused their efforts on two dimensions of leader behavior: initiating structure and consideration. **Initiating structure** involves an emphasis on the work to be done, a focus on the task, and production. Leaders who focus on initiating structure are concerned with how work is organized and on the achievement of goals. Leader behavior includes planning, directing others, and establishing deadlines and details of how work is to be done. For example, a nurse demonstrating the leader behavior of initiating structure could be a charge nurse who, at the beginning of a shift, makes out a patient assignment.

The dimension of **consideration** involves activities that focus on the employee and emphasize relating and getting along with people. Leader behavior focuses on consideration of the well-being of others. The leader is involved in creating a relationship that fosters communication and trust as a basis for respecting other people and their potential contribution. A nurse demonstrating consideration behavior will take the time to talk with coworkers, be empathetic, and show an interest in them as people.

The leader behaviors of initiating structure and consideration define leadership style. The various styles nurses use include:

- Low initiating structure, low consideration
- High initiating structure, low consideration
- High initiating structure, high consideration
- Low initiating structure, high consideration

The Ohio State University studies associate the high initiating structure/high consideration leader behaviors with better performance and satisfaction outcomes than the other styles. Nurses who use high initiating structure and high consideration leader behaviors will initiate and develop clear, well-structured assignments and work considerately with their staff to achieve quality outcomes. This leadership style is considered effective, although it may not be appropriate in every situation.

Another model based on two dimensions is the managerial grid developed by Blake and Mouton (1985).

Five styles identify the extent of structure, called *concern for production,* and consideration, called *concern for people,* demonstrated by the leader. Concern for both people and production can be low, moderate, or high (Figure 1-1).

Blake and Mouton's five leader styles are:

1. Impoverished leader for low production concern and low people concern
2. Authority compliance leader for high production concern and low people concern
3. Country club leader for high people concern and low production concern
4. Middle-of-the-road leader for moderate concern in both dimensions
5. Team leader for high production concern and high people concern

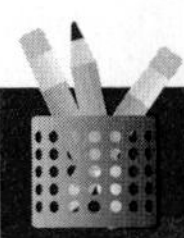

CASE STUDY 1-2

Among the individuals commonly identified as leaders (Table 1-2), can you identify a set of leadership traits, such as knowledge, self-confidence, determination, integrity, sociability, cognitive ability, caring, honesty, trustworthiness, flexiblity, desire to lead, and drive, that they all possess?

TABLE 1-2
Leaders Among Us: Past and Present

Mother Teresa	Martin Luther King, Jr.
Imogene King	John F. Kennedy
Hildegard Peplau	Sister Callista Roy
Rosa Parks	Franklin Delano Roosevelt
John Adams	Dorothea Orem
Barack Obama	Florence Nightingale
Pope Benedict	Peter Buerhaus
Mitt Romney	Hillary Clinton
Clara Barton	Virginia Henderson
Ida Androwich	Martha Rogers
Linda Aiken	Sister Rosemary Donley
Winston Churchill	Zenaida Corpuz

©Cengage Learning 2014

Now divide your class into groups. Have each group identify someone from this list whom they see as a leader. Describe the leader's traits and then have the groups share with the class who the leaders are and their traits.

Do the leaders demonstrate any traits such as drive, desire to lead, honesty and integrity, self-confidence, cognitive ability, or knowledge of their business?

When you work on the clinical unit, do you see any staff nurses displaying these leadership traits?

How can you develop these traits in yourself?

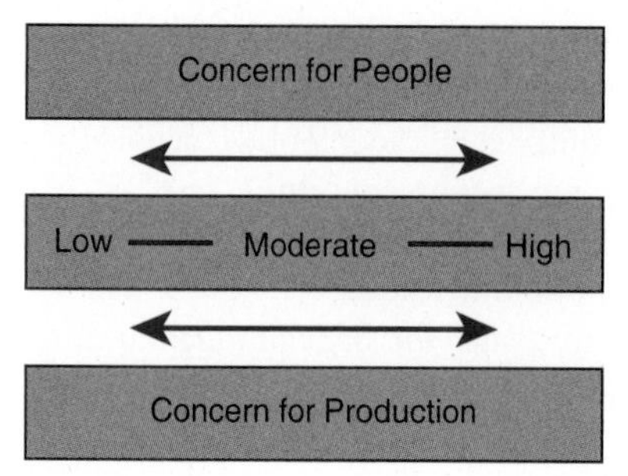

FIGURE 1-1

Key leadership dimensions.

(*Source:* Compiled with information from Blake, Mouton, and McCanse Leadership Grid from Leadership: Theory, Application, Skill Building by R. N. Lussier and C. F. Achua, 2000, Cincinnatti, OH: South-Western College.)

Contingency Approaches

Another approach to leadership is **contingency theory**. Contingency theory acknowledges that other factors in the environment influence outcomes as much as leadership style and that leader effectiveness is contingent upon something other than the leader's behavior. The premise is that different leader behavior patterns will be effective in different situations. Contingency approaches include Fielder's contingency theory, the situational theory of Hersey, Blanchard, and Johnson, path-goal theory, and the idea of substitutes for leadership.

FIELDER'S CONTINGENCY THEORY: Fielder (1967) is credited with the development of the contingency model of leadership effectiveness. Fielder's theory of leadership effectiveness views the pattern of leader behavior as dependent upon the interaction of the personality of the leader and the needs of the situation. The needs of the situation or how favorable the situation is toward the leader influences leader-member relationships, the degree of task structure, and the leader's position of power (Fielder, 1967).

Leader-member relations are the feelings and attitudes of followers regarding acceptance, trust, and credibility of the leader. Good leader-member relations exist when followers respect, trust, and have confidence in the leader. Poor leader-member relations reflect distrust, a lack of confidence and respect, and dissatisfaction with the leader by the followers.

Task structure refers to the degree to which work is defined, with specific procedures, explicit directions, and goals. High task structure involves routine, predictable, clearly defined work tasks. Low task structure involves work that is not routine, predictable, or clearly defined, such as creative, artistic, or qualitative research activities.

Position power is the degree of formal authority and influence associated with the leader. High position power is favorable for the leader and low position power is unfavorable. When all of these dimensions—leader-member relations, task structure, and position power—are high, the situation is favorable to the leader. When they are low, the situation is not favorable to the leader. In both of these circumstances, Fielder showed that a task-directed leader, concerned with task accomplishment, was effective. When the range of favorableness is intermediate or moderate in a situation, a human relations leader, concerned about people, was most effective. These situations need a leader with interpersonal and relationship skills to foster group achievement. Fielder's contingency theory is an approach that matches the organizational situation to the most favorable leadership style for that situation.

SITUATIONAL THEORY: Hersey, Blanchard, and Johnson's situational leadership theory (2008) addresses follower readiness as a factor in determining leadership style and considers *task behavior* and *relationship behavior.* High task behavior and low relationship behavior is called a *telling leadership* style. A high task, high relationship style is called a *selling leadership* style. A low task and high relationship style is called a *participating leadership* style. A low task and low relationship style is called a *delegating leadership* style.

Follower readiness, called maturity, is assessed in order to select one of the four leadership styles for a situation. For example, *telling leaders* define the roles and tasks of the follower and supervise them closely. Decisions are made by the leader and announced, so communication is largely one-way. *Selling leaders* still define the roles and tasks, but seek ideas and suggestions from the followers. Decisions remain the leader's prerogative but communication is much more two-way. *Participating leaders* pass day-to-day decisions, such as task allocation, to the followers. The leader facilitates and takes part in decisions but control is shared with the followers. *Delegating leaders* are still involved in decisions and problem solving but control is with the follower. The follower decides when and how the leader will be involved. An additional aspect of this model is the idea that the leader not only changes leadership style according to followers' needs, but also develops followers over time to increase their level of maturity (Lussier & Achua, 2013).

PATH-GOAL THEORY: In this leadership approach, the leader works to motivate followers and influence goal accomplishment. The seminal author on path-goal theory is Robert House (1971). By using the appropriate style of leadership for the situation (i.e., *directive, supportive, participative,* or *achievement-oriented),* the leader makes the path toward the goal easier for the follower. The *directive* style of leadership provides structure through direction and authority, with the leader focusing on the task and getting the job done. The *supportive style* of leadership is relationship oriented, with the leader providing encouragement, interest, and attention. *Participative* leadership means that the leader focuses on involving followers in the decision-making process. The *achievement-oriented* leadership style provides high structure and direction, as well as high support through consideration behavior.

In Path-Goal Theory, the leadership style is matched to the situational characteristics of the followers, such as the desire for authority, the extent to which the control of goal achievement is internal or external, and the ability of the follower to be involved. The leadership style is also matched to the situational factors in the environment, including the routine nature or complexity of the task, the power associated with the leader's position, and the work group relationship. This alignment of leadership style with the needs of followers is motivating and believed to enhance performance and satisfaction. The Path-Goal Theory is derived from expectancy theory, which suggests that people will be motivated if they think they are capable of performing their work, if they believe their efforts will result in a certain outcome, and if they believe that the payoffs for doing their work are worthwhile (Northouse, 2010).

SUBSTITUTES FOR LEADERSHIP: Substitutes for leadership are variables that may influence followers to the same extent as the leader's behavior. Kerr and Jermier (1978) investigated situational variables and identified some of these variables as substitutes that eliminate the need for leader behavior, and other variables as neutralizers that nullify the effects of the leader's behavior. Some of these variables include follower characteristics, such as the presence of structured routine tasks, the amount of feedback provided by the task, and the presence of intrinsic satisfaction in the work; and organizational characteristics, such as the presence of a cohesive group, a formal organization, a rigid adherence to rules, and low position power. For example, an individual's experience substitutes for task-direction leader behavior (Kerr & Jermier, 1978). This theory suggests that nurses and other professionals with a great deal of experience do not need direction and supervision to perform their work. Their knowledge serves as a leadership substitute. Another substitute for leader behavior is intrinsic satisfaction that emerges from just doing the work. Intrinsic satisfaction occurs frequently among nurses when they provide care to patients and families. Intrinsic satisfaction can substitute for the support and encouragement of relationship-oriented leader behavior.

Contemporary Approaches

Contemporary approaches to leadership address the leadership functions necessary to develop learning organizations and lead the process of transforming change. These approaches include charismatic leadership, transformational leadership theory, knowledge workers, emotional intelligence, and Wheatley's New Science of Leadership (Wheatley, 1999).

CHARISMATIC THEORY: A charismatic leader has an inspirational quality that promotes an emotional connection in followers. House (1971) developed a theory of charismatic leadership that described how charismatic leaders behave, as well as distinguishing characteristics and situations in which such leaders would be effective. Charismatic leaders display self-confidence and strength in their convictions, and communicate high expectations and confidence in others. These leaders have been described as emerging during a crisis, communicating vision, and using personal power and unconventional strategies (Conger & Kanungo, 1987). One consequence of this type of leadership is a belief in the charismatic leader that is so strong it takes on an almost supernatural sense and the leader is worshipped as if superhuman. Examples of charismatic leaders include Florence Nightingale, Winston Churchill, and Martin Luther King, Jr. Charisma seems to be a special and valuable quality that some people have and other people do not.

Transformational Leadership Theory: Burns (1978) defined transformational leadership as a process in which "leaders and followers raise one another to higher levels of motivation and morality" (p. 21). Transformational leadership theory is based on the idea of empowering others to engage in pursuing a collective purpose by working together to achieve a vision of a preferred future. This kind of leadership can influence both the leader and the follower to a higher level of conduct and achievement that transforms them both (Burns, 1978). Burns maintained that there are two types of leaders: the traditional manager concerned with day-to-day operations, called the **transactional leader**, and the leader who is committed to a vision that empowers others, called the **transformational leader**.

Transformational leaders motivate others by behaving in accordance with values, providing a vision that reflects mutual values, and empowering others to contribute. Bennis and Nanus (2003) describe this type of leader as a leader who "commits people to action, who converts followers into leaders, and who converts leaders into agents of change." According to research by Tichy and Devanna (1986), effective transformational leaders identify themselves as change agents; are courageous; believe in people; are value-driven; are lifelong learners; have the ability to deal with complexity, ambiguity, and uncertainty; and are visionaries. Yet transformational leadership may be demonstrated by anyone in an organization regardless of position (Burns, 1978). The interaction that occurs between individuals can be transformational and motivate both to a higher level of performance (Bass, 1985).

Transformational leadership at the organizational level is about innovation and change. The transformational leader uses vision which is based on shared values to align people and inspire growth and advancement. It is both the inspiration and the empowerment aspects of transformational leadership that lead to commitment beyond self-interest, commitment to a vision, and commitment to action that creates change. Transformational leadership theory suggests that the relationship between the leader and the follower inspires and empowers an individual toward commitment to the organization.

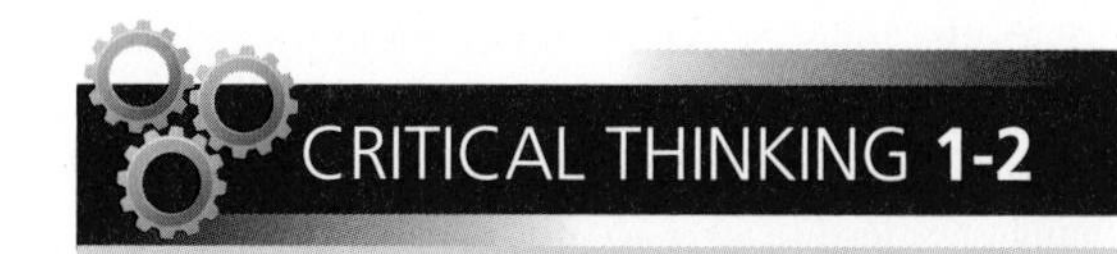

CRITICAL THINKING 1-2

As the nurse enters the room of a new postoperative patient with a radical laryngectomy, the patient begins to hemorrhage from his neck incision. The nurse applies direct pressure with one hand and calls for assistance. Help arrives and the patient is taken to surgery with the nurse still maintaining pressure on the hemorrhaging site. The patient lives and goes home a few days later.

How does good leadership on a patient care unit ensure positive nurse-sensitive patient outcomes in an emergency?

How can you develop your transformational leadership skills, such as belief in self as a change agent, belief in people, and being a lifelong learner to improve your ability to care for a group of patients and empower others to do so?

Nurse researchers have described nurse executives according to transformational leadership theory and have used this theory to measure leadership behavior among nurse executives and nurse managers (Leach, 2005; Dunham-Taylor, 2000; Wolf, Boland, & Aukerman, 1994; McDaniel & Wolf, 1992; Young, 1992). Additionally, transformational leadership theory has been the basis for nursing administration curriculum and for investigation of relationships such as between a nurse's commitment to an organization and productivity in a hospital setting (Leach, 2005; McNeese-Smith, 1997). Cassidy and Koroll (1998) explored the ethical aspects of transformational leadership, and Barker (1990) comprehensively discussed nursing in terms of transformational leadership theory.

Knowledge Workers: The organizations that nurses are a part of are changing. They reflect the advance and the promise of the technology that enables us to perform our work. Peter Drucker (1994) identifies the organization of the future as a knowledge organization composed of knowledge workers.

Knowledge workers are those workers who bring specialized, expert knowledge to an organization. They are valued for what they know. The knowledge organization will share, provide, and grow the information necessary to work efficiently and effectively. Drucker says that knowledge organizations, in which the knowledge worker is at the front lines with the expertise and the information to act, will become the dominant organizational type (Drucker, 1994; Helgesen, 1995). In organizations such as these, the ideas of leadership at the top and leadership equated with the power of a position are obsolete notions. Knowledge workers with the expertise and information to act are the organization's leaders. They provide the service, interact with the customer, represent the organization, and accomplish its goals. Leadership is needed at all levels within such an organization, not just at the top and not just with certain positions in the organization. Every nurse has knowledge and serves as a leader.

In the information age, it is the development of new knowledge and innovation and its meaningful interpretation and application that becomes the source for transactions with patients and staff. Nursing's transition to the information age is occurring within the context of rapidly advancing technology and nanotechnology and is influenced by three key trends. These trends have been termed *mobility, virtuality,* and *user-driven practices* (Porter-O'Grady, 2001).

Mobility refers to the ability to change skill sets as well as having the work dispersed among a variety of work locations, rather than work occurring at fixed sites (Bennis, Spreitzer, & Cummings, 2001). Nurses are working in many new settings today and are constantly adding to their knowledge as new technologies emerge.

Virtuality means working through virtual means using digital networks, where the worker may be far from the patient but present in a digital reality. Nurses are working in outpatient settings today where they carry a computer and are in instant communication with other practitioners and patients.

User-driven practices mean that the individual, at a time when digital media have given us more access to information and therefore more choices, acts more independently and is increasingly accountable for those choices and actions. Nurses are constantly assessing patients using traditional assessment methods as well as newer digital methods, for example, computerized vital sign monitors, and taking action to safeguard their patients and improve their care using these assessments.

Using Knowledge

Nurses can develop their leadership and management skills with continuing education and by increasing their knowledge and expertise in caring for a group of patients. Knowledgeable nursing leadership and management on a nursing unit fosters good patient care by providing a supportive environment for nurses to deliver care. A supportive leadership and management environment provides a clear chain of command, clear job descriptions, patient care standards, good staffing ratios, good Internet and library resources, continuing education support, and so on.

EMOTIONAL INTELLIGENCE: Emotional intelligence is a component of leadership and refers to the capacity for recognizing your own feelings and those of others, for motivating yourself, and for managing emotions well in yourself and in your relationships. It describes abilities distinct from, but complementary to academic intelligence. Many people who are "book smart" but lack emotional intelligence end up working for people who have lower IQs but excel in emotional intelligence skills (Goleman, 1998).

Emotional intelligence includes these five basic emotional and social competencies:

1. Self-awareness: Knowing what you are feeling in the moment, and using those preferences to guide your decision making; having a realistic assessment of your own abilities and a well-grounded sense of self-confidence
2. Self-regulation: Handling your emotions so that they facilitate rather than interfere with the task at hand, being conscientious and delaying gratification to pursue goals, and recovering well from emotional distress
3. Motivation: Using your deepest preferences to move and guide you toward your goals, to help you take initiative and strive to improve, and to persevere in the face of setbacks and frustrations
4. Empathy: Sensing what people are feeling, being able to take their perspective, and cultivating rapport and attunement with a broad diversity of people

5. Social skills: Handling emotions in relationships well and accurately reading social situations and networks; interacting smoothly; using these skills to persuade and lead, and negotiate and settle disputes, for cooperation and teamwork (Goleman, 1998)

Wheatley's New Science of Leadership: Margaret Wheatley, in *Leadership and the New Science* (1999), says, "There is a simpler way to lead organizations, one that requires less effort and produces less stress than the current practices." She presents us with a new view of leadership, one encompassing connectedness and self-organizing systems that follow a natural order of both chaos and uncertainty. This differs from a view that sees leadership as following a linear order in a hierarchy. Wheatley says that the leader's function is to guide an organization using vision, to make choices based on mutual values, and to engage in the culture to provide meaning and coherence. This type of leadership fosters growth within each of us as individuals and as members of a group. The notion of connection within a self-organizing system optimizes autonomy at all levels because the relationships between the individual and the whole are strong.

Wheatley (2005) discusses how people learn best when they are engaged in relationships with others and can exchange knowledge and expertise through informal, self-organized communities. Wheatley refers to these as "communities of practice" and encourages us to develop new leaders using such communities. Her notion of a community of practice represents several elements nurses are familiar with, that is, forming informal groups, using a group process of organizing, using principles of learning, and sharing information. What is unique in her description of these communities of practice is that they form via self-organization. They come together naturally. What makes these communities different from informal groups is Wheatley's characterization of a community built from relationships and participation in a way that connects nurses and allows the creation of meaning from information or the exchange of knowledge. In work done for the Center for Creative Leadership, communities of practice are described as being different from the ideas or experiences we have had with other groups and teams because communities of practice emerge from shared activity, shared knowledge, and ways of knowing that create meaning and thus facilitate a culture of engagement, participation, and relationships (Drath & Palus, 1994). Wheatley directs nurses to name these communities of practice that connect and bring people together, support these connections, nourish the community, and illuminate their work. These exciting notions hold great promise for health professionals as we learn how to collaborate within and across disciplines and countries to advance health care practices.

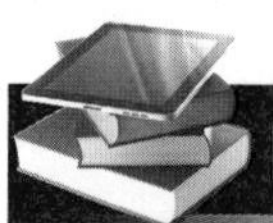

EVIDENCE FROM THE **LITERATURE**

Citation: Ridge, R. (2011). Future of nursing special: Practicing to potential. *Nursing Management, 42*(6), 32–37.

Discussion: The nursing profession must be transformed in terms of practice, education, and leadership to fulfill its role in the delivery of health care in the United States. The Institute of Medicine (IOM, 2010) report, *The Future of Nursing: Leading Change, Advancing Health*, addresses nursing at all practice levels, with the greatest emphasis on advanced practice. The report identifies barriers, describes new structures and opportunities, and provides an overall specific vision regarding the vital contribution of advanced practice nurses (APNs) to the health care system.

Implications for Practice: Drawing on previous IOM reports, the IOM report explores information technology (IT) as related to the provision of care and as an aid to documentation and decision making. Effective collaboration among and between multiple disciplines will require successful integration of information systems. Restructured teams with nurses at the forefront will be facilitated by expanded use of IT applications such as mobile workstations for nurses, remote biometric monitoring of patients, and streamlining of current work processes related to medication reconciliation, giving or receiving reports, and planning care.

MANAGEMENT

Management is defined as a process of planning, organizing and staffing, leading, and controlling actions to achieve goals. Planning involves setting goals and identifying ways to meet them. Organizing and staffing is the process of ensuring that the necessary human and physical resources are available to achieve the planning goals. Organizing also involves assigning work to the right person or group and specifying who has the authority to accomplish certain tasks. Leading is influencing others to achieve the organization's goals and involves energizing, directing, and persuading others to achieve those goals. Finally, controlling is comparing actual performance to a standard and revising the original plan as needed to achieve the goals (DuBrin, 2000).

Nurse managers often seem to work at a hectic pace and sustain that effort through long hours, frequently working without breaks. Yukl (1998) says that this reflects a preference by people in management positions for continuously seeking information and being constantly engaged in interactions with others who need information, help, guidance, or approval. The typical manager is always on the go. Research by McCall, Morrison, and Hanman (1978) showed that the daily activities of managers are diverse and fast paced with regular interruptions. Priority activities are integrated among inconsequential ones. In the scope of one morning, a nurse manager may engage in serious decisions about a critically ill patient, a staff or patient complaint, a shortage of nurse staffing, and so forth. A nurse manager's work is driven by problems that emerge in random order and that have a range of importance and urgency. These circumstances create an image of the nurse manager as a "firefighter" involved in immediate and operational concerns. A significant proportion of a manager's time is spent in interaction with others, and more of the work is concerned with handling information than in making decisions (McCall et al., 1978). Nurse managers constantly interact with other members of a health care team. This team can include nurses, various health care practitioners, unit staff, and staff from other departments who share information and assure that quality patient outcomes are achieved.

Management Roles

A frequently referenced taxonomy of managerial roles is from an in-depth, month-long study of five chief executives by Henry Mintzberg. A taxonomy is a system that groups or classifies principles. Mintzberg's observations led to the identification of three categories of managerial roles: (1) information processing roles, (2) interpersonal roles, and (3) decision-making roles (Mintzberg, 1973). A role includes behaviors, expectations, and recurrent activities within a pattern that is part of the organization's structure (Katz & Kahn, 1978).

The information processing roles identified by Mintzberg (1973) are those of monitor, disseminator, and spokesperson, each of which is used to manage the information needs that people have. The interpersonal roles consist of figurehead, leader, and liaison, and each of these is used to manage relationships with people. The decision-making roles are entrepreneur, disturbance handler, allocator of resources, and negotiator. Nurse managers take on these roles when they manage care.

The Management Process

In the early 1900s, an emphasis on management as a discipline emerged with a focus on the science of management and a view that management is an art of accomplishing things through people (Follet, 1924). Henri Fayol described the functions of planning, organizing, coordinating, and controlling as the management process (Fayol, 1916/1949). His work has become a classic in the way that we define the process of managing. Gulick and Urwick (1937) defined the management process according to seven principles. Their principles form the acronym POSDCORB, which stands for planning, organizing, staffing, directing, coordinating (CO), reporting, and budgeting (Gulick & Urwick, 1937; Henry, 1992). Their work is also considered to be a classic description of management functions and is still a relevant description of how the management process is carried out today.

More recently, Yukl (1998) and colleagues described 13 managerial role functions for managing the work and for managing relationships. The role functions for managing the work are planning and organizing, problem solving, clarifying roles and objectives,

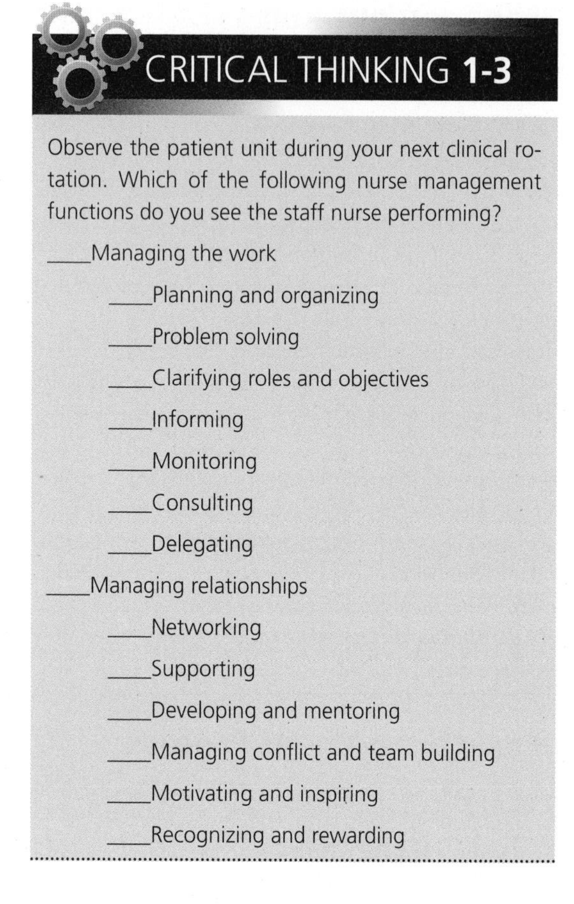

CRITICAL THINKING 1-3

Observe the patient unit during your next clinical rotation. Which of the following nurse management functions do you see the staff nurse performing?

____Managing the work

____Planning and organizing

____Problem solving

____Clarifying roles and objectives

____Informing

____Monitoring

____Consulting

____Delegating

____Managing relationships

____Networking

____Supporting

____Developing and mentoring

____Managing conflict and team building

____Motivating and inspiring

____Recognizing and rewarding

informing, monitoring, consulting, and delegating. The role functions for managing relationships are networking, supporting, developing and mentoring, managing conflict and team building, motivating and inspiring, and recognizing and rewarding.

The amount of time nurse managers spend on particular roles or functions varies by the level of their positions in organizations, ranging from first-level positions, to middle-level positions, to executive-level positions. The staff nurse manager may spend a large part of time both giving care and monitoring others as they deliver care, as well as monitoring the outcomes of care given. The next highest percentage of this nurse's time is spent in planning care, with other responsibilities such as coordinating, evaluating, negotiating, and serving as a multispecialist and generalist taking less than 10% each of this nurse's time.

In contrast, the middle-level nurse manager, such as the nurse manager of critical-care nursing, may spend less time in direct care and more time in each of the other functions, particularly planning, monitoring, and coordinating. At the highest level of the organization, usually described as the nurse executive level, planning and being a generalist are a greatly expanded role function, whereas direct patient care monitoring is not as primary a role function as it is in the other two levels. Nurses in executive-level roles in health care organizations often have the title of chief nurse executive or vice president of patient care services.

Organizational Management Perspectives

Much of our current understanding of organizational management is based on classical perspectives that were identified in the 1800s during the industrial age as factories developed. Since then many other perspectives have emerged (Shortell & Kaluzny, 2012; See Table 1-3).

Manager Resources

Nurse managers use four types of resources to accomplish their purpose (DuBrin, 2000). Nurse managers use human resources, such as the right staff on the health care team, to complete various assignments. They use financial resources wisely to help achieve organizational goals. Nurse managers also use physical resources such as patient care equipment to complete their work. Finally, nurse managers use information resources to stay up-to-date in delivering care to their patients.

Feedback

Because of their professional socialization and strong achievement needs, nurses want to deliver high-quality, excellent care to their patients. However, in order for them to know how well they are doing in this regard, they need high-quality information systems that provide feedback on a frequent basis. Such a system allows health care professionals to know not only how well they are doing, but also to enhance their confidence that they are doing things right (Kongstvedt, 2009).

TABLE 1-3
Major Organizational Management Perspectives

Perspective	Key Contributions
Bureaucratic Weber (1964)	Focuses on hierarchical superior-subordinate communication transmitted from top to bottom via a clear chain of command division of Uses explicit procedures, records, and files to govern activities Selects officeholders based on achievement Is endemic to all organizations Is less pronounced in small work groups and more pronounced in hospitals and large firms
Scientific Management Taylor (1911)	Uses time and motion studies to analyze a task into into its simplest components and then systematically improve a worker's performance of each component to maximize productivity and ensure conformity to a one best way of production
Classical School of Administration Gulick (1937) Gulick & Urwick (1937) Fayol (1949)	Includes unity of command (i.e., one boss); unity of direction (i.e., one objective, one plan, one boss); subordination of individual interest to general interest; centralization; authority; span of control (i.e., optimal number of people to supervise); and departmentalization
Human Relations Mayo (1945) McGregor (1960) Roethlisberger & Dickson (1947)	States that to improve productivity, management must focus on other things than monetary incentives and top-down control of work; managers must instead understand the informal organization of workers in groups and teams; the need of workers to be listened to and to participate in the design of their work (i.e., participation and self-governance); and understand the importance of morale and satisfaction as motivators of workers Hawthorne studies at Western Electric plant in Chicago led to the belief that human relations between workers and managers and among workers were the main determinants of efficiency The Hawthorne effect refers to the phenomenon of how being observed or studied results in a change in behavior Suggests that workers are less guided by financial incentives and more guided by humans (i.e., peer groups) Recognizes the interdependence of the organization and employees and seeks ways to achieve the goals of both
Contingency Bass (1981)	Highlights that the choice of a Theory X or Theory Y leadership style depends on key situational factors Theory X argues for greater structure, control, top-down decision making, and reliance on extrinsic rewards Theory Y argues for more participative management, self-governance, bottom-up decision making, and reliance on intrinsic rewards

(Continues)

TABLE 1-3 (Continued)

Perspective	Key Contributions
Decision-Making School Huber (1980)	Emphasizes unobtrusive controls over managerial decisions and behaviors Focuses on middle managers Uses controls including standard operating procedures, decision-making routines, socialization and training, organizational vocabularies and communication, and techniques to filter, process, edit, classify, and restrict the flow of information inside the firm
Open Systems and Resource Dependence Katz & Kahn (1978) Thompson, 1967 Lawrence & Lorsch, 1967 Blake & Mouton, 1964 Quinn, 1988 Pfeffer & Salancik, 1978	Emphasizes that organizations exist within an environment from which they must secure resources, support, and legitimacy in order to survive and operate States that organizations depend on other firms for critical resources and engage in strategies to protect themselves
Strategic Management March & Simon, 1958 Barney, 1991 Dyer & Singh, 1998 Ouchi (1980) Porter (1980)	Emphasizes industry structure and competitive forces as well as the firm's distinctive capabilities, resources, relational capabilities, and collaboration with upstream suppliers and downstream distributors and customers
Population Ecology or Organizational Ecology Aldrich (1979) Hannan & Freeman (1977) Hawley (1950) McKenzie (1968) Baum & Amburgey, 2005 Alexander & Amburgey, 1987 Wholey & Burns, 1993	States that the environment selects out and retains the most appropriate organizational form from an existing population of various forms Suggests that environmental forces make managerial choice and discretion very important for organizational survival and growth

(Continues)

TABLE 1-3 (Continued)

Perspective	Key Contributions
Institutional	Views organizations as organisms that adapt to pressures from without and within
Meyer & Rowan (1977)	
Selznik (1949)	States that firms take on a distinctive set of values, structures, and capacities as part of a natural history of development
DiMaggio & Powell (1983)	
Ruef & Scott (1998)	States that the firm becomes endued with values and goals from its environment as well as from its initial charter
Social Network	States that all behavior is social in nature , and that successful organizations will develop and use social networks to their advantage
Uzzi (1997,1999)	
Gulati (1995)	
Ahuja (2000)	
Burt (1992)	
Complex Adaptive System	Emphasizes that complex adaptive systems are open systems that are composed of of multiple, diverse, interconnected elements that the capability to change and learn from their experience
Dooley & Plsek (2001)	
Begun & White (1999)	
Nelson et al. (2008)	

Source: Compiled with information from Shortell, S. M., & Kaluzny, A. D. (2012). *Health Care Management* (6th ed.). Clifton Park, NY: Delmar Cengage Learning.

Feedback can be a powerful tool to assist managers in motivating behavior; however, there are several factors that should be considered to maximize feedback effectiveness. First, for feedback to have value, nurses must truly see that their behavior needs to change. Second, feedback needs to be frequent, timely, and given at precise time intervals to sustain new behaviors. Third, feedback must be usable, consistent, correct, and of sufficient diversity. It should contain various important patient care, staffing, utilization, financial, and quality-related information. Otherwise, behavior problems can intensify as rewards flow to improvements based on flawed feedback data (Charns & Smith Tewksbury, 1993). Last, managers should not portray the feedback as "good" or "bad." Professional nurses are knowledge workers and know when they have missed the goal (Shortell & Kaluzny, 2012).

MOTIVATION

The human relations perspective in organizational management grew from the conclusion that workers were motivated and their output was greater when the worker was treated humanistically. Motivation is not explicitly demonstrated by people but, rather, is interpreted from their behavior. **Motivation** is whatever influences our choices and creates direction, intensity, and persistence in our behavior (Hughes, Ginnett, & Curphy, 2006; Kanfer, 1990). Motivation is a process that occurs internally to influence and direct our behavior in order to satisfy needs (Lussier, 1999). Motivation theories are not management theories per se; however, they are frequently considered along with management theories (Figure 1-2, Table 1-4, and Figure 1-3).

Motivation theories are useful because they help explain why people act the way they do and how a manager can relate to individuals as people and workers. When you are interested in creating change, influencing others, and managing patient care outcomes, it is helpful to understand the motivations that are reflected in a person's behavior. Motivation is a critical part of leadership because we need to understand each other in order to lead effectively. See Table 1-5 for common motivation problems and potential solutions.

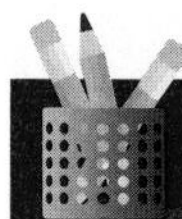

CASE STUDY 1-3

A patient fell at a local grocery store. Her husband insisted she go to the Emergency Department (ED). When the couple arrived at the ED, it was determined they did not speak English. The triage nurse asked the ED staff if anyone spoke Russian. In the meantime, the patient was sent to the X-ray department for X-rays of her chest and hip. A housekeeper was in the patient's room when the couple returned from the X-ray department. The housekeeper spoke Russian.

The doctor came into the room and asked the housekeeper to translate the following: "There is an area of hemorrhage on the patient's hip. She will be very sore and it will turn black and blue. There is no fracture. Here is a prescription for Vicodin to be used for pain, as needed. She should see her primary physician in a week."

The housekeeper translated this information by stating to the patient, "You will be turning black and blue and will develop a sore. This is a prescription for some type of medication. I am not sure what it is. The doctor said to use it for pain whenever you want." The couple shook their heads, indicated that they understood, smiled, and showed appreciation for both the care and translation of the information. The patient and husband were asked if they had any questions. They said "No." The patient was then discharged from the ED.

What do you see in this case that could have been done differently?

How might patient-centered care be applied to this case?

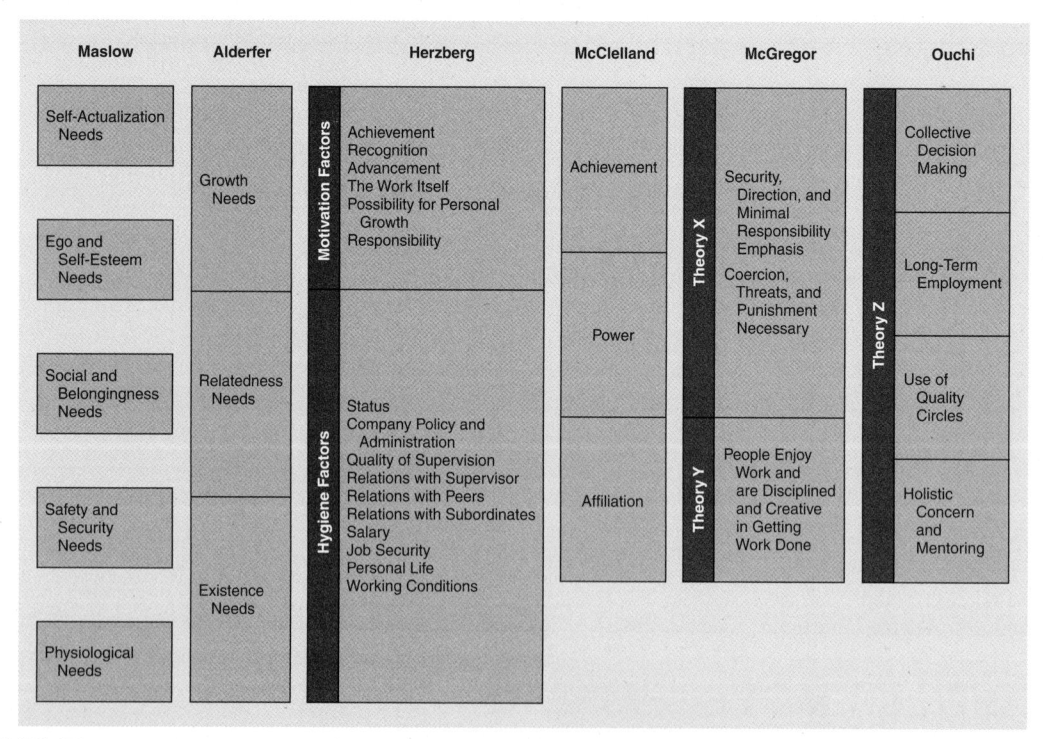

FIGURE 1-2

Selected theories of motivation.

(*Source:* Compiled with information from Shortell, S. M., Kaluzny, A. D. [2012]. *Health Care Management* [6th ed.]. Clifton Park, NY: Delmar Cengage Learning; and Leach, L. S., Leadership and management, from Kelly, P. L. [2012]. *Nursing Leadership & Management* [3rd ed.]. Clifton Park, NY: Delmar Cengage Learning.)

TABLE 1-4
Selected Motivation Theories

Main Contributors	Key Aspects
Abraham Maslow (1970) Hierarchy of Needs Theory	Motivation occurs when needs are not met. Certain needs have to be satisfied first, beginning with physiological needs, then safety and security needs, then social needs, followed by self-esteem needs and then self-actualization needs. Needs at one level must be satisfied before one is motivated by needs at the next higher level. See Figure 1-3.
Frederick Herzberg (1968) Two-Factor Theory (Hygiene and Motivation)	Hygiene factors include adequate salary, quality supervision, job security, safe and tolerable working conditions, and relationships with others. When these factors are absent, people are dissatisfied; when they are present, job dissatisfaction can be avoided. However, these factors alone will not motivate people and lead to job satisfaction. Motivation factors include satisfying and meaningful work, development and advancement opportunities, responsibility, and recognition. When these factors are present, people are motivated and satisfied with the job. When they are absent, people have a neutral attitude about the job and the organization.
Douglas McGregor (1960) Theory X	Theory X: Leaders must direct and control, as motivation results from reward and punishment. Employees prefer security, direction, and minimal responsibility, and need coercion and threats to get the job done.
Theory Y	Theory Y: Leaders must remove work obstacles, as workers have self-control and self-discipline; the workers' reward is their involvement in work and their opportunity to be creative.
William Ouchi (1981) Theory Z	Theory Z: Collective decision making, long-term employment, mentoring, holistic concern, and use of quality circles to manage service and quality are encouraged; this is a humanistic style of motivation based on Japanese organizations.

© Cengage Learning 2014

BENNER'S MODEL OF NOVICE TO EXPERT

Benner's (1984) Model of Novice to Expert provides a framework that can facilitate professional development of nursing leadership and management by building on the skill sets and experience of each practitioner. Benner's model acknowledges that there are tasks, competencies, and outcomes that practitioners can be expected to have acquired based on five levels of experience. Note that the 10-year rule states that it takes a decade of heavy labor to master any field (Ross, 2006).

Benner's Model of Novice to Expert is based on the Dreyfus and Dreyfus (1980) model of skill acquisition applied to nursing. There are five stages of Benner's model: novice, advanced beginner, competent, proficient, and expert. See Table 1-6.

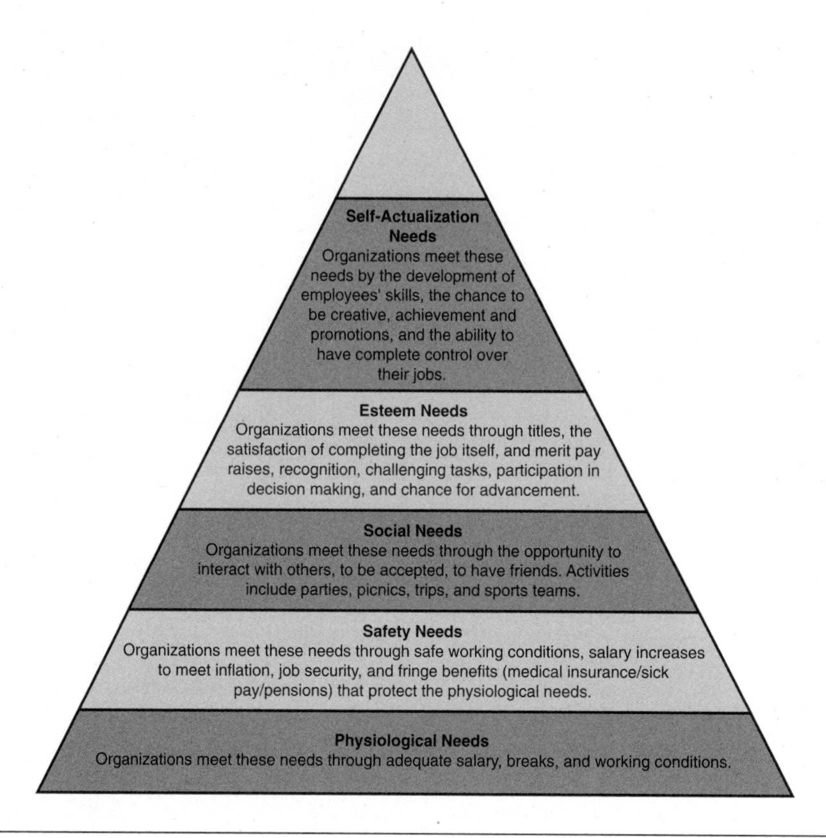

FIGURE 1-3

How organizations motivate with hierarchy of needs theory.

(*Source:* From Lussier/Achua, Leadership, 5e. © 2013 Cengage Learning.)

TABLE 1-5
Common Employee Motivation Problems and Potential Solutions

Motivational Problems	Potential Solutions
1. Inadequate performance definition, such as lack of goals, inadequate job descriptions, inadequate performance standards, inadequate performance assessment	–Well-defined job descriptions –Well-defined performance standards –Goal setting
2. Impediments to performance, such as bureaucratic or environmental obstacles, inadequate support or resources, poor employee-job matching, inadequate job information	–Feedback on performance –Enhanced hygiene factors, such as safe and clean environment, good salary and fringe benefits, job security, good staffing, time off from job, good equipment

(Continues)

TABLE 1-5 (Continued)

Motivational Problems	Potential Solutions
3. Inadequate performance-reward linkages, such as inappropriate or inadequate job rewards, poor timing of rewards, low probability of receiving rewards, inequity in distribution of rewards	–Pay for performance –Enhanced achievement or growth factors (i.e., employee involvement and participation, professional development opportunities, job redesign) –Enhanced esteem of power factors (i.e., autonomy or personal control, self management, modified work schedule, recognition, praise or awards, opportunity to display skills or talents, opportunity to mentor or train others, promotions in rank or position, information concerning organization or department, preferred work activities or projects, preferred work space) –Enhanced affiliation (i.e., work teams, task groups, social activities, professional and community group participation, personal communication or leadership style)

Source: Compiled with information from Shortell, S. M., & Kaluzny, A. D. (2012). *Health Care Management* (6th ed.). Clifton Park, NY: Delmar Cengage Learning.

TABLE 1-6
Benner's Model of Novice to Expert

Novice

Novice nurses have no experience with situations in which they are expected to perform. They see nursing as a series of tasks with specific rules. The novice tends to rigidly follow these rules to complete tasks rather than using judgment to apply the rules with discretion. Novice nurses work on handling pieces of the situation rather than focusing on handling the whole situation in the best way to meet patient needs.

Advanced Beginner

Advanced beginner nurses have a little more experience and they demonstrate marginally acceptable performance. They may have coped with enough real situations to note, or to have pointed out to them by a mentor, the important components of a situation. These important components require prior experience in actual situations for recognition. The advanced beginner nurses use principles based on their experience to guide their actions. They still need help setting priorities.

Competent

Competent nurses have been on the job in the same or similar situation for a few years. Competence develops when the nurse begins to see actions as part of long-range goals or plans. The conscious deliberate planning and critical thinking that are characteristic of this skill level help the competent nurse achieve efficiency and organization. The competent nurse lacks the speed and flexibility of the proficient nurse, but the competent nurse does have a feeling of mastery and the ability to prioritize and manage the many aspects of clinical nursing. Note that the 10-year rule states that it takes a decade of heavy labor to master any field (Ross, 2006).

(Continues)

TABLE 1-6 (Continued)

Proficient

Proficient nurses have a deep understanding of situations as a whole rather than seeing things as a series of tasks. Proficient nurses have learned from many experiences what typical events to expect in a given situation and how they need to modify their plans in response to these events. The proficient nurse can recognize when an expected situation does not materialize. This recognition improves the proficient nurse's decision making. Decision making becomes less labored because the proficient nurse quickly sees what is most important in a situation.

Expert

Expert nurses intuitively know what is going on with their patients. The expert nurse no longer relies on rules or guidelines. The expert nurse, with an enormous background of experience, has an intuitive grasp of each situation and zeroes in on the problem without wasteful consideration of a large range of unfruitful, alternative diagnoses and solutions. The expert nurse's performance is flexible and highly proficient. Expert nurses use their analytic ability in those situations where they have had no previous experience. If they get a wrong grasp of the situation and then find that events and behaviors are not occurring as expected, they can change course quickly. The expert nurse can also visualize what is possible in the future.

Source: Compiled with information from Benner, P. (1984). *From Novice to Expert.* Menlo Park, CA: Addison Wesley.

KEY CONCEPTS

- Nurses are leaders and make a difference to health care organizations through their contributions of expert knowledge and leadership. Leadership development is a necessary component of preparation as a health care provider.
- Leadership is a process that occurs between a leader and another individual; between the leader and a group; or between a leader and an organization, a community, or a society and that influences others, often by inspiring, enlivening, and engaging others to participate in the achievement of goals. Leadership can be formal or informal.
- Leadership and management are different.
- Leadership styles are described as autocratic, democratic, and laissez-faire, and have been studied by examining job-centered or task-oriented approaches as well as employee-centered or relationship-oriented approaches.
- Blake and Mouton's leadership model has five styles to address high or low people concerns and high or low production concerns.
- Contingency theories of leadership acknowledge that other factors in the environment in addition to the leader's behavior affect the leader's effectiveness.
- Substitutes for leadership are variables that eliminate the need for leadership or nullify the effect of the leader's behavior.
- Charismatic leadership theory describes leader behavior that displays self-confidence, passion, and communication of high expectations and confidence in others. This type of leader often emerges in a crisis with a vision, has an appeal based on personal power, and often uses unconventional strategies and emotional connections to succeed.
- Transformational leadership theory is a process in which "leaders and followers raise one another to higher levels of motivation and morality." Transformational leadership theory is based on the idea of

empowering others to engage in pursuing a collective purpose by working together to achieve a vision of a preferred future. Transformational leadership identifies two types of leaders (i.e., the transformational leader and the transactional leader).

- Nursing leadership in the future will be needed at all levels within an organization, not just at the top. Knowledge workers with specialized knowledge and expertise are both leaders and followers in knowledge organizations.
- Organizations are self-organizing systems in which, initially, what looks like chaos and uncertainty is indeed part of a larger coherence and natural order.
- Future directions for nursing knowledge workers in organizations will continue to be influenced by technology and by the notions of mobility, virtuality, and user-driven practices.
- Management is a process used to achieve organizational goals. It involves the management functions of planning, organizing and staffing, leading, and controlling actions to achieve goals.
- Management roles are classified as the information processing role, the interpersonal role, and the decision-making role.
- Managers use human, financial, physical, and information resources to achieve goals.
- Motivation is whatever influences our choices and creates direction, intensity, and persistence in our behavior.
- Benner's Model of Novice to Expert identifies five stages of nursing experience.Note that the 10-year rule states that it takes a decade of heavy labor to master any field (Ross, 2006).

KEY TERMS

autocratic leadership
consideration
contingency theory
democratic leadership
emotional intelligence
employee-centered leadership
formal leadership
high reliability organization
informal leadership
initiating structure
job-centered leaders
knowledge workers
laissez-faire leadership
leadership
leader-member relations
management
motivation
nursing-sensitive indicators
position power
substitutes for leadership
task structure
transactional leader

REVIEW QUESTIONS

1. Why is leadership important for nurses if they are not in a management position?
   A. It is not really important for nurses.
   B. Leadership is important at all levels in an organization because nurses have expert knowledge and are interacting with and influencing others.
   C. Nurse leaders leave their jobs sooner for other positions.
   D. Nurses who lead are less satisfied in their jobs.

2. Leadership is defined as which of the following?
   A. Being in a leadership position with authority to exert control and power over subordinates
   B. A process that occurs between a leader and another to participate in the achievement of goals
   C. Managing complexity
   D. Being self-confident and democratic

3. Management as a process that is used today by nurses in health care organizations is best described as which of the following?
   A. Scientific management
   B. Decision making
   C. Commanding and controlling others using hierarchical authority
   D. Planning, organizing, staffing, leading, and controlling actions to achieve goals

4. Motivation is whatever influences our choices. What motivation factors did Herzberg say would lead to job satisfaction?
   A. Being offered a substantial bonus when being hired
   B. Realizing that no one ever gets fired from the organization and that job security is high
   C. Having good relationships with colleagues and supervisors
   D. Being offered opportunities for achievement and advancement

5. A nurse on a medical-surgical unit presses the alert button to call a code for a patient experiencing a respiratory arrest. Which leadership style is most effective in this situation?
   A. Democratic
   B. Autocratic
   C. Laissez-faire
   D. Bureaucratic

6. Which of the following core competencies will an authentic leader require? Select all that apply.
   A. Self-knowledge
   B. Strategic vision
   C. Risk taking and creativity
   D. Interpersonal and communication effectiveness
   E. Use of inspiration
   F. Clinical skills

7. Which of the following is the best rationale for why nurse managers provide evaluation and feedback to nurses?
   A. Nurses will often change negative behavior when constructive feedback is provided.
   B. Patient care must be delivered at the highest level, which requires evaluation and feedback for those who provide it.
   C. The American Nurses Association suggests that nurses receive evaluation and feedback when patient care is compromised.
   D. A nurse's professional socialization and strong achievement needs encourage nurses to change with constructive feedback.

8. According to Ross, how long a period of heavy labor does it take to master any field?
   A. 10 days
   B. 12 months
   C. 5 years
   D. 10 years

9. What types resources does the chapter identify that managers use to achieve goals? Select all that apply.
   A. Human resources
   B. Financial resources
   C. Physical resources
   D. Information resources
   E. Thinking resources
   F. Psychological resources

10. Which of the following are stages of Benner's model? Select all that apply.
   A. Novice
   B. Advanced beginner
   C. Competent
   D. Thoughtful
   E. Proficient
   F. Expert

REVIEW ACTIVITIES

1. Take the opportunity to learn about yourself by reflecting on five predominant factors identified as being influential in a nurse's leadership development: self-confidence, innate leader qualities/tendencies, progression of experiences and success, influence of significant others, and personal life factors. Consider what reinforces your confidence in yourself. What innate qualities or traits do you have that contribute to your development as a nurse leader? Consider what professional experiences, mentors, and personal experiences or events can help you develop your leadership ability. How can you obtain these experiences?
2. Find the current written nursing policies and procedures on a patient care unit.
   Where is the information located?
   When was the last time the policies/procedures were updated?
   How are policy/procedure updates disseminated to the staff?
   How do nurses maintain high standards in their policies and procedures?
3. Rate each of these 12 job factors that contribute to job satisfaction by placing a number from 1 to 5 on the line before each factor. How important is the factor to you?

Very important		**Somewhat important**		**Not important**
5	4	3	2	1

______ 1. An interesting job I enjoy doing
______ 2. A good manager who treats people fairly
______ 3. Getting praise and other recognition and appreciation for the work I do
______ 4. A satisfying personal life at the job
______ 5. The opportunity for advancement
______ 6. A prestigious or status job
______ 7. Job responsibility that gives me freedom to do things my way
______ 8. Good working conditions (safe environment, nice office, cafeteria)

_______ 9. The opportunity to learn new things
_______ 10. Sensible company rules, regulations, procedures, and policies
_______ 11. A job I can do well and succeed at
_______ 12. Job security and benefits

Write the number from 1 to 5 that you selected for each factor in the appropriate column below. Total each column below for a score between 6 and 30 points. The closer to 30 your score is in each column below, the more important the factor (motivating or maintenance) is to you.

Motivating factors		Maintenance factors	
1.	_______	2.	_______
3.	_______	4.	_______
5.	_______	6.	_______
7.	_______	8.	_______
9.	_______	10.	_______
11.	_______	12.	_______
Totals	_______	Totals	_______

From *Leadership: Theory, Application, Skill Development* (pp. 15–16), by R. N. Lussier and C. F. Achua, 2013, Cincinnati, OH: South-Western College Publishing. 5th ed.

4. How does nursing leadership and management ensure quality patient care in an emergency?

5. What leadership projects are nurses in your work setting involved in? How is information about patient quality being used to improve nursing practice? What sources of evidence from nursing science are you exploring through reading journals, attending educational conferences, using the Internet, and participating in professional nursing associations?

EXPLORING THE WEB

Search the web, checking the following sites.

- Emerging Leader: *http://www.emergingleader.com*
- Leadership Directories—Who's who in the leadership of the United States: *http://www.leadershipdirectories.com*
- Leadership Skills Development: *http://www.impactfactory.com*
- LeaderValues: *http://www.leader-values.com*
- Don Clark's Big Dog Leadership: *http://www.nwlink.com/~Donclark*
- American Association of Critical-Care Nurses' Standards for Establishing and Sustaining Healthy Work Environments: *http://www.aacn.org.* Click Healthy Work Environments under Clinical Practice.
- American Organization of Nurse Executives Competencies: *http://www.aone.org.* Click Resources, and then Learning Tools, and then click AONE Nurse Exec Competencies.
- Analyze My Career: *http://analyzemycareer.com*
- American Nurses Association Magnet Status Hospitals: *http://www.nursingworld.org.* Search for ANCC.
- Nursing leaders: *http://www.google.com.* Search for nursing leader profiles.
- Joanna Briggs Institute: *http://www.joannabriggs.edu.* Search Evidence Based Practice Guidelines for leadership.

REFERENCES

Adeniran, R. K., Bhattacharya, A., & Adeniran, A. A. (2012). Professional excellence and career advancement in nursing: A conceptual framework for clinical leadership development. *Nursing Administration Quarterly, 36*(1), 41–51.

Ahuja, G. (2000). Collaboration networks, structural holes, and innovation: A longitudinal study. *Administrative Science Quarterly, 45*(3), 425–455.

Alderfer, C. P. (1972). Existence, relatedness, and growth; human needs in organizational settings. Free Press.

Aldrich, H. (1979). *Organizations and environments.* Englewood Cliffs, NJ: Princeton Hills.

Alexander, J. A., & Amburgey, T. L. (1987). The dynamics of change in the American hospital industry: Transformation or selection? *Medical Care Review, 44,* 279–321.

American Association of Critical-Care Nurses (AACN). (2005). AACN standards for establishing and sustaining healthy work environments: A journey to excellence. Retrieved January 1, 2012, from http://www.aacn.org/WD/HWE/Docs/HWEStandards.pdf

American Nurses Association (ANA). (2012). Nursing-Sensitive Indicators. Retrieved January 5, 2012, from http://www.nursingworld.org/MainMenuCategories/ThePracticeofProfessionalNursing/PatientSafetyQuality/Research-Measurement/The-National-Database/Nursing-Sensitive-Indicators_1.aspx

Amerson, R. (2010). The impact of service-learning on cultural competence. *Nursing Education Perspectives, 31*(1), 18–22.

Barker, A. (1990). *Transformational nursing leadership: A vision for the future.* Baltimore, MD: Williams & Wilkins.

Barney, J. (1991). Firm resources and sustained competitive advantage. *Journal of Management, 17,* 99–120.

Bass, B. (1981). *Stogdill's handbook of leadership.* New York, NY: Free Press.

Bass, B. (1985). *Leadership and performance beyond expectations.* New York, NY: Free Press.

Baum, J., & Amburgey, T. (2005). Organizational ecology. In J. Baum (Ed.), *The Blackwell companion to organizations* (pp. 304–326). Blackwell Business.

Begun, J. W., & White, K. R. (1999). The profession of nursing as a complex adaptive system: Strategies for change. In J. J. Kronenfeld (Ed.), *Research in the sociology of health care* (pp. 189–203). Greenwich, CT: JAI Press.

Benner, P. (1984). *From novice to expert.* Menlo Park, CA: Addison Wesley.

Bennis, W., & Nanus, B. (2003). *Leaders: The strategies for taking charge.* New York, NY: Harper & Row.

Bennis, W., Spreitzer, G. M., & Cummings, T. G. (2001). *The future of leadership.* San Francisco, CA: Jossey-Bass.

Bishop, V. (2010). Coalition in leadership. Politics: The big picture and the big game. *Journal of Research in Nursing, 15*(4), 291–293.

Blake, R., & Mouton, J. (1964). *The managerial grid: The key to leadership excellence.* Houston, TX: Gulf Publishing Co.

Blake, R., & Mouton, J. (1985). *The managerial grid III: The key to leadership excellence.* Houston, TX: Gulf Publishing Co.

Burns, J. M., (1978). *Leadership.* New York, NY: Harper & Row.

Burt, R. S. (1992). *Structural holes: The social structure of competition.* Cambridge, MA: Harvard University Press.

Cassidy, V., & Koroll, C. (1998). Ethical aspects of transformational leadership. In E. Hein (Ed.), *Contemporary leadership behavior.*

Charns, M., & Smith Tewksbury, L. (1993). *Collaborative management in health care.* San Francisco, CA: Jossey-Bass.

Comack, M. (January/March 2012). A journey of leadership: From bedside nurse to chief executive officer. *Nursing Administration Quarterly, 36*(1), 29–34.

Conger, J., & Kanungo, R. (1987). Toward a behavioral theory of charismatic leadership in organizational settings. *Academy of Management Review, 12,* 637–647.

Dahnke, M. (2009). The role of the American Nurses Association Code in ethical decision making. *Holistic Nursing Practice, 23*(2), 112–119.

DiMaggio, P. J., & Powell, W. W. (1983). The iron cage revisited: Institutional isomorphism and collective rationality in organizational fields. *American Sociological Review, 48,* 147–160.

Dooley, K., & Plsek, P. (2001). *A complex systems perspective on medication errors.* Working paper. Arizona State University.

Drath, W. H., & Palus, C. J. (1994). Making common sense: Leadership as meaning-making in a community of practice. Retrieved December 5, 2004, from http://www.ebookmall.com

Dreyfus, Stuart E., & Dreyfus, Hubert L. (February 1980). *A five-stage model of the mental activities involved in directed skill acquisition.* Washington, DC: Storming Media.

Drucker, P. F. (1994). *The post-capitalist society.* New York, NY: Harper & Row.

DuBrin, A. J. (2000). *The Active Manager.* Cincinnati, OH: South-Western College Publishing.

Dunham-Taylor, J. (2000). Nurse executive transformational leadership found in participative organizations. *Journal of Nursing Administration, 30*(5), 241–250.
Dyer, J. H., & Singh, H. (1998). The relational view: Cooperative strategies and sources of interorganizational competitive advantage. *Academy of Management Review, 23,* 660–679.
Fayol, H. (1949). (C. Storrs, Trans.). *General and industrial management.* London, England: Pitman.
Fielder, F. (1967). *A theory of leadership effectiveness.* New York: McGraw-Hill.
Follet, M. (1924). *Creative experience.* London, England: Longmans, Green.
Gladwell, M. (2008). Outliers. Little Brown.
Goleman, D. (1998). *Working with emotional intelligence.* New York, NY: Bantam Books.
Grossman, S., & Valiga, T. M. (2008). *The new leadership challenge: Creating the future of nursing.* Philadelphia, PA: F.A. Davis.
Gulati, R. (1995). Does familiarity breed trust? The implications of repeated ties for contractual choice in alliances. *Academy of Management Journal, 38,* 85–112.
Gulick, L. (1937). Notes on the theory of organization. Memo prepared for the President's Committee on Administrative Management.
Gulick, L., & Urwick, L. (Eds.). (1937). *Papers on the science of administration.* New York, NY: Columbia University Press.
Hannan, M. T., & Freeman, J. H. (1977). The population ecology of organizations. *American Journal of Sociology, 82,* 929–964.
Hawley, A. (1950). *Human ecology.* New York: Ronald Press.
Helgesen, S. (1995). *The web of inclusion: A new architecture for building organizations.* New York, NY: Doubleday Currency.
Henry, N. (1992). *Public administration and public affairs* (5th ed.). Englewood Cliffs, NJ: Prentice Hall.
Hersey, P., Blanchard, K., & Johnson, D. (2008). *Management of organizational behavior: Leading human resources* (9th ed.). Englewood Cliffs, NJ: Prentice Hall.
Herzberg, F. (1968, January/February). One more time: How do you motivate employees? *Harvard Business Review,* 53–62.
House, R. H. (1971). A path-goal theory of leader effectiveness. *Administrative Science Quarterly 16,* 321–338.
Huber, G. P. (1980). *Managerial decision making.* Glenview, IL: Scott, Foresman and Co.
Hughes, R. L., Ginnett, R. C., & Curphy, G. J. (2006). *Leadership: Enhancing the lessons of experience* (5th ed.). Boston, MA: McGraw-Hill.
Institute of Medicine (IOM). (2010). *The future of nursing: Leading change, advancing health.* Washington, DC: The National Academies Press.
Kanfer, R. (1990). Motivation theory in industrial and organizational psychology. In M. D. Dunnette & L. M. Hough (Eds.), *Handbook of industrial and organizational psychology: Vol. 1* (pp. 53–68). Palo Alto, CA: Consulting Psychologists Press.
Katz, D., & Kahn, R. L. (1978). *The social psychology of organizations* (2nd ed.). New York, NY: John Wiley.
Kelly, P. (2012). *Nursing leadership & management* (3rd ed.). Clifton Park, NY: Delmar Cengage Learning.
Kerr, S., & Jermier, J. (1978). Substitutes for leadership: Their meaning and measurement. *Organizational Behavior and Human Performance, 22,* 374–403.
Kirkpatrick, S. A., & Locke, E. A. (1991). Leadership: Do traits matter? *The Executive, 5,* 48–60.
Kongstvedt, P. R. (2009). *Managed care: What it is and how it works* (3rd ed.). Gaithersburg, MD: Aspen Publishers.
Kramer, M. (1990). The magnet hospitals: Excellence revisited. *Journal of Nursing Administration, 20*(9), 35–44.
Kramer, M., & Schmalenberg, C. E. (2005, July-Sep.). Best quality patient care: A historical perspective on magnet hospitals. *Nursing Administration Quarterly, 29*(3), 275–287.
Lawrence, P., & Lorsch, J. (1967). *Organization and environment.* Cambridge, MA: Harvard University Press.
Leach, L. S. (2005). Nurse executive leadership and organizational commitment among nurses. *Journal of Nursing Administration, 35*(5), 228–238.
Lewin, K. (1939). Field theory and experiment in social psychology: Concepts and methods. *Journal of Sociology, 44,* 868–896.
Lewin, K., & Lippitt, R. (1938). An experimental approach to the study of autocracy and democracy: A preliminary note. *Sociometry, 1,* 292–300.
Lewin, K., Lippitt, R., & White, R. (1939). Patterns of aggressive behavior in experimentally created social climates. *Journal of Social Psychology, 10,* 271–299.
Lussier, R. N. (1999). *Human relations in organizations: Applications and skill building* (4th ed.). San Francisco, CA: Irwin McGraw-Hill.
Lussier, R. N., & Achua, C. F. (2013). *Leadership: Theory, application, skill development* (5th ed.). Cincinnati, OH: South-Western College Publishing.
March, J., & Simon, H.A. (1958). *Organizations.* New York, NY: John Wiley & Sons.
Maslow, A. (1970). *Motivation and personality* (2nd ed.). New York, NY: Harper & Row.
Mayo, E. (1945). *The social problems of an industrial civilization.* Boston, MA: Harvard University Press.
McCall, M. W., Jr. (1998). *High flyers: Developing the next generation of leaders.* Boston, MA: Harvard Business School Press.

McCall, M. W., Jr., Morrison, A. M., & Hanman, R. L. (1978). *Studies of managerial work: Results and methods* (Tech. Rep.). Greensboro, NC: Center for Creative Leadership.

McClelland, D.C. (1988). *Human Motivation.* Cambridge University Press.

McClure, M., & Hinshaw, A. (Eds.). (2002). *Magnet hospitals revisited.* Washington, DC: American Nurses Publishing.

McClure, M., Poulin, M., Sovie, M., & Wandelt, M. (1983). *Magnet hospitals: Attraction and retention of professional nurses.* Kansas City, MO: American Nurses Association.

McDaniel, C., & Wolf, G. (1992). Transformational leadership in nursing service. *Journal of Nursing Administration, 12*(4), 204–207.

McGregor, D. (1960). *The human side of enterprise.* New York, NY: McGraw-Hill.

McKenzie, R. (1968). The scope of human ecology. In A. Hawley (Ed.), *On human ecology* (pp. 19–32). Chicago, IL: University of Chicago Press.

McNeese-Smith, D. (1997). The influences of manager behavior on nurses' job satisfaction, productivity, and commitment. *Journal of Nursing Administration, 27*(9), 47–55.

Meyer, J., & Rowan, B. (1977). Institutionalized organizations: Formal structure as myth ceremony. *American Journal of Sociology, 83,* 340–363.

Mills, E. (1964). Florence Nightingale and state registration. *International Nursing Review, 11,* 31–36.

Mintzberg, H. (1973). *The nature of managerial work.* New York, NY: Harper & Row.

Moorhead, G., & Griffin, R. W. (2001). *Organizational behavior: Managing people in organizations* (6th ed.). Boston, MA: Houghton Mifflin.

Murphy, L. (2005). Transformational leadership: A cascading chain reaction. *Journal of Nursing Management, 13,* 128–136.

Murphy, M., & DeBack, V. (1991). Today's nursing leaders: Creating the vision. *Nursing Administration Quarterly 16*(1), 71–80.

National League for Nursing. Core values. (2010). Retrieved September 26, 2010, from http://www.nln.org/aboutnln/corevalues.htm

Nightingale, F. (1859). *Notes on nursing: What it is, and What it is Not.* London, England: Harrison & Sons.

Nelson, E. C., et al. (2008). Clinical microsystems, part 1: The building blocks of health systems. *Joint Commission Journal on Quality and Patient Safety, 34,* 367–378.

Northouse, P. (2010). *Leadership: Theory and practice* (5th ed.). Thousand Oaks, CA: Sage.

Ouchi, W. G. (1980). Markets, bureaucracies, and clans. *Administrative Science Quarterly, 24,* 129–141.

Ouchi, W. G. (1981). *Theory Z: How American business can meet the Japanese challenge.* Reading, MA: Addison-Wesley.

Pfeffer, J., & Salancik, G. R. (1978). *The external control of organizations.* New York, NY: Harper & Row.

Porter, M. E. (1980). *Competitive strategy: Techniques for analyzing industries and competitors.* New York, NY: Free Press.

Porter-O'Grady, T. (2001). Profound change: 21st century nursing. *Nursing Outlook, 47*(1), 182–186.

Quinn, R. (1988). *Beyond rational management: Mastering the paradoxes and competing demands of high performance.* San Francisco, CA: Jossey-Bass.

Ridge, R. (2011). Future of nursing special: Practicing to potential. *Nursing Management, 42*(6), 32–37.

The Robert Wood Johnson Foundation and the Institute of Medicine initiative on the future of nursing. *The future of nursing: Leading change, advancing health.* (2010). Retrieved December 7, 2010, from http://www.rwjf.org/files/research/Future%20of%20Nursing_Leading%20Change%20Advancing%20Health.pdf

Roethlisberger, J. F., & Dickson, W. J. (1947). *Management and the worker.* Cambridge, MA: Harvard University Press.

Ross, P. E. (August, 2006). The expert mind. *The Scientific American, 8,* 64–71.

Ruef, M., & Scott, W. R. (1998). A multidimensional model of organizational legitimacy: Hospital survival in changing institutional markets. *Administrative Science Quarterly, 43*(4), 877–904.

Scott, J. G., Sochalski, J., & Aiken, L. (1999). Review of magnet hospital research: Findings and implications for professional nursing practice. *Journal of Nursing Administration*, 29(1), 9–19.

Selznick, P. (1948). Foundations of the theory of organizations. *American Sociological Review 13,* 25–35.

Shortell, S. M., & Kaluzny, A. D. (2012). *Health care management* (6th ed.). Clifton Park, NY: Delmar Cengage Learning.

Spector, P. E. (2006). *Industrial and organizational psychology: Research and practice* (4th ed.). Hoboken, NJ: John Wiley & Sons.

Spence Laschinger, H., Finegan, J., & Wilk, P. (2009). Context matters: The impact of unit leadership and empowerment on nurses' organizational commitment. *The Journal of Nursing Administration*, 39(5), 228–235.

Stodgill, R. M. (1948). Personal factors associated with leadership: A survey of the literature. *Journal of Psychology, 25,* 35–71.

Stodgill, R. M. (1974). *Handbook of leadership: Survey of theory and research.* New York, NY: Free Press.

Taylor, F. (1911). *The principles of scientific management.* New York, NY: W.W. Norton.

Thompson, J. D. (1967). *Organization in action.* New York, NY: McGraw-Hill.

Tichy, N., & Devanna, D. (1986). *Transformational leadership.* New York, NY: Wiley.

Uzzi, B. (1997). Social structure and competition in interfirm networks: The paradox of embeddedness. *Administrative Science Quarterly, 42*(1), 35–67.

Uzzi, B. (1999). Embeddedness in the making of financial capital: How social relations and networks benefit firms seeking financing. *American Sociological Review, 64,* 481–505.

Weber, M. (1964). *The theory of social and economic organization.* Glencoe, IL: Free Press.

Wheatley, M. J. (1999). *Leadership and the new science: Learning about organization from an orderly universe.* San Francisco, CA: Berrett-Koehler.

Wheatley, M. J. (2005). *Finding our way: Leadership for an uncertain time.* San Francisco, CA: Berrett-Koehler Publishers.

Wholey, D. R., & Burns, L. R. (1993). Organizational transitions: Form changes by health maintenance organizations. In S. Bacharach (Ed.), *Research in the sociology of organizations* (pp. 257–293). Greenwich, CT: JAI Press.

Wolf, G., Boland, S., & Aukerman, M. (1994). A transformational model for the practice of professional nursing: Part 1. *Journal of Nursing Administration, 24*(4), 51–57.

Wong, C., & Cummings, G. (2007). The relationship between nursing leadership and patient outcomes: A systematic review. *Journal of Nursing Management, 15,* 508–521.

Wong, C., & Cummings, G. (2009). Authentic leadership: A new theory for nursing or back to basics. *Journal of Health Organozation and Management, 23*(5), 522–538.

Young, S. (1992). Educational experiences of transformational nurse leaders. *Nursing Administration Quarterly, 17*(1), 25–33.

Yukl, G. (1998). *Leadership in organizations* (4th ed.). Upper Saddle River, NJ: Prentice Hall.

SUGGESTED READINGS

Akerjordet, K., & Severinsson, E. (2010). The state of the science of emotional intelligence related to nursing leadership: An integrative review. *Journal of Nursing Management, 18*(4), 363–382.

Bondas, T. (2010). Nursing leadership from the perspectives of clinical group supervision: A paradoxical practice. *Journal of Nursing Management, 18*(4), 425–439.

Carney, B. T., West, P., Neily, J., Mills, P. D., & Bagian, J. P. (2010). Differences in nurse and surgeon perceptions of teamwork: Implications for use of a briefing checklist in the OR. *AORN Journal, 91*(6), 722–729.

Cummings, G., Lee, H., Macgregor, I., Davey, M., Wong, C., Paul, L., & Stafford, E. (2008). Factors contributing to nursing leadership: A systematic review. *Journal of Health Services Research Policy, 13*(4), 240–248.

Ganann, R., Underwood, J., Mathews, S., Goodyear, R., Stamier, L., Meagher-Stewart, D., & Munroe, V. (2010). Leadership attributes: A key to optimal utilization of the community health nursing work force. *Nursing Leadership, 23*(2), 60–71.

Holden, L. M., Watts, D. D., & Walker, P. H. (2010). Communication and collaboration: It's about the pharmacists, as well as the physicians and nurses. *Quality & Safety in Health Care, 19*(3), 169–172.

Hyrkas, K., & Dende, D. (2008). Clinical nursing leadership: Perspectives on current topics. *Journal of Nursing Management, 16*(5), 495–498.

McBride, A. (2010). *The Growth and development of nurse leaders.* New York, NY: Springer.

O'Brien, M. E. (2011). *Servant leadership in nursing: Spirituality and practice in contemporary health care.* Burlington, MA: Jones & Bartlett Publishers.

Richardson, A., & Storr, J. (2010). Patient safety: A literature review on the impact of nursing empowerment, leadership and collaboration. *International Nursing Review, 57*(1), 12–21.

CHAPTER 2

The Health Care Environment

KATHLEEN KLEEFISCH, APRN, DNP, FNP-BC;
RONDA G. HUGHES, RN, PHD, MHS; AND
TANYA L. SLEEPER, GNP-BC, MSN, MSB

Fixing our health-care system as a whole is our primary challenge, and to make it happen you need to get engaged — to pound the pavement, get your hands dirty, endure real sacrifice, take on antiquated thinking, and help lead the public debate.

–SENATOR JOHN KERRY, 2011

OBJECTIVES

Upon completion of this chapter, the reader should be able to:

1. Discuss significant history and current influences on health care in the United States (U.S.).
2. Describe how the U.S. health care system is organized.
3. Review international perspectives on some high-income industrialized country's health care systems, e.g., France, Canada, and Japan.
4. Describe factors contributing to rising health care costs.
5. Outline the potential benefits of improving safety, quality, and access to health care.
6. Discuss improving health care quality through health professions education.

Tom worked as a manager for a corner grocery store that employed five people. Tom once asked the owner whether the employees could receive health insurance through their work. The owner said it was too expensive. Tom, his wife, and their three kids were uninsured. Tom's wife did not want to incur any medical bills and ignored a mole on her chest. After many months of delay, Tom insisted that she see a dermatologist. She was diagnosed with malignant melanoma, which had metastasized. She died two years later at the age of 37, leaving Tom to raise their three children.

What do you think of the occurrence of this type of scenario in the United States?

Explain how primary, secondary, and tertiary prevention might have changed the outcome for Tom's wife.

How can access to health care be assured for all patients regardless of the source of their insurance?

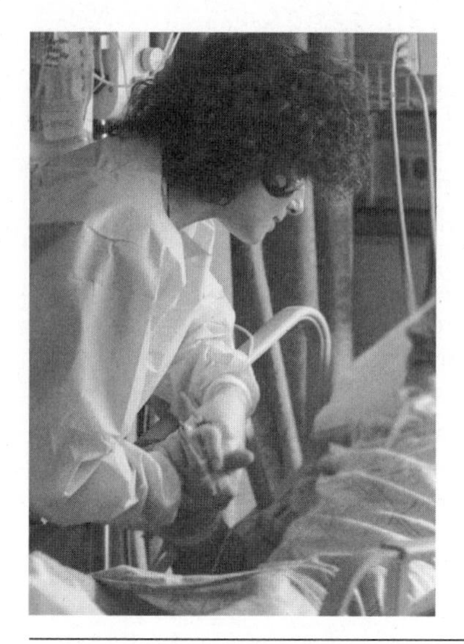

Source: Courtesy of Advocate Good Shepherd Hospital, Barrington, Illinois

Over 300 million Americans depend on the United States (U.S.) health care system to assist them in improving or maintaining their health. The high costs of this health care system present obstacles for a growing number of Americans who lack access to what is otherwise a superior system (National Coalition on Health Care [NCHC], 2008). Because of these high costs, 47 million Americans under the age of 65 lack access to health care because they do not have any form of health insurance (NCHC, 2008a). Countries such as France, Canada, Japan, Germany, and the United Kingdom provide universal health care (UHC) programs to their citizens. In these countries, per capita spending is considerably less than in the United States, yet health care outcomes for such things as infant mortality, immunization rates, and life expectancy in the United States are poorer by comparison (Nolte & McKee, 2008).

Throughout the history of the United States, efforts to implement a UHC program have been resisted, with costly social and economic consequences. Americans who lack health coverage are not likely to benefit from the care needed for health promotion, illness prevention, early detection, and health restoration programs. To avoid the financial burden of health care costs, Americans who lack health insurance often delay obtaining care. Their contact with the health care system is episodic and usually occurs in acute care settings. Even after their symptoms have progressed and are well advanced, uninsured Americans are more likely to obtain only irregular, sporadic care. This means that they lack consistent care from a health care provider whom they see regularly, whether for health promotion, illness prevention, or treatment. Inability to pay for recommended treatments and medications also compromises their adherence to health care recommendations, which in turn affects their recovery. A cascading effect then occurs, with soaring costs and progressively worsening health outcomes. A growing number of working Americans is affected by this dilemma, putting health for all into sharp focus on the national agenda.

Using the insights of Florence Nightingale, this chapter begins by providing a brief overview of historical and current influences on the U.S. health care system. The organization, funding, and quality of health care are reviewed. International perspectives on some other high-income industrialized countries' health care systems, e.g., France, Canada, and Japan, are reviewed. Factors contributing to rising health care costs and the potential benefits of improving safety, quality, and access to health care are reviewed. Improving health care quality through health professions education and the challenges and opportunities for nurses in the future are discussed.

HISTORY OF U.S. HEALTH CARE

One hundred years ago, illnesses such as tuberculosis or pneumonia required lengthy hospitalizations and were often catastrophic for individuals and families. Today, such illnesses are preventable and are often easily treated. Handwashing and vaccination programs have been used extensively to prevent the spread of communicable diseases. Additionally, surgical interventions in hospitals, for example, tonsillectomies, appendectomies, and reproductive procedures, have improved to treat otherwise debilitating or mortal conditions (Mayo, 2007). Health care is delivered by professional nursing and medical practitioners who are science-based and use evidence-based practice. It is primarily directed at preventing and treating chronic and behavioral diseases. Health care advances have extended life expectancy with the consequence of more elderly people requiring more health care for chronic and complex health problems. The majority of clinical care is still provided in hospitals, but length of stay in hospitals is much shorter and a variety of innovative models of care are now used to provide cost-effective care for people with acute, community, and long-term clinical needs (Health Workforce Solutions LLC & Robert Wood Johnson Foundation, 2008).

Florence Nightingale observed that noise, food, rest, light, fresh air, and cleanliness were instrumental in health and illness patterns. Thus, she maintained, the aim of nursing was to put the patient in the best condition for nature to act upon her or him (Nightingale, F. 1860). Nightingale also discovered the link between adverse patient outcomes and a lack of cleanliness and handwashing. The surprising lack of adherence by health care providers to handwashing accounts for 2 million hospital-acquired infections, is attributable for up to 90,000 deaths, and burdens the health care system with a cost of up to $29 billion annually (Jarvis, 2006). The most prevalent and preventable hospital-acquired infections are bloodstream infections, pneumonia, and surgical site and urinary tract infections (Gaynes et al., 2001). The highest rates of infection have been found to occur in burn intensive care units (ICUs), neonatal ICUs, and pediatric ICUs, areas where infections can easily be fatal (Agency for Healthcare Research and Quality [AHRQ], 2007b; Center for Health Design, 2005; Hamilton, 2003; National Nosocomial Infections Surveillance [NNIS], 1998).

Structuring Hospitals around Nursing Care

Nightingale also described the importance of structuring hospitals around nursing care. The initial design of hospitals followed that advice by building large wards where nurses could easily monitor and observe their patients. Later, hospital design evolved so that patient rooms surrounded centrally located nursing stations. Then, as today, the physical environment of hospitals could create stress for patients, their families, and clinical staff. In 1946, the Hospital Survey and Construction Act was enacted by Congress, which accelerated the building of hospitals and public health centers nationwide (Hospital Survey and Construction Act, 1946). This legislation, also known as the Hill-Burton Act, solidified the corporatization of health care delivery. Today, research is finding links between the physical environment and patient outcomes, patient safety, and patient and staff satisfaction (Hamilton, 2003). Studies show that elements of hospital design such as exposure to natural light, private rooms, and facilities that are staff friendly and have less noise contribute to improved patient outcomes (Ulrich, R. S., C. Zimring, A. Joseph, X. Quan, and R. Choudhary. 2004. The role of the physical environment in the hospital of the 21st century: A once-in-a-lifetime opportunity. Concord, CA: The Center for Health Design).

Although little is known about how to best design the hospital environment to facilitate clinical advances and care delivery, billions of dollars are being expended for new hospital construction across the United States. The Robert Wood Johnson Foundation, the nation's largest philanthropy devoted exclusively to health and health care, has provided funding to the Center for Health Design, a nonprofit research organization, for the Designing the 21st Century Hospital Project, which is the most extensive review of the evidence-based approach to hospital design ever conducted. See www.healthdesign.org.

Collecting Data

Nightingale also astutely recognized the importance of collecting and using data to assess the quality of health care. She employed coxcomb diagrams to present visual images of the number of preventable deaths during the Crimean war and then later in London hospitals. Today, data is collected from numerous sources—patient records, surveys, clinical trials and other health research, administrative systems, government agencies, and policy institutes. A focus on clinical performance, outcome measures, and quality improvement brought about the beginning of formalized measurement in the 1970s (Dunefsky, 2008). From this formalized measurement of clinical performance, outcome measures, and quality improvement, reports are developed, such as the Centers for Disease Control and Prevention (CDC) National Vital Statistics Reports (Martin, Hamilton, Sutton, & Ventura, 2006); The National Healthcare Disparities Report (NHDR) (Agency for Healthcare Research and Quality [AHRQ], 2007a); and other reports from the Institute of Medicine (IOM, 1999, 2001) and the Surgeon General's office. Additionally, private philanthropic organizations such as the Commonwealth Fund, the Kaiser Family Foundation (KFF), and the Robert Wood Johnson Foundation also analyze health care data and publish reports related to the health care needs of America. Locally, data is available from each state department of health. Internationally, organizations such as the World Health Organization (WHO) and the Pan American Health Organization report on global health trends and issues. To make informed decisions and set goals, health policy makers rely on the data and findings documented by such organizations. Table 2-1 lists several health data websites.

Influence of External Forces on Health Care

Recognizing the influence of external forces on care delivery and scope of practice, Nightingale also kept informed of the activities of practitioners and government policy makers (Dossey, Selanders, & Beck, 2005). Every action and decision that influences health and health systems should be important to nurses. Nurses must become more adept at using politics to influence health care policy and patient quality and safety. With health care being the largest sector of our economy, insurance companies, pharmaceutical companies, and health care technology and equipment companies, as well as employers, clinicians, managers, and patients all have a vested interest in proposed changes to health care financing, organization, and the responsibilities and scope of practice for clinicians.

Political Influences on Health Care

In 1912, considerations by President Theodore Roosevelt's administration to adopt a modified workers' health insurance plan were swept aside when President Woodrow Wilson took office. Physicians and the life insurance industry supported this move through the early 1930s, as they were opposed to government regulation and they were motivated to avoid any restraint on the

TABLE 2-1
Websites for Health Data Sources

Websites for Health Data Sources
Agency for Healthcare Research and Quality: www.ahrq.gov
Centers for Disease Control and Prevention: www.cdc.gov
Commonwealth Fund: www.commonwealthfund.org
The Institute for Healthcare Improvement: www.ihi.org
Institute of Medicine: www.iom.edu
Joint Commission: www.jointcommission.org
Kaiser Family Foundation: www.kff.org
Robert Wood Johnson Foundation: www.rwjf.org
Surgeon General's Office: www.surgeongeneral.gov
World Health Organization: www.who.int

© Cengage Learning 2014

fees and premiums they charged. The need for more equitable health insurance was highlighted with the onset of the Depression in the 1930s. At this time, growing medical costs associated with hospital care, technological advances, and increased physician fees meant that vast numbers of previously well-to-do people could no longer afford to pay for the medical attention they required. In response to this national dilemma, the American Medical Association organized the Committee on the Cost of Medical Care, which attempted to organize the health care system and curb its costs. The work completed by this Committee was fraught with social and political divisions, and, in response, President Franklin Roosevelt formed the Committee on Economic Security. The "New Deal" program was implemented at this time and included federal relief programs, social services, and aid for the elderly. The Social Security Act of 1935 was also introduced, which defined the role of the federal government in the delivery and financing of health care (Maville & Huerta, 2007; Ross, 2002).

In 1965, an amendment to the Social Security Act was signed by President Lyndon Johnson, which introduced Medicare, a health insurance program for the elderly, and Medicaid, a health insurance program for the needy, both paid for with government funds. Due to rising health care costs in the 1990s, health care reform was again on the national agenda and President Bill Clinton introduced the Health Security Act. This Act failed to achieve political approval.

In 2010, President Obama signed the Affordable Care Act (ACA), into law. Key health coverage provisions of the ACA included:

- an expansion of Medicaid for individuals under age 65
- the creation of health insurance exchanges through which individuals who do not have access to public coverage or affordable employer coverage are able to purchase insurance more affordably
- new regulations on all health plans that prevents health insurers from denying coverage to people for any reason and from charging higher premiums based on health status and gender
- the requirement that most individuals have health insurance beginning in 2014
- a penalty to employers that do not offer affordable coverage to their employees, with exceptions for small employers (THE HENRY J. KAISER FAMILY FOUNDATION (2012)).

U.S. health care continues to operate within a free market system, which means that it is a health care system controlled by private individuals and corporations rather than by a government. This free market system exerts control over health care delivery and financing. Payment for health care in this free market system stems primarily from multiple third-party payers. Health care services are provided to the patient (first party) by the health care provider and hospital (second party). These providers and hospitals (second party) bill their services to multiple insurance companies and health care programs (third-party). This third-party payer system leads to high administrative costs in the U.S. system (Figure 2-1).

ORGANIZATION OF HEALTH CARE

Health care systems have three simple components: structure, process, and outcome (Donabedian, 2005). The **structure** component of health care includes resources or structures needed to deliver quality health care, for example, human and physical resources, such as nurses and nursing and medical practitioners; hospital buildings; medical records; and pharmaceuticals. Providing a mechanism whereby access to health care is made possible is also a necessary structural component. The **process** component of health care includes the quality activities, procedures, tasks, communications, and processes performed within the health care structures, such as hospital admissions, surgical operations, and nursing and medical care delivery following standards and guidelines to achieve quality outcomes. Referrals to specialized providers, treatments, and the provision of evidence-based care from health care providers, as well as discharge procedures, are also illustrations of health care processes. The **outcome** component of health care refers to the results of good care delivery achieved by using quality structures and quality processes and includes the achievement of outcomes such as patient satisfaction, good health and functional ability, and the absence of health care-acquired infections

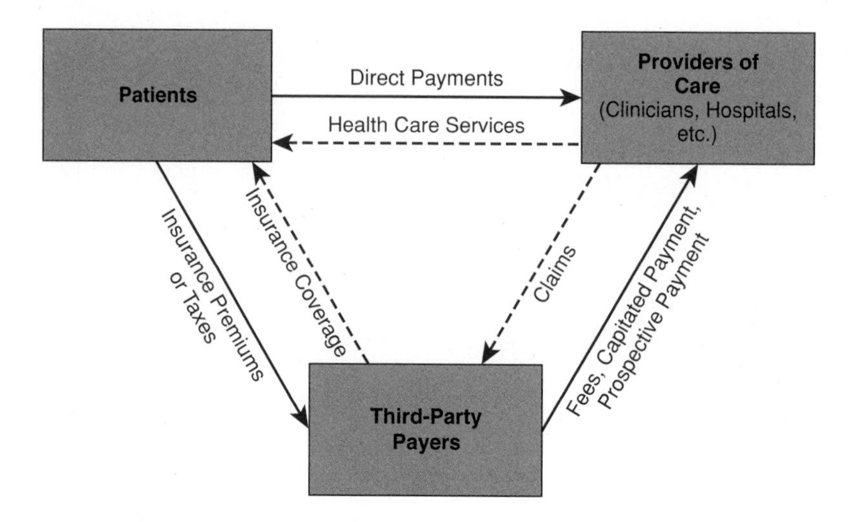

FIGURE 2-1

Economic relationships in the health care delivery system.
(*Source:* Adapted from Jönsson B. (1989, Dec.) What can Americans learn from Europeans? Health Care Financing Review. Spec No: 79–93; discussion 93–110.)

and morbidity. Measuring patient length of stay and the factors contributing to increasing or decreasing patient admissions, and recruitment and retention of the health care workforce are also important outcome measures. Table 2-2 offers examples of structure, process, and outcome performance measures in clinical care, financial management, and human resources management.

The World Health Organization (WHO) has put forth three primary goals for what good health care should do:

1. Ensure that the health status of everyone is the best that is possible across the lifespan.
2. Respond to patients' expectations of respectful treatment and include a focus on patients by health care clinicians.
3. Provide financial protection for everyone regardless of ability to pay (WHO, 2000).

Consistent with these goals, Healthy People 2020 has also developed overarching goals to increase quality and years of healthy life and eliminate health disparities. These goals are:

- Attain high-quality, longer lives free of preventable disease, disability, injury, and premature death.
- Achieve health equity, eliminate disparities, and improve the health of all groups.
- Create social and physical environments that promote good health for all.
- Promote quality of life, healthy development, and healthy behaviors across all life stages (USDHHS, 2010a).

U.S. Health Care Rankings

Most U.S. citizens believe that they live in a nation that delivers the most comprehensive health care in the entire world. This is not true. Although state-of-the-art health care is available in the United States, access is limited to those who can afford the high costs associated with such care. The United States spends more money on health care than any other nation, yet health status and outcomes are significantly lower than in other industrialized or high-income nations. Infant mortality rate (IMR) and life expectancy at birth (LEB) are two measures of the health of a nation that reflect the quality of the health care delivery system. According to the U.S. Central Intelligence Agency (2012), the United States ranks 174 in IMR among the nations of the world and 51 in LEB. Note that differences in data collecting methods and protocols can shape the way estimates are made of the data from countries across the world.

A study of health care systems conducted by Schoen, Osborn, Doty, Bishop, Peugh, and Murukutla (2007), found that, among adults in seven countries, United States adults reported the highest overall error

TABLE 2-2
Examples of Performance Measures by Category

	Clinical Care	Financial Management	Human Resources Management
Structure	*Effectiveness* ◆ Percent of nurses and physicians who are certified ◆ JC (formerly JCAHO) accreditation ◆ Presence of Magnet recognition	*Effectiveness* ◆ Qualifications of administrators in finance department ◆ Presence of an integrated financial and clinical information system and clinical decision-making technology	*Effectiveness* ◆ Ability to attract desired nursing and medical practitioners ◆ Competitive salary and benefits ◆ Quality staff education
Process	*Effectiveness* ◆ Ratio of medication errors ◆ Ratio of complications *Productivity* ◆ Ratio of total patient days to total full-time equivalent (FTE) nursing and medical practitioners *Efficiency* ◆ Average cost per admission ◆ Average cost per surgery	*Effectiveness* ◆ Days in accounts receivable ◆ Market share *Productivity* ◆ Ratio of collections to FTE financial staff ◆ Ratio of new capital acquisitions to fund-raising staff *Efficiency* ◆ Debt/equity ratio	*Effectiveness* ◆ Number and type of staff grievances ◆ Organizational climate *Productivity* ◆ Ratio of front-line staff to managers *Efficiency* ◆ Recruitment costs
Outcome	*Effectiveness* ◆ Severity-adjusted mortality ◆ Patient satisfaction ◆ Patient functional health status ◆ Medical errors	*Effectiveness* ◆ Return on assets ◆ Operating margins	*Effectiveness* ◆ Staff turnover rate ◆ Staff satisfaction

Source: Compiled with information from Shortell, S. M., & Kaluzny, A. D. (2006). *Health Care Management* (5th ed.). Clifton Park, NY: Delmar Cengage Learning.

rates, including medication and lab errors. One-third of patients with chronic disease reported a lab or medical error in the past two years, compared with 26% of patients in Australia and 28% in Canada. The error rate was highest among patients seeing multiple practitioners for comorbid conditions.

This is not a new problem; in 1918 Anna Harkness founded The Commonwealth Fund with the mandate that it should "do something for the welfare of mankind." Throughout its history, The Commonwealth Fund has been instrumental in implementing projects and communicating their results to influential audiences. In 2006, The Commonwealth Fund Commission developed the National Scorecard on U.S. Health System Performance. The Scorecard measures the health system across 42 key indicators of health care including: quality, access, efficiency, equity, and healthy lives. In 2006, the U.S. health care system scored an average of 66 out of a maximum 100. In 2008, a score of 65 was achieved. Of greatest concern in 2008 was that access to health care had significantly declined. In 2011, the U.S. health care system achieved a score of 64 out of 100 (The Commonwealth Fund, 2011) (Figure 2-2).

Some major findings from the U.S. Scorecard include the following:

- **Infant Mortality.** The U.S. infant mortality rate is 7.0 deaths per 1,000 live births, compared with 2.7 deaths in the top 3 countries.
- **Health Disparities.** 51% of U.S. adults received preventive and screening tests according to guidelines for their age and sex.
- **Childhood Obesity.** Nearly one-third of children ages 10 to 17 were overweight or obese as of 2007. Unless there is an improvement in healthy eating and weight control, obesity and related health problems are likely to rise and could wipe out recent health gains from declining smoking rates.
- **Safe Care.** In a sign that safety concerns extend beyond the hospital, in 2007 one-quarter of elderly Medicare beneficiaries were prescribed a drug that is potentially inappropriate for older people. Wider use of electronic systems that alert clinicians of such risks may help improve safety in the future.
- **Patient-Centered, Timely, Coordinated Care.** In 2008, only 43% of U.S. adults with health problems were able to rapidly secure an appointment with a physician when they were sick, about half the rate in the best country. Nineteen percent of U.S. patients reported undergoing duplicate tests, almost five times the rate in the benchmark country (The Commonwealth Fund, 2011).

Universal Health Care

Universal health care (UHC) is a government-sponsored system that ensures health care coverage for all eligible residents of a nation regardless of income level or employment status. UHC varies widely in its structure and funding mechanisms, particularly in the degree to which it is publicly funded. Typically, most UHC costs are met by the population via compulsory

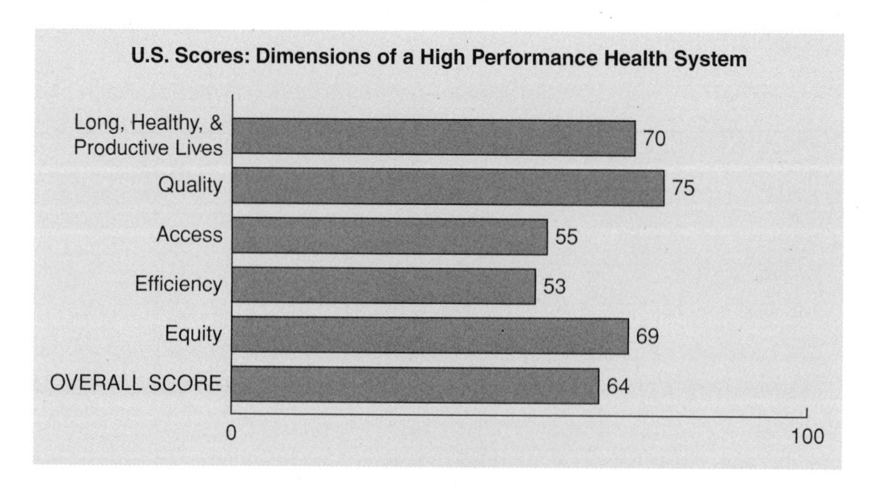

FIGURE 2-2

U.S. scorecard on health system performance.

(*Source:* Commonwealth Fund National Scorecard on U.S. Health System Performance. [2011]. Retrieved November 27, 2011. from http://www .commonwealthfund.org/Publications/Fund-Reports/2011/Oct/Why-Not-the-Best-2008.aspx?page=all)

health insurance or taxation or a combination of both. In some cases, government involvement in UHC also includes being the single payer and directly managing the health care system, though many countries use mixed public/private payment systems to deliver universal health care. According to the Institute of Medicine (Insuring America's Health: Principles and Recommendations, 2004), the United States is the only wealthy, industrialized nation that does not provide universal health care. Access to health care for most Americans is tied directly to having health insurance. As a result, serious gaps in health care coverage leave millions of people in the United States uninsured, thus placing them at risk of being sicker and dying younger than the insured (Muenning et al., 2005, pp. 2–34). In 2007, 53% of the United States had employer health insurance. Four percent had individual health insurance, thirteen percent had Medicaid, twelve percent had Medicare, and fifteen percent had no insurance (Kaiser Family Foundation, 2008a).

The U.S. Patient Protection and Affordable Care Act (PPACA)

With the passage of The U.S. Patient Protection and Affordable Care Act (PPACA), legislation to improve health care coverage for all, and the Health Care and Education Reconciliation Act (HCERA) in 2010, these figures will change. PPACA is a United States federal statute signed into law by President Barack Obama on March 23, 2010. Together with the Health Care and Education Reconciliation Act, it is a significant regulatory overhaul of the U.S. health care system. PPACA is aimed primarily at decreasing the number of uninsured Americans and reducing the overall costs of health care. It provides a number of mechanisms—including mandates, subsidies, and tax credits—to employers and individuals in order to increase the health care coverage rate. (Krugman, 2010; Pear, 2012). PPACA moves to improve health care outcomes, streamline the delivery of health care, and require insurance companies to cover all applicants and offer the same rates regardless of preexisting conditions or gender (Hearst, 2012; The Week, 2012). The Congressional Budget Office has projected that PPACA will lower future deficits (Elmendorf, 2011a) and Medicare spending (Elmendorf, 2011b). On June 28, 2012, the United States Supreme Court upheld the constitutionality of most of PPACA in the case National Federation of Independent Business v. Sebelius (Barrett, 2012).

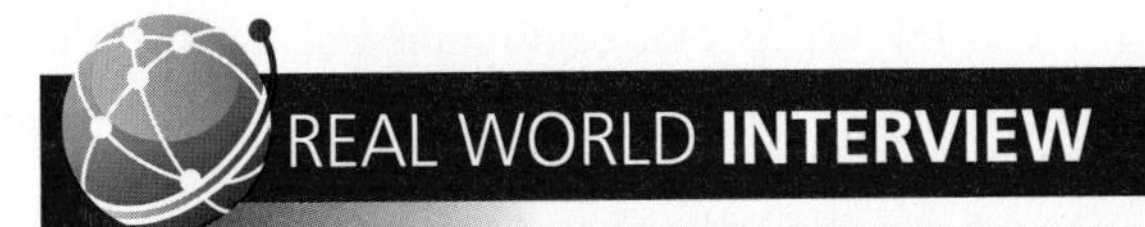

REAL WORLD INTERVIEW

As a nurse practitioner, there are many things about the American health care system that I really value. There are minimal wait times and there are lots of specialties. I like that a patient whom I refer with a serious diagnosis can be seen by a specialist within two weeks. We develop and make top-notch technology available and we have great health care standards. For all of these reasons, we keep the world on track and it follows our lead. I'm also aware every day of the shortcomings of the health care system. It's far too expensive, there are too many special interest groups, and it's all going to collapse under its own weight, a classic example of capitalism gone amuck. For example, health insurance companies have too much power, and I hate how all the insurance hoops prevent me and my colleagues from giving the best care to our patients.

We need a national health policy, and if the American people make enough noise, politicians will get behind it, too. I'm in favor of a national health plan, one that will ensure that all Americans have access to care. It needs to be one that incorporates what we already do best with what's useful from other countries such as Japan and Canada. We have a lot to learn from what they do well that we don't do.

NADINE LAMOREAU, MSN, APRN, FNP-C
Fort Fairfield, Maine

Emphasis on Hospital Care

The number of acute care hospital beds in the United States is 2.7 per 1,000 people. This number is lower than the average of 3.9 acute care hospital beds per 1,000 people in other countries such as France, Canada, and Japan. Since 1980, hospital bed use and length of stay have decreased in the United States, which corresponds to an increase in the use of outpatient and day-surgery facilities (Health System Change, 2006; Organisation for Economic Co-operation and Development, 2008). In the United States, the emphasis on acute health care services has driven health care costs higher, but has not necessarily improved the quality of care or patient outcomes (Werner & Bradlow, 2006; Jeffrey & Newacheck, 2006). Considering what health care services are needed by patients to improve their health status, only 8 out of 1,000 people will benefit from hospitalization, something that seems odd when considering where the research dollars are targeted and where the majority of health care dollars are devoted, that is, acute care settings in hospitals. When you look at a group of 1,000 people, it is estimated that 800 of them will experience symptoms of some disease or condition. Of this group of 800, 265 will be seen in a practitioner's office, hospital outpatient department or emergency department, or use home health care. Only eight will eventually be hospitalized. The majority do not need hospitalization and would benefit from more resources available for primary health care delivery outside the hospital (Green, Gryer, Yawn, Lanier, & Dovery, 2000). Note that a consistent focus on illness and injury, often referred to as a downstream focus, means fewer dollars are invested in upstream efforts. A focus on upstream efforts directed at keeping the population well through health promotion and illness prevention strategies would be less costly.

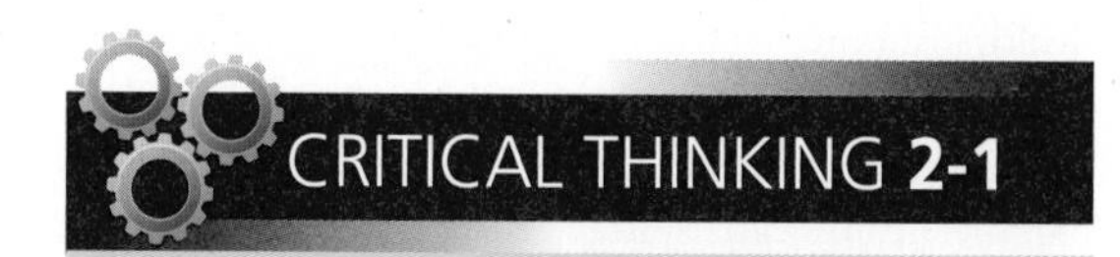

Dalen and Alpert (2008) maintain that the United States needs only to follow its own Medicare model to implement a viable national health care program. They state, "Medicare pays the private sector to deliver quality health care to more than 44 million Americans. Those who stick with traditional Medicare have free choice of physicians and hospitals. Nearly every U.S. physician and nearly every hospital in the United States has elected to participate in Medicare. The administrative costs of Medicare are only 2% compared to costs of 12% with for-profit health insurers" (p. 554).

Is a national health care plan the solution to our health care problems?

What are the positions of your state board of nursing and the American Nurses Association on this? Visit their websites to review their position statements.

Need for Primary Health Care

Given that the majority of patient needs and patient care delivery occurs outside acute care settings, primary care "which provides integrated, accessible health care services by clinicians who are accountable for addressing a large majority of personal health care needs, developing a sustained partnership with patients, and practicing in the context of family" (IOM, 1996, p. 1), should be better understood and appreciated for the role it has in improving patients' health status and health outcomes. The key foundations of primary care (Starfield, 1998) can be applied across the health care continuum and across organizational settings because primary care emphasizes seven important features: care that is continuous, comprehensive, coordinated, community oriented, family centered, culturally competent, and begun at first contact with the patient. According to Starfield (1998), patients and clinicians need to work together to appropriately utilize services based on the following four foundations of primary care:

- First Contact: Conduct the initial evaluation and define the health dysfunctions, treatment options, and health goals.
- Longitudinally: Sustain a patient-clinician relationship continuously over time, throughout the patient's illness, acute need and disease management.
- Comprehensive: Manage the wide range of health care needs, across health care settings, and among different health care professionals.

- Coordination: Build upon longitudinally. Care received through referrals and other providers is followed and integrated, averting unnecessary services and duplication of services.

Primary care clinicians, who include both medical and nursing practitioners, can be a patient's greatest asset in negotiating the health care system and improving patient outcomes. It is through understanding the patient's past and present that future health care needs can be anticipated. Primary care interventions, such as health promotion and timely preventive care and medication administration, can reduce the need for hospitalizations, improve the health of patients, and avert adverse morbidity and mortality outcomes. Patients and their families can communicate with clinicians to understand their health and how to partner with clinicians to improve decision making. This is what patient-centered care is based on, both primary care and patient decision making.

The World Health Report (WHO, 2008), Primary Health Care: Now More than Ever, underscores the need for primary health care. The report cites a disproportionate focus on specialist hospital care, fragmentation of health systems, and the proliferation of unregulated commercial care. The World Health Organization (2010) has also identified key elements in improving health status through primary care strategies aimed at reducing disparities through universal access, enhancing coordination and delivery of care, and increasing stakeholder participation at multiple levels.

Public Health versus Individual Health Care

The health care system in America has been described as an industry consisting of a "sprawling set of activities and enterprises" (Knickman & Kovner, 2008, p. 4), with "profit-making as its objective" (Demaro, 2008). Use of the term *health care system* is misleading, as it suggests an organized system with knowledgeable individuals and concerned agencies working together to achieve health goals for the population through appropriate public health and medical care—ideal, but not the case in the United States. The difference between public health care for the entire population and health care for individuals who can pay for it is an important distinction to understand with respect to the organization and delivery of health care in the United States.

Public health care activities are directed toward keeping communities and the population healthy. Individual health care consists of activities that assist in restoring health of individuals after the onset of symptoms of an illness or injury. Public health care, which receives less than 4% of national health spending (Hunt & Knickman, 2008), is provided by a diverse group of health care professionals including public health nursing and medical practitioners. Public health care promotes and protects public health through programs directed toward healthier lifestyles, immunization, disease prevention, environmental protection, and ensuring safe food and water; this can be provided in clinics, work sites, and other public forums. Conversely, individual health care, provided after the onset of symptoms primarily by individual nursing and medical practitioners, is available in clinics and hospitals. With a focus on short-term acute care treatment, individual health care costs much more than public health care. A persistent emphasis on short-term individual health care fails at keeping the population well through ongoing disease prevention efforts and demonstrates where American health care priorities rest (Figure 2-3).

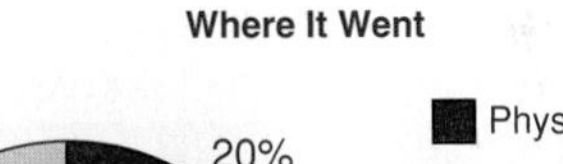

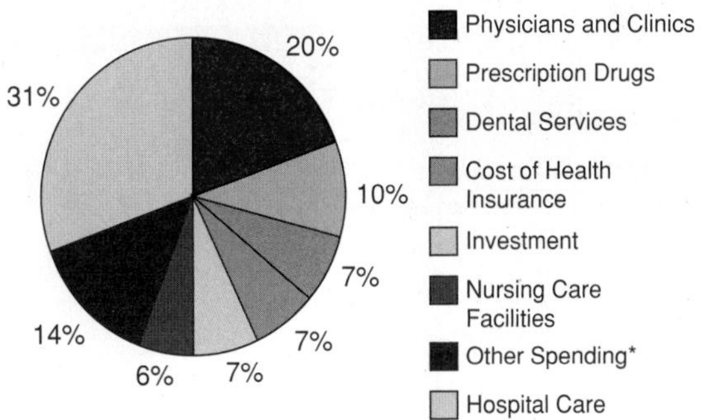

*Other spending includes government public health activities, home health care, and other health, residential, and personal care.

FIGURE 2-3

The nation's health dollar, calendar year 2009: Where it went.

(*Source:* Centers for Medicare & Medicaid Services, Office of the Actuary National Health Statistics Group. (2009). Retrieved November 14, 2011, from https://www.cms.gov/NationalHealthExpendData/downloads/PieChartSourcesExpenditures2009.pdf)

The U.S. health care system is defined by other features as well (Knickman & Kovner, 2008). The role of institutions in delivering care includes the organization of acute, long-term, and community health care. Each respective institution has evolved with its own roles and traditions to meet different health care needs. A diverse group of health professionals is responsible for organizing and delivering health care. Physicians, nurses, administrators, policy makers, business leaders, physical therapists, social workers, researchers, and technicians all hold vested interests in how care is delivered, and the differing ideologies may pose tensions between groups.

The Federal Government

The federal government provides for the general welfare of the population through the collection and allocation of money for the oversight and administration of health care programs. Several organizations and divisions of the federal government are specifically involved in health care programs. The U.S. Department of Health and Human Services (USDHHS) is the largest such organization. A visit to the website of the HHS (www.hhs.gov/about/index.html) demonstrates that this federal body oversees the functioning of several subdivisions and agencies, including:

- Agency for Healthcare Research and Quality (AHRQ)
- Centers for Disease Control and Prevention (CDC)
- Centers for Medicare & Medicaid Services (CMS)
- Food and Drug Administration (FDA)
- Health Resources and Services Administration(HRSA)
- Indian Health Services (IHS)
- National Institutes of Health (NIH)
- Substance Abuse and Mental Health Services Administration (SAMHSA)

Other arms of the federal government and other departments such as the Department of Housing and Urban Development, the Department of Justice, the Department of Labor, and the Department of Defense also assume some responsibility for the health and well-being of the population.

State and Local Governments

Public health services at the state and local levels of government are delivered by boards of health and state and local health departments. The ability of public

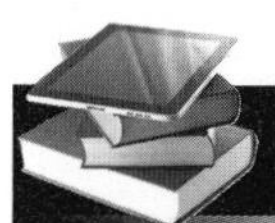

EVIDENCE FROM THE **LITERATURE**

Citation: Coddington, J. A., & Sands, L. P. (2008). Cost of health care and quality outcomes of patients at nurse-managed clinics. *Nursing Economics, 26*(2), 75–83.

Discussion: Lack of health insurance is a critical factor in access to appropriate health services and is directly associated with increased morbidity and mortality, lack of continuity of care, and rising health care costs. Nurse-managed clinics (NMCs) can serve as an important safety net in the health care delivery system by offering needed health services to populations of people affected by poverty and lack of insurance. NMCs remove barriers to care, improve health care access, and foster therapeutic relationships with nurse practitioners who provide primary care to vulnerable people. Much evidence also exists that nurse-managed clinics improve the use of preventive services, aid in the promotion of health, increase compliance with treatment, improve patient satisfaction, and reduce emergency room visits and re-hospitalizations.

Implications for Practice: The opportunity to provide quality care to vulnerable populations through NMCs is excellent. Overcoming the challenge of policies that restrict third-party reimbursement for nurse practitioners would allow an increased number of patients to be seen at NMCs.

health services to improve the health of the public is potentially great but has been limited in the United States Efforts for bioterrorism and disaster preparedness have brought the nation's public health infrastructure desolation to light. There has been a recent increase in funding for U.S. disaster preparedness efforts but little money has been focused on public health care funding and infrastructure.

Home Health Care

The location of care delivery is continually changing to adapt to technologies and patient needs, for example the use of home health care services in the community setting in lieu of institutional care. According to the National Health Care Expenditure Projections (Center for Medicare & Medicaid Services [CMC], 2010), home health care expenditures grew to 11.7 percent of national health care expenditures in 2009, and spending reached $72.2 billion. This increase has been primarily driven by higher growth in Medicaid spending partly due to Medicaid's continued shifting of long-term care from institutional to home settings. In light of an aging population, home health care services will continue to serve an integral role in health care delivery.

Health Care Disparities

Health care disparities are persistent inequalities between the health outcomes of people in one group versus another group, due to such variables as gender, sexuality, age, ethnicity, socioeconomic group, lifestyle, and/or health care access. These health care disparities have been recognized as great influences on health. The 2011 Centers for Disease Control and Prevention (CDC) Health Disparities and Inequities Report highlights disparities in health care access, exposure to environmental hazards, morbidity, mortality, behavioral risk factors, disability status, and social determinants of selected health problems at the national level.

Not enough health care delivery and attention are directed toward the top underlying causes of death in the United States (i.e., tobacco, poor diet, physical inactivity, alcohol consumption, microbial agents, toxic agents, motor vehicle accidents, firearms, sexual behavior, and illicit drug use) (Mokdad, Marks, Stroup, & Gerberding, 2004).

Analysis of large data sets illustrates that as one ages, more health care services are utilized; women use health care services more frequently then men, and whites have greater health care access, and therefore higher utilization rates, than do patients of color (National Healthcare Disparities Report [NHDR], 2005; National Healthcare Quality Report [NHQR], 2005).

Healthy People 2020

Figure 2-4, Healthy People 2020 Framework, highlights health care determinants and identifies overarching goals for nurses and other health care workers to work toward, in order to achieve the goal of improved health of a diverse society where all people live long, healthy lives. (U.S. Department of Health and Human Services [USDHHS], 2010).

HEALTH CARE SPENDING

Currently, the U.S. health care system consists of a mix of health care providers from either nonprofit or for-profit organizations in both the public and private sectors. Reimbursement for health care services is paid in one or a combination of these four ways:

- Private insurers
- Publicly funded payers
- Charitable entities
- Direct payment by consumers

In 2009, as indicated in Figure 2-5, 71% of health care financing came from health insurance, both public and private, and 29% came from other sources.

Many gaps exist in these private and public programs, including incomplete health care coverage, need for co-payments and deductibles, lack of provider choice, need for pre-authorizations, and other difficulties in maneuvering through the requirements. **Co-payments** are a fixed health care fee paid by the patient to the health care provider at the time of service; co-payments are paid by patients in addition to the money the health care provider will receive from the insurance company. **Deductibles**

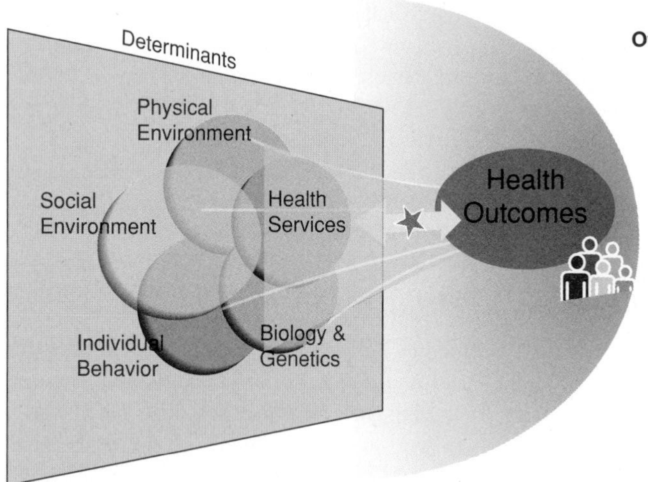

FIGURE 2-4

Healthy People 2020 framework.

(*Source:* From U.S. Department of Health and Human Services (HHS). (2010c). Healthy People 2020 Framework, accessed May 20, 2012, at http://healthypeople.gov/2020/Consortium/HP2020Framework.pdf)

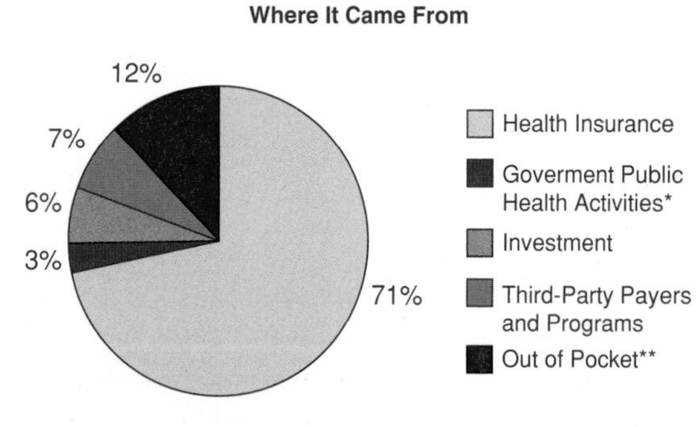

* Includes worksite health care, other private revenues, Indian Health service, worker's compensation assistance, maternal and child health, vocational rehabilitation, Substance Abuse and Mental Health Services Administration, school health, and other federal and local programs

** Includes co-payments, deductibles, and any amounts not covered by health insurance.

FIGURE 2-5

The nation's health dollar, calendar year 2009: Where it came from.

(*Source:* Centers for Medicare & Medicaid Services, Office of the Actuary National Health Statistics Group. [2009]. Retrieved November 14, 2011, from https://www.cms.gov/NationalHealthExpendData/downloads/PieChartSourcesExpenditures2009.pdf)

are a predetermined out-of-pocket fee paid by a patient for health care services before reimbursement through health insurance begins to be paid. For example, if an insurance plan has a $50 co-payment and a $1,000 deductible, the patient is responsible for paying the $50 co-payment at each health care visit plus paying the first $1,000 (deductible) of health care costs, after which costs will be reimbursed as allowed by the patient's health insurance plan. **Pre-authorization** requires that approval be obtained from the insurance company before care or treatment such as hospitalization or diagnostic testing is initiated if such services are to be reimbursed by the patient's health insurance plan.

Rising Health Care Costs

Health care costs are measured as part of the U.S. gross domestic product (GDP). The **gross domestic product (GDP)** is an economic measure of a country's national income and output within a year and reflects the market value of goods and services produced within the country. The GDP is used as a barometer of the national economy. Internationally, the United States spends more of its GDP on health care than any other wealthy country, all of which provide health care insurance for all their citizens. Health care costs in the United States are increasing 2.5 percentage points faster than the annual U.S. GDP. Employer-based health care premiums have doubled since 2000, yet those who are insured incur greater financial burdens as they pay for more out-of-pocket expenses. U.S. national health care expenditures were $1.9 trillion in 2004 (Kaiser Family Foundation [KFF] & Health Research and Education Trust, 2007). A staggering 16% of the GDP was spent on health care. From 1960 to 2000, the GDP for health care grew nearly fifteen-fold, from approximately $526 billion to the trillions of dollars spent today. It is projected that health care spending will rise to $4 trillion by 2015 (Borger et al., 2006). Health care spending continues to increase and is growing at 2.5 percentage points faster than the growth of the GDP (Centers for Medicare & Medicaid Services [CMS], 2006). In 2000, the percentage of GDP for health care was 15.3%, and analysts project this number to keep rising to 20% (Borger et al., 2006).

Medical debt is now the number one reason for personal bankruptcy. The majority of people declaring bankruptcy because of medical debt are employed and have health insurance (Himmelstein, Warren, Thorne, & Woolhandler, 2005). Spending on health care services is concentrated in disproportionate ways, which adds to the inflation of health care costs. For example, 10% of people account for 60% of spending on health care services; 20% of health care expenditures are spent on 1% of the population, indicating that a small percentage of the population absorbs a tremendous amount of health care services and spending. On the other side of the health care spectrum, 50% of the population contributes to 3% of health care expenditures. From another perspective, 44% of health care expenses are concentrated in the treatment of five predominant health problems: heart conditions, cancer, trauma, mental health disorders, and pulmonary conditions (Kaiser Family Foundation, 2007a; Stanton, 2006).

Health Care Insurance

In the United States, health care insurance is one of the most significant factors in facilitating access to health care services. The United States has a mix of publicly and privately financed insurance, supported by varying mixes of premiums and taxes. Publicly funded health insurance programs such as Medicare, Medicaid, and State Children's Health Insurance Program (SCHIP) provide health care coverage to people who qualify on the basis of low income, disability, or age (children and the elderly), leaving an estimated 46 million people or 15.3% of the population uninsured. This estimate includes 9 million children (Robert Wood Johnson Foundation, 2008). The Kaiser Family Foundation (2008b) estimates that this figure increases to 77 million people who go without health insurance coverage for all or part of the year. The 2010 passage of The Patient Protection and Affordable Care Act and the Health Care and Education Reconciliation Act is an attempt to improve health care coverage for all.

In the past, American health insurance companies have routinely rejected applicants with a preexisting condition. The insurance companies often denied claims. If a customer was hit by a truck and faced big medical bills, the insurance company dug through the records searching for grounds to cancel the policy, often while the victim was still in the hospital (Reid, 2008). Foreign health insurance companies, in contrast, must accept all applicants, and they can't cancel insurance as long as you pay your premiums. Everyone is mandated to buy insurance to give the plans an adequate pool of rate payers. The key difference is that foreign health insurance plans exist only to pay people's medical bills, not to make a profit. The United States is the only developed country that lets insurance companies profit from basic health coverage. In many ways, foreign health care models are not really foreign to America, because our health system uses elements of all of them. See information later in this chapter on selected foreign health care systems.

State Regulation of Health Insurance

Three key pieces of federal legislation set forth national standards that the individual states use to regulate health insurance. First, the Employee Retirement

Income Security Act (ERISA) of 1974 provides a framework for states to regulate health insurers. Second, the Consolidated Omnibus Budget Reconciliation Act (COBRA) of 1985 ensures that employees who resigned, were laid off, were terminated, or lost their job due to family-related reasons can retain their health insurance coverage for up to 18 months and, in some cases, up to a maximum of 36 months, if they are deemed qualified and pay the full premium. A third piece of legislation, the Health Insurance Portability and Accountability Act (HIPAA) of 1996 imposes restrictions on limitations and exclusions of insurance coverage for those with preexisting conditions and restricts other attempts to exclude employees from insurance coverage. It also provides protection of insurance coverage as employees change employers, and it provides tax exclusions for medical savings accounts.

INTERNATIONAL PERSPECTIVES ON HEALTH CARE

To the extent that the United States is similar economically and sociopolitically to countries such as France, Canada, and Japan, an examination of the health systems in those countries is useful. The differences between allocation of health care spending in the United States as compared to other Organisation for Economic Co-operation and Development (OECD) countries are graphically displayed in Figure 2-6.

France

France, ranked as having the best health care system in the world (Nolte & McKee, 2008), spends 11.1% of its gross domestic product on health care

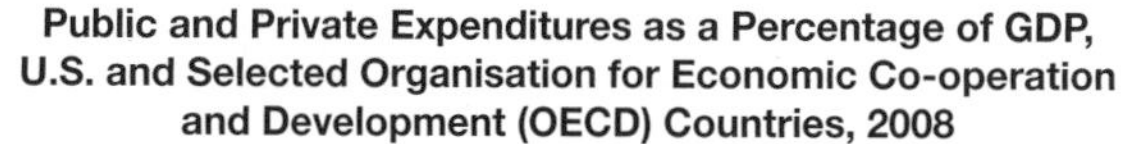

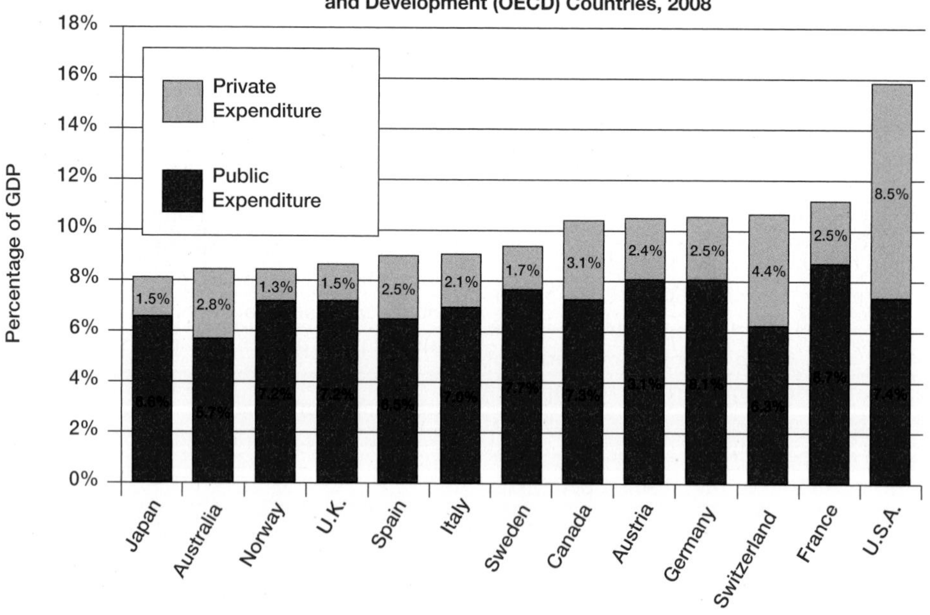

FIGURE 2-6

Public and private health expenditures as a percentage of GDP; U.S. and Kaiser Family Foundation (KFF). (2011). Selected organisation for economic co-operation and development (OECD) countries, 2008.

Note that over the last three decades, the United States has seen increased spending by both the public and private sectors. This figure illustrates how the United States has had a faster rate of both sources of spending than other countries included in this analysis.

(*Source:* Snapshot - Health Care Spending in the United States and Selected OECD Countries, April 2011", The Henry J. Kaiser Family Foundation, April 2011. This information was reprinted with permission from the Henry J. Kaiser Family Foundation. The Kaiser Family Foundation, a leader in health policy analysis, health journalism and communication, is dedicated to filling the need for trusted, independent information on the major health issues facing our nation and its people. The Foundation is a nonprofit private operating foundation, based in Menlo Park, California.)

(Organisation for Economic Co-operation and Development, 2008). This is approximately one-half of what the United States spends on health care.

Canada

Annually, the Canadian government spends 10% of its gross domestic product on its national health care system. Canada has the eighth largest global health care budget in the world (Organisation for Economic Co-operation and Development, 2008). The Canadian health care system is administered by each Canadian provincial or territorial government. Seventy percent of health spending is publicly funded through federal and provincial taxation of individuals and corporations, and the remaining thirty percent is paid through private and out-of-pocket sources for additional services such as prescription medications or dental and vision care (Canadian Institute for Health Information, 2006). All Canadians have equal access to the same quality and quantity of health care. Under the Canada Health Act of 1984, comprehensive health care is publicly administered, portable between provinces, and accessible to all. Primary care is provided by physicians and nurse practitioners, who may work in private clinics or public institutions. These health care providers are reimbursed on a fee-for-service basis, which allows them to be reimbursed by each provincial or territorial health plan for each health care service rendered to a patient.

Unlike the privatized health care system in the United States, extra billing, deductibles, and co-payments are not allowed. The health care provider bills the provincial or territorial health plan and is reimbursed with an agreed upon amount for each health service given. No additional charges or costs can be billed to or recovered from the patient. With only one insurance payer, referred to as a single-payer system, many of the problems embedded within the American health care system are eliminated. There are some problems, however. Only one-quarter (26%) of U.S. and Canadian patients reported same-day access to doctors when they were sick—and one-fourth or more reported long waits. In contrast, about half or more of Dutch (60%), New Zealand (54%), and United Kingdom (48%) patients were able to get a same-day appointment.

U.S. patients were the most likely to find it very difficult to get after-hours care without going to an emergency room: 40 percent said it was very difficult, compared with only 15 percent in the Netherlands and Germany, the lowest rates of any country on this measure. In the past two years, 59 percent of U.S. patients visited an emergency room; only Canada had higher rates (64%). In both countries, one in five said they went to the ER for a condition that could have been cared for by a regular doctor if one had been available (Commonwealth Fund, 2008b).

Wait times in Canada are circumvented based on the gravity of a patient's condition, but this solution aggravates the waiting time for less urgent cases. In a geographically vast country with a small population compared to the United States, some Canadians in rural or isolated locales often travel long distances to obtain specialized services.

As an example of the comprehensiveness and affordability of the Canadian health care service, a 51-year-old Canadian nurse working in the United States recently returned with her spouse and 15-year-old child to her home province of Alberta for one year. During that time, the family enrolled in the Alberta Health Care Insurance Plan for a cost of $88 per month (Alberta Health and Wellness, 2004). Health care for the nurse included an annual physical examination, lab tests, mammogram, bone density testing, and a routine colonoscopy. The colonoscopy required a five-month wait. Her husband underwent elective day surgery, which was booked seven months in advance. Her daughter was immunized at school, and she was once treated at a community health center for a persistent respiratory infection. Beyond payment of their monthly premium, the family was issued no bills for the health care they received.

Japan

To pay for its national health care system, Japan spends 8.2% of its gross domestic product on health care. This is less than France, Canada, or the United States, and Japan enjoys the longest life expectancy of all, that is, 82.4 years (Organisation for Economic Co-operation and Development, 2008). Membership in either of two broad health insurance programs is mandatory in Japan. The Employee Health Insurance

Program provides health care coverage for people employed by medium to large companies, national or local government, or private schools. The National Health Insurance Program covers self-employed and unemployed persons, as well as those employed in agriculture, forestry, or the fisheries industry. Payment toward each health insurance plan varies, but in both programs, patients share in paying for their health care costs up to a certain level, after which the insurance plan provides full coverage (National Coalition on Health Care, 2008c).

The Japanese health care system provides comprehensive care and is one of the most advanced in the world. Physicians and hospitals are predominantly run as private businesses, and costs for care are reimbursed through the national health care system. Patients' health care costs are reimbursed at a fixed amount determined by the government. Refusal of coverage by insurers is impossible, and personal medical debt is nonexistent. Because health care providers are reimbursed for the number of services provided, Japan leads other countries in the number of drugs prescribed, the number of tests ordered per patient, and patient length of stay in a hospital. The Japanese average 16 consultations with a health care provider per year, 3 to 4 times the rate of consultations in the United States.

Factors contributing to lower health care costs in Japan include healthier diets and lifestyles with a lower incidence of chronic diseases. Reimbursement rates for health care services are low, but reimbursement strategies for quantity rather than quality of services erodes the advantage a healthier lifestyle might have in terms of curbing costs. Despite cost containment efforts, health care expenses are increasing. A shortage of physicians also means the wait time to access the health system is an issue. Additionally, with an aging population and shrinking workforce, concerns as to how access, affordability, and quality will continue in the future are being voiced (National Coalition on Health Care, 2008c; Reid, 2008).

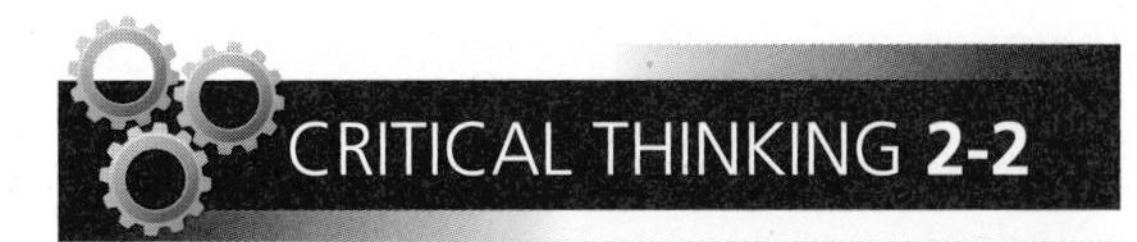

Starting in January of 2012, the Centers for Medicare & Medicaid Services (CMS) are implementing a new health care model, Accountable Care Organizations (ACOs). Federally approved ACOs will be eligible to care for Medicare patients. The basic ACO model starts with a lead group of health care providers. CMS rules also allow rural clinics and federally qualified health centers to lead an ACO, including hospitals, specialists, and long-term care facilities. Unlike much of the current health care system, in which health care providers make money only when treating sick people, ACOs may reward health care providers with a share of the cost savings achieved by retaining or improving patient health. Conversely, health care providers may see financial losses if they don't meet benchmarks in patient outcomes and care coordination, according to the CMS. ACOs differ from HMOs, their proponents say, as patients are free to visit care providers outside the organization, and costs can't be cut at the expense of quality care. Note that CMS reports more than half of Medicare beneficiaries have five or more chronic conditions.

How might ACOs provide better health care to individuals with chronic conditions?

What role will nursing have in ACOs?

FACTORS CONTRIBUTING TO RISING HEALTH CARE COSTS

Many factors contribute to the rising costs of health care. Some of these factors include the aging of the population with growth in the demand for health care, increased utilization of pharmaceuticals, expensive new technologies, rising hospital care costs, practitioner behavior, cost shifting, and administrative costs (Thorpe, Woodruff, & Ginsburg, 2005).

Aging and Pharmaceutical Use

According to the Administration on Aging (2010), by 2030, 72.1 million Americans will be age 65 and older and will comprise approximately 19 percent of the population. Although the aging population continues to grow, trends in nursing home utilization have declined in recent years as more and more seniors are receiving care within the community setting. In 2004, the number of nursing homes in the

United States fell to 16,100 in comparison to 17,208 nursing homes in 1996. In addition, the number of available nursing home beds decreased (CDC, 2011). On average, annual per capita expenditures on those patients aged 65 and older is $11,089, significantly higher than the annual expenditure of $3,352 for those aged 19 to 64 (Keehan, 2004).

Prescription medications are used by 92% of seniors and 61% of nonelderly adults (Woo, Ranji, Lundy, & Chen, 2007). These medication costs add 10% to national health care expenditures. Prescription drug use increased among the elderly after Medicare Part D, a prescription drug benefit plan, was introduced in 2006 (Catlin, Cowan, Hartman, Heffler, & National Health Expenditure Accounts Team, 2008). Currently, individuals are eligible for prescription drug coverage under a Part D plan if they are entitled to benefits under Medicare. Not all drugs are covered at the same level, giving participants incentives to choose certain drugs over others (Kaiser Family Foundation, 2010). Several pharmacies, for example Walgreens, CVS, Target, etc., have made some inexpensive generic medications available to patients at reduced cost.

Technology and Rising Hospital Costs

Although technological advances have facilitated earlier diagnoses and better treatment of disease, factors such as the greater availability of new technology drive per capita expenditures higher (Boddenheimer, 2005b). Treatment for the five most expensive health conditions, heart disease, cancer, trauma, mental disorders, and pulmonary conditions (Stanton, 2006), requires the use of expensive medications and technologies. While use of some technologies such as electronic record keeping may reduce costs, the presumed success of sophisticated drugs and technologies shapes consumer expectations of what the health care system can deliver. Health care consumers, including both patients and providers, also contribute to the cost of health care. These consumers' demands for intense services despite the lack of definite clinical need or evidence of efficacy strain health care spending. As an example, the United State performs more than three times (83) the number of magnetic resonance imaging (MRI) scans per person than does Canada (25.5) or Great Britain (19) (Canadian Institute for Health Information, 2006). Yet the United States lags behind these same countries with respect to patient care outcomes (Commonwealth Fund, 2006; Commonwealth Fund, 2008a).

Today, there are almost 6,000 hospitals nationwide. Hospital services contribute to the rise in health care costs due to the increased utilization of expensive technologies, high labor costs, rising malpractice premiums, and increased costs of hospitalization. Given the aging hospital infrastructure and increases in hospital reimbursements, future building of new hospital beds will also increase health care costs (Bazzoli, Gerland, & May, 2006).

Practitioner Behavior

A shortage of frontline health care providers, most noticeably among registered nurses (RNs), also adds to the cost of health care. With 10.5 nurses per 1,000 members of the population, the number of RNs in the United States is slightly greater than among other wealthy countries, which average 9.7 nurses per 1,000 members of the population (Organisation for Economic Co-operation and Development, 2008). Additionally, the median age of nurses is 46. More than 50% of the nursing workforce is close to retirement. Recent reforms in health care will give millions of people access to the health care system. More nurses and health professionals are needed.These factors, combined with an anticipated strengthening of the future economy, will create a renewed critical shortage for nurses.

The number of physicians per person in the United States is less than in other wealthy countries such as France, Canada, or Japan (Organisation for Economic Co-operation and Development, 2008). This shortage is most pronounced in certain practice specialties, for example, family practice physicians and geriatric physicians. Physician shortages are also apparent in rural areas. In addition, American physicians earn more than their counterparts in other countries. A physician specialist who makes $300,000 in the United States or a family physician whose income is $175,000 per year in the United States would, on average, earn approximately 25% to 50% less in Canada (Eisenberg, 2006). Defensive medicine and the high cost of medical malpractice insurance all add to increasing physician costs. Malpractice claims in the United States are filed 50% more often than in Great Britain and 350% more often than in Canada (Anderson, Hussey, Frogner, & Waters, 2005). Two-thirds of claims in the United States are dropped, which results in a similar distribution of claim settlements among these countries. Regardless, the need for medical malpractice insurance to protect American physicians against such claims contributes to the cost of physician care.

Cost Shifting and Administrative Costs

The practice of **cost shifting**, whereby health care providers raise prices for the privately insured to offset the lower health care payments from both Medicare and Medicaid as well as the often nonpayment of health care premiums from the uninsured, continues to raise the cost of health care. Medicare and Medicaid payments are less than 50% of what private insurers pay. Health care providers shift charges for health care costs to the private insurance sector. Some estimates of the cost shift are being valued at $6 billion annually. Costs to the public for these programs continue to increase. While the intent of the Medicaid program has been to ensure access to health care for mainly low-income pregnant women and children, over 72% of Medicaid's $295.9 billion dollars in expenditures in 2004 went toward care of the disabled and dual-eligibles. Dual-eligibles are the elderly who are eligible for both Medicaid and Medicare, and they are the fastest growing proportion enrolled in Medicaid (Holahan & Cohen, 2006).

According to Boddenheimer (2005a), the cost of administration of U.S. health care in 1999 was 24% of the nation's health care expenditures. In an attempt to reduce these costs, providers such as practitioner's offices, clinics, and hospitals have invested in information technology (IT). Because of the increased demand for such systems, the administrative cost of implementation has gone up, though efficient use of these systems in the future has the potential to decrease costs.

Other Factors Contributing to Rising Health Care Costs

Ongoing attention to healthy lifestyles, such as eating healthy foods, engaging in regular exercise, maintaining a healthy weight, living smoke-free, and limiting alcohol intake, reduces the health care required to manage the chronic disease conditions associated with the absence of such behaviors. However, as indicated by Knickman and Kovner (2008), these healthy lifestyle strategies have failed to reduce overall health care costs. Because rising health care costs are based on utilization, it is important to understand other factors that can both increase and decrease utilization, as listed in Table 2-3.

HEALTH CARE QUALITY, SAFETY, AND ACCESS

The Institute of Medicine (IOM), established in 1970 under the charter of the National Academy of Science, provides independent, objective, evidence-based advice to policy makers, health professionals, the private sector, and the public. The IOM report *To Err Is Human*, confronted health care clinicians and managers with concerns about the poor quality of health care attributable to misuse, overuse, and underuse of resources and procedures, which was responsible for thousands of deaths (IOM, 1999). The IOM report *Crossing the Quality Chasm* (IOM, 2001) and several other large studies (McGlynn et al., 2003; Thomas et al., 2000) have shown that the quality of health care in the United States is at an unexpected low level given the amount of money the United States spends on health care. The United States needs to set guidelines for health care improvement (Table 2-4).

A complete listing of IOM reports is available at www.iom.edu/Reports.aspx. Other phases of the IOM quality initiatives focus on operationalizing the vision of a future health system described in the *Quality Chasm* report. These phases have generated several publications, including *Patient Safety: Achieving a New Standard for Care* (2003a), *Keeping Patients Safe: Transforming the Work Environment of Nurses* (2003b), *Health Professions Education: A Bridge to Quality* (2003c), *Priority Areas for National*

TABLE 2-3
Forces That Affect Overall Health Care Utilization

Force	Factors That May Decrease Health Services Utilization	Factors That May Increase Health Services Utilization
◆ Financial incentives that reward practitioners and hospitals for performance (e.g., pay for performance [P4P] programs that reward quality practice)	◆ Changes in clinician practice patterns (e.g., encouraging patient self-care and healthy lifestyles; reduced length of hospital stay)	◆ Changes in clinician practice patterns (e.g., more aggressive treatment of the elderly)
◆ Increased accountability for performance	◆ Consensus documents or guidelines that recommend decreases in utilization	◆ Consensus documents or guidelines that recommend increases in utilization
◆ Technological advances in the biological and clinical sciences	◆ Better understanding of the risk factors of diseases and prevention initiatives (e.g., smoking-prevention programs, cholesterol-lowering drugs)	◆ New procedures and technologies (e.g., hip replacement, stent insertion, magnetic resonance imaging [MRI]) ◆ New drugs, expanded use of existing drugs ◆ Increased supply of services (e.g., ambulatory surgery centers, assisted living residences)
◆ Increase in chronic illness	◆ Discovery/implementation of treatments that cure or eliminate diseases ◆ Public health/sanitation advances (e.g., quality standards for food and water distribution)	◆ More functional limitations associated with aging ◆ More illness associated with aging ◆ More deaths among the increased number of elderly
◆ Increased ethnic and cultural diversity of the population	◆ Lack of insurance coverage ◆ Low income	◆ Growth in national population ◆ Efforts to eliminate disparities in access and outcomes
◆ Changes in the supply and education of health professionals	◆ Decreased supply (e.g., hospital closures, large numbers of nurses and medical and nursing practitioners retiring) ◆ Shifts to other sites of care may cause declines in utilization of staff at the original sites (e.g., ambulatory surgery, assisted living)	◆ Increase in chronic conditions ◆ Growth in national populations

(Continues)

TABLE 2-3 (Continued)

Force	Factors That May Decrease Health Services Utilization	Factors That May Increase Health Services Utilization
◆ Social morbidity (e.g., drugs, violence, disasters)	◆ Disparities in access to health services and outcomes	◆ New health problems (e.g., HIV/AIDS, bioterrorism)
◆ Access to patient information	◆ Changes in consumer preferences (e.g., home birthing, more self-care, alternative medicine)	◆ Changes in consumer demand
◆ Globalization and expansion of the world economy	◆ Growth in uninsured population	◆ Growth in national populations
◆ Cost control and competition for limited resources	◆ Insurance payer pressures to reduce costs	◆ Increased health insurance coverage ◆ Consumer/employee pressures for more comprehensive insurance coverage ◆ Changes in consumer preferences and demand (e.g., cosmetic surgery, hip and knee replacements, direct marketing of pharmaceuticals)

Source: Adapted from Bernstein, A. B., Hing, E., Moss, A. J., Allen, K. F., Siller, A. B., & Tiggle, R. B. (2003). *Health care in America: Trends in utilization.* Hyattsville, MD: National Center for Health Statistics; and Shortell, S. M., & Kaluzny, A. D. (2006). *Health care management* (5th ed.). Clifton Park, NY: Delmar Cengage Learning.

Action: Transforming Health Care Quality (2003d), *Performance Measurement: Accelerating Improvement* (2005), *Preventing Medication Errors* (2006a), *Rewarding Provider Performance: Aligning Incentives in Medicare* (2006b), and many others.

Health Care Variation

Groundbreaking research beginning in the 1970s has demonstrated that significant variation in utilization of specific health care services associated with geographic location, provider preferences and training, type of health insurance, and patient-specific factors such as age and gender exists (Wennberg & Gittelsohn, 1973; Leape, 1992; Adams, Fraser, & Abrams, 1973; Safran, Rogers, Tarlov, McHorney, & Ware, 1997; Greenfield et al., 1992; Williams, Eckert, L'italien, Lapuerta, & Weinberger, 2003). Utilization rates of health care services have been found to be associated with availability of services and technologies, for example, MRIs, hospital beds, practitioners (Joines, Hertz-Picciotto, Carey, Gesler, & Suchindran, 2003), prevalence and severity of morbidities (Dunn, Lyman, & Marx, 2005; National Healthcare Quality Report, 2005), race/ ethnicity (National Healthcare Quality Report, 2005), patient adherence, health-seeking behaviors of patients (Calvocoressi et al., 2004), and many other factors. Variation in the delivery and quality of health services is also associated with sociodemographics; hospital types, for example, urban/ rural or teaching/non-teaching; and clinical areas, for example heart disease, diabetes, pneumonia, and clinical preventive services. According to Fisher, Goodman, & Chandra (2008), hospitalization for medical conditions such as worsening diabetes or heart failure increases the risk of medical error and complications, both of which entail more costs. Findings from a study by the Dartmouth Atlas Project revealed that the supply of services, not how sick people were, was more likely

TABLE 2-4
Goals and Guidelines for Health Care Improvement

Six Goals for an Improved Health Care System

1. Safe: Avoid injuries from care intended to help patients.
2. Effective: Provide services based on scientific knowledge to all who could benefit and refrain from providing services to those not likely to benefit (Avoid overuse and underuse).
3. Patient Centered: Provide respectful and responsive care to individuals; patient preferences, needs, and values must guide clinical decision making.
4. Timely: Reduce wait time and harmful delays for those who receive and give care.
5. Efficient: Avoid waste of equipment, supplies, ideas, energy, and other costly resources.
6. Equitable: Provide care consistent in quality irrespective of gender, ethnicity, geographical, and socioeconomic factors.

Guidelines for Redesigning Care

1. Offer care based on continuous healing relationships: Make care available every day through face-to-face visits, telephone, Internet, and other means.
2. Customize care based on patient needs and values: Provide care responsive to patient needs and preferences.
3. Have patient as source of control: Foster patient empowerment and autonomy through information and shared decision making.
4. Share knowledge and free flow of information: Facilitate patient access to his or her own medical information and to available clinical knowledge.
5. Use evidence-based decision making: Provide consistent quality of care based on best available scientific knowledge.
6. Develop safety as a systems property: Develop systems of safety that mitigate or reduce error, promote patient safety, and reduce risk of injury.
7. Be transparent: Make information available to patients and families about health plans, hospitals, clinical practice, and alternative treatment options, including performance related to their safety, evidence-based practice, and patient satisfaction.
8. Anticipate needs: Anticipate patient needs rather than respond to events.
9. Continuously decrease waste: Use limited resources wisely.
10. Cooperate among clinicians: Collaborate and coordinate care between clinicians and institutions.

Source: Compiled from the Institute of Medicine. (2001). *Crossing the quality chasm: A new health system for the 21st century.* Washington, DC: National Academy Press; and Berwick, D. M. (2002). A user's manual for the IOM's 'Quality Chasm' report. *Health Affairs, 2* (3), 80–90.

to determine the resources used (Fisher, Goodman, & Chandra, 2008). Regions of the country and health care providers with more resources have higher rates of use and cost. Efforts to decrease the variation of health care practices through standardization of care with quality, evidence-based guidelines are important to improve clinical decision making care delivery, health outcomes, and cost efficiency. Achieving health care transparency, that is, truth in reporting health care practice preferences and truth in reporting health care error, is often hampered by the fear of litigation or reprisal against the health care provider. The Patient Safety and Quality Improvement Act of 2005 (see www.ahrq.govqual/pso-act.htm) addresses such concerns by encouraging health care providers to participate in developing and implementing evidence-based improvement initiatives. The Act also highlights the importance of recognizing and responding to underlying hazards and risks to patient safety. Establishing national health benchmarks, such as those in Healthy People 2020 (USDHHS, 2010) is another strategy by which to achieve and measure quality improvement. Performance is monitored between states and reflects the health trends and improvements among groups demonstrated to be disadvantaged or vulnerable (AHRQ, 2008b).

Evidence-Based Practice

Health care practitioners want to provide only that care that makes a positive difference in the lives of their patients. However, the history of health care does not well represent a process specifically devoted to achieving clinical practice based on fact (Sackett, Straus, Richardson, Rosenberg, & Haynes, 2000). Evidence-based practice is not a new concept. Archie

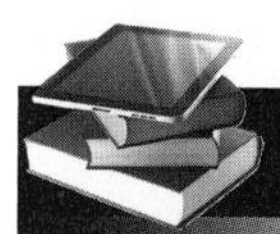

EVIDENCE FROM THE **LITERATURE**

Citation: Newhouse, R. P., Weiner, J. P., Stanik-Hutt, J., White, K. M., Johantgen, M., Steinwachs, D., Zangaro, G., Aldebron, J., & Bass, E. (2011). Advanced practice nurses as a solution to the workforce crisis: Implications of a systematic review of their effectiveness. *Nursing Economics, 29*(5), 230–250.

Discussion: Advanced practice registered nurses (APRN) have assumed an increasing role as providers in the health care system. This is particularly true in the underserved populations. APRNs practicing in APRN roles include certified registered nurse anesthetists (CRNAs), nurse practitioners (NPs), clinical nurse specialist (CNSs), and certified nurse midwives (CNMs). The aim of this systematic review was to answer the following question: Compared to other providers (physicians or teams without advanced practice registered nurses, are APRN patient outcomes of care similar? This systematic review appraised published studies between the years of 1990 and 2008. Results of these studies demonstrated that patient outcomes of care provided by certified nurse midwives and nurse practitioners in collaboration with physicians are similar to and in some ways better than care provided by physicians alone for the patients. Use of clinical nurse specialists can reduce Results of these studies demonstrated that patient outcomes length of stay and reduce hospital costs. These results extend what is known about APRN outcomes from previous reviews by assessing all types of APRNs over a span of 18 years, using a systematic process with an intentionally broad inclusion of patient populations, outcomes, and settings. The results indicate APRNs provide effective and high-quality patient care, have an important role in improving quality of patient care in the United States, and aid in addressing concerns about whether care provided by APRNs can safely augment the physician supply to support reform efforts aimed at expanding access to care.

Implications for Practice: The ideal health care system incorporates multiple practitioners who communicate with and are accountable to each other and the patient in the delivery of evidence-based care. This systematic review presents a high level of evidence that APRNs provide safe, effective care to a number of specific populations in a variety of settings. APRNs in coordination with other providers provide health promotion and evidence-based care. As Americans move forward with health reform, health care practitioners need to move forward with collaborative models of care delivery to attain unified national health goals.

Cochrane, a British epidemiologist, wrote and published articles on the importance of research supporting clinical practice (Mechanic & Dobson, 1996). Evidence-based practice is the integration of best evidence with clinical expertise together with patient choice (Sackett et al., 2000). Technology has now made it possible for practitioners to begin to focus on collecting reliable, sufficient data to determine best clinical practice. Although the amount and quality of clinical research has increased, and more research content has been threaded throughout educational programs, awareness and use of research by practicing health care providers remains poor (Camiah, 1997; Jolley, 2002). It can take as long as seventeen years to translate research findings into practice (Balas & Boren, 2000).

Recently, it was noted that when simple evidence-based changes of administering aspirin and beta-blockers are made, thus changing the processes of care for patients who have had a myocardial infarction, health care dollars can be lowered and lives saved. This is true even if it is because aspirin use is being measured to assess provider performance (Williams, Schmaltz, Morton, Koss, & Loeb, 2005). Such change in the processes of care delivery based on evidence could change the list of the top ten causes of death, that is, heart disease, cancer, cerebrovascular disease, chronic pulmonary disease, accidents, diabetes mellitus, influenza and pneumonia, Alzheimer's disease, kidney disease, and septicemia (CDC, 2005).

Transforming Care at the Bedside

The Robert Wood Johnson Foundation (RWJF) and the Institute for Healthcare Improvement (IHI) agreed to work together on an initiative called Transforming Care at the Bedside (TCAB) to improve care on medical-surgical units and improve staff satisfaction. The framework for TCAB change on the medical-surgical units was built around improvements in four main categories:

- Safe and Reliable Care
- Vitality and Teamwork
- Patient-Centered Care
- Value-Added Care Processes

Over the course of several years, participating hospitals tested, refined, and implemented change ideas within each of the four categories, many with very promising early results. Examples of TCAB initiatives include the following:

- Use of rapid response teams to "rescue" patients before a crisis occurs
- Specific communication models that support consistent and clear communication among caregivers
- Professional support programs such as preceptorships and educational opportunities
- Redesigned workspaces that enhance efficiency and reduce waste

Since 2008, a number of hospital teams across the United States have joined the 10 initial participants in applying TCAB principles and processes to dramatically improve the quality of patient care on medical and surgical units. These teams are from more than 70 hospitals in IHI's IMPACT Network's Learning and Innovation Community on Transforming Care at the Bedside and 67 hospitals in the American Organization of Nurse Executives(AONE) TCAB program, as well as from individual hospitals and health systems that have downloaded TCAB "How-to Guides," tools, and resources to launch their own medical-surgical transformations. For more information, please visit http://www.ihi.org, and search for TCAB.

Performance and Quality Measurement

Performance and quality measurements are essential components of health improvement efforts. Performance and quality are measured to determine resource allocation, organize care delivery, assess clinician competency, and improve the health care delivery process. The 2008 National Health Care Quality Report (AHRQ, 2009) revealed areas in which health care performance has improved over time. It also found that, across the process of care measures tracked in the report, patients received recommended care less than 60 percent of the time. Nursing leaders have also recognized the need to establish classification systems that can be used to measure nursing care performance (Table 2-5).

TABLE 2-5
Selected Classification Systems

North American Nursing Diagnosis Association (NANDA): www.nanda.org
Home Health Care Classification (HHCC): www.sabacare.com
PeriOperative Nursing Data Set: www.aorn.org
National Quality Forum-endorsed Nursing-sensitive Consensus Standards: www.qualityforum.org
Omaha System: www.omahasystem.org
ABC Codes: www.alternativelink.com
Logical Observation Identifiers Names and Codes: www.loinc.org
Patient Care Data Set: e-mail: judy.ozbolt@vanderbilt.edu
SNOMED CT: www.snomed.org
International Classification of Nursing Practice: www.icn.ch
Nursing Interventions Classification: www.nursing.uiowa.edu
Nursing Outcomes Classification: www.nursing.uiowa.edu
National Database of Nursing Quality Indicators (NDNQI): www.nursingworld.org. Search for NDNQI.

© Cengage Learning 2014

Note that setting standards for appropriate care and guideline development should have a basis in validated measures of quality, using reliable performance data, and making appropriate adjustments in care delivery. However, it is important to know that the majority of quality care is not measurable using current methods (Epstein, 1995; Smith, Atherly, Kane, & Pacala, 1997). Reliable methods and measures need to be developed and tested. Also, practitioners have been resistant to their care delivery being measured because they have believed that it would interfere with their professionalism and autonomy. If this belief persists, the majority of health care delivery will not be measured.

Malcolm Baldridge National Quality Award

Health care organizations are eligible to consider another framework for health care quality and to apply for the Malcolm Baldridge National Quality Award. The Baldridge Award highlights the importance of leadership; strategic planning; and a customer focus in building a quality health care system. Baldridge also stresses the importance of measurement, analysis, and knowledge management; workforce focus; operations focus; and results (Baldridge Health Care Criteria Program, 2011–2012; Available at http://www.nist.gov/baldrige/publications/hc_criteria.cfm.).

Outcome Measurement

In health care, the term outcome measurement is used to define the collection and reporting of information about an observed event in relation to a care delivery process or health promotion action. Outcome measurement necessitates identification of valid and reliable outcome indicators, the selection of appropriate measurement, and the assurance of timeliness of data collection and reporting. The usefulness and efficacy of outcome measurement is affected by:

- The timing of data collection;
- The quality of data;

- The consistency and accuracy of the data collection process; and
- The commitment and ability of those collecting the data and making decisions on the findings (Melnyk & Fineout-Overholt, 2005).

Outcome measurements can be made indicating an individual's clinical state, such as his severity of illness, course of illness, and the effect of interventions on his clinical state. Outcome measures involving a patient's functional status evaluate his ability to perform activities of daily living (ADLs). These can include outcome measures of physical health in terms of function, cost of care, health care access, and general health perceptions. The outcome measures can distinguish the concepts of physical and mental health and identify the five outcome indicator categories of clinical status, functioning, physical symptoms, emotional status, and patient/family evaluation and perceptions about quality of life. Selected quality-of-life outcome measures include quality-adjusted life years (QALY), quality-adjusted life expectancy (QALE), and quality-adjusted healthy life years (QUALY) (Drummond, Stoddart, & Torrance, 1994).

The Medical Outcomes Study (MOS) "Short Form 36" Health Survey is one of the many health indices that have been developed since 1950. The SF-36, as it is commonly known (Ware & Sherbourne, 1992), measures physical functioning, role limitations due to physical health, bodily pain, social functioning, general mental health, role limitations due to emotional problems, vitality, and general health perceptions.

Other health status measurement surveys in use today include the Quality of Life Index (Spitzer, 1998), developed to measure the general health and well-being of terminally ill individuals; the COOP Charts for primary care practice patients; the functional status questionnaire (Jette & Cleary, 1987), a self-administered general health and social well-being survey for ambulatory patients; the Duke Health Profile (Parkerson, Broadhead, & Tse, 1990), which evaluates health status in primary care patients; the Sickness Impact Profile (Bergner, Bobbit, Carter, & Gilson, 1981), which was developed to measure changes in an individual's behavior as a result of illness; and the Nottingham Health Profile (Hunt, McKenna, McEwen, Williams, & Papp, 1981), developed as a measure of perceived general health status for primary care patients and general population health surveys.

Public Reporting of Health Care Outcomes

Transparency of health care outcome performance through public reporting based on national standards and methods is integral to reforming health care to improve patient outcomes, cost efficiency, and access to health care, particularly for vulnerable populations. Public reporting of health care outcomes encourages consumers to make informed choices about the quality and cost of health services. Likewise, health care practitioners, who are often reimbursed for the volume of patients that they see rather than the quality of care that they provide, may be motivated and rewarded to improve quality. Public reporting can be used to determine where inefficient and ineffective care exists. It can also influence reimbursement policies in which payment is linked to the ability to achieve standards and benchmarks, for example, payment for quality performance (Dudley & Rosenthal, 2006). **Balanced scorecards** are used to monitor and report customer perspectives; financial perspectives; internal processes and human resources; and learning and growth (Kaplan & Norton, 2004) for strategic management and as a way to examine performance throughout the organization. A review of balanced scorecards allows the organization to review multiple key areas of performance, selected on the basis of their importance to the organization's strategic plan for quality.

Other National Public Quality Reports

Several key national public quality reports and items of interest for health care and nursing leaders and managers for purposes of performance measurement and benchmarking or comparison are as follows:

- *AHRQ National Healthcare Quality Report (2010):* Available at http://www.ahrq.gov/qual/nhqr10/nhqr10.pdf
- *AHRQ National Healthcare Disparities Report (2010):* Available at http://www.ahrq.gov/qual/nhdr10/nhdr10.pdf

- *Healthy People 2020:* Accessible at http://www.healthypeople.gov
- *Health Grades for Hospital and Physicians:* Available at http://www.healthgrades.com
- *Leapfrog*: Available at http://www.leapfroggroup.org
- Agency for Healthcare Research and Quality's Key Quality Initiatives, https://www.talkingquality.ahrq.gov/content/resources/keyinitiatives.aspx
- Agency for Healthcare Research and Quality's (AHRQ's) Patient Safety and Quality Indicators, http://www.qualityindicators.ahrq.gov/
- Aligning Forces for Quality (AF4Q), http://forces4quality.org/
- Ambulatory Care Quality (AQA) Alliance, http://www.aqaalliance.org/
- The Hospital Quality Alliance, https://www.cahps.ahrq.gov/Surveys-Guidance/Hospital/About-Hospital-Survey/Development-Hospital-Survey/The-Hospital-Quality-Alliance.aspx
- *Crossing the Quality Chasm: The IOM Health Care Quality Initiative*: http://www.iom.edu/Global/News%20Announcements/Crossing-the-Quality-Chasm-The-IOM-Health-Care-Quality-Initiative.aspx

Public reporting of quality performance has been shown to influence declines in cardiac surgery mortality (Peterson, DeLong, Jollis, Muhlbaier, & Mark, 1998); improvements in the processes of obstetrics care (Bost, 2001); and employee enrollment and desire to switch health care providers (Beaulieu, 2002). While providers and policymakers do seek out these public quality reports, the general public typically does not search them out, does not understand them, distrusts them, and fails to make use of them (Marshall, Hiscock, & Sibbald, 2002).

In many respects, hospitals are providing quality care. Data to assess clinical performance from the Joint Commission (JC), formerly known as the Joint Commission on Accreditation of Healthcare Organizations, core measures program, which uses standardized, evidence-based measures, and data from the Medicare program show improvements in the quality of care in hospitals (Williams et al., 2005; Jencks, Huff, & Cuerdon, 2003). Yet, at hospitals that do not meet the sample-size requirement for national comparisons, quality performance remains mediocre (Jha, Li, Orav, & Epstein, 2005).

Disease Management

According to the Disease Management Association of America (DMAA) (2010), disease management is a system of coordinated health care interventions and communications for patient populations with chronic conditions in which the need for patient self-care is significant. What makes caring for patients with chronic disease problematic is that the patients usually have multiple chronic conditions, for example, the patient with congestive heart failure who also has hypertension, diabetes, emphysema, urinary incontinence, and chronic pain. Chronic diseases, such as heart disease, stroke, cancer, chronic respiratory disease, stroke, cancer, and diabetes, are by far the leading cause of mortality in the world, representing 60 percent of all deaths (World Health Organization, 2010). Because of this, management of a single disease will not be successful, given the likelihood of the presence of other diseases or co morbidities. The efforts of many disease management programs have been successful in improving patient outcomes and providing high quality, cost effective care (DePalma, 2006). In a recent study evaluating the impact of both pay for performance programs and public reporting programs in hospitals, the results found that both these programs led to great improvements in all measures of quality (Lindenauer, et al., 2007).

Accreditation and Patient Safety

Health care accreditation is a mechanism used to ensure that organizations meet certain national standards. Hospitals and other organizations seek accreditation to demonstrate their abilities to meet national quality standards. In the United States, numerous groups provide accreditation for various health care organizations, including the Community Health Accreditation Program (CHAP), the Joint Commission (JC), Healthcare Facilities Accreditation Program (HFAP), Accreditation Commission for Health Care (ACHC), the Healthcare Quality Association on Accreditation (HQAA), and many others.

Let's look at two of these nationally recognized accrediting organizations: The Joint Commission (JC) and the Healthcare Facilities Accreditation Program (HFAP). Each organization's review processes are extensive, and payments to a hospital by government insurers of health care (Centers for Medicare & Medicaid Services) are dependent on the hospital's ability to meet the standards of JC or HFAP with a high degree of compliance.

The Joint Commission is a not-for-profit organization which accredits and certifies more than 19,000 health care organizations and programs in the United States (The Joint Commission, 2012). One of the greatest forces for quality improvement efforts in hospitals is the Joint Commission's patient safety requirements, in large part due to hospital's fears of possibly losing accreditation if the JC standards are not achieved and sustained. ORYX® is the Joint Commission's performance measurement and improvement initiative, first implemented in 1997. Hospitals are required to collect and transmit data to the Joint Commission for a minimum of four core measure sets or a combination of applicable core measure sets and non-core measures. See http://www.jointcommission.org/core_measure_set/.

Because of health care errors that became apparent through JC and other national reporting mechanisms, National Patient Safety Goals (NPSG) were established by the JC in 2003. The 2012 National Patient Safety Goals for Hospitals, Ambulatory Health Care, Behavioral Health Care, Critical Access Hospitals, Disease-Specific Care, Home Care, Laboratories, Long-Term Care, Office-Based Surgery, and other are available at http://www.jointcommission.org/standards_information/npsgs.aspx.

Magnet Program

The Magnet Recognition Program of the American Nurses Credentialing Center is a tool for establishing an environment that recognizes excellence in nursing services in a health care system (Magnet Recognition Program [MRP], 2005). Research continues to demonstrate positive implications of the MRP, relating magnet characteristics to nurse job satisfaction and retention, prevention of job burnout, and improvement in perceived quality of care (Aiken, Havens, & Sloane, 2000; Friese, 2005; Lake & Friese, 2006).

IMPROVING QUALITY THROUGH HEALTH PROFESSIONS EDUCATION

To begin to realize the quality agenda set forth by the IOM (IOM, 2001), a subsequent report, *Health Professions Education: A Bridge to Quality* (IOM, 2003), delineates a needed "overhaul" of the curriculum of health professionals education to transform current skills and knowledge (IOM, 2003, p. 1). The five IOM Core Competencies Needed for Health Care Professionals are identified as:

1. *Ability to provide patient-centered care*
2. *Ability to effectively work in interdisciplinary teams*
3. *Ability to understand evidence-based practices*
4. *Ability to measure the quality of care*
5. *Ability to use health information*

The IOM's Report *Keeping Patients Safe*, emphasizes the connections among nursing, patient safety, and quality of care. It sets forth the work structures and work processes that health care workers use in the delivery of care and emphasizes the need to design the nurses' environment to promote the practice of safe nursing (IOM, 2003). The importance of organizational management practices, strong nursing leadership, and adequate nursing staffing for providing a safe care environment is critical (Laschinger & Leiter, 2006).

In 2008, the American Association of Colleges of Nursing (AACN) and the National League for Nursing (NLN) embraced the inclusion of quality improvement, systems thinking, change strategies, and patient safety into undergraduate and graduate nursing education curricula.

Quality and Safety Education for Nurses (QSEN)

In 2005, the Robert Wood Johnson Foundation funded the University of North Carolina at Chapel Hill School of Nursing for a long-term project aimed at increasing the inclusion of quality and safety in nursing education and the development of well-prepared faculty to teach the quality and safety competencies recommended by the Institute of Medicine (IOM)

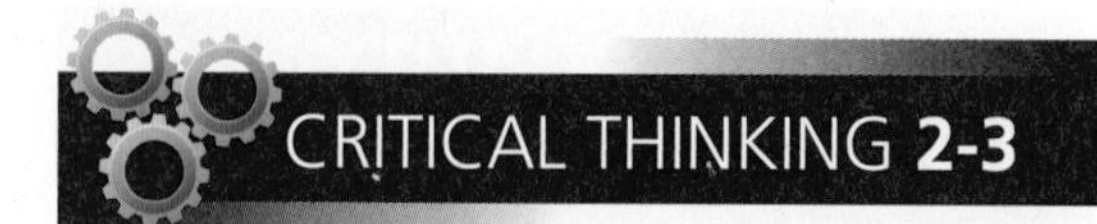

CRITICAL THINKING 2-3

Go to the website http://qsen.org/. Click on Quality/Safety competencies. Select one of the competencies, i.e., Patient-Centered Care, Teamwork & Collaboration, Evidence-Based Practice, Quality Improvement, Safety, or Informatics. Note the definition of the competency, and then click on the pre-licensure knowledge, skills and attitudes (KSAs) for the competency. What did you find there? How can use use this information to improve patient care?

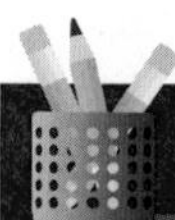

CASE STUDY 2-1

Review the ratings of hospitals in your area of the country at these sites:

www.healthgrades.com

www.solucient.com

www.100tophospitals.com

www.leapfroggroup.org

www.consumerreports.org/health/doctors-hospitals/hospital-ratings.htm

http://health.usnews.com/best-hospitals

www.hospitalcompare.hhs.gov

What kinds of ratings are given to hospitals in your area?

Review the criteria and evaluation system used to rate the hospitals at each site. Are they valid and reliable?

Will you choose a hospital for your own family's care using a rating system like this?

to make health care safe, effective, patient centered, timely, efficient, and equitable (IOM, 2001). This project, the Quality and Safety Education for Nurses (QSEN) project, was supported by AACN in 2009 (Kovner et al., 2010). The QSEN website, http://www.qsen.org/, is now a comprehensive resource for teaching strategies, etc., for the development of quality and safety knowledge, skill, and attitiude related to competency in Patient-Centered Care, Teamwork & Collaboration, Evidence-Based Practice, Quality Improvement, Safety, and Informatics in nursing. Faculty from 15 nursing education programs participated in the QSEN Learning Collaborative in Phase II.

CHALLENGES AND OPPORTUNITIES FOR NURSES

Eight principles are integral to health care reform as envisioned by the Institute of Medicine (IOM. (2008). These eight principles are accountability, efficiency, objectivity, scientific rigor, consistency, feasibility, responsiveness, and transparency. These principles are consistent with a professional nursing agenda, which states that all persons are entitled to affordable, quality health care services (American Nurses Association [ANA], 2008).

Individual nurses can help achieve this agenda and influence a renewed health care system by doing the following:

- Keep abreast of current issues affecting patients and their access to affordable, quality health care. Newspaper, television, radio, and Internet sources publicize numerous items related to health care.
- Dispel the myths and opinions that often shape the misguided beliefs about health care, its consumers, and the direction the system needs to take. Decipher what is reliable and valid information from what is biased, shocking, or fear-filled. Clarify such matters with colleagues, family, and friends who may be less informed.
- Pay attention to the quality measures employed at your workplace. Speak up about what is working well, where safety is risked, or where waste is occurring.
- Heighten awareness of the health care issues you encounter in your practice related to the health care crisis. Craft letters to newspapers or legislators and write opinion editorials or blogs to convey why health care reform is needed.

- Get involved professionally. Become a member of your state nursing association and determine what is being done at the state and national level to address health care reform.
- Health care and health care reform are political issues. Be informed about the political process, with all of its stakeholders and vested interests. Identify what your elected representatives are doing at the state and national level to address concerns about the health care system. Are their efforts sustainable and moving toward a high quality health plan, or do they add to the patchwork approach that currently characterizes the health care system?
- Talk about nursing and the work you do as a health care provider. Be vocal about the expertise nurses have as affordable, caring, and competent clinicians and as agents for health care renewal.
- Support colleagues and promote their talent. Prompt others who show interest and aptitude to pursue nursing as a career. Encourage colleagues to consider advanced nursing roles, whether as clinicians, educators, administrators, researchers, or perhaps even as potential legislators.
- Volunteer in the ways you can to assist the leaders in health care whom you trust and respect.

This list is but a beginning of the many opportunities in which all nurses can be involved. Change in the health care system is ongoing and inevitable, but with more nurses actively engaged, the process is far more likely to meet the goal of providing quality health care for all.

KEY CONCEPTS

- Historically and currently, there are many influences on health care in the United States.
- Health care reports provide invaluable information that emphasizes the successes and failures of health care throughout our nation.
- Evidence of significant disparities and low quality continues to demonstrate the need for significant health care improvement.
- Health care systems have three simple components: structure, process, and outcome.
- The United States is one of only a few large countries in the world without a universal system of health care.
- In the United States, the emphasis on acute care health care services has successfully driven health care costs higher, but has not necessarily improved the quality of care or patient outcomes.
- Many high income industrialized countries' health care systems, e.g., France, Canada, and Japan, deliver health care to all their citizens efficiently.
- There are many factors that contribute to rising health care costs in the United States.
- There are many potential benefits of improving safety, quality, and access to health care in the United States.
- Primary care provides integrated, accessible health care services by clinicians who are accountable for addressing a large majority of personal health care needs, developing a sustained partnership with patients, and practicing in the context of family and community.
- The federal government is a major driver of health care organization and delivery in the United States.
- Inequalities in income, insurance coverage, gender, race or ethnicity, and geography affect a person's ability to have access to health care in the United States.
- Many factors contribute to the rising costs of health care. The key factors include the aging of the population with growth in the demand for health care, increased utilization of pharmaceuticals, expensive new technologies, rising hospital care costs, practitioner behavior, cost shifting, and administrative costs.

- The health care report *Crossing the Quality Chasm* (IOM, 2001) and several large studies (McGlynn et al., 2003; Thomas et al., 2000) have shown that the quality of health care in the United States is at an unexpected low level given the amount of money the United States spends on health care and that it needs improvement in many dimensions.
- Health care performance and quality are measured to determine resource allocation, organize care delivery, assess clinician competency, and improve health care delivery processes and outcomes.
- Several key reports of interest for health care and nursing leaders and managers for purposes of performance measurement and benchmarking are available.
- Evidence-based practice involves supplementing clinical expertise with the judicious and conscientious implementation of the most current and best evidence along with patient values and preferences to guide health care decision making.
- Health care accreditation is a mechanism used to identify if organizations meet certain national standards.
- On March 23, 2010, the Patient Protection and Affordable Care Act (PPACA) was signed into law by President Obama. The PPACA (along with the Health Care and Education Reconciliation Act [HCERA] of 2010) was the principal health care reform legislation of the 111th United States Congress.
- In 2009, the American Association of Colleges of Nursing lent its support to the Quality and Safety Education for Nurses (QSEN) project.
- The Magnet Recognition Program of the American Nurses Credentialing Center is a tool for establishing an environment that recognizes excellence in nursing services in a health care system.
- There is a need to focus on retooling the health care workforce with new knowledge and requisite skills to function in better, redesigned health care systems.
- The quality and safety education for nurses (QSEN) project is moving to improve health care quality through improvements in nursing education related to teamwork and collaboration, informatics, patient-centered care, evidence-based practice, quality improvement, and safety.
- There are many challenges and opportunities for nurses in the future.

KEY TERMS

balanced scorecards
co-payments
cost shifting
deductibles
gross domestic product (GDP)
health care disparities
outcome
pre-authorization
process
structure
universal health care (UHC)

REVIEW QUESTIONS

1. The nurse arrives for the day shift; her patient is upset to learn he will be receiving a bill for services received at the hospital. He states that in his native country he would be receiving the best health care in the world and occur no additional cost. The nurse realizes that the patient is referring to which country?
   A. Canada
   B. France
   C. Japan
   D. Africa

2. The nurse understands that this type of program can be used as a tool for establishing an environment that recognizes excellence in nursing services in a health care system.
   A. The Malcolm Baldridge Program
   B. The Quality of Life Index Program
   C. The Magnet Recognition Program
   D. The Joint Commission's Patient Safety Program

3. Sandy is a nurse volunteering at a food pantry. She realizes that people who lack health insurance or are underinsured are more likely to do which of the following?
   A. Seek health care as soon as illness symptoms occur
   B. Postpone health care, resulting in higher morbidity, mortality, and cost
   C. Buy organic produce to improve health through nutrition
   D. Travel to other countries where health care is provided by the government

4. The nurse is working the night shift on a medical/surgical floor. Before he begins his shift, he washes his hands thoroughly. Who is the nurse that has been credited for discovering the link between adverse patient outcomes and lack of cleanliness and handwashing?
   A. Walt Whitman
   B. Clara Barton
   C. Patricia Benner
   D. Florence Nightingale

5. The nurse understands that health care systems have three components. Which health care component includes the work of hospital admissions, surgical operations, and nursing care delivery following standards and guidelines to achieve quality outcomes?
   A. Structure
   B. Process
   C. Outcome
   D. Discharge

6. While studying health care, the nurse discovers that this is the top underlying cause of health care disparity in the United States.
   A. Socioeconomic status
   B. Age
   C. Geographic location
   D. Chronic illness

7. Which of the following organizations is a full service professional organization representing the nation's entire registered nurse population?
   A. American Association of Colleges of Nursing (AACN)
   B. National League for Nursing (NLN)
   C. American Nurses Association (ANA)
   D. Quality and Safety Education for Nurses (QSEN)

8. Nursing practice that is guided by supplementing clinical expertise with judicious implementation of the current evidence along with patient values and preferences is called which of the following?
   A. Patient-centered practice
   B. Evidence-based practice
   C. Medical model practice
   D. Clinical guideline practice

9. Because the United States does not have universal health care, community health nurses design these types of programs to help fill in the gap.

A. Public Health Care Programs
B. Cost Shifting Programs
C. Prospective Payment Programs
D. Capitation Programs

10. Mrs. Brown has Type 2 diabetes, primary hypertension, and congestive heart failure. The nurse is coordinating health care interventions and communication strategies to help Mrs. Brown cope and manage her chronic diseases. The nurse is using what health care strategy?

A. Disease Management
B. Primary Care Management
C. Health Insurance Portability and Accountability Act Management
D. Hill-Burton Act Management

11. Key factors contributing to rising health care costs in the United States include which of the following? Select all that apply.

A. An aging population
B. Advancements in technology
C. Increased utilization of pharmaceuticals
D. Rising costs of hospitals
E. Increasing administrative costs
F. Diminishing value of the dollar

12. The Patient Protection and Affordable Care Act provides comprehensive health care reform through a number of initiatives including which of the following? Select all that apply.

A. Expanding health insurance coverage
B. Decreasing insurance coverage of pre existing conditions
C. Targeting fraud, abuse, and waste in health care
D. Decreasing access to primary care services
E. Promoting prevention health strategies
F. Increasing costs for those more able to pay

REVIEW ACTIVITIES

1. Although it is difficult to modify the structure of health care, what could you do to implement a system to continually modify the process of health care delivery to improve health care quality in your organization?
2. What are strategies to ensure patient access to appropriate health care services in public and private health care agencies?
3. How can the five IOM health professions competencies for quality care be achieved in the current workplace?

EXPLORING THE WEB

- Alliance for Health Reform: *http://www.allhealth.org*
- Centers for Medicare & Medicaid Services (CMS): *http://www.cms.gov*
- Department of Defense (DOD) TRICARE program: *http://www.tricare.mil*
- Health Resources and Services Administration (HRSA): *http://www.hrsa.gov*
- National Center for Health Statistics (NCHS): *http://www.cdc.gov* Search for National Center for Health Statistics.

- National Institutes of Health (NIH): *http://www.nih.gov*
- Substance Abuse and Mental Health Services Administration (SAMHSA): *http://www.samhsa.gov*
- Veterans Health Administration (VHA): *http://www.va.gov*
- Joint Commission (JC): *http://www.jointcommission.org*
- National Committee for Quality Assurance (NCQA): *http://www.ncqa.org*
- National Quality Forum (NQF): *http://www.qualityforum.org*
- Malcolm Baldridge Quality Award (MBQA): *http://www.quality.nist.gov*
- Press Ganey Patient Satisfaction Surveys: *http://www.pressganey.com*
- Quality and Safety Education for Nurses (QSEN): *http://www.qsen.org*
- Healthcare Facilities Accreditation Program (HFAP): *http://www.hfap.org*
- Community Health Accreditation Program (CHAP): *http://www.chapinc.org*
- Accreditation Commission for Health Care (ACHC): *http://www.achc.org*
- Healthcare Quality Association on Accreditation (HQAA): *http://www.hqaa.org*
- DNV Healthcare: *http://www.dnvaccreditation.com*
- Accreditation Association for Ambulatory Health Care (AAAHC): *http://www.aaahc.org*

REFERENCES

Adams, D. R., Fraser, D. B., & Abrams, H. L. (1973). The complications of coronary arteriography. *Circulation, 48*(3), 609–618.

Agency for Healthcare Research and Quality (AHRQ). (2007a). *National Healthcare Quality & Disparities Report.* Rockville, MD: Author.

Agency for Healthcare Research and Quality (AHRQ). (2007b). *Transforming hospitals: Designing for safety and quality.* Rockville, MD: Author. Retrieved from www.ahrq.gov/qual/ transform.pdf

Agency for Healthcare Research and Quality (AHRQ). (2008). The Patient Safety and Quality Improvement Act of 2005. Overview, June 2008. Rockville, MD. Retrieved from http://www.ahrq.gov/qual/psoact.htm. accessed October 28, 2012.

Agency for Healthcare Research and Quality (AHRQ). (2008a). *National Healthcare Disparities Report.* Rockville, MD: Author. Retrieved from www.ahrq.gov/qual/qrdr07.htm

Agency for Healthcare Research and Quality (AHRQ). (2008b). *National Healthcare Quality Report.* Rockville, MD: Author. Retrieved from www.ahrq.gov/qual/qrdr07.htm#toc

Agency for Healthcare Research and Quality (AHRQ). (2009). National Healthcare Quality Report, 2008. Rockville, MD: Author. Retrieved from http://www.ahrq.gov/qual/nhqr08/nhqr08.pdf

Aiken, L. H., Havens, D. S., & Sloane, D. M. (2000). The magnet nursing services recognition program. *American Journal of Nursing, 100*(3), 26–36.

Alberta Health and Wellness. (2004). Health care insurance plan. Edmonton, Alberta: Author. Retrieved from www.health.alberta.ca

American Nurses Association (ANA). (2008). Health system reform agenda. Retrieved from www.nursingworld.org/MainMe-nuCategories/HealthcareandPolicyIssues/HSR/ANAsHealthSystemReformAgenda.aspx

Anderson, G. R., Hussey, P. S., Frogner, B. K., & Waters, H. R. (2005). Health spending in the United States and the rest of the industrialized world. *Health Affairs, 24*(4), 903–914.

Balas, E. A., & Boren, S. A. (2000). *Managing clinical knowledge for healthcare improvements* (pp. 65–70). Germany: Schattauer Publishing Company.

Baldridge Health Care Criteria Program, (2011–2012); Retrieved from http://www.nist.gov/baldrige/publications/hc_criteria.cfm

Barrett, P. M. (2012, June 28). Supreme Court supports Obamacare, bolsters Obama. *Bloomberg Business week.* Retrieved June 30, 2012.

Bazzoli, G. J., Gerland, A., & May, J. (2006). Construction activity in U.S. hospitals. *Health Affairs, 25*(3), 783–791.

Beaulieu, N. D. (2002). Quality information and consumer health plan choices. *Journal of Health Economics, 21*(1), 43–63.

Bergner, M., Bobbit, R. A., Carter, W. B., & Gilson, B. S. (1981). The sickness impact profile: Development and final revision of a health status measure. *Medical Care, 19*(8), 787–805.

Bernstein, A. B., Hing, E., Moss, A. J., Allen, K. F., Siller, A. B., & Tiggle, R. B. (2003). Health care in America, trends in utilization. U.S. Department of Health and Human Services. Centers for disease control and prevention. National center for health statistics. Hyattsville, MD. Retrieved from www.cdc.gov/nchs/data/misc/healthcare.pdf

Berwick, D. M. (2002). A user's manual for the IOM's "Quality Chasm" report. *Health Affairs, 21*(3), 80–90.

Boddenheimer, T. (2005a). High and rising health care costs. Part 1: Seeking an explanation. *Annals of Internal Medicine, 142*(10), 847–854.

Boddenheimer, T. (2005b). High and rising health care costs. Part 2: Technologic innovation. *Annals of Internal Medicine, 142*(11), 932–937.

Borger, C, Smith, S., Truffer, C, Keehan, S., Sisko, A., Poisal, J., et al. (2006). Health spending projections through 2015: Changes on the horizon. *Health Affairs, 25*(2), 61–73.

Bost JE. (2001). Managed care organizations publicly reporting three years of HEDIS measures. Managed care interface. September;*14*(9):50-4.

Calvocoressi, L., Kasl, S. V., Lee, C. H., Stolar, M., Claus, E. B., & Jones, B. A. (2004). A prospective study of perceived susceptibility to breast cancer and nonadherence to mammography screening guidelines in African American and white women ages 40 to 79 years. *Cancer Epidemiology Biomarkers Preview, 13*(12), 2096–2105.

Camiah, S. (1997). Utilization of nursing research in practice and application strategies to raise awareness amongst nurse practitioners: A model for success. *Journal of Advanced Nursing*, 26, 1193–1202.

Canadian Institute for Health Information (2006). CIHI looks at how Canada measures up in health spending. Ottawa, Ontario: Author. Retrieved from www.cihi.ca/cihiweb/en/downloads/Dir_Wint06_ENG.pdf

Catlin, A., Cowan, C, Hartman, M., Heffler, S., & National Health Expenditure Accounts Team. (2008). National health spending in 2006: A year of change for prescription drugs. *Health Affairs, 27*(1), 14–29.

Center for Health Design. (2005). Scorecards for evidence based design. Retrievedcomp: from www.healthdesign.org/research/reports/documents/scorecard_12_05.pdf

Centers for Disease Control and Prevention (CDC). (2005). Leading causes of death. Atlanta, GA: Author. Retrieved from www.cdc.gov/nchs/FASTATS/lcod.htm

Centers for Medicare & Medicaid Services (CMS). (2006). Historical national health expenditure data. Retrieved from www.cms.hhs.gov/NationalHealthExpendData/02_NationalHealthAccountsHistorical.asp#TopOfPage

Centers for Medicare & Medicaid Services (CMS). (2010). National health expenditures projections 2009–2019. Retrieved from http://www.cms.gov/NationalHealthExpendData/downloads/pdfj2009.pdf

Centers for Medicare & Medicaid Services, Office of the Actuary National Health Statistics Group. (2009). Retrieved from https://www.cms.gov/NationalHealthExpendData/downloads/PieChartSourcesExpenditures2009.pdf November 14, 2011.

Central Intelligence Agency (2012). The World Factbook. Retrieved from https://www.cia.gov/library/publications/the-world-factbook/geos/us.html, accessed October 28, 2012.

Coddington, J. A., & Sands, L. P. (2008). Cost of health care and quality outcomes of patients at nurse-managed clinics. *Nursing Economics, 26*(2), 75–83.

Commonwealth Fund. (2007). Mirror, Mirror on the Wall: An International Update on the Comparative Performance of American Health Care. Retrieved from http://www.commonwealthfund.org/Publications/Fund-Reports/2007/May/Mirror--Mirror-on-the-Wall--An-International-Update-on-the-Comparative-Performance-of-American-Healt.aspx, accessed October 28, 2012.

Commonwealth Fund. (2008a). Why not the best? Results from the national scorecard on U.S. health system performance, 2008. The Commonwealth Fund Commission on a High Performance Health System. Retrieved from www.commonwealthfund.org/publications/

Commonwealth Fund. (2008b). Retrieved from http://www.commonwealthfund.org/News/News-Releases/2008/Nov/New-International-Survey--More-Than-Half-of-U-S-Chronically-Ill-Adults-Skip-Needed-Care-Due-to-Cost.aspx

Commonwealth Fund. (2008c). Schoen, C., Osborn, R., How, S., Doty, M., & Peugh, J. (2008). In chronic condition experiences of patients with complex healthcare needs in eight countries. Health affairs web exclusive, November 13, 2008.

Craig, D.J., Ullian, J. & Fitzgerald, B. (2005). Convocation speakers share life lessons learned firsthand. B.U. Bridge. June 3, 2005· Vol. VIII, No. 31. Retrieved from http://www.bu.edu/bridge/archive/2005/06-03/convocation.html,accessed October 28, 2012.

Cunningham, P.W. (2012). Supreme Court upholds Obama's health care overhaul . The Washington Times. June 28, 2012. Retrieved from http://www.washingtontimes.com/news/2012/jun/28/supreme-court-upholds-rules-obamas-health-care-ove/?page=all

Dalen, J. E., & Alpert, J. S. (2008). National health insurance: Could it work in the U.S.? American Journal of Medicine, 121(7), 553–554.

Davis, K. (2005). Ten points for transforming the U.S. health care system. Retrieved from www.cmwf.org/aboutus/aboutus_show.htm?doc_id=259233

Davis, K., Schoen, C., Schoenbaum, S. C., Doty, M. M., Holmgren, A. L., Kriss, J. L., & Shea, K. K. (2007). *Mirror, mirror on the wall: An international update on the comparative performance of American health care.* New York, NY: The Commonwealth Fund.

Demaro, R. A. (2008). Posted in bill Moyers journal. Retrieved from www.pbs.org/moyers/journal/05092008/PROFILE.

DePalma, J. (2006). Disease management: Evidence support. *Home Health Care Management and Practice, 18*(3), 223–234.

Department of Health & Human Services. Administration on Aging. (2011). Aging Statistics. Retrieved from http://www.aoa.gov/aoaroot/aging_statistics/index.aspx, accessed October 28, 2012.

Devers, K. J., Pham, H. H., & Liu, G. (2004). What is driving hospitals' patient-safety efforts? *Health Affairs, 23*(2), 103–115.

Disease Management Association of America (DMAA). (2010). Population health. Retrieved from http://www.dmaa.org/dm_definition.asp

Donabedian, A. (2005). Evaluating the quality of medical care. *Milbank Quarterly, 20*(1) 137–141.

Dossey, B., Selanders, L., & Beck, D. (2005). *Florence Nightingale today: Healing, leadership, global action.* Washington, DC: American Nurses Publishing.

Drummond, M. F., Stoddart, F. L., & Torrance, G. W. (1994). *Methods for the economic evaluation of health care programmes.* Oxford, England: Oxford University Press.

Dudley, R. A., & Rosenthal, M. B. (2006). *Pay for performance: A decision guide for purchasers* (AHRQ Pub. No. 06-0047). Rockville, MD: Agency for Healthcare Research and Quality.

Dunefsky, F. (2008). Quality health care. In R. Kearney-Nunnery (Ed.), *Advancing Your Career* (4th ed.). Philadelphia, PA: Davis.

Dunn, W. R., Lyman, S., & Marx, R. G. (2005). Small area variation in orthopedics. *Journal of Knee Surgery, 18*(1), 51–56.

Education Trust & Health Research and Kaiser Family Foundation (KFF). (2006). Kaiser Family Foundation (KFF). (2008a). Health Coverage for the Uninsured. Retrieved from www.statehealthfacts.org/comparecat.jsp?cat=3

Education Trust & Health Research and Kaiser Family Foundation (KFF). (2006). Employer health benefits: 2006 annual survey. Publication number 7527. Retrieved October, 2006, from www.kff.org.

Eisenberg, M. J. (2006). An American physician in the Canadian health care system. *Archives of Internal Medicine, 166,* 281–282.

Elmendorf, D. W. (2011a, March 30). CBO's Analysis of the Major Health Care Legislation Enacted in March 2010 (pdf). Washington, DC: Congressional Budget Office. Retrieved July 15, 2012.

Elmendorf, D. W. (2011b, June). CBO's 2011 Long-Term Budget Outlook (pdf). Washington, DC: Congressional Budget Office. Retrieved from http://www.cbo.gov/sites/default/files/cbofiles/attachments/06-21-Long-Term_Budget_Outlook.pdf, accessed October 28, 2012.

Epstein, A. M. (1995). Performance reports on quality—prototypes, problems, and prospects. *New England Journal of Medicine, 333,* 57–61.

Fisher, E. S., Goodman, D. C, & Chandra, A. (2008). *Disparities in health and health care among Medicare beneficiaries: A brief report of the Dartmouth Atlas Project.* Dartmouth Institute for Health Policy and Clinical Practice/Robert Wood Johnson Foundation. Retrieved from www.dartmouthatlas.org/af4q/AF4Q_Disparities_ Report.pdf

Friese, C. R. (2005). Nurse practice environments and outcomes: Implications for oncology nursing. *Oncology Nursing Forum, 32*(4), 765–772.

Gaynes, R., Richards, C., Edwards, J., Emori, T., Horan, T., Alonso-Eschanove, J., et al. (2001, March–April). Feeding back surveillance data to prevent hospital acquired infections. *Emerging Infectious Diseases, 7*(2), 295–298.

Green, L. A., Gryer, G. E., Yawn, B. P., Lanier, D., & Dovery, S. M. (2000). The ecology of medical care revisited. *New England Journal of Medicine, 344,* 2021–2025.

Greenfield, S., Nelson, E. C., Zubkoff, M., Manning, W., Rogers, W., Kravitz, R. L., et al. (1992). Variations in resource utilization among medical specialties and systems of care. Results from the medical outcomes study. *Journal of the American Medical Association, 267*(12), 1624–1630.

Hamilton, D. K. (2003). The four levels of evidence based practice. *Healthcare Design, 3,* 18–26.

Health System Change. (2006). Tracking health care costs: Spending growth remains stable at high rate in 2005. *Data Bulletin, 33.* Retrieved from www.hschange.org

Health Workforce Solutions LLC, & Robert Wood Johnson Foundation. (2008). Innovative care models. Retrieved from www.innovativecaremodels.com/about/about

Hearst, Steven R. (June 28, 2012). "Supreme Court Upholds. Cunningham, P.W. (2012). Supreme Court upholds Obama's health care overhaul. The Washington Times. June 28, 2012. Retrieved from http://www.washingtontimes.com/news/2012/jun/28/supreme-court-upholds-rules-obamas-health-care-ove/?page=all

The Henry J. Kaiser Family Foundation (2012). Summary of Coverage Provisions in the Affordable Care Act. Retrieved from http://www.kff.org/healthreform/upload/8023-R.pdf, accessed October 28, 2012.

Himmelstein, D. U., Warren, E., Thorne, D., & Woolhandler, S. (2005, February 2). Illness and injury as contributors to bankruptcy. Health Affairs Web Exclusive, pp. W5–63. Retrieved from content.healthaffairs.org/cgi/content/abstract/hlthaff.w5.63v1

Holahan, J., & Cohen, M. (2006). *Understanding the recent changes in Medicaid spending and enrollment growth between 2000–2004.* Issue Paper. Kaiser Commission on Medicaid and the Uninsured. Retrieved from www .kff.org/medicaid/ upload/7499.pdf

Hospital Survey and Construction Act. (1946). *Canadian Medical Association Journal, 55,* 616.

Hunt, K. A., & Knickman, J. R. (2008). Financing health care. In A. R. Kovner & J. R. Knickman (Eds.), *Jonas and Kovner's Health Care Delivery in the United States* (9th ed.). New York, NY: Springer.

Hunt, S. M., McKenna, P., McEwen, J., Williams, J., & Papp, E. (1981). The Nottingham health profile: Subjective health status and medical consultations. *Social Science and Medicine, 15*(3, Pt. 1), 221–229.

Institute of Medicine (IOM). (1996). *Primary care: America's health in a new era.* Washington, DC: National Academy Press.

Institute of Medicine (IOM). (1999). *To err is human: Building a safer healthcare system.* Washington, DC: National Academy Press.

Institute of Medicine (IOM). (2001). *Crossing the quality chasm: A new health system for the 21st century.* Washington, DC: National Academy Press.

Institute of Medicine (IOM). (2003a, November 20). *Patient safety: Achieving a new Standard for Care.* Retrieved from www.iom.edu/?id=35961

Institute of Medicine (IOM). (2003b, November 4). *Keeping patients safe: Transforming the Work Environment of Nurses.* Retrieved from www.iom .edu/?id=35961

Institute of Medicine (IOM). (2003c, April 8). *Health professions Education: A Bridge to Quality.* Retrieved from www.iom.edu/?id=35961

Institute of Medicine (IOM). (2003d, January 7). *Priority areas for National Action: Transforming Health Care Quality.* Retrieved from www.iom. edu/?id=35961

Institute of Medicine (IOM). (2005, December 1). *Performance measurement: Accelerating Improvement.* Retrieved from www.iom.edu/CMS/2955.aspx?show=0;3#LP3

Institute of Medicine (IOM). (2006a, July 20). *Preventing medication Errors: Quality Chasm Series.* Retrieved from www.iom.edu/?id=35961

Institute of Medicine (IOM). (2006b). Rewarding Provider Performance: Aligning Incentives in Medicare. Retrieved from http://www.iom.edu/Reports/2006/Rewarding-Provider-Performance-Aligning-Incentives-in-Medicare .aspx, accessed October 28, 2012.

Jarvis, W. R. (2006). The state of the science of health care epidemiology, infection control, and patient safety. Infection Control Association (Singapore). Retrieved from www.icas.org.sg/images/StateofScience.pdf

Jeffrey, A. E., & Newacheck, P. W. (2006). Role of insurance for children with special health care needs: A synthesis of the evidence. *Pediatrics, 778*(4), 1027–1038.

Jencks, S. R., Huff, E. D., & Cuerdon, O. (2003). Change in the quality of care delivered to Medicare beneficiaries. *Journal of the American Medical Association, 289,* 305–312.

Jette, A. M., & Cleary, P. D. (1987). Functional disability assessment. *Physical Therapy, 67,* 1854–1859.

Jha, A. K., Li, Z., Orav, E. J., & Epstein, A. M. (2005). Care in U.S. hospitals: The hospital quality alliance program. *New England Journal of Medicine, 353*(3), 265–274.

Joines, J. D., Hertz-Picciotto, I., Carey, T. S., Gesler, W., & Suchindran, C. (2003). A spatial analysis of count-level variation in hospitalization rates for low back problems in North Carolina. *Social Science and Medicine, 56*(12), 2541–2553.

The Joint Commission. (2012). Accreditation Standards. Retrieved from http://www.jointcommission.org/, accessed october 28, 2012.

Jolley, S. (2002). Raising research awareness: A strategy for nurses. *Nursing Standard, 16*(33), 33–39.

Jönsson B. (1989). What can Americans learn from Europeans? *Health Care Financing Review.* December; Spec No: 79-93; discussion 93–110.

Kaiser Family Foundation (KFF). (2007). Trends in health care costs and spending. Menlo Park, CA: Kaiser Family Foundation. Retrieved from www.kff.org/insurance/upload/7692.pdf

Kaiser Family Foundation (KFF). (2008a). Health Coverage for the Uninsured. Retrieved from www.statehealthfacts.org/comparecat.jsp?cat=3

Kaiser Family Foundation (KFF). (2008b). Covering the uninsured in 2008: Key facts about current costs, sources of payment, and incremental costs. Menlo Park CA: Author. Retrieved from www.kff.org/uninsured/upload/7810.pdf

Kaiser Family Foundation (KFF).(2010). Focus on health reform. Summary of new health reform law, Patient Protection and Affordable Care Act (P.L. 111-148). Retrieved from http://www.kff.org/healthreform/8061 .cfmMarch 26, 2010.

Kaiser Family Foundation (KFF). (2011). Selected Organisation for Economic Co-operation and Development (OECD) Countries, 2008. Retrieved from Organisation for Economic Co-operation and Development (2010), "OECD Health Data", OECD Health Statistics (database). doi: 10.1787/data-00350-en (Retrieved on 14 February 2011).

Kaplan, R. S., & Norton, D. P., (2004). *Strategy maps.* Boston, MA. Harvard Business School Press.

Keehan, S. (2004). Health spending by age. *Health Affairs, 23*(6), 280–281.

Knickman, J. R., & Kovner, A. R. (2008). Overview: The state of health care delivery in the United States. In A. R. Kovner & J. R. Knickman (Eds.), *Jonas and Kovner's Health Care Delivery in the United States* (9th ed., pp. 3–11). New York, NY: Springer.

Knowing What Works in Health Care: A Roadmap for the Nation. National Academies Press. Retrieved from http://books.google.com/books?id=Y8Z2Qgh7kRAC&pg=PA155&lpg=PA155&dq=iom,+accountability,+transparency,+efficiency,+scientific+rigor&source=bl&ots=wbB7QA_xDk&sig=RankKXl08NG2zQA0NMjGyVwHKTk&hl=en&sa=X&ei=NweQUPCbAYzO0QHMioHoBg&ved=0CEgQ6AEwBg#v=onepage&q=iom%2C%20accountability%2C%20transparency%2C%20efficiency%2C%20scientific%20rigor&f=false, accessed October 28, 2012.

Kovner, C.T., Brewer, C.S., Yingrengreung, S., et al. (2010, January 31). New Nurses' views of quality improvement education. The Joint Commission Journal on Quality and Patient Safety, 36(1), 29–35.

Krugman, P. (2010, January 31 Krugman calls Senate health care bill similar to law in Massachusetts. Retrieved from PolitiFact.com August 29, 2012.

Lake, E. T., & Friese, C. R. (2006). Variations in nursing practice environments: Relation to staffing and hospital characteristics. *Nursing Research, 55*(1), 1–9.

Leape, L. L. (1992). Unnecessary surgery. *Annual Review of Public Health, 13,* 363–383.

Leiter, M. P., & Laschinger, H. K. S. (2006). A work environment to support professional nursing practice: Implications for burnout. *Nursing Research. 55,* 137–146

Lindenauer, P., Roman, S., Rothenberg, M., Benjamin, E., Ma, A., & Bratzler, D. (2007). Public reporting and pay for performance in hospital quality improvement. *The New England Journal of Medicine, 365*(5), 486–496.

Magnet Recognition Program (MRP). (2005).*Force of magnetism statement of evidence* (pp. 32–45). Silver Spring, MD.American Nurses Credentialing Center.

Marshall, M. N., Hiscock, J., & Sibbald, B. (2002). Attitudes to the public release of comparative information on the quality of general practice care: A qualitative study. *British Medical Journal,* 325(7375), 1278.

Martin, J. A., Hamilton, B. E., Sutton, P. D., & Ventura, S. J. (2006). Births: Final data for 2004. *National vital statistics reports (Vol.* 55, No. 1). Hyattsville, MD: National Center for Health Statistics.

Maville, J. A., & Huerta, C. G. (2007). *Health promotion in nursing* (2nd ed.). Clifton Park, NY: Delmar Cengage Learning.

Mayo, T. W. (2007). U.S. health care timelines. Southern Methodist University, Dedman School of Law. Retrieved from faculty.smu.edu/tmayo/health%20care%20timeline.htm

McGlynn, E. A., Asch, S. M., Adams, J., Keesey, J., Hicks, J., DeCristofaro, A., & Kerr, A. (2003). The quality of health care delivered to adults in the United States. *New England Journal of Medicine, 348,* 2635–2645.

Mechanic, R. E. & Dobson, A. (1996). The impact of managed care on clinical research: A preliminary investigation. Health affairs *15*(3); 72–89.

Melnyk, B. M., & Fineout-Overholt, E. (2005). *Evidence-based practice in nursing & healthcare.* Philadelphia, PA: Lippincott William & Wilkins.

Mokdad, A. H., Marks, J. S., Stroup, D. R., & Gerberding, J. L. (2004). Actual causes of death in the United States, 2000. *Journal of American Medical Association, 291*(10), 1238–1245.

Muenning, P., Franks, P., Jia, H., Lubetkin, E., & Gold, M. R. (2005). The income-associated burden of disease in the United States. Social Science Medicine, 61 (9), 2018–2026.

National Coalition on Health Care (NCHC). (2008). Facts on health care costs. Retrieved from www.nchc.org/facts/costs.shtml

National Healthcare Disparities Report (NHDR). (2005). Agency for Healthcare Research and Quality, Rockville, MD. Retrieved from www.ahrq.gov/qual/nhdr05/nhdr05.htm

National Healthcare Quality Report (NHQR). (2005). Agency for Healthcare Research and Quality, Rockville, MD. Retrieved fromwww.ahrq.gov/qual/nhqr05/nhqr05.htm

The National Institute of Standards and Technology (NIST). (2012). The 2011-2012 Health Care Criteria for Performance Excellence. Retrieved from http://www.nist.gov/baldrige/publications/hc_criteria.cfm, accessed October 28, 2012.

National Nosocomial Infections Surveillance (NNIS) System Report. (1998, October). Data summary from October 1986–April 1998, issued June 1998. *American Journal of Infectious Control, 26*(5), 522–533.

Newhouse, R. P., Weiner, J. P., Stanik-Hutt, J., White, K. M., Johantgen, M., Steinwachs, D., Zangaro, G., Aldebron, J., & Bass, E. (2011). Advanced practice nurses as a solution to the workforce crisis; Implications of a systematic review of their effectiveness. Nursing Economics, 29(5), 230–250.

New International Survey: More Than Half of U.S. Chronically Ill Adults Skip Needed Care Due to Costs. Retrieved from http://www.commonwealthfund.org/Search.aspx?search=chronically+ill+skip+care+due+to+cost&filefilter=1

Nightingale, F. (1860). *Notes on nursing.* Princeton, PA: Vertex.

Nightingale, F. (1860). Notes on nursing. What it is, and what it is not. New York, NY: D. Appleton and Company.

Nolte, E., & McKee, C. M. (2008). Measuring the health of nations: Updating an earlier analysis. *Health Affairs, 27*(1), 58–71.

Organisation for Economic Co-operation and Development. (2008). OECD Health Data 2008: How does Japan compare. Paris, France: Author. Retrieved from www.oecd.org/document/46/0,3343,en _2649_33929_34971438_1_1_1_1,00.html

Parkerson, G. R., Jr., Broadhead, W. E., & Tse, C.-K. J. (1990). The Duke health profile: A 17 item measure of health and dysfunction. *Medical Care, 28,* 1056–1072.

Pear, R. (2012, July 7). Health law critics prepare to battle over insurance exchange subsidies. *New York Times.* Retrieved July 7, 2012. Retrieved from http://www .nytimes.com/2012/07/08/us/critics-of-health-care-law-prepare-to-battle-over-insurance-exchange-subsidies .html?_r=0

Peterson, E. D., DeLong, E. R., Jollis, J. G., Muhlbaier, L. H., & Mark, D. B. (1998). The effects of New York's bypass surgery provider profiling on access to care and patient outcomes in the elderly. *Journal of the American College of Cardiology, 32*(4), 993–999.

Reid, T. R. (2008). Japanese pay less for more health care. Washington, DC: National Public Radio. Retrieved from www.npr.org/templates/story/story.php?storyid=89626309.Robertwood Johnsonfoundation

Robert Wood Johnson Foundation. (2008). Cover the uninsured. Retrieved from covertheuninsured.org/

Ross, J. S. (2002). The committee on the costs of medical care and the history of health insurance in the United States. *Einstein Quarterly Journal of Biological Medicine,* 19, 129–134.

Sackett, D. L., Straus, S. E., Richardson, W. S., Rosenberg, W., & Haynes, R. B. (2000). *Evidence-based medicine: How to practice and teach EBM*. London, England: Churchill Livingstone.

Safran, D. G., Rogers, W. H., Tarlov, A. R., McHorney, C. A., & Ware, J. E., Jr. (1997). Gender differences in medical treatment: The case of physician-prescribed activity restrictions. *Social Science Medicine, 45*(5), 711–722.

Schoen, C., Osborn, R., Doty, M.M., Bishop, M., Peugh, J., & Murukutla , N. The Commonwealth Fund. (2007). Toward Higher-Performance Health Systems: Adults' Health Care Experiences in Seven Countries, 2007. November 1, 2007: Volume 92. Retrieved from http://www.commonwealthfund.org/Publications/In-the-Literature/2007/Nov/Toward-Higher-Performance-Health-Systems--Adults-Health-Care-Experiences-in-Seven-Countries--2007.aspx, accessed October 29, 2012.

Shortell, S. M., & Kaluzny, A. D. (2006). *Health Care Management* (5th ed., p. 9). Clifton Park, NY: Delmar Cengage Learning.

Smith, M. A., Atherly, A. J., Kane, R. L., & Pacala, J. T. (1997). Peer review of the quality of care: Reliability and sources of variability for outcome and process assessment. *The Journal of the American Medical Association, 278,*1573–1578.

Spitzer, W. O. (1998). Quality of life. In D. Burley & W. H. W. Inman (Eds.), *Therapeutic risk: Perception, measurement, and management.* New York, NY: Wiley.

Stanton, M. W. (2006). The high concentration of U.S. health care expenditures. *Research in Action, 19,* 1–11. Retrieved from www.ahrq.gov/research/ria2019/expendria.pdf

Starfield, B. (1998). *Primary care: Balancing health needs, services, and technology.* New York, NY: Oxford University Press.

Thomas, E. J., Studdert, D. M., Burstin, H. R., Orav, E. J., Zeena, T., Williams, E. J., et al. (2000). Incidence and types of adverse events and negligent care in Utah and Colorado. *Medical Care, 38,* 261–271.

Thorpe, K., Woodruff, R., & Ginsburg, P. (2005). Factors driving cost increases. Retrieved from www.ahrq.gov/news/ulp/costs/ulpcosts1.htm

Tilson, H., & Berkowitz, B. (2006). The public health enterprise: Examining our twenty-first century policy challenges. *Health Affairs, 25*(4), 900–910.

Ulrich, B., Quan, X., Zimring, C., Joseph, A., & Choudhary, R. (2004). *The role of the physical environment in the hospital of the 21st Century.* Concord, CA: Center for Health Design. Retrieved from www.rwjf.org/files/publications/other/Role of the PhysicalEnvironment.pdf.

U.S. Department of Health and Human Services. (2010a). Healthy People 2020. Retrieved from http://www .healthypeople.gov/2020/default.aspx

U.S. Department of Health and Human Services (USDHHS) (2010b). Administration on Aging. Retrieved from http://www.aoa.gov/

U.S. Department of Health and Human Services (USDHHS) (2010b). Healthy People 2020 Framework. Retrieved from http://healthypeople .gov/2020/Consortium/HP2020Framework.pdf. May 20, 2012.

U.S. scorecard on health system performance. (Source: Commonwealth Fund National Scorecard on U.S. Health System Performance. [2008]. Retrieved from http://www.commonwealthfund.org/Publications/Fund-Reports/2011/Oct/Why-Not-the-Best-2011.aspx

Ware, J. E., & Sherbourne, C. D. (1992). The MOS 36-item shortform health survey I: Conceptual framework and item selection. *Medical Care, 30,* 473–478.

The Week. (2012). ObamaCare survives the Supreme Court: 5 takeaways. June 28, 2012. Retrieved June 30, 2012.Retrieved from http://theweek.com/article/index/229985/obamacare-survives-the-supreme-court-5-takeaways

Wennberg, J. E., & Gittelsohn, A. M. (1973). Small area variations in health care delivery. *Science, 182*(117), 1102–1108.

Werner, R. M., & Bradlow, E. T. (2006). Relationship between Medicare's hospital compare performance measures and mortality rates. *Journal of American Medical Association, 296*(22), 2694–2702.

Williams, L. S., Eckert, G. J., L'italien, G. J., Lapuerta, P., & Weinberger, M. (2003). Regional variation in healthcare utilization and outcomes in ischemic stroke. *Journal of Stroke and Cerebrovascular Disease, 12*(6) 259–265.

Williams, S. C., Schmaltz, S. P., Morton, D. J., Koss, R. G., & Loeb, J. M. (2005). Quality of care in U.S. hospitals as reflected by standard measures, 2003–2004. *New England Journal of Medicine, 353*(3), 255–264.

Woo, A., Ranji, U., Lundy, J., & Chen, F. (2007). Prescription drug costs. Menlo Park, CA: Kaiser Family Foundation. Retrieved from www.kaiseredu.org/topics_im.asp?id=352&aparentID=68 &aimID=1

World Health Organization (WHO). (2000). The world health report 2000—Health systems: Improving performance. Geneva, Switzerland: Author.

World Health Organization (WHO). (2008). The world health report: 2008 primary health care—Now more than ever. Retrieved from http:www.who.int/whr/2008/whr08_en.pdf

World Health Organization (WHO). (2010). Primary health care. Retrieved from http://www.who.int/topics/primary_health_care/en/

SUGGESTED READINGS

Agency for Healthcare Research and Quality(AHRQ). (2009*). National healthcare disparities report, 2008.* Rockville, MD: U.S. Department of Health and Human Services.

American Association of Colleges of Nursing (AACN). (2008). Nursing shortage fact sheet. Washington, DC: Author. Retrieved from www.aacn.nche.edu/Media/pdf/NrsgShortageFS.pdf

American College of Physicians. (2008). Achieving a high-performance health care system with universal access: What the United States can learn from other countries. *Annals of Internal Medicine, 148(*1), 55–75.

American Hospital Association. (2007). *Fast facts on U.S. hospitals.* Retrieved from http://aha.org/aha/resource-center/Statistics-andStudies/fast-facts.html

American Hospital Association. (2009*). American Hospital Association underpayment by Medicare and Medicaid fact sheet.* Retrieved from http://www.americanhealthsolution.org/asssets/Uploads/Blog/09medicunderpayment1.pdf

An, J., Saloner, R., & Ranji, U. (2008). U.S. health care costs. Menlo Park, CA: Kaiser Family Foundation. Retrieved from www.kaiseredu.org/topics_im.asp?imID=1&aparentID=61&id=358

Anderson, R. M., Rice, T. H., & Kominski, G. F. (2007). *Changing the U.S. health care system: Key issues in health services policy and management* (3rd ed.). San Francisco, CA: Jossey-Bass.

Baker, S. (2008). *U.S. National Health Spending, 2006.* University of South Carolina, Arnold School of Public Health, Department of Health Services Policy and Management, HSPM J712. Retrieved from hspm.sph.sc.edu/Courses/Econ/Classes/nhe06/hspm.sph.sc.edu/Courses/Econ/nhe06/

Boivin, J., & Domrose, C. (2009). Healthcare reform needs you: Nursing-led innovations carry country toward prevention-focused care. *Nurse.com-The Digital Edition, 6,* 21–24. Retrieved from http://www.nxtbook.com/nxt/gannetthg/nursecom_200909/#/20

Centers for Disease Control and Prevention (CDC). (2011). Health, U.S. 2011, with special emphasis on socioeconomic status and health. Nursing homes, beds, residents, and occupancy rates, by state: United States, selected years 1995 -2010. Retrieved from http://www.cdc.gov/nchs/data/hus/hus11.pdf#120, accessed October 28, 2012.

Centers for Disease Control and Prevention. (2011). CDC Health Disparities & Inequalities Report – United States, 2011, Retrieved from http://www.cdc.gov/minorityhealth/CHDIReport.html, accessed October 28, 2012.

Cover the Uninsured. (2008). Robert Woods Johnson Foundation. Retrieved from covertheuninsured.org/

DeNavas-Walt, C., Proctor, B. D., & Smith, J. C. (2010). *U.S. Census Bureau, Current Population Reports, P60–238. Income, poverty, and health insurance coverage in the United States: 2009.* Washington, DC: U.S. Government Printing Office.

DMAA. (2008). DMAA definition of disease management. Washington, DC: DMAA: The Care Continuum Alliance. Retrieved from www.dmaa.org/contact_us.asp

Health Care and Education Reconciliation Act. (2010). Pub. L. 111–152, 124stat. 1029.

Ho, K., Brady, J., & Clancy, C. M. (2008). Improving quality and reducing disparities: The role of nurses. *Journal of Nursing Care Quality, 23*(3), 185–188.

Indian Health Service (IHS). (2006). Indian health service fact Sheet. Retrieved from info.ihs.gov/Files/IHSFacts-June2006.pdf

Institute of Medicine (IOM). (2004). *Insuring America's health: Principles and recommendations.* Washington, DC: National Academies Press.

Institute of Medicine (IOM). (2008). *Knowing what works in health care: A roadmap for the nation.* Washington, DC: National Academies Press.

Institute of Medicine (IOM). (2011). *The future of nursing: Leading change, advancing health.* Washington, DC: National Academies Press.

Kaiser Family Foundation (KFF). (2007). The uninsured, a primer: Key facts about Americans without health insurance. Washington, DC: Kaiser Family Foundation. Retrieved from www.kff.org/uninsured/upload/7451–03.pdf

Kaiser Family Foundation. (2009). *Medicaid and the uninsured.* Washington, DC: Kaiser Family Foundation.

Kleinpell, R. M. (2007). Advanced practice nurses: Invisible champions? *Nursing Management, 38* (5), 18–22.

Knox, R., & Poole, J. W. (2008, August 2). Health care for all: Massachusetts steps forward on health coverage. Washington, DC: National Public Radio. Retrieved from www.npr.org/templates/story/story.php?storyId=92758148

Massachusetts Nurses Association. (2008). Single payer health care. Retrieved from www.massnurses.org/single_payer/singlepay.htm

Miller, K. (Producer). (2008, May 9). Bill Moyers Journal: California Nurses Association. Washington, DC: Public Broadcasting Service. Retrieved from www.pbs.org/moyers/journal/05092008/profile.html

Montalvo, I. (2007). The national database of nursing quality indicators (NDNQI). *Online Journal of Issues in Nursing, 12*(3). Retrieved from www.nursingworld.org/MainMenuCategories/ANAMarketplace/ANAPeriodicals/OJIN/Tableof-Contents/Volume122007/No3Sept07/NursingQuality-Indicators .aspx

Nabili, S. (2010). What is a hospitalist? Retrieved from http://www.medicinenet.com/script/main/art.asp?articlekey=93946

National Practitioner Data Bank-Health Integrity and Protection Data Bank. (2009). Healthcare integrity and protection data bank. Retrieved from http://www.npdb-hipdb.hrsa.gov/hipdb.html

O'Neil, E. (2008). Centering on a nursing leadership agenda for a new health care age. The Center for the Health Professions, University of California, San Francisco. Retrieved from www.futurehealth.ucsf.edu/from_the_director_ 0308.html

Patient Protection and Affordable Care Act. (2010). Pub. L. 111–148, 124 stat. 119.

Schoen, C., Collins, S. R., Kriss, J. L., & Doty, M. M. (2008). How many are underinsured? Trends among U.S. adults, 2003 and 2007. New York: Commonwealth Fund. Retrieved from www. commonwealthfund.org/publications/publications_show.htm?doc_id=688615

Teenier, P. (2008). 2008 refinements to the Medicare home health prospective payment system. *Home Healthcare Nurse, 26(3),* 181–184.

U.S. Department of Health and Human Services. (2008a). Annual update of the HHS poverty guidelines. Retrieved from aspe.hhs.gov/poverty/08Poverty.shtml

U.S. Department of Health and Human Services. (2008b). Medicare and you, 2008. Centers for Medicare & Medicaid Services. Baltimore, MD: Author. Retrieved from www.cms.hhs.gov

CHAPTER 3

Nursing Today

KATHLEEN M. MCPHAUL, RN, PHD, MPH; PATRICIA M. SCHOON, RN, MPH; CAROLYN CHRISTIE-MCAULIFFE, FNP, PHD; AMY ANDROWICH O'MALLEY, RN, MSN; RINDA ALEXANDER, RN, CS, PHD; IDA M. ANDROWICH, RN, BC, PHD, FAAN; AND PATRICIA KELLY, RN, MSN

Each day brings you opportunities to raise important questions, speak to higher values, and surface unresolved conflicts. Every day you have the chance to make a difference in the lives of people around you.

–RONALD A. HEIFETZ AND MARTY LINSKY, 2002

OBJECTIVES

Upon completion of this chapter, the reader should be able to:

1. Relate the impact of one milestone in nursing's history to your practice today.
2. Describe one aspect of your work that is consistent with one or more elements of a profession.
3. Discuss how participation and membership in professional nursing organizations demonstrate professionalism.
4. Discuss the contributions of members of the inter-professional team in hospital, community, and primary care settings.
5. Develop an evidence-based practice question from a clinical issue.
6. Describe how your organization collects information on nurse-sensitive quality indicators.
7. Describe one implication of population-based care for hospital nurses and managers

The profession of nursing has kept pace with changes in society that reflect changes in women's roles. In addition, men are increasingly choosing nursing, and nursing jobs are expanding as health care expands to meet the increased demands of an older United States (U.S.) population. The Future of Nursing Report (Institute of Medicine, 2010) maps out a blueprint for nursing, and Regional Action Groups are implementing the blueprint (Future of Nursing Campaign for Action, 2011). As the Affordable Care Act of 2010 is implemented, it is likely that the health care system will undergo both expected and unexpected changes.

How has history shaped the profession of nursing?

What changes do you hope to see as a result of the Future of Nursing 2010 Report?

How will the Affordable Care Act influence the work of nurses?

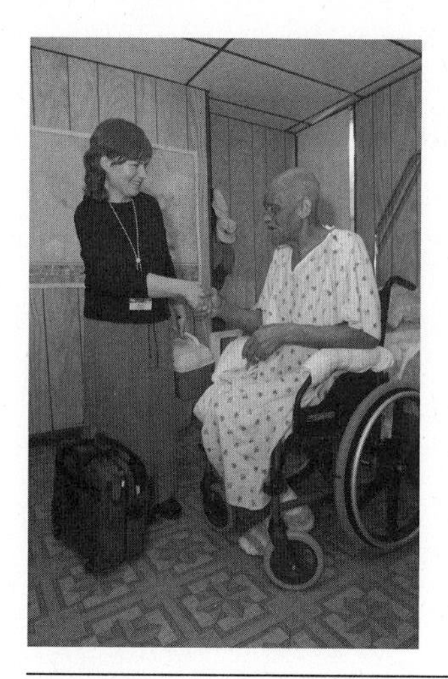

© Cengage Learning 2014

Registered nurses are the major professional group providing citizens with health care today. There are more than 3 million licensed RNs, and approximately 2 million are employed in the profession (Health Service Resource Administration, 2010). Nurses deliver expert, highly skilled, caring, and evidence-based nursing services in hospitals, primary care settings, and community settings. These nursing services promote health and healing through acute, palliative, and preventive care. Nursing practice has evolved for thousands of years with a long history of serving society and conducting research that provides a scientific basis for nursing care. Nurses are often members of professional nursing organizations and have developed quality indicators and health care systems to document and measure nursing practice provided to individuals and groups or populations of patients.

The 2010 Future of Nursing Report (IOM, 2010) together with the historic 2010 Patient Protection and Affordable Care Act (PPACA, 2010) provide a framework for nursing practice to participate in improved accountability for patient care outcomes throughout the lifespan of a patient population. Grounding nursing practice in evidence-based processes increases the likelihood that nursing care will improve patient outcomes and help control costs. Nursing-sensitive outcomes represent important measures for nurses to use when monitoring nursing care. Nursing today represents a kaleidoscope of professional roles as well as a diversity of educational backgrounds including associate, bachelor's, master's and doctoral degrees. Currently, nurses and other health professionals are educated separately from each other. Nurses work with and appreciate the scope of practice of many health care professionals.

This chapter reviews nursing's history and its relation to practice today. It examines nursing professionalism and evidence-based care. The chapter discusses the contributions of members of the interprofessional team in the hospital, community, and primary care setting. It notes how organizations collect information on nurse-sensitive quality indicators and discusses population-based care.

EVOLUTION OF NURSING

The evolution of nursing dates back to 4000 BC to primitive societies in which mother-nurses worked with priests. Modern nursing was founded by Florence Nightingale, with the opening of the first Training School of Nurses, St. Thomas's Hospital, London, in 1860. Table 3-1 outlines some significant events in the history of nursing. Each milestone and historical event in nursing's evolution has impacted the education, the career, and the future of today's nurse.

Since Florence Nightingale's innovative approach to nursing education arrived in the United States

TABLE 3-1
Selected Events Influencing the Evolution of Nursing

Date	Event
1859	Nightingale's *Notes on Nursing* published in England
1860	First Nightingale School of Nursing, St. Thomas's Hospital, London
1871	New York State Training School for Nurses, Brooklyn Maternity, Brooklyn, New York
1872	New England Hospital for Women: 1-year program for nurses
1873	First three Nightingale schools in United States: Bellevue (New York City), Connecticut, and Massachusetts General
1899	Founded: International Council of Nurses (ICN)
	First postgraduate courses for nurses at Teachers College, Columbia University
1900	*American Journal of Nursing* (AJN) begins publication
1901–1912	Founded: American Federation of Nurses
1903	North Carolina: passed first state nurse registration law
	Founded: Army Nurse Corps
1905	American Federation of Nurses joined ICN
1908	National Association of Colored Graduate Nurses (NACGN)
	Founded: Navy Nurse Corps
1909	Founded: first 3-year diploma school in a university setting at University of Minnesota
1911	Founded: American Nurses Association (ANA), formerly the Associated Alumnae
1912	ANA represented American nurses at ICN
1920	Congress passed the federal suffrage amendment
1921	Women earned right to vote
1943	Founded: Federal Cadet Nurse Corps to train nurses for World War II
1948	Brown Report: *Future of Nursing*
1956	Hughes study: *20,000 Nurses Tell Their Stories*
1964	Nurse Training Act
1965	First nurse practitioner program, pediatrics
	ANA position paper on entry into practice
1970	Secretary's commission to study extended roles for nurses
1983	Institute of Medicine Committee on Nursing and Nursing Education study
1999	Institute of Medicine (IOM) Report: *To Err is Human: Building A Safer Health System*
1999	California Safe-Staffing Law mandating minimum RN ratios became law
2004	IOM Report: *Keeping Patients Safe, Transforming the Work Environment of Nurses*
2010	IOM Report: *The Future of Nursing: Leading Change, Advancing Health*
2010	Passage of the Patient Protection and Affordable Care Act

Source: Adapted from DeLaune, S. C. & Ladner, P. K. (2011). *Fundamentals of Nursing* (4th ed.). Clifton Park, NY: Delmar Cengage Learning.

in 1871, professional nursing has kept pace and evolved with society's and women's roles and rights. Nurses have advocated for improved access to health care, have conducted patient care research, and have engaged in political and legal activity to enhance and protect the profession of nursing and the rights of patients. Increasingly, the safety of patients in U.S. hospitals relies on the systems of care that preserve the ability of nurses to work to the highest level of their education and be full partners on the health care delivery team. From the political action of the California nurses who insisted upon minimum safe-staffing ratios for patient care (Institute for Health and Socioeconomic Policy, 2001) to the acquitted whistle-blower nurses in Winkler County, Texas, who dared to report a physician's unsafe practices (Winkler County Nurses Update, 2010), nursing today and in the future is about advancing and translating scientific knowledge, utilizing innovative technology, engaging in political activism, and being a full partner on inter-professional teams.

Nursing Theorists

Many nursing theorists contributed to the development of modern nursing (Table 3-2).

PROFESSION OF NURSING

Registered nurses today have a diversity of educational backgrounds including an associate's degree, a bachelor's degree, a master's degree, and a doctoral degree. The recent Institute of Medicine Report, *The Future of Nursing*: Leading Change, Advancing Health, recommends that the minimum preparation for a nurse be a bachelor's degree. Advanced nursing roles, such as nurse managers, nurse specialists, nurse primary care providers, and nurse researchers, have master's degrees and, increasingly, doctoral degrees. Currently, the professional education system of nurses is distinct from medicine, physical therapy, dentistry, pharmacy, and social work, but increasingly, there are calls for greater integration of professional education in the nursing, medical, and health disciplines. The following attributes describe a profession:

- Professional status is achieved when an occupation involves a unique practice that carries individual responsibility and is based on theoretical knowledge.
- The privilege to practice is granted only after the individual has completed a standardized program of

TABLE 3-2
Selected Nursing Theorists and Their Models

Theorist	Model
Nightingale (1859)	Environmental Theory
Orem (1971)	Self-Care Deficit Theory
Peplau (1952)	Interpersonal Process
Roy (1976)	Adaptation Model
Henderson (1955)	Basic Needs
Paterson and Zderad (1976)	Humanistic Nursing
Levine (1969)	Conservation Theory
Neuman (1972/1995)	Systems Model
Rogers (1970)	Science of Unitary Beings
Watson (1979/1989)	Human Caring Theory
King (1971)	Goal Attainment Theory
Parse (1981/1995)	Human Becoming Theory

Source: Compiled with information from Nursing Theories (2011). Retrieved May 18, 2011, from http://currentnursing.com/nursing_theory/introduction.html

highly specialized education and has demonstrated an ability to meet the standards for practice.
- The body of specialized knowledge is continually developed and evaluated through research.
- The members are self-organizing and collectively assume the responsibility of establishing standards for education in practice. They continually evaluate the quality of service provided in order to protect the individual members and the public.

The guiding blueprint for the profession of nursing for the next decade is the recent IOM Report, *The Future of Nursing: Leading Change, Advancing Health.* In this Report, there are four recommendations:

1. Nurses should practice to the full extent of their education and training.
2. Nurses should achieve higher levels of education and training through an improved educational system that promotes seamless academic progression.
3. Nurses should be full partners with physicians and other health care professionals in redesigning health care in the United States.
4. Effective workforce planning and policy making require better data collection and information.

These recommendations are widely expected to shape the profession of nursing in the coming years. Through Regional Action Committees, nurse leaders are planning immediate and long-term goals in states across the United States (Future of Nursing Campaign for Action, 2011). Table 3-3 and Table 3-4 and Table 3-5 and Table 3-6 identify the characteristics of a profession, the characteristics of a professional, a plan for professionalism, and steps for developing a professional style.

TABLE 3-3
Characteristics of a Profession

Flexner, 1915

- Professional activity is based on intellectual action along with personal responsibility
- The practice of a profession is based on knowledge, not routine activities
- There is practical application in a profession rather than just theorizing
- There are techniques that can be taught
- A profession is organized internally
- A profession is motivated by altruism, with members working in some sense for the good of society

Pavalko, 1971

- Work based on systematic body of theory and abstract knowledge
- Work has social value
- Length of education is required for specialization
- Service to public
- Autonomy
- Commitment to profession
- Group identity and subculture
- Existence of a code of ethics

(Continues)

TABLE 3-3 (Continued)

Manthey, 2002

- An identifiable body of knowledge that can best be transmitted via formal education
- Autonomous decision making
- Peer review of practice
- Identification with a professional organization as the standard setter and arbiter of practice

Public Law 93-360 on Collective Bargaining

- Predominantly intellectual work
- Varied work requirements
- Discretion and judgment required
- Results not standardized over time
- Advanced instruction and study required

Compiled with information from: Mitchell, G. M., & Grippando, P. R. (1994). *Nursing Perspectives and Issues* (5th ed.). Clifton Park, NY: Delmar Cengage Learning; and Manthey, M. (2002). *The Practice of Primary Nursing: Relationship-Based, Resource-Driven Care Delivery* (2nd ed.). Minneapolis, MN: Creative Healthcare Management, Inc.

TABLE 3-4
Characteristics of a Professional

Professional Values		
Caring	Freedom	Justice
Altruism	Esthetics	Truth
Equality	Human dignity	Ethical
Nonjudgmental		

Professional Behaviors and Attributes	
Appearance	Participation in nursing research/evidence-based practice
Time-management skills	Effective teamwork, communication, and collaboration
Self-discipline	Stress management
Maintenance of licensure/certification	Self-evaluation
Participation in institutional/community activities	Initiative
Participation in continuing education	Motivation
Political awareness	Creativity
Reading professional journals	Participation in patient-centered care, quality improvement, safety, and informatics activities

Source: From Mitchell, G. M., Grippando, P. R. (1994). *Nursing Perspectives and Issues* (5th ed.). Clifton Park, NY: Delmar Cengage Learning.

TABLE 3-5
Plan for Professionalism

Behavior/Attribute	1-Year Goals	5-Year Goals
Appearance		
Time-management skills		
Self-discipline		
Licensure/certification		
Institutional/community activity participation		
Education		
Political awareness		
Professional journals		
Nursing research/Evidence-based practice participation		
Stress management		
Exercise		
Initiative		
Motivation		
Creativity		
Teamwork, effective communication, and collaboration		
Participation in patient-centered care activities		
Participation in quality improvement activities		
Participation in safety activities		
Participation in informatics activities		

Developed with information from U.S. Department of Health and Human Services. National Heart, Lung, and Blood Institute. Calculate Your Body Mass Index. Retrieved December 7, 2011, from http://www.nhlbisupport.com/bmi/bminojs.htm; and Centers for Disease Control and Prevention. (2011b). Physical Activity for Everyone. Retrieved December 7, 2011, from http://www.cdc.gov/physicalactivity/everyone/guidelines/adults.html; and Kelly, P. Unpublished manuscript. (2012).

Professional Nursing Organizations

Professional nursing organizations allow nurses the opportunity to network with other nurses, share research and evidence-based findings, receive mentoring, conduct political advocacy, and participate in continuing education. Professional associations such as the American Nurses Association (ANA) also set and maintain professional standards and create a Code of Ethics. (ANA, 2011). According to the ANA, it "advances the nursing profession by fostering high standards of nursing practice, promoting the rights of nurses in the workplace, projecting a

TABLE 3-6
Developing a Professional Style

1. Assess your current education and experience.
2. As you start your new nursing role, review the following on your unit.
   Most common:
   - Medical diagnoses
   - Nursing diagnoses
   - Medications and IV solutions
   - Diagnostic tests
   - Laboratory tests
   - Nursing and medical interventions and treatments
3. Set goals for any additional education and experience that you may need specific to the patient care unit you are working on and the community that you serve.
4. Review your own job description and the roles and job descriptions of nursing and other health care and medical staff you work with.
5. Identify the names and contact information of all nursing, medical, and health care staff you work with.
6. Discuss delegation with your preceptor, and observe how the preceptor delegates to others.
7. Observe the impact of delegation on both the delegator and the person delegated to.
8. Remember the Golden Rule: Do unto others as you would want them to do unto you.
9. Recognize that, under the law, the RN holds the responsibility and accountability for nursing care.
10. Communicate assertively. Work at being direct, open, and honest in your new role.
11. Exercise your power with kindness to all. Participate in professional committees at work.
12. Hold others accountable for their responsibilities as spelled out in their job descriptions.
13. Be open to performance improvement feedback about your personal delegation style.
14. Modify your communication approach to fit the needs of patients, staff, and yourself.
15. Monitor your care. Assure that your patients receive high-quality, evidence-based patient-centered care and that your care continuously improves in quality.
16. Monitor the literature so you are up to date on evidence-based care for patients.
17. Use informatics. Monitor data that shows that your patients are safe, satisfied, and pain-free; feel cared about; are complication-free; and have no nurse-sensitive outcomes.
18. Offer professional nursing service to your patients and community.
19. Speak up about the important role that nurses play in preventing patient complications.
20. Network with other professionals and join your professional organization.
21. Utilize a team approach to your work, develop rapport, and collaborate with other members of the inter-professional team.

(Continues)

TABLE 3-6 (Continued)

22. Receive professional salary and benefits.
23. Take good care of yourself and strive for professional and personal balance. Maintain a healthy diet and exercise program.
24. Dress like a professional. This tends to convey a higher level of knowledge and a sincere interest in advancement. A disheveled appearance may give the impression of a disinterested, marginal performer.
25. Communicate pride in being a nurse. Expect to be treated like a professional!
26. Refuse to be part of horizontal violence—e.g., bullying, gossiping, criticism, innuendo, scapegoating, undermining, intimidation, withholding information, insubordination, ostracizing, and physical, verbal, and passive aggression—toward other nurses and health care workers.

© Cengage Learning 2014

positive and realistic view of nursing, and by lobbying the Congress and regulatory agencies on health care issues affecting nurses and the public" (ANA, 2011). ANA is the primary association representing all nurses regardless of level of practice or specialty. Membership in ANA includes membership in a state affiliate where local issues are addressed. State affiliates send delegates to ANA's biannual House of Delegates to democratically determine ANA's position on issues of interest to nursing and patients. A related organization, The American Nurses Credentialing Center (ANCC), provides credentialing services for specialties and for Magnet hospitals.

Other associations such as Sigma Theta Tau, the nursing honor society, promote specialized interests such as nursing research and scholarship. Table 3-7 lists various nursing professional associations. Nurses often belong to more than one professional nursing organization. These organizations develop standards and offer continuing education to their members.

The Inter-Professional Team

Professional nurses, whether in hospitals, homes, or other community settings, are partners and members of inter-professional teams. Team functioning and communication are under increasing scrutiny in health care. Sentinel events, medical errors, and patient care quality are often linked to ineffective team communication in the hospital. Outside the hospital, there is increasing concern that lack of communication, collaboration, and coordination of care is resulting in preventable readmissions to hospital care, e.g., readmissions of patients discharged after an acute myocardial infarction.

In 1999, the Institute of Medicine (IOM) reported that 44,000 to 98,000 people die yearly from preventable medical errors. The need for safe, patient-centered care was identified. Some of the initiatives that have subsequently been developed to provide safe, patient-centered care in hospitals are identified in Table 3-8.

EVIDENCE-BASED PRACTICE

Evidence-based practice (EBP) is defined as "a problem-solving approach to clinical decision making ... that integrates the best available scientific evidence with the best available experiential (patient and practitioner) evidence" (Newhouse et al., 2007). The body of evidence supporting clinical practice is steadily growing. However, even when evidence-based quality care guidelines are available for numerous conditions, for example, diabetes, congestive heart failure, and asthma, they have not been fully implemented in actual patient care, and variation in clinical practice is abundant (Timmermans & Mauck, 2005; McGlynn et al., 2003; Kitson, 2007). EBP uses evidence-based resources to guide the development of appropriate strategies to deliver quality, cost-effective care (Table 3-9). Outcomes provide evidence about

TABLE 3-7
Selected Professional Health Care Organizations

Organization	Website
Selected Nursing Organizations	
American Nurses Association	http://www.nursingworld.org
International Council of Nurses	http://www.icn.ch
National Student Nurses Association	http://www.nsna.org
Selected Nursing Specialty Associations	
American Association of Critical-Care Nurses	http://www.aacn.org
American Association of Occupational Health Nurses	http://www.aaohn.org
American College of Nurse Midwives	http://www.midwife.org
American Nursing Informatics Association	http://www.ania.org
Association of Nurses in AIDS Care	http://www.anacnet.org
Emergency Nurses Association	http://www.ena.org
Selected Academic, Educational, and Honor Societies	
American Academy of Nursing	http://www.nursingworld.org/aan
American Association of Colleges of Nursing	http://www.aacn.nche.edu
American Academy of Nurse Practitioners	http://www.aanp.org
National League for Nursing	http://www.nln.org
Sigma Theta Tau International	http://www.nursingsociety.org
Selected Inter-professional Associations	
American Association of Diabetes Educators	http://www.diabeteseducator.org
American Dietetic Association	http://www.eatright.org
American Medical Association	http://www.ama-assn.org
American Pharmacists Association	http://www.pharmacist.com
American Public Health Association	http://www.apha.org
American Physical Therapy Association	http://www.apta.org
Selected Minority Professional Associations	
American Assembly of Men in Nursing	http://www.aamn.org
National Association of Hispanic Nurses	http://www.thehispanicnurses.org
National Black Nurses Association	http://www.nbna.org

© Cengage Learning 2014

benefits, risks, and results of treatments so individuals can make informed decisions and choices to improve their quality of life. Select journal sources for evidence-based practice are listed in Table 3-10.

Evidence-Based Practice Model

Nurses seeking to increase the use of evidence in the nursing care on their clinical units may want to apply the Practice Question, Evidence, and Translation

TABLE 3-8
Patient-Centered Care Safety Initiatives

Initiative	Example	Sponsoring Organization
Medication Safety	Avoid abbreviations that are associated with frequent misinterpretation and medication errors, e.g., q.d., MS, PCA.	Institute for Safe Medication Practice http://www.ismp.org/tools/default.asp
Core Measures	Provide all patients with heart failure with discharge instructions that include medications (dose and schedule), activity goals, weight goals, diet, symptoms to report, and plan for follow-up.	The Joint Commission http://www.jointcommission.org
Communication	Use a standardized format for patient report handoffs in patient care.	Institute for Healthcare Improvement http://www.IHI.org
Hand Hygiene	Encourage patients to ask their health care providers to practice hand hygiene.	Centers for Disease Control and Prevention http://www.cdc.gov
Safe Patient Handling	Improve the caregiver's posture and prevent injury during patient ambulation by using gait belts and handles.	Association of Safe Patient Handling Professionals http://www.asphp.org
Suicide Prevention	Be alert to signs of suicidal ideation in patients with established risk factors.	U.S. Preventive Services Task Force http://www.uspreventiveservicestaskforce.org/uspstf/uspssuic.htm
Rapid Response Team	Request additional assistance from specially trained health care team when a patient's condition appears to be worsening.	Institute for Healthcare Improvement http://www.IHI.org
Surgical Care Improvement Project	Use a safer method (electric clippers or hair removal cream—not a razor) to remove hair from surgical patients needing hair removal from the surgical area before surgery.	Centers for Medicare and Medicaid Services http://www.hospitalcompare.hhs.gov
Environmental Safety	Know how to access and use the information on Material Safety Data Sheets pertinent to your unit.	Occupational Safety & Health Administration http://www.osha.gov
Staffing Guidelines	Use the Nursing Hours per Patient Day model to determine the number of nurses required for care within a specific unit.	American Nurses Association National Database of Nursing Quality Indicators http://www.nursingquality.org

(Continues)

TABLE 3-8 (Continued)

Initiative	Example	Sponsoring Organization
Workplace Bullying (Lateral or Horizontal Violence)	Confronting bullies may be uncomfortable, but the only mistake you can make is to avoid the situation altogether.	Center for American Nurses http://www.navigatenursing.org
Health Care Rankings	Prevent high cholesterol with a healthy diet, maintaining a healthy weight, exercising regularly, and eliminating tobacco use.	United Health Foundation http://www.americashealthrankings.org

Source: Compiled with unpublished information from Rovinski-Wagner, C, and Mills, P., contributors to Patient Safety and Quality of Care by Kelly, P., Vottero, B., and Christie-McAuliffe, C. (2013). Clifton Park, NY: Delmar Cengage Learning. Mitchell, G. M. & Grippando, P. R. (1994). Nursing Perspectives and Issues (5th ed.). Clifton Park, NY: Delmar Cengage Learning. and Kelly, P. Unpublished manuscript, (2012).

TABLE 3-9
Evidence-Based Resources

National Guideline Clearinghouse	http://www.guideline.gov
Agency for Health Care Research and Quality	http://www.ahrq.gov
Sigma Theta Tau International	http://www.nursingsociety.org
Global Evidence Mapping Initiative	http://www.evidencemap.org
Cochrane Collaboration	http://www.cochrane.org
Joanna Briggs Institute for Evidence-Based Nursing and Midwifery	http://www.joannabriggs.edu.au
Sarah Cole Hirsh Institute for Best Nursing Practices Based on Evidence	http://www.fpb.case.edu. Search for *Hirsh Institute*.
Centre for Evidence-Based Nursing	http://www.york.ac.uk. Search for *Evidence-Based Nursing*.
Registered Nurses' Association of Ontario	http://www.rnao.org
Gerontological Nursing Interventions Research Center (GNIRC)	http://www.nursing.uiowa.edu
Research Centre for Transcultural Studies in Health	http://www.mdx.ac.uk
Academic Center for Evidence-Based Nursing (ACE)	http://www.acestar.uthscsa.edu
Cumulative Index to Nursing and Allied Health (CINAHL)	http://www.cinahl.com
Evidence-Based Nursing Journal	http://www.evidencebasednursing.com
McGill University Health Centre, Clinical and Professional Staff Development, Research & Clinical Resources for Evidence-Based Nursing	http://www.muhc-ebn.mcgill.ca
MEDLINE via PubMed, free resource provided by the National Library of Medicine	http://www.ncbi.nlm.nih.gov/pubmed

(Continues)

TABLE 3-9 (Continued)

Netting the Evidence—A ScHARR Introduction to Evidence-Based Practice on the Internet	http://www.shef.ac.uk
PubMed Tutorial (NLM), an in-depth tutorial from the National Library of Medicine	http://www.nlm.nih.gov
University of Minnesota evidence-based nursing site tutorial	http://www.evidence.ahc.umn.edu
Nursing Knowledge International	http://www.nursingknowledge.org
Virginia Henderson International Nursing Library	http://www.nursinglibrary.org

© Cengage Learning 2014

TABLE 3-10
Selected Journal Sources for Evidence-Based Practice

Advances in Nursing Science	Journal of Nursing Scholarship
American Journal of Nursing	Journal of Transcultural Nursing
American Journal of Public Health	New England Journal of Medicine
Applied Nursing Research	Nursing Clinics of North America
Clinical Nursing Research	Nursing Economics
Clinical Effectiveness in Nursing	Nursing Policy Forum
Hastings Report	Nursing Research
Health Affairs	Nursing Science Quarterly
Health Care Management Review	Oncology Nursing Forum
Health Services Research	Online Journal of Knowledge Synthesis for Nursing
Heart and Lung	Qualitative Health Research
Hospice Journal	Research in Nursing and Health
International Journal of Nursing Studies	Scholarly Inquiry in Nursing Practice
Journal of Advanced Nursing	Social Science and Medicine
Journal of Health Economics	Western Journal of Nursing Research
Journal of The American Medical Association	Worldviews on Evidence-Based Nursing

© Cengage Learning 2014

(PET) Model developed by The Johns Hopkins Hospital Nursing Department in collaboration with The Johns Hopkins University School of Nursing (Figure 3-1). This PET Model uses an inter-professional team approach, and nursing leadership and facilitation are key to this. Collaboration with a school of nursing or the nursing research department of a hospital can help ensure adequate assessment of the

The Johns Hopkins Nursing Evidence-based Practice

PET (Practice Question, Evidence, and Translation)

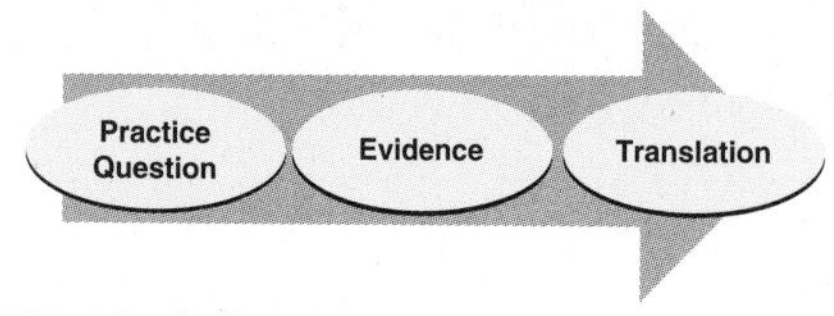

PRACTICE QUESTION

Step 1: Recruit interprofessional team
Step 2: Develop and refine the EBP question
Step 3: Define the scope of the EBP question and identify stakeholders
Step 4: Determine responsibility for project leadership
Step 5: Schedule team meetings

EVIDENCE

Step 6: Conduct internal and external search for evidence
Step 7: Appraise the level and quality of each piece of evidence
Step 8: Summarize the individual evidence
Step 9: Synthesize overall strength and quality of evidence
Step 10: Develop recommendations for change based on evidence synthesis

- Strong, compelling evidence
- Good evidence, consistent results
- Good evidence, conflicting results
- Insufficient or absent evidence

TRANSLATION

Step 11: Determine fit, feasibility, and appropriateness of recommendation(s) for translation path
Step 12: Create action plan
Step 13: Secure support and resources to implement action plan
Step 14: Implement action plan
Step 15: Evaluate outcomes
Step 16: Report outcomes to stakeholders
Step 17: Identify next steps
Step 18: Disseminate findings

FIGURE 3-1

The Johns Hopkins nursing evidence-based practice model.
(*Source:* Courtesy of The Johns Hopkins Hospital/The Johns Hopkins University Nursing Department, Baltimore , MD.)

scientific literature. A research evidence appraisal tool (Table 3-11) and a non-research evidence appraisal tool (Table 3-12) provide basic templates for nurses and evidence-based project team leaders to evaluate the research and nonresearch sources of evidence. Note that nonresearch sources of evidence must be considered and weighed along with the research evidence.

Nurse-Sensitive Patient Outcomes

The existence of professional nursing benefits patients who develop lower rates of nurse-sensitive outcomes, including lower death rates from one of the following life-threatening complications: hospital-acquired infections, such as pneumonia, urinary tract- or central line-associated blood infections, pressure ulcers, and failure to rescue patients, to name a few (ANA, 2011). Nurses combine caring with professional expertise to prevent these nurse-sensitive outcomes.

RAPID-RESPONSE TEAMS

Rapid-response teams have been developed in health care facilities to rescue patients whose condition deteriorates suddenly while hospitalized. Such teams have become a widely used patient safety intervention due in large part to their inclusion in the Institute for Healthcare Improvement's "100,000 Lives Campaign" in 2005. Patients often exhibit warning signs of deterioration (e.g., abnormal vital signs) in the hours before experiencing a bad outcome (e.g., cardiac arrest). In contrast to standard cardiac-arrest teams, which are summoned only after cardiopulmonary arrest occurs, rapid-response teams bring trained nursing and medical practitioners to the bedside early and may prevent poor outcomes for patients (http://psnet.ahrq.gov/resource.aspx?resourceID=3228).

Health Care Ratings

Thomson Reuters has reviewed the performance of hospitals of all types and sizes. It publishes a listing of the 100 top hospitals nationally (http://100tophospitals.com/top-national-hospitals/). *U.S. News and World Report* annually publishes a list of the top hospitals nationally (http://health.usnews.com/best-hospitals). See also the health care ratings at Health Grades (www.healthgrades.com), Leapfrog Hospital Quality and Safety (http://www.leapfroggroup.org/cp), and at the Department of Health & Human Services Hospital Compare site (http://www.hospitalcompare.hhs.gov).

Importance of Evidence, Outcomes, and Ratings

Why are evidence-based practice (EBP), monitoring outcomes, and using rating systems important? Few

TABLE 3-11
Research Evidence Appraisal Tool

Johns Hopkins Nursing Evidence-based Practice

Research Evidence Appraisal Tool

Evidence Level and Quality:______________________

Article Title:	Number:
Author(s):	Publication Date:
Journal:	
Setting:	Sample (Composition & size):

Does this evidence address my EBP question?	☐Yes	☐No Do not proceed with appraisal of this evidence

Level of Evidence (Study Design)			
A. Is this a report of a single research study? ***If no, go to B.***		☐Yes	☐No
1. Was there an intervention? 2. Was there a control group? 3. Were study participants randomly assigned to the intervention and control groups?		☐Yes ☐Yes ☐Yes	☐No ☐No ☐No
If yes to all three, this is a randomized controlled trial (RCT) or experimental study →	☐ LEVEL I		
If yes to #1 and #2, or yes to #1 and no to #2 and #3 this is a quasi Experimental study (some degree of investigator control, some manipulation of an independent variable, lacks random assignment to groups, may have a control group) →	☐ LEVEL II		
If yes to #1 only or no to #1, #2, and #3, this is a non-experimental study (no manipulation of independent variable; can be descriptive, comparative, or correlational; often uses secondary data) **or a qualitative study** (exploratory in nature such as interviews or focus groups, a starting point for studies for which little research currently exists, has small sample sizes, may use results to design empirical studies) →	☐ LEVEL III		
NEXT, *COMPLETE THE BOTTOM SECTION ON THE NEXT PAGE,STUDY FINDINGS THAT HELP YOU ANSWER THE EBP QUESTION.*			

(Continues)

TABLE 3-11 (Continued)

Johns Hopkins Nursing Evidence-based Practice

Research Evidence Appraisal Tool

B. Is this a summary of multiple research studies? ***If no to both A and B, go to Non-Research Evidence Appraisal Form.***		☐Yes	☐No
1. Does it employ a comprehensive search strategy and rigorous appraisal method (**Systematic Review**)? ***If no, use Non-Research Evidence Appraisal Form; if yes:***		☐Yes	☐No
a. Does it combine and analyze results from the studies to generate a new statistic (effect size)? (**Systematic review with meta-analysis**)		☐Yes	☐No
b. Does it analyze and synthesize concepts from qualitative studies? (**Systematic review with meta-synthesis**)		☐Yes	☐No
If yes to either a or b, go to 2 below.			
2. For Systematic Reviews and Systematic Reviews with meta-analysis or meta-synthesis:			
a. Are all studies included RCTs? →	☐ LEVEL I		
b. Are the studies a combination of RCTs and quasi-experimental or quasi-experimental only? →	☐ LEVEL II		
c. Are the studies a combination of RCTs, quasi-experimental and non-experimental or non-experimental only? →	☐ LEVEL III		
d. Are any or all of the included studies qualitative? →	☐ LEVEL III		
COMPLETE THE NEXT SECTION, STUDY FINDINGS THAT HELP YOU ANSWER THE EBP QUESTIONS.			
Study findings that help you answer the EBP question:			

NOW COMPLETE THE NEXT PAGE, *QUALITY APPRAISAL OF RESEARCH STUDY,* AND ASSIGN A QUALITY SCORE TO YOUR ARTICLE.

(Continues)

TABLE 3-11 (Continued)

Johns Hopkins Nursing Evidence-based Practice

Research Evidence Appraisal Tool

Quality Appraisal of Research Studies			
• Does the researcher identify what is known and not known about the problem and how the study will address any gaps in knowledge?	☐Yes	☐No	
• Was the purpose of the study clearly presented?	☐Yes	☐No	
• Was the literature review current (most sources within last 5 years or classic)?	☐Yes	☐No	
• Was sample size sufficient based on study design and rationale?	☐Yes	☐No	
• If there is a control group:			
o Were the characteristics and/or demographics similar in both the control and intervention groups?	☐Yes	☐No	☐NA
o If multiple settings were used, were the settings similar?	☐Yes	☐No	☐NA
o Were all groups equally treated except for the intervention group(s)?	☐Yes	☐No	☐NA
• Are data collection methods described clearly?	☐Yes	☐No	
• Were the instruments reliable (Cronbach's α [alpha] ≥ 0.70)?	☐Yes	☐No	☐NA
• Was instrument validity discussed?	☐Yes	☐No	☐NA
• If surveys/questionnaires were used, was the response rate ≥ 25%?	☐Yes	☐No	☐NA
• Were the results presented clearly?	☐Yes	☐No	
• If tables were presented, was the narrative consistent with the table content?	☐Yes	☐No	☐NA
• Were study limitations identified and addressed?	☐Yes	☐No	
• Were conclusions based on results?	☐Yes	☐No	

Quality Appraisal of Systematic Review with or without Meta-Analysis or Meta-Synthesis		
• Was the purpose of the systematic review clearly stated?	☐Yes	☐No
• Were reports comprehensive, with reproducible search strategy?	☐Yes	☐No
o Key search terms stated		
o Multiple databases searched and identified		
o Inclusion and exclusion criteria stated		
• Was there a flow diagram showing the number of studies eliminated at each level of review?	☐Yes	☐No
• Were details of included studies presented (design, sample, methods, results, outcomes, strengths, and limitations)?	☐Yes	☐No
• Were methods for appraising the strength of evidence (level and quality) described?	☐Yes	☐No
• Were conclusions based on results?	☐Yes	☐No
o Results were interpreted		
o Conclusions flowed logically from the interpretation and systematic review question		
• Did the systematic review include both a section addressing limitations and how they were addressed?	☐Yes	☐No

QUALITY RATING BASED ON QUALITY APPRAISAL

A **High quality:** consistent, generalizable results; sufficient sample size for the study design; adequate control; definitive conclusions; consistent recommendations based on comprehensive literature review that includes thorough reference to scientific evidence

B **Good quality:** reasonably consistent results; sufficient sample size for the study design; some control, and fairly definitive conclusions; reasonably consistent recommendations based on fairly comprehensive literature review that includes some reference to scientific evidence

C **Low quality or major flaws:** little evidence with inconsistent results; insufficient sample size for the study design; conclusions cannot be drawn

Source: Courtesy of The Johns Hopkins Hospital/The Johns Hopkins University Nursing Department, Baltimore, MD.

TABLE 3-12
Non-Research Evidence Appraisal Tool

The Johns Hopkins Nursing Evidence-based Practice

Non-Research Evidence Appraisal Tool

Evidence Level & Quality:________________

Article Title:	Number:
Author(s):	Publication Date:
Journal:	

Does this evidence address the EBP question?	☐Yes	☐No Do not proceed with appraisal of this evidence

☐ **Clinical Practice Guidelines:** Systematically developed recommendations from nationally recognized experts based on research evidence or expert consensus panel. **LEVEL IV**

☐ **Consensus or Position Statement:** Systematically developed recommendations based on research and nationally recognized expert opinion that guides members of a professional organization in decision making by presenting a particular issue of concern. **LEVEL IV**

• Are the types of evidence included identified?	☐Yes	☐No
• Were appropriate stakeholders involved in the development of recommendations?	☐Yes	☐No
• Are groups to which recommendations apply and do not apply clearly stated?	☐Yes	☐No
• Have potential biases been eliminated?	☐Yes	☐No
• Were recommendations valid (reproducible search, expert consensus, independent review, current, and level of supporting evidence identified for each recommendation)?	☐Yes	☐No
• Were the recommendations supported by evidence?	☐Yes	☐No
• Are recommendations clear?	☐Yes	☐No

☐ **Literature Review:** Summary of published literature without systematic appraisal of evidence quality or strength. **LEVEL V**

• Is subject matter to be reviewed clearly stated?	☐Yes	☐No
• Is relevant, up-to-date literature included in the review (most sources within last 5 years or classic)?	☐Yes	☐No
• Is there a meaningful analysis of the conclusions in the literature?	☐Yes	☐No
• Are gaps in the literature identified?	☐Yes	☐No
• Are recommendations made for future practice or study?	☐Yes	☐No

☐ **Expert Opinion:** Opinion of one or more individuals based on clinical expertise. **LEVEL V**

• Has the individual published or presented on the topic?	☐Yes	☐No
• Is author's opinion based on scientific evidence?	☐Yes	☐No
• Is the author's opinion clearly stated?	☐Yes	☐No
• Are potential biases acknowledged?	☐Yes	☐No

(Continues)

TABLE 3-12 (Continued)

The Johns Hopkins Nursing Evidence-based Practice

Non-Research Evidence Appraisal Tool

Organizational Experience:

☐ **Quality Improvement:** Cyclical method to examine organization-specific processes at the local level. **LEVEL V**

☐ **Financial:** Economic evaluation that applies analytic techniques to identify, measure, and compare the cost and outcomes of two or more alternative programs or interventions. **LEVEL V**

Setting:	**Sample (composition/size):**	
• Was the aim of the project clearly stated?	☐Yes	☐No
• Was the method adequately described?	☐Yes	☐No
• Were process or outcome measures identified?	☐Yes	☐No
• Were results adequately described?	☐Yes	☐No
• Was interpretation clear and appropriate?	☐Yes	☐No
• Are components of cost/benefit analysis described?	☐Yes	☐No ☐N/A

☐ **Case Report:** In-depth look at a person, group, or other social unit. **LEVEL V**

• Is the purpose of the case report clearly stated?	☐Yes	☐No
• Is the case report clearly presented?	☐Yes	☐No
• Are the findings of the case report supported by relevant theory or research?	☐Yes	☐No
• Are the recommendations clearly stated and linked to the findings?	☐Yes	☐No

Community Standard, Clinician Experience or Consumer Experience:

☐ **Community Standard:** Current practice for comparable settings in the community **LEVEL V**

☐ **Clinician Experience:** Knowledge gained through practice experience **LEVEL V**

☐ **Consumer Experience:** Knowledge gained through life experience **LEVEL V**

Information Source(s):	Number of Sources:	
• Source of information has credible experience.	☐Yes	☐No
• Opinions are clearly stated.	☐Yes	☐No ☐N/A
• Identified practices are consistent.	☐Yes	☐No ☐N/A

Findings that help you answer the EBP question:

(Continues)

TABLE 3-12 (Continued)

The Johns Hopkins Nursing Evidence-based Practice

Non-Research Evidence Appraisal Tool

QUALITY RATING FOR CLINICAL PRACTICE GUIDELINES, CONSENSUS OR POSITION STATEMENTS (LEVEL IV)

A **High quality:** officially sponsored by a professional, public, private organization, or government agency; documentation of a systematic literature search strategy; consistent results with sufficient numbers of well-designed studies; criteria-based evaluation of overall scientific strength and quality of included studies and definitive conclusions; national expertise is clearly evident; developed or revised within the last 5 years.

B **Good quality:** officially sponsored by a professional, public, private organization, or government agency; reasonably thorough and appropriate systematic literature search strategy; reasonably consistent results, sufficient numbers of well-designed studies; evaluation of strengths and limitations of included studies with fairly definitive conclusions; national expertise is clearly evident; developed or revised within the last 5 years.

C **Low quality or major flaws:** not sponsored by an official organization or agency; undefined, poorly defined, or limited literature search strategy; no evaluation of strengths and limitations of included studies, insufficient evidence with inconsistent results, conclusions cannot be drawn; not revised within the last 5 years..

QUALITY RATING FOR ORGANIZATIONAL EXPERIENCE (LEVEL V)

A **High quality:** clear aims and objectives; consistent results across multiple settings; formal quality improvement/financial analysis methods used; definitive conclusions; consistent recommendations with thorough reference to scientific evidence

B **Good quality:** clear aims and objectives; consistent results in a single setting; reasonably consistent recommendations with some reference to scientific evidence

C **Low quality or major flaws:** unclear or missing aims and objectives; inconsistent results; poorly defined quality improvement/financial analysis method; recommendations cannot be made

QUALITY RATING FOR LITERATURE REVIEW, EXPERT OPINION, COMMUNITY STANDARD, EXPERIENCE (LEVEL V)

A **High quality:** expertise is clearly evident; draws definitive conclusions; provides scientific rationale; thought leader in the field

B **Good quality:** expertise appears to be credible; draws fairly definitive conclusions; provides logical argument for opinions

C **Low quality or major flaws:** expertise is not discernable or is dubious; conclusions cannot be drawn

Source: Courtesy of The Johns Hopkins Hospital/The Johns Hopkins University Nursing Department, Baltimore, MD.

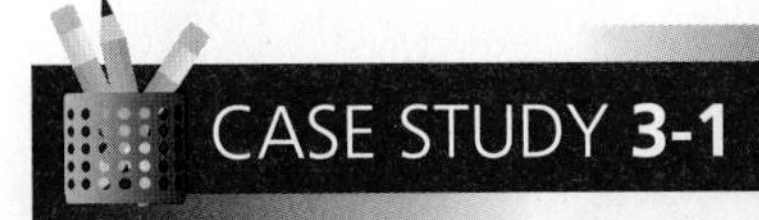

CASE STUDY **3-1**

Note the websites for evidence-based resources in Table 3-9. Search the National Guideline Clearinghouse for diabetes. What resources for Diabetes Self-Management Education will assist your patient? Check some of the other websites in the Table. Did you find any good resources to help with your current patient care?

clinician actions have been demonstrated to be supported by scientific evidence. Many actions are not needed or are potentially harmful. Often, patients do not receive care which corresponds to present scientific evidence. Consequently, there is nothing more important to patients and professional nursing than evidence-based clinical interventions that can be linked to clinical outcomes and used as a basis for rating care.

Generally speaking, nursing, medicine, health care institutions, and health policy makers recognize EBP as care based on a method of collecting, reviewing, interpreting, critiquing, and evaluating research and other relevant literature for direct application to patient care. EBP uses evidence from the following: research; performance data; quality improvement studies such as hospital or nursing report cards, program evaluations, and surveys; national and local consensus recommendations of experts; rating systems; and clinical experience. The EBC process further involves the integrating of both clinician-observed evidence and research-directed evidence. This then leads to state-of-the-art integration of available knowledge and evidence in a particular area of clinical concern that can be evaluated and measured through outcomes of care.

Nursing Work Environment

Consistent with the principles of EBP is the relationship between the nursing work environment and the nurse's health and patient safety and quality (Hughes, 2008). For example, nurses and other health care staff suffer injuries, infections, and exposure to chemicals in addition to violence from patients, stress, emotional demands, and long working hours. These occupational hazards have been well studied and impact nurses' health and also impact patient care. The health care industry has the highest rate of occupational musculoskeletal injuries when compared to other employment sectors (Trinkoff et al., 2008).

In 2011, the National Prevention, Health Promotion, and Public Health Council announced the National Prevention Strategy (Figure 3-2), a comprehensive plan that will help increase the number of Americans who are healthy at every stage of life. The National Prevention Strategy recognizes that good health comes not just from receiving quality medical care, but also from clean air and water, safe outdoor spaces for physical activity, safe worksites, healthy foods, violence-free environments, and healthy homes. Prevention should be woven into all aspects of our lives, including where and how we live, learn, work, and play. The first National Prevention Strategy encompasses four strategic directions. They are:

- Building healthy and safe community environments
- Expanding quality preventive services in both clinical and community settings
- Empowering people to make healthy choices, and
- Eliminating health disparities.

These strategic directions will focus on the following seven leading causes of preventable illness and death.

- Tobacco-free living
- Drug-free living and proper alcohol use
- Healthy eating
- Active living
- Injury and violence-free living
- Reproductive and sexual health
- Mental and emotional well-being

More information about the National Prevention Strategy and the National Prevention Council can be found at http://www.healthcare.gov/prevention/nphpphc/index.html.

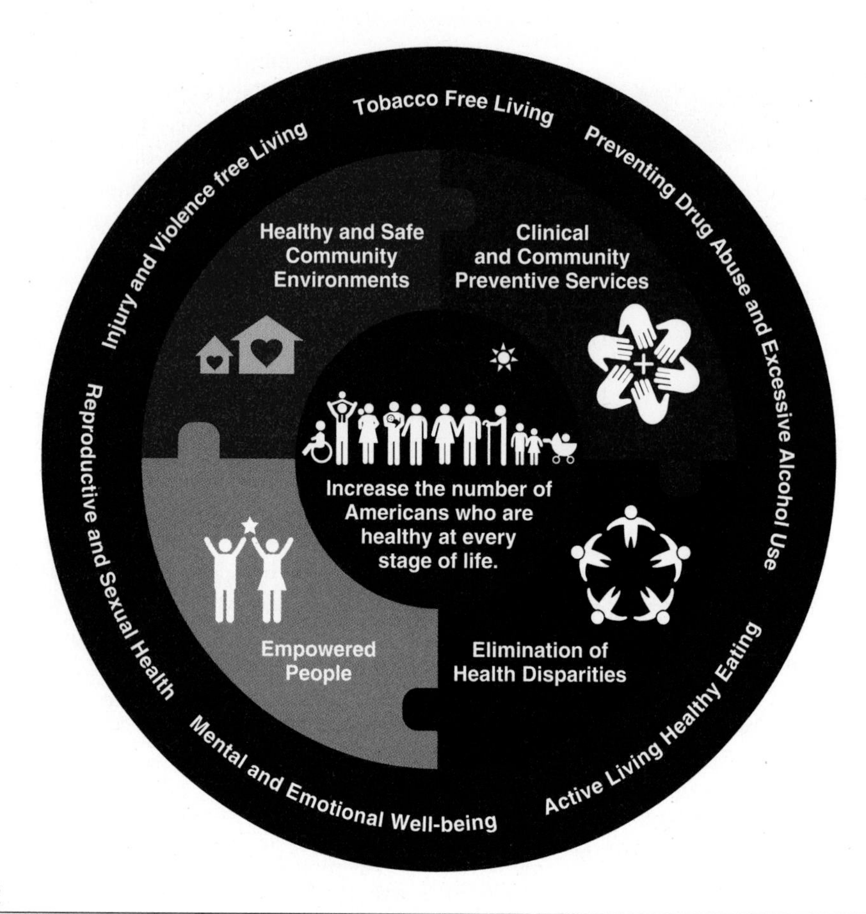

FIGURE 3-2

The national prevention strategy: America's plan for better health and wellness.
(*Source:* Courtesy of http://www.healthcare.gov/prevention/nphpphc/strategy/introduction.pdf. Retrieved January 11. 2012.)

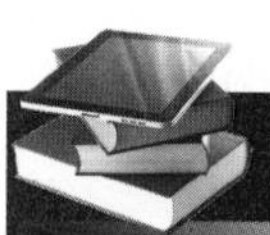

EVIDENCE FROM THE **LITERATURE**

Citation: Newhouse, R. P., Dearholdt, S. L., Poe, S. S., Pugh, L. C., & White, K. M. (2007). The *Johns Hopkins Nursing Evidence-Based Practice Model and Guidelines.* Sigma Theta Tau International, Indianapolis, IN. Appendix A. p.196.

Discussion: Developing an evidence-based question from a clinical concern or issue takes a systematic approach. Several evidence-based practice (EBP) models as well as guidance for the evidence-based process exist to assist clinicians. Newhouse points out that practice problems arise because of safety or risk-management concerns, poor patient outcomes, use of nonstandard clinical approaches to care, concerns that a process or practice takes too long, or the use of clinical practice without a scientific base (Newhouse et al., 2007).

(Continues)

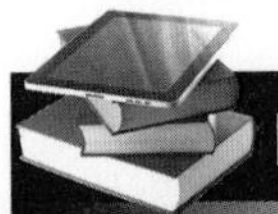

EVIDENCE FROM THE **LITERATURE** (CONTINUED)

Nurse managers create EBP teams and facilitate staff nurses' participation in EBP teams or committees. If the EBP is on-going, everyone in the organization becomes part of the learning process. EBP questions begin with clinical issues and may apply to practice, education, or administration. They may affect an individual, a patient population, or an organization.

Nurses use the PICO process to guide the start of the EBP process by asking a well-focused question in their literature search, that is:

- P stands for Patient, Population, or Problem;
- I stands for Intervention;
- C stands for Comparison with other treatments; and
- O stands for the Outcome.

For example,

(P) In a group of patients over the age of 60,

(I) how does early ambulation on the day of surgery,

(C) versus ambulation the next morning,

(O) improve patient outcomes?

Key terms from the PICO-based approach can be entered in library databases to identify key references. Review the steps of evidence-based practice at http://www.biomed.lib.umn.edu/learn/ebp/mod01/index.html. This PICO-based approach can be applied to both clinical and organizational situations and can lead to improvement of care and function.

Without a well-focused question, it can be very difficult and time consuming to identify appropriate resources and literature to guide the EBP process. Using the PICO framework helps the clinician articulate the important parts of the clinical question most applicable to a patient and facilitates the literature-searching process by identifying the key concepts for an effective search strategy. After a thorough search of the literature using the terms directed by PICO, reviewing current practice and standards, consulting experts and patients, looking at clinical experience, and considering costs, a researchable question is developed in narrow, manageable terms.

Implications for Practice: Nurses practicing in the 21st century must embrace the principles of evidence-based practice as an approach to clinical care and professional accountability.

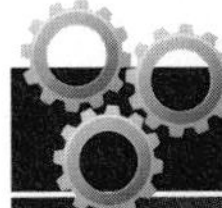

CRITICAL THINKING **3-1**

Go to the website http://www.sandiego.edu. Search for "nursing theorists." How does nursing theory influence your practice as a professional? Pick one of the theories, and comment on how your practice of nursing may fit with the theory.

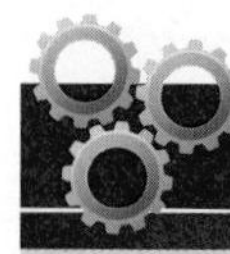

CRITICAL THINKING 3-2

Go to this site at the University of Minnesota: http://www.biomed.lib.umn.edu/learn/ebp/mod01/index.html. Take the tutorial. Note that the practice of evidence-based practice includes five fundamental steps:

Step 1: Formulating a well-built question

Step 2: Identifying articles and other evidence-based resources that answer the question

Step 3: Critically appraising the evidence to assess its validity

Step 4: Applying the evidence

Step 5: Reevaluating the application of evidence and areas for improvement

What did you learn about EBP and PICO from the site?

Be sure to work through the case studies at the site.

Construct a PICO question when you are done, and do a search for the key PICO terms in http://www.ncbi.nlm.nih.gov/pubmed/.

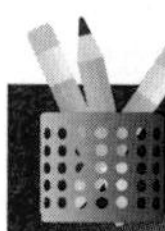

CASE STUDY 3-2

Foundations such as the Macy Foundation and the Robert Wood Johnson Foundation bring stakeholders together to envision a health professional educational system that facilitates inter-professional team effectiveness. During a conference of the American Association of Medical Colleges (2011), Donald M. Berwick, the outgoing administrator of the Centers for Medicare & Medicaid Services (CMS), framed this scenario: "Before the Affordable Care Act, if Mrs. Jones [a hypothetical older patient] has congestive heart failure, diabetes, and a touch of depression, she's going to see five doctors, take six medications, and visit seven health care facilities." Under that scenario, the cardiologist might not talk to the diabetes specialist or the nurse, and no one realizes that Mrs. Jones has forgotten to take her medication to control high blood pressure. As a result, Mrs. Jones has a rise in blood pressure, suffers a stroke, and must be admitted to a nursing home.

Berwick urged the conference attendees to "imagine the same scenario 10 years in the future. Mrs. Jones receives care from a team that communicates effectively and coordinates the care she needs at the right time with the right provider and the right intervention." Even if Mrs. Jones forgets to take her pills, the team deals with it in a timely manner. Berwick continues, "As a result, her blood pressure never rises to a dangerous level, and she doesn't suffer a stroke. Everyone is better off because Mrs. Jones is at home."

What potentially expensive outcomes are averted when missed medications are recognized in a timely manner?

In the future, how will hospital nurses work to prevent unnecessary hospitalizations?

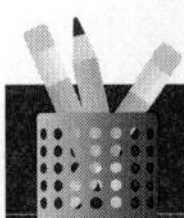

CASE STUDY 3-3

Review the *Healthy People 2020* Overarching Goals at http://www.healthypeople.gov/2020/about/default.aspx. Click on several of the four foundation health measures you find there namely:

- General health status
- Health-related quality of life and well-being
- Determinants of health
- Disparities

Note the measures of health that you find there. How can this data be used to improve the health of populations?

POPULATION-BASED HEALTH CARE

Nurses today are working increasingly in population-based health care practices. **Population-based health care practice** is the development, provision, and evaluation of inter-professional health care services to population groups experiencing increased health risks or disparities. It works in partnership with health care consumers and the community, to improve the health of the community and its diverse population groups. Vulnerable population groups are subgroups of a community that are powerless, marginalized or disenfranchised, and experiencing health disparities. Table 3-13 has examples of population-based recommendations from the community preventive services guide for the seven priority areas of the National Prevention Strategy. Table 3-14 has examples of population-based public health intervention programs. Table 3-15 highlights evaluation of population-based nursing practice. Research into health and illness recognizes the contribution of social, economic, and environmental factors to health.

The Patient Protection and Affordable Care Act (PPACA) of 2010 requires nonprofit hospitals and health systems to conduct regular community assessments which will lead to the identification and prioritization of community health care needs. Furthermore, due to certain financing aspects of the Act, population care strategies such as disease management, patient-centered medical homes, and other strategies to prevent hospital readmissions and unnecessary medical care are becoming more widespread (PPACA, 2010; McCall & Cromwell, 2011).

The following take place: restoration of property with rebuilding, replacing lost or damaged property, returning to school and work, and continuing without those lost in the disaster; reconstitution, where the life of the community returns to normal; and mitigation, i.e., future-oriented activities to prevent or minimize the effects of future disasters takes place.

DISASTER PREPAREDNESS AND RESPONSE

Since the terrorist attack on the World Trade Center in New York on September 11, 2001, disaster preparedness and management have been ongoing priorities of the United States. Nurses, as the largest group of health care professionals, have a key role to play in disaster relief (Langan & James, 2005).

REAL WORLD INTERVIEW

It amazes me that people still think private insurance is better than government insurance. I work in a doctor's office and deal with insurance companies daily. I talk to both government and private health insurance representatives. I have fewer problems with Medicare government insurance than I do with the for-profit private insurance companies like Anthem Blue Cross/Blue Shield, United HealthCare, or others. The private health insurance companies require prior approval from them before a patient can proceed with surgery or scans. These prior approvals require many hours for office staff to obtain them. When there is a need for me to call and follow up on a denied insurance company claim, 80 percent of the time the insurance company's customer service representative is in a foreign country. These calls usually take more time due to language differences and many times do not resolve the problem. Often, these call centers will have to finally transfer me to a higher authority representative to resolve the problem. When this is done, I am transferred to a call center in America. I understand now that some of the private insurance companies have realized that the extra time it takes to remedy the problem translates into higher wages and that some insurance companies are moving the insurance company call centers back to America.

I don't think people understand how many people are hurting and losing their homes and savings just to pay their health care bills. Many of our patients have insurance with a $10,000 deductible. This is what one simple outpatient surgery, (e.g., appendectomy, laparoscopic cholecystectomy), would cost, so right away they would have a $10,000 bill before their insurance even kicks in. One patient told us that, after losing his job and health insurance, he could no longer keep his home and he had to move in with his parents. He was a man in his 50s and he told us that was why he would not be able to pay his bill. I have received letters from spouses of patients dealing with terminal cancer stating that they have no resources left to pay their health care bills after exhausting their insurance and losing their source of income as the ill patient could no longer work. Other patients have taken out loans or tapped into their 401K plans to pay their health care bills. How many times have you seen an article in the paper telling about a spaghetti supper for someone who has cancer to help them defray their exorbitant health care bills? I don't think that Americans should become destitute after incurring health care problems.

People think that government insurance would ration or control the care of a patient. They fail to see that, to a degree, private insurance companies already do this, deciding what and where tests may be performed, if the insurance company considers a procedure is medically necessary, and so on, etc. Private insurance companies also dictate which doctors their patients can see in their insurance network. If their patients are allowed to go out of their insurance network to see another doctor, patients pay a larger co-pay and deductible.

I know that a single-payer health care system would not be without problems, but it would be a start toward giving everyone the same quality and availability of health care.

MARGARET ZAK
Highland, Indiana

A **disaster** is defined as an incident where human suffering and needs cannot be managed or alleviated by the victims without assistance and that requires extraordinary efforts beyond those needed for everyday emergencies (American Red Cross, 1975; Noji, 1997). Whether dealing with a randomly occurring natural disaster or an accidental or purposeful man-made disaster, nurses must be ready to participate in disaster relief efforts. Natural disasters include events such as epidemics, famine, hurricanes, floods, earthquakes, volcanic eruptions, landslides, snowstorms, and droughts. Accidental man-made disasters include events such as multiple-vehicle accidents, plane crashes, fires, industrial chemical spills or

TABLE 3-13
Examples of Population-Based Recommendations from the Community Preventive Services Guide for the Seven Priority Areas of the National Prevention Strategy

Strategic Goals/Priority Area	Example of Population-Based Recommendation
Tobacco-free living	Raising the price of tobacco products Mass media campaigns in combination with other inventions http://www.thecommunityguide.org/tobacco/initiation/index.html
Drug-free living and proper alcohol use	Enforcement of laws prohibiting sales to minors Maintaining limits on days of sale http://www.thecommunityguide.org/alcohol/index.html
Healthy eating	Multicomponent coaching or counseling interventions for obesity Improving access to healthy foods (e.g., changing cafeteria options and vending machine content) at work http://www.thecommunityguide.org/obesity/workprograms.html
Active living	Social support interventions in community settings Enhanced school-based physical education http://www.thecommunityguide.org/pa/behavioral-social/index.html
Injury and violence-free living	Early childhood home visitation to prevent child maltreatment Laws mandating safety seats for children in cars http://www.thecommunityguide.org/violence/home/index.html http://www.thecommunityguide.org/mvoi/childsafetyseats/index.html
Reproductive and sexual health	Community-wide campaigns to promote the use of folic acid supplements Interventions to fortify food products with folic acid http://www.thecommunityguide.org/birthdefects/index.html
Mental and emotional well-being	Collaborative care for the management of depressive disorders Home-based depression care management for older adults http://www.thecommunityguide.org/mentalhealth/index.html

Source: Minnesota Department of Health, Section of Public Health Nursing. (2001). Public Health Interventions-Application for Public Health Nursing Practice. St. Paul, MN: Minnesota Department of Health.

TABLE 3-14
Examples of Population-Based Public Health Intervention Programs

Individual/Family Level of Practice	Example
Referral and Follow-Up:	Vulnerable older adults discharged from emergency department to home were referred for public health nursing home visits (Kelly, 2005).
Social Marketing: College campus initiative	Social marketing with a "grateful head" theme was used to increase helmet use among cyclists on a college campus (Ludwig, Buchholz, & Clarke, 2005).
Community Level of Practice	
Coalition Building: Chicago Southeast Diabetes Community Action Coalition Screening	Coalition building was used as a strategy to reduce diabetic health disparities in a Chicago community Giachello et al., 2003).
County of San Diego TB Control Program	County-level screening of recent immigrants and refugees for pulmonary tuberculosis was used to identify those with a positive Mantoux (LoBue & Moser, 2004).
Systems Level of Practice	
Collaboration: Health disparities collaborative	Collaboration among health care providers improved diabetic care in community health centers (Chin et al., 2004).
Consultation and Delegated Functions: School-based health clinics	Use of POTS (plain old telephone system) to link school nurses with other health care providers improved school health services (Young & Ireson, 2003).

Source: Minnesota Department of Health, Section of Public Health Nursing. (2001). Public Health Interventions-Application for Public Health Nursing Practice. St. Paul, MN: Minnesota Department of Health.

TABLE 3-15
Program Evaluation of Population-Based Nursing Practice

Access	Did we find the high-risk, underserved, vulnerable population groups in the community or service area and provide timely and accessible services?
	Did we offer service regardless of age, gender, race, ethnicity, health care status, or location?
Quality	Did our services meet the greatest unmet health needs of the community or the at-risk, vulnerable, underserved population groups?
	Did their health status improve?
	Were their health risks reduced?
	Were they satisfied with the services they received?

(Continues)

TABLE 3-15 (Continued)

Cost	Were patients able to afford what we had to offer? Did we manage to stay within our budget? Are we reducing the cost of care over time?
Equity	Did we use our resources in a way that met the priority health needs of all of our high-risk patient groups? Did we target our services and use our resources to improve the health status of those who were the most underserved? Did we have enough resources left over to meet the essential health needs of lower-risk population groups?

Source: © The Johns Hopkins Hospital/ The Johns Hopkins University

radiation leaks, community-wide food poisoning, and mass power outages.

Purposeful man-made disasters include terrorism and war. Weapons of terrorism and war include conventional weapons (bombs, guns, grenades) and nonconventional weapons (chemical, biological, and nuclear). There are five stages in a disaster cycle that warrant action:

- Non-Disaster Stage—Disaster threat is in the future and there is time for planning, preparation, and mitigation, that is, preventing or reducing the harmful effects of a disaster.
- Pre-Disaster Stage—Evidence of an impending disaster is known and actions include warning, preimpact mobilization, and evacuation as appropriate.
- Impact Stage—Disaster has occurred and the community experiences immediate effects; rapid assessment of damages, injuries, and population needs is completed.
- Emergency Stage—There is immediate and long-term need for assistance including first aid, search and rescue, emergency medical assistance, establishment and restoration of transportation and communication, assessment of infectious diseases and mental health problems, and evacuation of residents as needed.
- Reconstruction or Recovery Stage—The following take place: restoration of property with rebuilding; replacing lost or damaged property; returning to school and work; continuing without those lost in the disaster; reconstitution, where the life of the community returns to normal; and mitigation, i.e., future-oriented activities to prevent or minimize the effects of future disasters takes place.

The Centers for Disease Control and Prevention (CDC) has identified six public health, emergency action-based preparedness, disaster goals (Langan & James, 2005).

- Detect—Identify the cause and distribution of potential threats to the public's health through epidemiologic, laboratory, and intelligence agency surveillance.
- Control—Provide medical countermeasures and health guidance to those affected by threats to the public's health.
- Maintain—Assure continuity of essential services during a public health emergency.
- Recover—Restore public health services and assure environmental safety following threats to the public's health.
- Plan—Complete and refine key public health response plans.
- Train and Exercise—Improve the ability of the public health workforce to respond to emergencies.

Two types of preparedness are critical to an effective disaster response: public health preparedness and medical preparedness. Nurses may be involved in both efforts.

- **Public health preparedness** is the ability of the public health system, community, and individuals to prevent, protect against, quickly respond to, and recover from health emergencies, particularly those in which scale, timing, or unpredictability threaten to overwhelm routine capabilities.
- **Medical preparedness** is the ability of the health care system to prevent, protect against, quickly respond to, and recover from health emergencies, particularly those whose scale, timing, or unpredictability threaten to overwhelm routine capabilities. Medical preparedness generally is the responsibility of agencies other than the CDC (CDC, 2010).

Nine comprehensive disaster preparedness strategies have been identified by the International Federation of Red Cross and Red Crescent Societies (2000). These strategies include:

- Hazard, risk, and vulnerability assessments
- Response mechanisms and strategies
- Preparedness plans
- Coordination
- Information management
- Early-warning systems
- Resource mobilization
- Public education, training, and rehearsals
- Community-based disaster preparedness.

Every local, state, or national community and health care facility should have a disaster plan. Actions that nurses may want to take in order to prepare themselves for potential disasters include:

- Formation of a family disaster plan
- Continuing education in disaster preparedness
- Disaster preparedness training at work
- Obtaining information about rights and responsibilities in the employment setting and under state law
- Becoming a volunteer for local or national disaster relief organizations.

Visit some of the following websites for information on how to develop a family disaster plan:

- http://www.ready.gov
- http://emergency.cdc.gov/preparedness
- http://www.getreadyforflu.org/newsite.htm

You may also want to think about how you can prepare yourself to respond to a disaster as part of your professional nursing role. Visit the International Nursing Coalition for Mass Casualty Education, Nursing Curriculum for Emergency Preparedness, at http://www.nursing.vanderbilt.edu/incmce/modules.html

ACCREDITATION

Nurses today work in accredited health care organizations. The Joint Commission (JC) is the current national organization that develops standards and accredits health care organizations. This accreditation is important to hospitals because meeting safety and quality standards is important to consumers and is also required for federal reimbursement of Medicare and Medicaid patient care services.

As many as 50 percent of the JC's hospital accreditation standards were written to correspond with Medicare's Conditions of Participation, a comprehensive set of criteria that hospitals and other care providers must meet to qualify for reimbursement. The JC's adherence to the Conditions stems from its "deemed" status with Medicare, which means that JC-accredited hospitals are assumed to have met the Medicare participation standards. Hospitals paid an average of $46,000 for a JC survey in 2010 (Joint Commission, 2011). Table 3-16 outlines the list of chapters in the JC Accreditation Manual. Each chapter highlights how quality is reviewed. All hospitals and long-term care organizations seeking JC accreditation monitor patient outcomes and use a performance measurement system to provide data about these patient outcomes and other indicators of care. Nurses today monitor accreditation standards and the other forces influencing health care (Table 3-17).

TABLE 3-16
Hospital Accreditation Standards Overview

- Environment of care
- Emergency management
- Human resources
- Infection prevention and control
- Information management
- Leadership
- Life safety
- Medication management
- Medical staff
- National patient safety goals
- Nursing
- Provision of care, treatment, and services
- Performance improvement
- Record of care, treatment, and services
- Rights and responsibilities of the individual
- Transplant safety
- Waived testing

Source: Joint Commission Resources. (2008). *CAMH: 2008 comprehensive accreditation manual of hospitals.* Oakbrook Terrace, IL: Joint Commission on Accreditation of Healthcare Organizations. Retrieved from http://www.jointcommission.org

TABLE 3-17
Nine Forces Influencing Health Care Delivery and Their Implications for Nursing Management

External Force	Nursing Management Implications
1. Financial incentives that reward superior performance	◆ Need to monitor quality, safety, cost, clinical outcomes ◆ Redesign patient care delivery ◆ Avoid patient hospital readmissions ◆ Increased growth of accountable care organizations
2. Increased accountability for performance	◆ Information systems that facilitate patient-centered care across episodes of illness and "pathways of wellness" ◆ Effective implementation of clinical practice guidelines and related care management processes ◆ Ability to demonstrate continuous improvements of all functions and processes
3. Technological advances in the biological and clinical sciences	◆ Expansion of the use of informatics for electronic record systems, decision making, clinical alerts, etc. ◆ Increased capacity to manage care across organizational boundaries and in different settings ◆ Need to confront new ethical dilemmas

(Continues)

TABLE 3-17 (Continued)

4. Aging of the population and associated increase in chronic illness	◆ Increased demand for primary care,, wellness, health promotion services, and chronic care management ◆ Challenge of managing ethical issues associated with prolongation of life
5. Increased ethnic and cultural diversity of the population	◆ Greater difficulty in meeting patient expectations ◆ Meeting the challenge of eliminating disparities in care provision and outcomes ◆ Challenge of managing an increasingly diverse health services workforce
6. Changes in the supply and education of health professionals	◆ Need for creative approaches in meeting the population's need for disease prevention, health promotion, and chronic care management services ◆ Need to compensate for shortages in some categories of health professionals (e.g., physical therapy, pharmacy, and some areas of nursing) ◆ Need to develop effective teams of caregivers across multiple care delivery sites ◆ Need to develop work settings conducive to recruitment and retention
7. Socioeconomic factors (unemployment, low wages, poor educational system, terrorism, new surprises)	◆ Patient populations may be stressed, violent, depressed, or addicted, increasing the complexity of care. ◆ Need for increased social support systems and chronic care management ◆ Need to work effectively with public health community agencies to address "preparedness" issues
8. Information technology	◆ Training the health care workforce in new information technologies ◆ Increased ability to coordinate care across sites ◆ Challenge of managing an increased pace of change due to more rapid information transfer ◆ Challenge of dealing with confidentiality issues associated with new information technologies
9. Globalization and expansion of the world economy	◆ Need to manage cross-national and cross-cultural patient care referrals ◆ Increasing competitiveness and productivity of the American labor force ◆ Managing global strategic alliances, particularly in the areas of biotechnology and new technology development ◆ Meeting the challenge of new and reemerging infectious diseases

Source: Adapted from Shortell, S. M., & Kaluzny, A. D. (2006). *Health Care Management* (5th ed.). Clifton Park, NY: Delmar Cengage Learning, and Kelly, P. U published manuscript. (2012).

KEY CONCEPTS

- ✦ Nursing has evolved from early times into the highly skilled, educated discipline of today.
- ✦ Nurses must strive to ensure that their approach to their nursing career includes activities that reflect the elements of a profession.
- ✦ Professional organizations are vehicles for maintaining the status of nursing as a profession.
- ✦ Nurses are full partners on the inter-professional patient care delivery team.
- ✦ The focus of evidence-based practice can be expected to remain a driving force in the health care arena in the foreseeable future.
- ✦ The nurse's work environment is a key factor in nurse and patient safety.
- ✦ Strong and effective voices in the inter-professional health care team reduce nursing and medical errors.
- ✦ Nursing-sensitive indicators have been developed to document and measure the impact of nursing care.
- ✦ Nursing can make significant contributions to the advancement of evidence-based practice
- ✦ The Affordable Care Act promotes population-based care.
- ✦ The goals of population-based health care are access, quality, cost containment, and equity.
- ✦ The Joint Commission is a major national organization that accredits health care organizations. This accreditation is one of the ways hospitals are accountable for patient safety and quality.

KEY TERMS

disaster
evidence-based practice (EBP)
medical preparedness
population-based health care practice
public health preparedness

REVIEW QUESTIONS

1. Which of the following is the major purpose of evidence-based care (EBC)?
   A. To increase variability of care
   B. To cause a link to be missing in clinical care
   C. To determine what medical models can be applied by nursing
   D. To provide a problem-solving approach to clinical decision making using the best available evidence

2. Which of the following are used for program evaluation in population-based nursing practice?
   A. Access, cost, empowerment, equity
   B. Access, cost, equity, resilience
   C. Access, cost, equity, quality
   D. Cost, equity, resilience, quality

3. Working conditions impact patient care and nurse health. Which of the following are possible hazards associated with health care work?
   A. Patient assaults and back injuries from lifting and moving patients
   B. Plantar fasciitis due to standing
   C. Lung cancer from smoking
   D. Congestive heart failure from stress

4. The National Prevention Strategy has prioritized seven areas of health. Which of the following is NOT identified as one of the seven areas?
   A. Tobacco-free living and active living
   B. Drug-free living and proper alcohol use
   C. Healthy eating and mental and emotional well-being
   D. Safe driving and wearing bike helmets

5. Which of the following is NOT a nursing theorist listed as having contributed to the development of modern nursing?
   A. Roy
   B. Orem
   C. King
   D. Shortell

6. Which of the following identifies health care ratings for the United States Department of Health & Human Services?
   A. Health Grades
   B. Leapfrog
   C. Hospital Compare
   D. *U.S. News and World Report*

7. Which of the following is NOT a nurse-sensitive hospital-acquired patient outcome? Select all that apply.
   A. Pneumonia
   B. Pressure ulcers
   C. Failure to rescue
   D. Myocardial infarction
   E. Central line associated blood infection

8. Which of the following is NOT considered a necessary professional behavior and attribute? Select all that apply.
   A. Stress management
   B. Membership in a union
   C. Time-management skills
   D. Maintenance of licensure
   E. Participation in nursing research
   F. Participation in community activities

9. Vulnerable older adults are discharged from an emergency department to home and are referred for public health nursing home visits. This is an example of which of the following types of population-based public health intervention programs?
   A. Federal level of practice
   B. Systems level of practice
   C. Community level of practice
   D. Individual or family level of practice

10. Which of the following are forces influencing health care delivery and nursing management? Select all that apply.
   A. Aging population
   B. Cultural diversity
   C. Information technology
   D. Supply and education of nurses
   E. Increased accountability for performance

REVIEW ACTIVITIES

1. Compare and contrast individual-focused nursing practice with population-based nursing practice. What nursing knowledge and skills do you need to practice population-based nursing care?
2. Many believe that nurses should adopt a global framework for the empowerment of women to reduce health disparities. Discuss what you think this framework could include. How could you become a nursing advocate for this at the local, national, and international levels?
3. Review Pavalko's characteristics of a profession in Table 3-3. Is nursing a profession?

EXPLORING THE WEB

- Where could you find information to help serve the health care needs of immigrants?
  National Immigration Law Center, Health Care
  http://www.nilc.org
- Visit the Oncology Nursing Society's online evidence-based practice resource area:
  http://www.ons.org
- What sites could you recommend to patients and families seeking information about self-help, research summaries, and clinical practice guidelines, for example, the National Library of Medicine , the Agency for Healthcare Research and Quality, and Medline Plus at the National Library of Medicine?
  http://www.nlm.nih.gov/medlineplus
  http://www.ahrq.gov
  http://www.centerwatch.com
  http://www.guideline.gov
  http://www.cdc.gov
  http://www.netdoctor.co.uk
  http://www.health.gov
- Go to the site for the Malcolm Baldridge National Quality Award. What information did you find there?
  http://www.nist.gov/baldrige
- Go to the site for the American Nurses Credentialing Center. What information did you find there?
  http://www.nursecredentialing.org
- Search these sites: Medicare,
  National Institutes of Health, American Nurses Association, National League for Nursing, American Cancer Society, American Heart Association, American Diabetes Association, and Cengage Learning. What did you find?
  http://www.medicare.gov
  http://www.nih.gov
  http://www.nursingworld.org
  http://www.nln.org
  http://www.cancer.org
  http://www.americanheart.org
  http://www.diabetes.org
  http://www.cengage.com/us
- Go to PubMed. What did you find there? Can you access nursing and medical journals? Would you recommend this site to patients?
  http://www.ncbi.nlm.nih.gov

- ✦ What are some helpful sites for nurses?
  http://www.nursingworld.org
  http://www.allnurses.com
  http://www.jointcommission.org
  http://www.continuingeducation.com
  http://www.hotnursejobs.com
  http://www.hospitalsoup.com
  http://www.cdc.gov

REFERENCES

Affordable Care Act. (2011). Retrieved December 26, 2011, from http://www.healthcare.gov/law/full/index.html

American Association of Medical Colleges. (2011). *Team-Based competencies: Building a shared foundation for education and practice.* Conference Proceedings, February 16–17, 2011. Washington, DC. Retrieved December 27, 2011, from https://www.aamc.org/download/186752/data/team-based_competencies.pdf

American Nurses Association. (2011). Scope and standards of practice. Retrieved December 26, 2011, from http://www.nursingworld.org/scopeandstandardsofpractice

American Nurses Association (2012). Nursing sensitive indicators. Retrieved October 31, 2012, from http://www.nursingworld.org/MainMenuCategories/ThePracticeofProfessionalNursing/PatientSafety Quality/Research-Measurement/The-National-Database/Nursing-Sensitive-Indicators_1

American Physical Therapy Association. (2009). Model definition of physical therapy for state practice acts. Retrieved December 6, 2011, from http://www.apta.org/uploadedFiles/APTAorg/About_Us/Policies/BOD/Practice/ScopeofPractice.pdf

American Red Cross. (1975). *Disaster relief program, 2235.* Washington, DC: Author.

Centers for Disease Control and Prevention (CDC). (2010). Emergency preparedness and response. Retrieved September 25, 2010, from http://emergency .cdc.gov/cdc/

Chin, M., Cook, S., Drum, M., Guillen, J., Humikowski, C., Koppert, J., Harrison, J., Lippold, S., Schaefer, C. (2004). Improving diabetes care in midwest community health centers with the health disparities collaborative. *Diabetes Care, 27*(1), 2–8.

Cochrane Library at McMaster University. (2000, March). Using Medline to search for evidence. Retrieved from http://www.londonlinks.ac.uk/evidence_ strategies/coch_search.htm

DeLaune, S. C., & Ladner, P. K. (2011). *Fundamentals of nursing* (4th ed.). Clifton Park, NY: Delmar Cengage Learning.

Dunnion, M.E. & Kelly, B. (2005). From the emergency department to home. *Journal of Clinical Nursing, 14,* 776–785.

Future of Nursing Campaign for Action. Retrieved December 26, 2011, from http://thefutureofnursing.org/content/regional-action-coalitions

Giachello, A., Arrom, J., Davis, M., Sayad, J., Ramirez, D., Nandi, C., & Ramos, C. (2003). Reducing diabetes health disparities through community-based participatory action research: The Chicago southeast diabetes community action coalition. *Public Health Reports, 118*(4), 309–323.

Health Service Resource Adminstration. (2010). The registered nurse population: Findings from the 2008 national sample survey of registered nurses. Retrieved December 26, 2011, from http://bhpr.hrsa.gov/healthworkforce/rnsurvey2008.html

Heifetz, R. A., & Linsky, M. (2002). *Leadership on the line.* Boston, MA: Harvard Business School Press.

Institute for Health and Socioeconomic Policy (IHSP). (2001). AB 394: California and the demand for safe and effective nurse-to-patient staffing ratios.Retrieved from http://nurses.3cdn.net/a985cdaf1305cc6478_f3m6b0kw8.pdf.

Institute of Medicine (IOM). (2002). *Unequal treatment confronting racial and ethnic disparities in health care.* Institute of Medicine Report. Washington, DC: National Academies Press.

Institute of Medicine (IOM). (2010). *The future of nursing: Leading change, advancing health.* Institute of Medicine Report. Washington, DC: National Academies Press.

International Federation of Red Cross and Red Crescent Societies. (2000). Disaster preparedness training programme: Introduction to disaster preparedness. Retrieved October 31, 2012, from http://www.ifrc.org/Global/Publications/disasters/all.pdf

Joint Commission. (2011). Cost of accreditation. Retrieved July 5, 2012, from http://www.jointcommission international.org/Cost-of-Accreditation/

Joint Commission Resources. (2008). *CAMH: 2008 comprehensive accreditation manual of hospitals.* Oakbrook Terrace, IL: Joint Commission on Accreditation of Healthcare Organizations. Retrieved from http://www.jointcommission.org

Kitson, A. (2007). What influences the use of research in clinical practice? *Nursing Research,* 56(4), Supplement 1:S1—S3.

Langan, J., & James, D. (2005). *Preparing nurses for disaster management.* Upper Saddle River, NJ: Pearson Prentice Hall.

LoBue, P. A., & Moser, K. S. (2004, December). Screening of immigrants and refugees for pulmonary tuberculosis in San Diego County, California. *Chest, 126*(6), 1777–1782.

Lowes, R. (2011). Texas physician pleads guilty in whistle-blowing nurses' case. Medscape Medical News. Retrieved from http://www.medscape.com/viewarticle/753029?src=ptalk

Ludwig, T., Buchholz, C., & Clarke, S. (2005). Using social marketing to increase the use of helmets among bicyclists. *Journal of American College Health, 4*(1), 51–58.

Manthey, M. (2002). *The Practice of Primary Nursing: Relationship-Based, Resource-Driven Care Delivery* (2nd ed.). Minneapolis, MN: Creative Healthcare Management, Inc.

McCall, M., & Cromwell, J. (2011). Results from the Medicare health support disease-management pilot program. *New England Journal of Medicine, 365,* 1704–1712.

McGlynn, E. A., Asch, S. M., Adams, J., Keesey, J., Hicks, J., DeCristofaro, A., et al. (2003). The quality of health care delivered to adults in the United States. *New England Journal of Medicine,* 348, 2635–2645.

Mitchell, G. M. & Grippando, P. R. (1994). *Nursing perspectives and issues* (5th ed.). Clifton Park, NY: Delmar Cengage Learning.

National Prevention Council. (2011). *National prevention strategy.* Washington, DC: U.S. Department of Health and Human Services, Office of the Surgeon General.

Newhouse, R. P., Dearholdt, S. L., Poe, S. S., Pugh, L. C., & White, K. M. (2007). *The Johns Hopkins nursing evidence-based practice model and guidelines* (Appendix A, p. 196). Indianapolis, IN: Sigma Theta Tau International.

Nightingale, F. (1914). Florence Nightingale to her nurses: A selection from Miss Nightingale's addresses to probationers and nurses of the Nightingale School at St. Thomas's Hospital (p. 1; Address in May 1872). London, England: Macmillan.

Noji, E. K. (1997). The nature of disaster: General characteristics and public health effects. In E. K. Noji (Ed.), *The public health consequences of disasters* (pp. 3–20). New York, NY: Oxford University Press.

Public Law 11-148. (2010). Patient protection and affordable care. Retrieved December 5, 2011, from http://docs.house.gov/energycommerce/ppacacon.pdf

Robert Wood Johnson Foundation. (2011). The future of nursing campaign for action. Retrieved from http://www.thefutureofnursing.org

Shortell, S. M., & Kaluzny, A. D. (2006). *Health care management* (5th ed.). Clifton Park, NY: Delmar Cengage Learning.

Timmermans, S., & Mauck, A. (2005). The promises and pitfalls of evidence-based medicine. *Health Affairs, 24*(1), 18–28.

Trinkoff, A. M., Geiger-Brown, J., Caruso, C. C., Lipscomb, J. A., Johantgen, M., Nelson, A., Sattler, B., Selby, V. (2008). Personal safety for nurses. In R. Hughes (Ed.), *Patient safety and quality: An evidence-based handbook for nurses.* Rockville, MD: AHRQ Publication No. 08-0043, April 2008. Retrieved from http://www.ahrq.gov/qual/nurseshdbk

Winkler County Nurse Update, Texas Nurses Association. (2010). Retrieved December 26, 2011, from http://www.texasnurses.org/displaycommon.cfm?an=1&subarticlenbr=509

Young, T., & Ireson, C., (2003). Effectiveness of school-based telehealth care in urban and suburban elementary schools. *Pediatrics, 112*(5), 1088–1094.

SUGGESTED READINGS

American Nurses Association. (2001). *Code of ethics for nursing with interpretive statements.* Washington, DC: American Nurses Publishing.

American Nurses Association. (2008). Professional role competence position statement. Retrieved December 27, 2011, from http://gm6.nursingworld.org/MainMenuCategories/Policy-Advocacy/Positions-and-Resolutions/ANAPositionStatements/Position-Statements-Alphabetically/Professional-Role-Competence.html

American Nurses Association. (2010a). *Nursing's Scope and standards of practice,* (2nd ed.). Silver Spring, MD: Nursesbooks.org.

American Nurses Association. (2010b). *Nursingís social policy statement: The essence of the profession.* Silver Spring, MD: Nursesbooks.org.

Gordon, S. (Ed.). (2010). *When chicken soup isn't enough: Stories of nurses standing up for themselves, their patients, and their profession.* Ithica, NY, and London, England: ILR Press.

Hardcastle, L., Record, K. L., Jacobson, P. D., & Gosten, L. O. (2011). Improving the population's health: The Affordable Care Act and the importance of integration. *Journal of Law, Medicine & Ethics, 39,* 317–327.

Heifetz, R. A., & Linsky, M. (2002). *Leadership on the line.* Boston, MA: Harvard Business School Press.

Institute of Medicine. (2010). *The future of nursing: Leading change, advancing health.* Washington, DC: National Academies Press.

Newhouse, R. P., Dearholdt, S. L., Poe, S. S., Pugh, L. C., & White, K. M. (2007). *The Johns Hopkins nursing evidence-based practice model and guidelines.* Sigma Theta Tau International, Indianapolis, IN. Appendix A. p. 196.

Schoon, P. (2008). Population-Based health care practice. In P. Kelly (Ed.), *Nursing leadership & management.* Clifton Park, NY: Delmar Cengage Learning.

Styles, M. M., Schumann, M. J., Bickford, C., & White, K. M. (2008). *Specialization and credentialing in nursing revisited.* Silver Spring, MD: Nursesbooks.org.

Wu, Y., Larrabee, J. H., & Putnam, H. P. (2006, January-February). Caring behaviors inventory. *Nursing Research, 55*(1), 18–25.

CHAPTER 4

Decision Making, Critical Thinking, Technology, and Informatics

JANICE TAZBIR, RN, MS, CS, CCRN, CNE; SHARON LITTLE-STOETZEL, RN, MS, CNE; BARBARA K. FANE, MS, RN, APRN-BC; JOSETTE JONES, RN, PHD; AND LESLIE H. NICOLL, RN, PHD, MBA, BC

> *Man is man because he is free to operate within a framework of his destiny. He is free to deliberate, to make decisions, and to choose between alternatives.*
>
> –MARTIN LUTHER KING, JR. 1959
> (HISTORY LEARNING SITE, 2011)

OBJECTIVES

Upon completion of this chapter, the reader should be able to:

1. Apply the decision-making process to patient-centered care.
2. Explain how problem solving, critical thinking, reflective thinking, and intuitive thinking relate to decision making.
3. Examine tools to improve decision making.
4. Identify how technology can help with decision making.
5. Discuss individual versus inter-professional team decision making.
6. Discuss relevant technology and informatics used in health care today.

You are a new nurse on a medical-surgical unit and have just come from a unit meeting. At the meeting, your nurse manager reported the results of the patient satisfaction survey from the previous year. Patient satisfaction has steadily declined, and for the past three months, only 20 percent of patients were satisfied. The manager selected a task force to investigate potential solutions to this problem and appointed you to the committee. The survey identified some reasons for the dissatisfaction: long waiting periods after pushing the nurse call light, not being informed about tests and procedures being performed, and being treated in an impersonal manner.

What should be the first step of the task force?

How can critical thinking, the decision-making process, and technology help the group solve the situation?

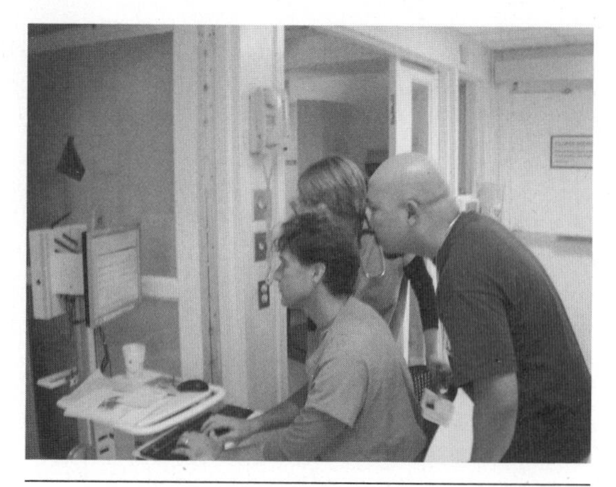

© Cengage Learning 2014

Rapid changes in the health care environment have expanded the decision-making role of the nurse. Decision making and critical thinking by nurses are necessary for safe patient-centered care. Patient care is becoming complex, and acuity is rising. Effective decisions using critical thinking about patient care must be made in a timely manner. Technology can help with this. Computers, technology, and the Internet have changed the way we communicate, obtain information, work, entertain, and make important health decisions. Pew Internet, a project of the Pew Research Center, reports that seventy-five percent of adults and ninety-five percent of teens have access to the Internet. One in five Americans have gone online to find people with similar health care concerns (Comsti, 2011). Peer-to-peer health care, or seeking and sharing advice about health, is nothing new. What is new is the ability to do it with Internet speed and scale. One problem with this is most people do not know how to discern if the information they are retrieving is reliable. Nurses need to help patients sift through the overwhelming amount of information that is available at their fingertips and decipher what is accurate and reliable. This chapter explores the decision-making process and the critical-thinking process. It also examines advantages of and limitations to group decision making, as well as the use of technology in decision making. The use of technology and informatics as they evolve in health care are also discussed.

DECISION MAKING

In everyday practice, nurses make decisions about patient-centered care. DeLaune and Ladner (2011) define **decision making** as "considering and selecting interventions from a repertoire of actions that facilitate the achievement of a desired outcome" (p. 89). Problem solving and critical, reflective, and intuitive thinking (Table 4-1) may be used during the decision-making process, as illustrated in Figure 4-1. Experience precedes expertise in decision making. Beginning nurses use procedures and protocols to clinically reason and come up with clinical actions. Competent nurses move away from protocols and are able to draw on past experiences, good and bad, to analyze and interpret to determine actions. Proficient nurses think beyond the planned, using complex thought processes, and can see the "whole picture" (Benner, Hughes, & Sutphen, 2008).

Although decisions are unique to different situations, the same decision-making process can be applied to most all situations. The decision-making process consists of five steps (Table 4-2).

In the following clinical application, the decision-making process is applied to a clinical problem-solving situation.

TABLE 4-1
Review of Terms

Decision making	Considering and selecting interventions from a repertoire of actions that facilitate the achievement of a desired outcome (DeLaune & Ladner, 2011).
Critical thinking	Thinking about your thinking while you are thinking in order to make your thinking better (Paul, 1992).
Reflective thinking	Watching or observing ourselves as we perform a task or make a decision about a particular situation (Pesut & Herman, 1999). Journal writing assists with reflective thinking.
Intuitive thinking	An innate feeling that nurses develop that helps them to act in certain situations (Gardner, 2003). Intuitive thinking has been described as a "gut" feeling assessment that something is right or wrong.
Problem solving	An active process that starts with a problem and ends with a solution.

© Cengage Learning 2014

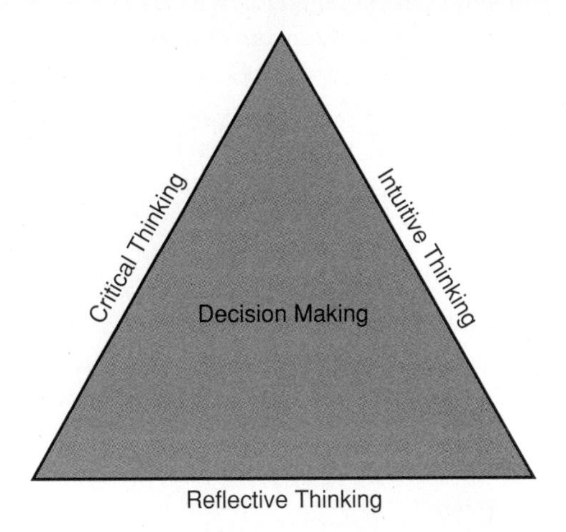

FIGURE 4-1
Critical thinking, intuitive thinking, and reflective thinking are incorporated throughout the decision-making process.
© Cengage Learning 2014

TABLE 4-2
The Decision-Making Process

Step 1: Identify the need for a decision.
Step 2: Determine the goal or outcome.
Step 3: Identify alternatives or actions along with the benefits and consequences of each action.
Step 4: Decide which action to implement.
Step 5: Evaluate the decision.

Source: Little-Stoetzel, S., & Fane, B.K. (2012). Decision making and critical thinking. In P. Kelly, (Ed.), *Nursing leadership and management* (3rd ed.). Clifton Park, NY: Delmar Cengage Learning.

Problem Solving

You are the night shift nurse caring for Mr. Cintas. In the morning, Mr. Cintas is scheduled for a permanent pacemaker insertion to replace his temporary pacemaker, which is still functioning. Hospital policy states that no visitor may stay all night with a patient unless that patient is very critically ill. Mr. and Mrs. Cintas are both requesting that Mrs. Cintas stay all night in a chair beside Mr. Cintas's bed because both are anxious about his upcoming procedure. Use your decision-making and problem-solving skills to help you decide what to do.

- Step 1: Identify the need for a decision. Gather data and identify key participants. Should you let Mrs. Cintas spend the night? Consider all the information (the evidence, hospital policy, the patient's and Mrs. Cintas's wishes, anxiety level, and so on).

- Step 2: Determine the goal or outcome. Questions to consider include the following: Can an exception to hospital policy be made? Is the goal to alleviate Mr. and Mrs. Cintas's anxiety? Will Mr. Cintas's level of anxiety adversely affect the outcome of the surgery? Will Mr. and Mrs. Cintas be satisfied? Are there other goals?
- Step 3: Identify all alternative actions and the benefits and consequences of each. If you enforce hospital policy, the benefits are that all patients are treated equally and the written policy supports the decision. Possible consequences are that Mr. Cintas's anxiety level increases, perhaps adversely affecting the outcome of his surgery, and Mr. and Mrs. Cintas will not be advocates for the health center. The other alternative is to allow Mrs. Cintas to stay all night. Potential benefits are that Mr. Cintas's level of anxiety will decrease, and Mr. and Mrs. Cintas will be satisfied customers. The consequence is that a precedent is set that may make it difficult to enforce the existing hospital policy.
- Step 4: Decide which action to implement. Consider the two alternatives and the benefits and consequences of each. Then implement the decision.
- Step 5: Evaluate the decision. Was the goal achieved?

From the beginning of their careers, new graduate nurses are faced with the responsibility of making decisions regarding patient centered care. When nurses are faced with a difficult clinical decision, they often benefit by consulting with the inter-professional team as early as possible. These may include other RNs on the unit or supervisors.

Limitations to Effective Decision Making

What are obstacles to effective decision making? Past experiences, values, personal biases, and preconceived ideas affect the way people view problems and situations. DeLaune and Ladner (2011) have identified criteria that may negatively affect the decision-making or problem-solving processes:

- Jumping to conclusions without examining the situation thoroughly
- Failing to obtain all of the necessary information
- Choosing decisions that are too broad, too complicated, or lack definition
- Failing to choose and communicate a rational solution
- Failing to intervene and evaluate the decision or solution appropriately

CRITICAL THINKING

What does it mean to be a critical thinker? Paul (1992) defines **critical thinking** as "thinking about your thinking while you're thinking in order to make your thinking better" (p. 7). Critical thinking applies knowledge and experience to identify patient-centered problems and use clinical judgment resulting in optimal patient outcomes (Benner, Hughes, & Sutphen, 2008).

A good critical thinker is able to examine situations from all sides and make decisions, taking into account research and the best evidence and various points of view. A good critical thinker does not say, "We've always done it this way," and refuse to consider alternate ways. The critical thinker thinks "out of the box" and generates new ideas and alternatives when making decisions. The critical thinker asks "why?" questions about a situation to arrive at the best decision. Four basic skills—critical reading, critical listening, critical writing, and critical speaking—are necessary for the development of critical-thinking skills. These skills are part of the process of developing and using thinking for decision making. Ability in these four areas can be developed by using the universal intellectual standards illustrated in Table 4-3.

As you begin to apply critical thinking to nursing, use these universal intellectual standards when you are reading material from a textbook, listening to an oral presentation, writing a paper, answering test questions, or presenting ideas in oral form. Ask yourself whether the ideas are clear or unclear, precise or imprecise, specific or vague, accurate or inaccurate. Are they relevant or irrelevant, logical or illogical, deep or superficial, complete or incomplete, significant or insignificant, adequate or inadequate, and fair or unfair? You will improve your critical-thinking skills over time with practice.

Reflective Thinking

Pesut and Herman (1999) describe **reflective thinking** as watching or observing ourselves as we perform a task or make a decision about a particular situation. We have two selves, the active self and the reflective self. The reflective self watches the active self as it engages in activities. The reflective self acts as observer and offers suggestions about the activities. To be a good

TABLE 4-3
The Spectrum of Universal Intellectual Standards

Clear	Unclear
Precise	Imprecise
Specific	Vague
Accurate	Inaccurate
Relevant	Irrelevant
Logical	Illogical
Deep	Superficial
Detailed	General
Significant	Insignificant
Adequate	Inadequate
Fair	Unfair

Source: Adapted with permission from the Foundation for Critical Thinking. Please see website: http://www.criticalthinking.org.

CRITICAL THINKING 4-1

Use the decision-making process in Table 4-2 and ask yourself the critical-thinking questions inspired by Table 4-3 when you are making decisions. Have I gathered the best available evidence to help with the decision? Is my information clear or unclear, precise or imprecise, specific or vague, accurate or inaccurate? Is it relevant or irrelevant, logical or illogical, deep or superficial, complete or incomplete, significant or insignificant, adequate or inadequate, and fair or unfair? Apply these critical-thinking questions and review the best available evidence at each step.

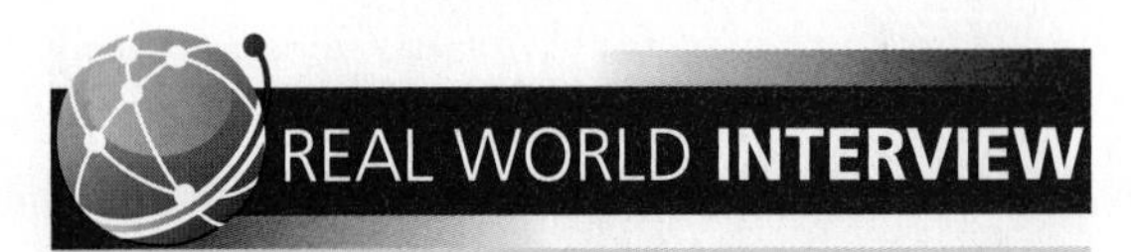

REAL WORLD INTERVIEW

The Computerized Patient Record System (CPRS) is the electronic health record in use at all Department of Veterans Affairs (VA) Medical Centers. CPRS is a computerized program that presents the patient's health data in an organized, user-friendly way to support clinical decision making. CPRS allows VA health care providers to review, document, and update a patient's electronic health record. CPRS includes the ability to place orders for medications, special procedures, X-rays, nursing interventions, consults, diets, laboratory tests, and much more. Clinical staff can also access a veteran's electronic health record at any other VA site across the country within seconds. This ensures that the clinician has access to all clinically relevant data available at VA facilities.

Additional CPRS capabilities include:

A check system for ordering that alerts clinicians when a possible problem could exist when an order is placed; these include clinical events such as duplicate drug orders and critical drug interactions, or when the patient's allergy assessment has not been documented.

A notification system alerts clinicians about clinically significant events such as critical lab values or abnormal imaging results.

A patient posting system, displayed on every CPRS screen, that shows significant information related specifically to each individual patient. This includes crisis notes that make staff aware of any precarious situations involving the patient, and clinical warnings, such as suicide ideation or isolation precautions. The posting system also displays patient-specific adverse drug reactions and advance directive information.

A clinical reminder system that allows clinicians to track and improve preventive health care for patients and ensure timely clinical interventions, such as reminding clinicians that their diabetic patient is due for an annual eye exam or that their patient is due for a colon cancer screening.

VistA Imaging provides access to medical images, including X-rays, scanned documents, exam results, photos, endoscopies, and so forth.

(Continues)

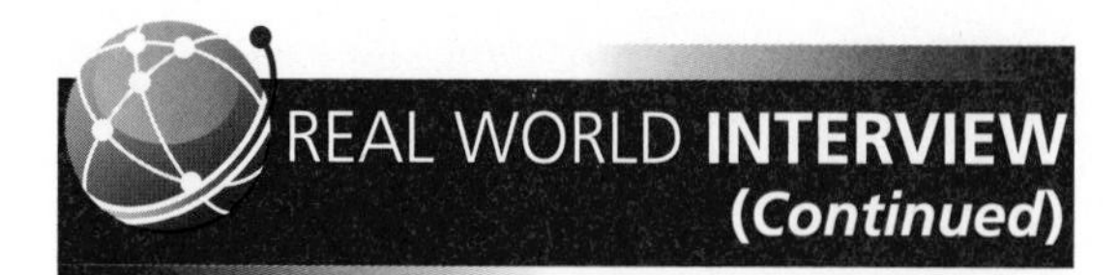

A Bar Code Medication Administration (BCMA) system that electronically validates and documents the administration of inpatient medications to ensure that the right patient receives the right medication in the right dose, at the right time, via the right route; BCMA will alert the staff nurse if all of these are not correct.

The VistA software is available to the public under a law called the Freedom of Information Act (FOIA). For more information, log on to http://www.hardhats.org/foia.html.

Laurie Blum-Eisa, RN

CPRS Clinical Applications Coordinator

Jesse Brown VA Medical Center

Chicago, Illinois

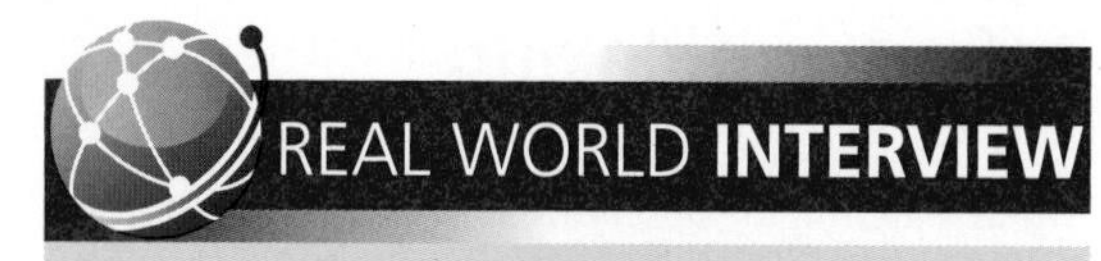

I was in a situation where I just didn't think my patient looked good. I decided to go ahead and start two new IV sites, just in case. The patient arrested two hours later, and we really needed those IV sites. I felt good about my decision.

CHERYL BUNTZ, RN

New Graduate

Independence, Missouri

critical thinker, one must practice reflective thinking. Reflection upon a situation or problem after a decision is made allows the individual to evaluate the decision. Students can become better reflective thinkers through the use of clinical journals. In the clinical setting, debriefing is often used to promote reflective thinking after a situation, such as cardiac arrest. It allows team members to analyze the situation and see what was

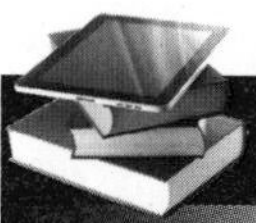

EVIDENCE FROM THE **LITERATURE**

Citation: Henneman, E. A., Cunningham, H., Roche, J. P., & Curnin, M. E. (2007). Human patient simulation: Teaching students to provide safe care. *Nurse Educator, 32*(5), 212–217.

Discussion: The use of human patient simulation as a teaching methodology for nursing students has become popular. It effectively demands paying careful attention to the details of the simulation, debriefing staff after use, and employing good evaluation processes. Our experience in designing simulation experiences and evaluating student behaviors confirms the resource-intensive nature of human patient simulation and the need for clear, measurable objectives. When used properly, human patient simulation offers a unique opportunity to teach nursing students important patient safety principles and strengthen teamwork. For example, one simulator model allows the insertion of a chest tube or the application of a trauma or wound care kit. Such features support educators' abilities to create learning situations that address a variety of specific clinical problems or needs. Human patient simulation can also provide clinicians an opportunity to care for a simulated patient with other acute clinical problems, such as airway obstruction, cardiac arrest, hemorrhage, or shock.

Implications for Practice: Working with patient simulators allows students to solve problems, utilize teamwork, and communicate effectively with the inter-professional team. Role-playing provides an opportunity to practice teamwork and collaboration, improve communication, and enhance patient safety. By integrating concepts related to patient safety—such as human factors engineering, staff management, and situational awareness—participants learn approaches and concepts related to patient safety and develop clinical skills that reduce the potential for errors. Patient safety and avoidable medical errors are a concern in any institution. The Institute of Medicine report *To Err Is Human: Building a Safer Health System* recommends simulation training as one strategy to prevent errors in the clinical setting.

done correctly and what could be improved to ultimately improve care and patient outcomes.

Intuitive Thinking and Problem Solving

Intuition and **intuitive thinking** are described as an innate feeling that nurses develop that helps them to act in certain situations (Gardner, 2003). It has also been described as a "gut" feeling that something is wrong. Intuitive thinking may result from unconscious assessment and analysis of data based on an individual's past experience. Nurses may make decisions about patient care based, in part, on intuitive thinking. This may seem contrary to using the logical, evidenced-based practice with reasoning that is so prevalent in nursing literature. Intuition guides expert nurses to use a small amount of clinical information and arrive at a conclusion drawing from the ability to recognize patterns and themes from past experiences in a very short time period.

Pretz and Folse (2011) studied intuition in nursing and found more experienced nurses reported using intuition than those with little experience. Benner et al. (2009) support this by saying, "intuition constitutes a significant part of everyday practice of expert nurses" (p. 210).

Problem solving is an active process that starts with a problem and ends with a solution. Nurses address multiple needs and problems of patients on an hourly basis. Some problems are uncomplicated and require one simple solution. Other problems may be complex and require more analysis by the nurse.

DECISION-MAKING TOOLS AND TECHNOLOGY

Sometimes, when a decision is made, the outcome is certain. Other times, a nurse will need to make a decision without having all of the information needed to ensure a good outcome. Decision making in both certain and uncertain times can be improved by using various tools. Figure 4-2 shows a decision-analysis tree for choosing whether to go back to school. See Figure 4-3 for a decision-analysis tree for a patient who smokes.

A decision-making grid may help to separate the multiple factors that surround a situation. Figure 4-4 illustrates use of a decision-making grid by a unit that was told it had to reduce the workforce by two full-time equivalents (FTEs). This grid is useful in this example to visually separate the factors of cost savings, effect on job satisfaction of remaining staff, and effect on patient satisfaction.

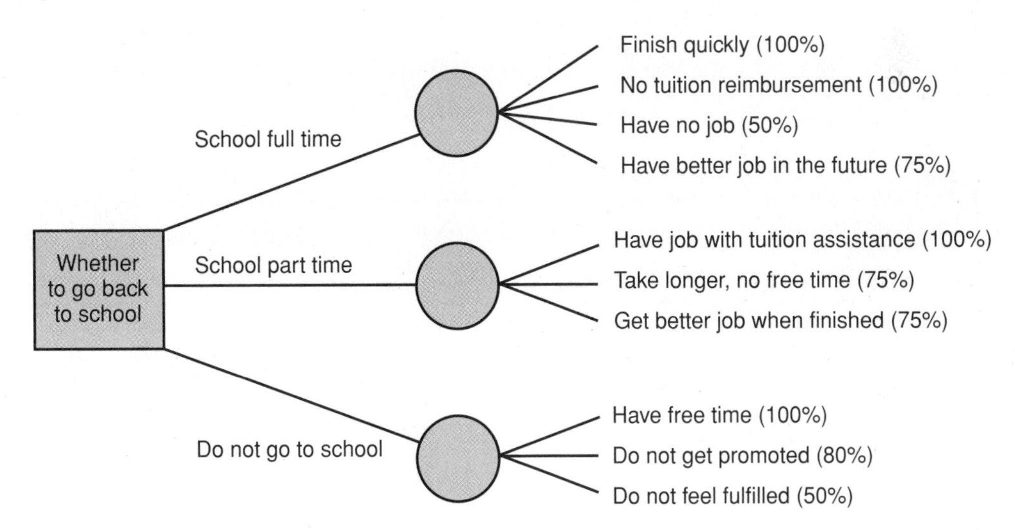

FIGURE 4-2

Decision tree for choosing whether to go back to school.

© Cengage Learning 2014

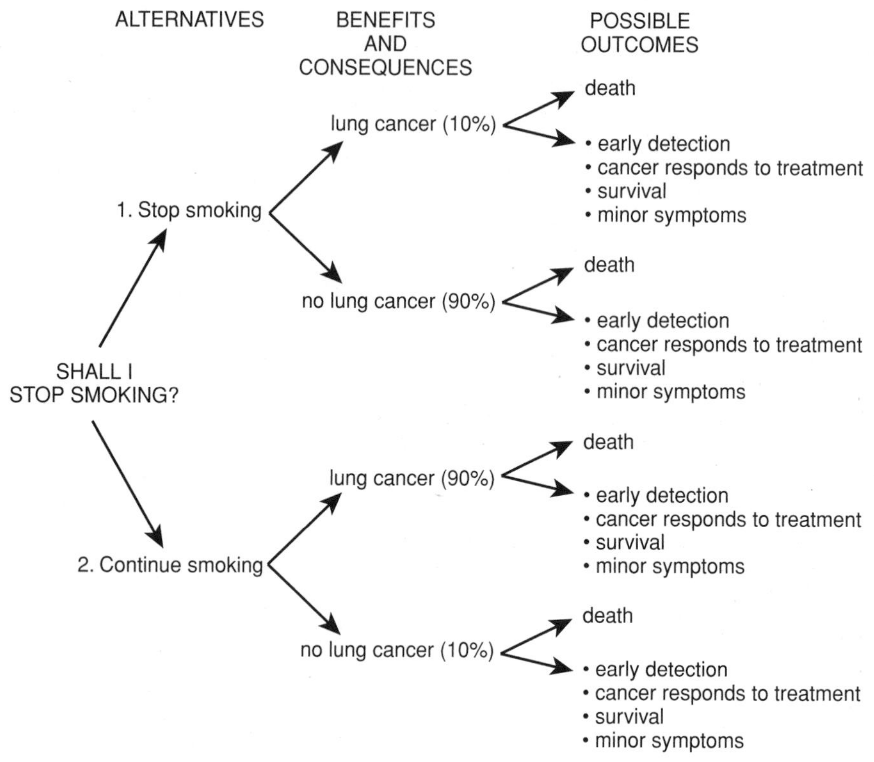

FIGURE 4-3

Decision-analysis tree for a patient who smokes.

© Cengage Learning 2014

Methods of Reduction	Cost Savings	Effect on Job Satisfaction	Effect on Patient Satisfaction
Lay off the two most senior full-time employees	$93,500	Significant reduction	Significant reduction
Lay off the two most recently hired full-time employees	$63,200	Significant reduction	Moderate reduction
Reduce by staff attrition	$78,000	Minor reduction	Minor reduction

FIGURE 4-4

Sample decision-making grid.

© Cengage Learning 2014

A decision-making grid is also useful when a nurse is trying to decide between two choices. Figure 4-5 is an example of a decision-making grid used by a nurse deciding between working at hospital A or hospital B.

The Program Evaluation and Review Technique (PERT) is useful in determining timing of decisions. The PERT flowchart provides a visual picture depicting the sequence of tasks that must take place to complete a project. Jones and Beck

Elements	Importance Score (out of 10)	Likelihood Score (out of 10)	Risk (multiply scores)
Work at hospital A			
Learning experience	10	10	100
Good mentor support	8	8	64
Financial reward	6	6	36
Growth potential	8	8	64
Good location	10	10	100
Total			364
Work at hospital B			
Learning experience	8	8	64
Good mentor support	7	7	49
Financial reward	8	8	64
Growth potential	9	9	81
Good location	6	6	36
Total			294

FIGURE 4-5

Sample decision-making grid for employment choices.

© Cengage Learning 2014

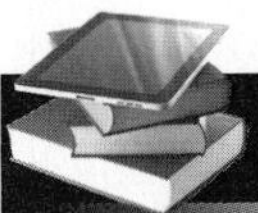

EVIDENCE FROM THE **LITERATURE**

Citation: Fineout-Overholt, E., Mazurek Melynk, B., Stillwell, S. B., & Williamson, K. M. (2010, March). Evidence-Based practice step by step: Implementing an evidence-based practice change. *American Journal of Nursing. 111*(3):54–60.

Discussion: This is the ninth article in a series of articles that began in November 2009 from the Arizona State University College of Nursing and Health Innovation's Center for the Advancement of Evidence-Based Practice. Evidence-based practice (EBP) is a problem-solving approach to the delivery of health care that integrates the best evidence from studies and patient care data with clinician expertise and patient preferences and values. When delivered in a context of caring and in a supportive organizational culture, the highest quality of care and best patient outcomes can be achieved. The purpose of this series is to give nurses the knowledge and skills they need to implement EBP consistently, one step at a time. Articles appear every other month to allow time to incorporate information as readers work toward implementing EBP at their institutions. Also, the authors have scheduled "Chat with the Authors" calls every few months to provide a direct line to the experts to help readers resolve questions.

Implications for Practice: Practicing nurses, nursing faculty, and students will want to review this series of articles that reviews various elements of EBP (e.g., use of PICO, rapid critical appraisal of research). The articles can assist in planning continuing education opportunities and in designing nursing curricula that prepare nurses for use of EBP and twenty-first century professional practice.

(1996) provide an example of a PERT flow diagram depicting from beginning to end an implementation of case management (Figure 4-6). The chart shows the amount of time required to complete the project and the sequence of events necessary to complete the project. A Gantt chart (Figure 4-7) can also be useful for decision makers to illustrate a project from beginning to end.

The vice president for nursing plans to change all units to include case managers. She believes that this can be accomplished within a year and a half. In order for this to be achieved, the following activities and events have to occur:

Activity Symbol	Activity Descriptions	Immediate Predecessor
A.	Form a multidisciplinary advisory group	None
B.	Agree upon definitions	A
C.	Notify members of subcommittees	B
D.	Write job descriptions	C
E.	Advertise for candidates for case manager	D
F.	Review qualifications of candidates	E
G.	Select candidates for case manager	F
H.	Review patient charts	None
I.	Write patient care maps	H
J.	Meet with case managers	None
K.	Orient case managers	J
L.	Orient unit and hospital staff	K
M.	Utilize case management process	L

Events

1.	Project begins
2.	Meeting of multidisciplinary committee
3.	Formation of subcommittees
4.	Subcommittee for description meets
5.	Subcommittee for patient care maps meets
6.	Candidates for case managers are interviewed
7.	Candidates are hired
8.	Subcommittee for patient care maps meets to finalize maps
9.	Orientation begins
10.	Implementation begins
11.	Project is evaluated

Expected Time Calculations

Activity	*Duration*
A	0.5 month
B	1 month
C	0.5 month
D	1 month
E	1 month
F	2 months
G	1 month
H	1 month
I	2 months
J	1 month
K&L	1 month
M	3 months

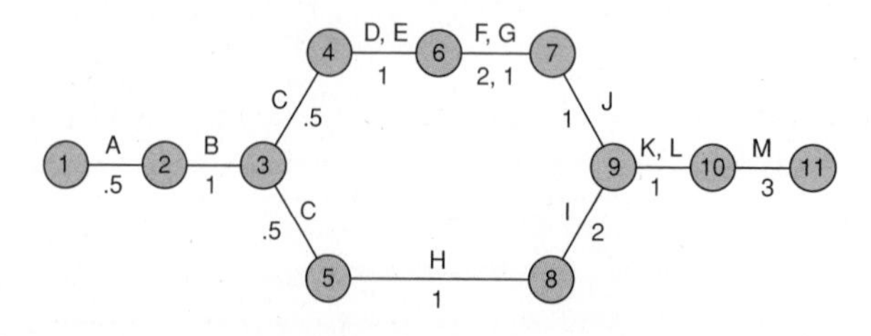

FIGURE 4-6

PERT diagram with critical path for implementation of case management.

© Cengage Learning 2014

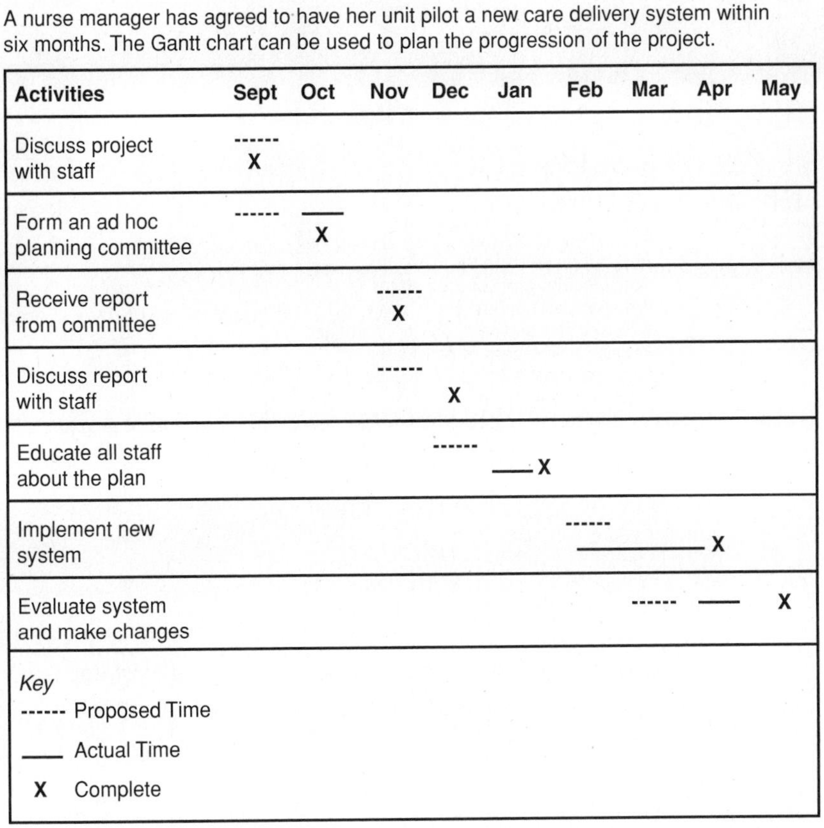

A nurse manager has agreed to have her unit pilot a new care delivery system within six months. The Gantt chart can be used to plan the progression of the project.

Activities	Sept	Oct	Nov	Dec	Jan	Feb	Mar	Apr	May
Discuss project with staff	------ X								
Form an ad hoc planning committee	------	—— X							
Receive report from committee			------ X						
Discuss report with staff			------	X					
Educate all staff about the plan				------	—— X				
Implement new system						------ ——	——	—— X	
Evaluate system and make changes							------	——	X

Key
------ Proposed Time
—— Actual Time
X Complete

FIGURE 4-7
Gantt chart: Implementation of care delivery system.
© Cengage Learning 2014

Dos and Don'ts of Decision Making

A foundation for good decision making comes with experience and learning from those experiences. Table 4-4 gives the student some additional tips to consider when making decisions.

GROUP DECISION MAKING

Certain situations may call for group decision making. A group may offer innovative alternatives and decisions and afford some protection from mistakes because it uses the combined knowledge of all its members. Today's leadership and management styles include people in the decision-making process who will be most affected by the decision. The effectiveness of a group depends greatly on the group's members. The size of the group and the personalities of group members are important considerations when choosing participants. More ideas can be generated with groups, thus allowing for more communication and more choices. This increases the likelihood of higher-quality outcomes.

A major disadvantage of group decision making is the time involved. Without effective leadership, groups can waste time and be nonproductive. Group decision making can be more costly and it can also lead to conflict. Groups can be dominated by one person or become the battleground for a power struggle among assertive members.

TABLE 4-4
Dos and Don'ts of Decision Making

DO	DON'T
Identify why the decision needs to be made.	Feel pressure to make a decision too quickly.
Gather all information necessary to make the decision.	Doubt your ability to make a decision.
Consider all the possible outcomes.	Procrastinate; delaying choices can have negative implications.
	Make a decision purely by your emotions.

Source: Adapted from Yao, B. H. (2010). The dos and don'ts of successful decision making. *Ezine@rticles.* Retrieved September 29, 2011, from http://ezinearticles.com/? The-dos-and-donts-of-successful-decision-making&id=4873870

TABLE 4-5
Individual Versus Group Decision Making

1. Does the individual have all the information and resources needed to make the best decision?
2. Does the group have supplementary information needed to make the best decision?
3. Will individual personalities within the group work well together?
4. Is it absolutely critical that the group be involved in the decision and accept the decision prior to implementation?
5. Will the group accept a decision made by an individual? By the group?
6. Is there time for a group decision?
7. Will the course of action chosen make a difference to the organization?
8. Do the group and individuals have the best interest of the organization foremost in mind when considering the decision?
9. Will the decision cause undue conflict within the group?

Source: Adapted from Vroom, V., & Yetton, P. (1973). *Leadership and Decision Making* (pp. 21–30). Pittsburgh, PA: University of Pittsburgh Press.

Group decision making may, however, increase the acceptance of the decision by all members. Vroom and Yetton (1973) identified elements individuals should consider before making a decision alone or with a group. See Table 4-5.

Techniques of Group Decision Making

There are various techniques of group decision making. The *nominal group technique, Delphi technique,* and *consensus building* are different methods to facilitate group decision making.

Nominal Group Technique

The nominal group technique was developed by Delbecq, Van de Ven, and Gustafson in 1971. The word *nominal* refers to the nonverbal aspect of this approach. In the first step, there is no discussion; group members write out their ideas or responses to the identified issue or question posed by the group leader. The second step involves presentation of the ideas to the group members, along with the advantages and disadvantages of each. These ideas are presented on a chart or using available technology. The third phase offers an opportunity for discussion to clarify and evaluate the ideas. The fourth phase includes private voting on the ideas. The ideas receiving the highest number of votes are the solutions implemented.

Delphi Group Technique

The Delphi technique differs from the nominal technique in that group members are not meeting face to face. Questionnaires are distributed to group members for their opinions, and the responses are then summarized and disseminated to the group members. This process continues for as many times as necessary for the group members to reach consensus. An advantage of this technique is that it can involve a large number of participants and thus a greater number of ideas.

Consensus Building

Consensus is defined by the Merriam-Webster's Online Dictionary (2011) as "a general agreement; the judgment arrived at by most of those concerned." A common misconception is that consensus means everyone agrees with the decision 100 percent. Contrary to this misunderstanding, **consensus** means that all group members can live with and fully support the decision regardless of whether they totally agree. Building consensus is useful with groups because all group members participate and can realize the contributions each member makes to the decision. A disadvantage to the consensus strategy is that decision making requires more time.

CASE STUDY 4-1

You have been working on a medical-surgical unit. As you complete your nursing program, you begin to interview at several hospitals.

Set up a decision-making grid to help you analyze your choices. What factors are most important to you as you begin to consider your decision? Use Figure 4-5.

USE OF TECHNOLOGY IN DECISION MAKING

The best source of clinical decision making and judgment is the professional practitioner. However, computer technology offers many ways to record and retrieve information to support the evidence-based needs and actions of nurses.

These include:

- Electronic health records
- Patient-decision support tools, clinical- and business-related
- Laboratory and X-ray results, reporting and viewing systems
- Computerized prescribing and order entry, including barcoding
- Community and population health management and information
- Communication, patient classification staffing systems, and administrative systems
- Evidence-based practice and information retrieval systems
- Quality improvement data collection/data summary systems
- Documentation and care planning
- Patient monitoring and problem alerts
- Inventory control

A specific example of how technology is attempting to improve safety and quality in the hospital setting is by the use of the HyGreen™ system to improve hand-hygiene compliance. This technology uses sensors on name badges to record when health care personnel wash their hands using sanitizer solution outside the patient room. Once in the patient room, another sensor detects if the person has used sanitizer and indicates that by a green light. If the person has not used sanitizer, the badge will vibrate to remind the person to sanitize before touching the patient (see http://www.hygreeninc.com/solution/).

Simulation

Simulation is a safe, nonthreatening way to hone critical thinking and clinical decision-making skills. Simulation is widely used in the academic setting and is being used more frequently in the hospital setting.

In the Institute of Medicine (IOM) report *To Err is Human: Building a Safer Health Care System* (Kohn, Corrigan, & Donaldson, 2000), simulation training is recommended as one strategy that can be used to prevent errors in the clinical setting. The report states that "health care organizations and teaching institutions should participate in the development and use of simulation for training novice practitioners, problem solving, and crisis management, especially when new and potentially hazardous procedures and equipment are introduced" (p. 179). The use of simulation as a teaching strategy can contribute to patient safety and optimize outcomes of care, providing learners with opportunities to experience scenarios and intervene in clinical situations within a safe, supervised setting without posing a risk to a patient (Durham & Alden, 2008).

Simulation promotes teamwork, effective communication, develops critical thinking and clinical decision-making skills. Simulation is utilized for staff development while introducing new equipment or protocols to give nurses a safe way to practice skills until proficient (Durham & Alden, 2008). Reflection is used as part of simulation and is an effective tool to objectively review situations, actions, communication, and outcomes. It is a nonthreatening way to further critical-thinking skills without the potential for patient harm.

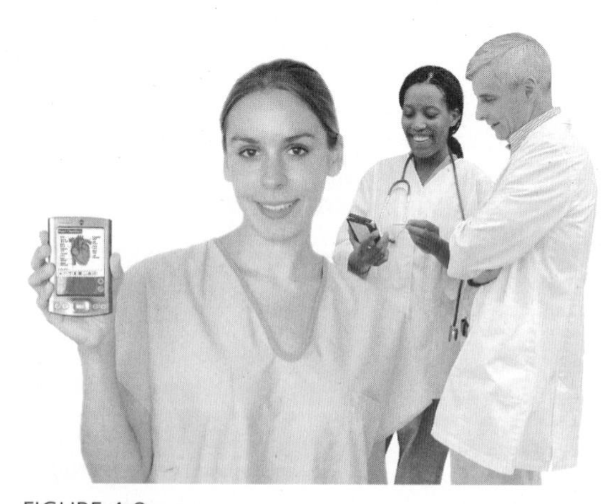

FIGURE 4-8

Nurse with a PDA.

(*Source:* Courtesy PEPID, Heather Hautman)

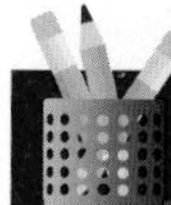

CASE STUDY **4-2**

You have been hired in a large teaching hospital with state-of-the-art technology in all realms of care. As a beginning professional nurse, how will technology influence the care you provide?

What types of technology will you have to master during your orientation to independently provide care?

What resources are available to you?

Joint Commission National Patient Safety Goals

Several other forces have highlighted the need for increased patient technology. The Joint Commission (JC) has set National Patient Safety Goals for 2011, many of which require the use of technology, including:

- Eliminate transfusion errors related to patient misidentification
- Use a two-person verification process or a one-person verification process accompanied by automated identification technology, such as bar coding
- Reduce the likelihood of patient harm associated with the use of anticoagulant therapy when heparin is administered intravenously and continuously; use programmable pumps in order to provide consistent and accurate dosing
- Implement evidence-based practices to prevent health care-associated infections due to multidrug-resistant organisms in acute care hospitals
- Conduct periodic risk assessments (in time frames defined by the hospital) for multidrug-resistant organism acquisition and transmission
- Implement a surveillance program for multidrug-resistant organisms based on the risk assessment
- Measure and monitor multidrug-resistant organism prevention processes and outcomes, including the following:
  - Multidrug-resistant organism infection rates using evidence-based metrics

- Compliance with evidence-based guidelines or best practices
- Evaluation of the education program provided to staff and licensed independent practitioners
- Implement evidence-based practices to prevent central line-associated bloodstream infections
- Conduct periodic risk assessments for central line-associated bloodstream infections, monitor compliance with evidence-based practices, and evaluate the effectiveness of prevention efforts (The risk assessments are conducted in time frames defined by the hospital, and this infection surveillance activity is hospital-wide, not targeted.)
- Provide central line-associated bloodstream infection rate data and prevention outcome measures to key stakeholders, including leaders, licensed independent practitioners, nursing staff, and other clinicians
- Use a catheter checklist and a standardized protocol for central venous catheter insertion
- Implement evidence-based practices for preventing surgical site infections

As part of the effort to reduce surgical site infections:

- Conduct periodic risk assessments for surgical site infections in a time frame determined by the hospital
- Select surgical site infection measures using best practices or evidence-based guidelines
- Monitor compliance with best practices or evidence-based guidelines
- Evaluate the effectiveness of prevention efforts
- Measure surgical site infection rates for the first 30 days following procedures that do not involve inserting implantable devices and for the first year following procedures involving implantable devices (The hospital's measurement strategies follow evidence-based guidelines.)
- Provide process and outcome (e.g., surgical site infection rate) measure results to key stakeholders (www.joint-commission.org. Click on *National Patient Safety Goals*)

Attainment of these goals requires the consistent use of technology.

Leapfrog Group

The Leapfrog Group is another force advocating for technology. Leapfrog is a voluntary program aimed at using employer purchasing power to alert America's health industry that big leaps in health care safety, quality, and customer value will be recognized and rewarded. Among other initiatives, Leapfrog works with its employer members to encourage transparency and easy access to health care information, as well as rewards for hospitals that have a proven record of high quality care. Leapfrog measures how hospitals are doing with multiple indicators, including:

- Computerized practitioner order entry (CPOE) into computers linked to error-prevention software
- Evidence-based hospital performance on five high-risk procedures and care for two high-risk neonatal conditions
- Progress on National Quality Forum Safe Practices *Source:* http://www.leapfroggroup.org. Data support services are offered to Leapfrog by Thomson Medstat (see www.medstat.com).

The Department of Health and Human Services is requiring mandatory reporting of preventable infection data starting in 2010 for all hospitals that participate in the Centers for Medicare and Medicaid Services (CMS) pay-for-reporting program. Tracking, reporting multiple safety indicators, and making the information available are becoming the new norm for hospitals because of the availability of the technology to track, increased consumer demand, and payment concerns.

The National Quality Forum

The National Quality Forum (NQF) is a not-for-profit membership organization created to develop and implement a national strategy for health care quality measurement and reporting. The NQF believes that attaining quality is a three-step process. The first step is to define quality with uniform standards and measures that apply to the many facets of patient care. The second step is to report findings and see where patient care falls short. Lastly is the examination of the information and use of it to improve care (National Quality Forum, 2011).

The NQF formed a National Priority Partnership and published a report in 2010 that identified eight priorities with the greatest potential to eradicate disparities, reduce harm, and remove waste from the American health care system:

- Patient and family engagement
- Safety
- Care coordination
- Palliative and end-of-life care
- Equitable access
- Elimination of overuse
- Population health
- Infrastructure supports

A shared sense of urgency about the impact of health care quality on patient outcomes, workforce productivity, and health care costs has prompted leaders in the public and private sectors to create the NQF as a mechanism to bring about national change.

The Specialty of Nursing Informatics

The Americans Nurses Association Nursing Informatics has been recognized as a specialty for RNs since 1992.

Several nursing and health informatics scholarly journals, such as *Computers, Informatics, and Nursing* (www.cinjournal.com) and *Journal of the Medical Informatics Association* (www.jamia.org), provide essential nursing informatics education. The American Nurses Credentialing Center (ANCC) offers certification examinations for a variety of specialties in nursing, including informatics (www.nursingworld.org/ancc).

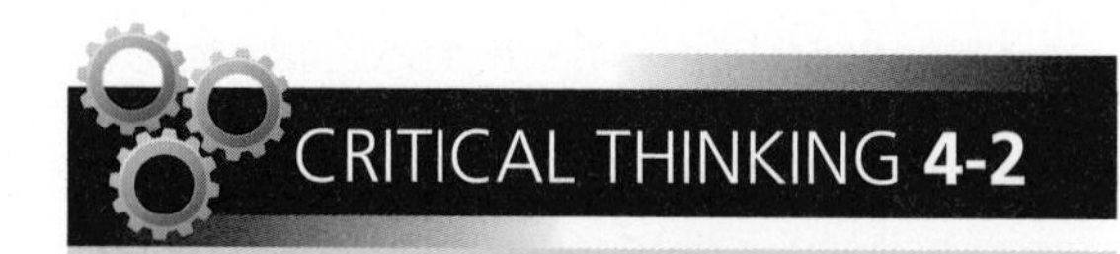

CRITICAL THINKING **4-2**

Visit the American Nurses Credentialing Center at www.nursingworld.org. Click on "careers and credentialing/certification." Choose a specialty in which a nurse can be certified and compare it to the certification in informatics. How are they similar? How are they different?

The definition of **nursing informatics** agreed upon by the International Medical Informatics Association–Nursing Informatics (IMIA-NI), Special Interest Group, at their General Assembly in Stockholm in 1997 (amended for clarity in Seoul, 1998), is: the integration of nursing, its information, and information management with information processing and communication technology to support the health of people worldwide. The focus of IMIA is to foster collaboration among nurses and others who are interested in nursing informatics (www.imia.org) (Jones & Nicoll, 2012). Some common elements of nursing informatics (NI) include the following (DeLaune & Ladner, 2011):

- Computerized order entry
- Electronic health records
- Patient-decision support tools, clinical and business related

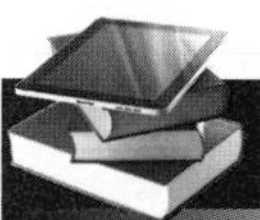

EVIDENCE FROM THE **LITERATURE**

Citation: Kelley, T. F., Brandon, D. H., & Docherty, S. L. (2011). Electronic nursing documentation as a strategy to improve quality of patient care. *Journal of Nursing Scholarship, 43*, 154–162. doi: 10.1111/j.1547-5069.2011.01397.x

Discussion: This integrative review of the literature examined the relationship between nurses' electronic documentation and the quality of care given to hospitalized patients. Most U.S. hospitals are currently switching from paper-based to electronic documentation, anticipating improved quality. The extent to which nurses' electronic documentation improves the quality of care to hospitalized patients remains unknown because of the lack of effective comparisons with nurses' paper-based documentation.

Implications for Practice: Future research needs to investigate the day-to-day relationship between nurses' electronic documentation and the quality of care provided to patients in the hospital.

- Laboratory and X-ray results, reporting as well as picture retrieval and viewing systems
- Electronic prescribing, order entry, and medication administration systems including barcoding
- Community and population health management and information
- Communication using Internet, intranet, and e-mail; staffing; and administrative systems, e.g., billing
- Evidence-based knowledge and information-retrieval systems with access to remote library and Internet resources
- Quality improvement of data-collection and data-summary systems, and of business intelligence
- Documentation and care planning
- Putting patient monitoring for vital signs and other measurements directly into the patient's record
- Problem alerts for vital signs and other measurements
- Electronic bed boards to review bed status and availability
- Data-mining techniques for sifting through large amounts of data to discover knowledge
- Disease surveillance systems
- Web pages to personalize information
- Computer-generated nursing care plans, critical pathways, and patient documentation, such as discharge instructions and medication information.
- Access to computer-archived patient data from previous patient encounters
- Collaboration with patients, other nurses, and health care providers

Nursing informatics continues to grow in need and broaden in scope.

The TIGER Initiative and Quality and Safety Education for Nurses (QSEN)

The Technology Informatics Guiding Educational Reform (TIGER) Initiative aims to enable practicing nurses and nursing students to fully engage in the unfolding electronic era in health care. The TIGER Initiative is working to catalyze a dynamic, sustainable, and productive relationship between the Alliance for Nursing Informatics (ANI), with its 20 nursing informatics professional societies, and the major nursing organizations including the American Nurses Association (ANA), the Association of Nurse Executives (AONE), the American Association of Colleges of Nursing (AACN), and others which collectively represent over 2,000,000 nurses (TIGER, 2009). The TIGER Initiative is focused on using informatics tools, principles, theories, and practices to enable nurses to make health care safer, more effective, efficient, patient centered, timely, and equitable (TIGER, 2009). Collaborative teams have researched best practices from both nursing education and practice within nine key topic areas, so that this knowledge can be shared through information technology. The nine topic areas are:

- Standards and interoperability
- National health information technology (IT) agenda
- Informatics competencies
- Education and faculty development
- Staff development
- Usability and clinical application design
- Virtual demonstration center
- Leadership development
- Consumer empowerment and personal health records

(*Source:* Technology Informatics Guiding Education Reform [TIGER], 2009. Nursing informatics competencies are available on the TIGER website and the Quality and Safety Education for Nurses website [http://www.qsen.org].)

QSEN is a comprehensive resource for quality and safety education for nurses. This website is a place to learn and share ideas about educational strategies that promote quality and safety competency development in nursing (Jones & Nicoll, 2012).

Relevant Technology Used in Health Care Today

Nurses are not immune to the changes that computers are bringing to both everyday life and nursing practice. By 2015, use of a certified electronic health record (EHR) is mandated under the Health Information Technology for Economic and Clinical Health (HITECH) Act (CMS, 2010). HITECH created new

Medicare and Medicaid incentive payment programs totaling as much as $27 billion to help eligible physicians, other professionals, and hospitals as they transition from paper-based medical records to EHRs. The Medicare and Medicaid EHR Incentive Programs provide a financial incentive to health care providers for the "meaningful use" of certified EHR technology to achieve health and efficiency goals. By putting into action and meaningfully using an EHR system, providers need to show they are using certified EHR technology in ways that can be measured significantly in quality and in quantity, for example, to improve the quality of health care and/or to submit information about clinical quality and other measures. Providers will reap benefits beyond financial incentives such as a reduction in errors, improved availability of records and data, increased clinical reminders and alerts, support for clinical decisions, and increased use of e-prescribing/refill automation (Jones & Nicoll, 2012). To demonstrate meaningful use successfully, eligible professionals and hospitals are required to report information about clinical quality measures specific to them (CMS, 2010). Providers who do not meet the requirements and become "meaningful users" of EHR by 2015 will have their reimbursement reduced (CMS, 2010). EHR can provide many benefits for providers and patients with more complete and accurate health information and better access to the EMR. As professionals, information technology can help achieve the goals of quality patient-centered care and increased patient safety (Jones & Nicoll, 2012). To clarify the terminology, electronic medical records (EMRs) are the computerized, legal, clinical records created in hospitals and physicians' offices. Essentially, the EMR is the legal record of what happened to the patient in these environments. Electronic health records (EHRs) comprise data summaries of the EMR that are shared between different stakeholders including the government and the patients themselves. Often these terms are used interchangeably. The CMS (2011) clarifies that it uses the term EHR and provides payment only to hospitals that use certified EHR technology. In the United States, EHRs will ride on the proposed National Health Information Network.

The National Quality Forum created the Quality Data Model (QDM), an "information model," that clearly defines concepts used in quality measures and clinical care that are related to the automation of EHR use. It provides a way to describe or define clinical concepts in a standardized format, so those monitoring clinical performance and outcomes can clearly communicate information. The QDM provides the potential for more precisely defined, universally adopted, electronic quality measures to automate measurement and compare and improve quality using electronic health information. Use of the QDM will enable more standardized, less burdensome quality measurement and reporting and more consistent use and communication of EHRs for direct patient care. In addition to enabling comparisons across performance measures, the QDM can promote delivery of more appropriate, consistent, and evidence-based care through clinical decision support applications (National Quality Forum, 2011).

The Veterans Affairs Department is currently using Veterans Health Information Systems and Technology Architecture (VistA), supporting more than 150 hospitals and 887 ambulatory care facilities (Lipowicz, 2011). VistA is considered a world-class electronic health record system, yet the Veterans Affairs Department is currently in the process to update and modernize the system.

The Healthcare Information and Management Systems Society (HIMSS) (2008) published information of the use of EHRs in Germany, the Netherlands, Greece, England, Wales, Denmark, Norway, India, New Zealand, Malaysia, Hong Kong, Singapore, Israel, Canada, and the United States. It appears that all countries are aware of the importance of EHRs and the potential of global EHR integration. Problems that arise include the differences in each countries' healthcare system, the national EHR status, the approach, the type of government, and the technology resources (HIMSS, 2008). Some countries, like Canada, are clearly ahead of the United States, and approximately 50 percent of Canadians have EHRs available to authorized professionals who provide care. Other countries, such as India, though technologically savvy, do not have a mandatory, comprehensive EHR plan in place yet.

Nurses in hospitals and clinics document nursing care and patient data in the EHR. The main purpose of documentation is facilitating information flow that supports safety, quality, and continuity of care (Keenan et al., 2008). Computerized charting strives to streamline the documentation process, ensure that quality matters are tracked and safe care is provided. There does not appear to be any data to support the accuracy of electronic charting, nor that what is charted has been clinically completed. Checking a box requires little effort, while providing patient care does.

Whether you are a nursing student learning a clinical procedure using a computer-based instruction program; a nurse on the floor using electronic devices such as ventilators, intravenous pumps, telemetry, and the electronic health record; a nursing administrator using a spreadsheet and database to plan a budget; or a nursing researcher or clinician keeping updated with the latest evidence-based nursing care, it is evident that information technology has become an essential part of professional nursing practice, both on the individual and institutional levels (Jones & Nicoll, 2012).

Electronic health record systems provide better protection of confidential health information than do paper-based systems, because they have controls to ensure that only authorized users with legitimate uses have access to health information. Security functions address the confidentiality of private health information and the integrity of the data. Security functions must be designed to ensure compliance with applicable laws, regulations, and standards. Security systems and users must ensure that access to data is provided only to those who are authorized and have a legitimate purpose for using the data and must provide a means to detect inappropriate access. Importantly for staff nurses, nurses should access information only for patients they are actively caring for. Nurses looking up information on any patient not in their care or allowing another member of the health care team to look up patient information can be considered a breach of security. One should always log off when walking away from the computer to avoid potential security breaches. Three important terms are used when discussing security: privacy, confidentiality, and security. It is important to understand the differences among these concepts (Jones & Nicoll, 2012):

- *Privacy* refers to the right of individuals to keep information about themselves from being disclosed to anyone. If a patient had an abortion and chose not to tell a health care provider this fact, the patient would be keeping that information private.
- *Confidentiality* refers to the act of limiting disclosure of private matters. After a patient has disclosed private information to a health care provider, the provider has a responsibility to maintain the confidentiality of that information.
- *Security* refers to the means of controlling access and protecting information from accidental or intentional disclosure to unauthorized persons and from alteration, destruction, or loss. When private information is placed in a confidential EHR, the system must have controls in place to maintain the security of the system and not allow unauthorized persons access to the data.

A forgotten aspect of security that should be considered is disaster planning. Natural disasters, such as earthquakes and floods, as well as man-made disasters, like broad attacks on an individual

CRITICAL THINKING **4-3**

Go to http://www.qsen.org. Look for the "informatics" section in Quality/Safety Competencies. Then, look for the Website Evaluation Exercise. Identify the learning needs of a patient to whom you are assigned. Search for websites that address these learning needs. Use either of the two resources listed under Strategy Overview, in the Website Evaluation Exercise. Evaluate the quality of the websites. Complete the Web evaluation form (pdf) at the site (Day & Smith, 2007). Compile a list of high-quality websites that can be shared with nurses on the unit. In discussion with the patient and family, present the information you have found and describe the evaluation criteria that should be used when searching for health information on the Internet.

company, on a network, or on the nation's Internet infrastructure, may also impact the security of mobile health devices and the systems that run them (Jones & Nicoll, 2012). Portable devices are particularly at risk, being small and easy to steal or lose. A back-up plan for documentation should be in place at all facilities in case of an emergency as well as a mechanism for reporting a stolen or lost device.

The P-F-A Assessment

One strategy to search the Internet that can be utilized by health care workers and taught to patients and families is to conduct a "purpose-focus-approach" (P-F-A) assessment. To determine your purpose, ask yourself why you are doing the search and why you need the information. Consider questions such as the following:

- Is it for personal interest?
- Do you want to obtain information to share with coworkers or a patient?
- Are you verifying information given to you by someone else?
- Are you preparing information to give to patients or families?

Based on the purpose, the focus may be as follows:

- Broad and general (basic information for yourself)
- Lay-oriented (to give information to a patient) or professionally oriented (for colleagues)
- Narrow and technical with a research orientation (Nicoll, 2003)

Information literacy is a necessary skill for extracting evidence from research and practice resulting in evidence-based practice (EBP). EBP is the process of systematically finding, appraising, and using contemporaneous research findings as the basis for clinical decisions. Evidence-based health care asks questions, finds and appraises the relevance based on accurate analysis of current nursing knowledge and practice, and harnesses that information for everyday clinical practice. The primary sources for this type of information are Web-based resources such as online databases (e.g., Medline, CINAHL) (Jones & Nicoll, 2012) (see Table 4-6). To search the evidence you must have a clear, clinical question from a patient's problem, search for the best available evidence relevant to the intervention at hand, and evaluate the evidence for its validity and usefulness before implementing findings in clinical practice.

TABLE 4-6
List of Favorite Health Care Websites

Websites	Databases
www.ahrq.gov	CINAHL
www.americanheart.org	Cochrane Library
www.arthritis.org	Gale Health and Wellness Resource Center
www.cancer.org	Health Consumer: Nursing
www.cancernet.nci.nih.gov	The Joanna Briggs Institute (JBI COnNect+)
www.cdc.gov	Journals@OVID
www.clinicaltrials.gov	Medline (EBSCO)
www.cms.hhs.gov	Medline (OVID)
www.diabetes.org	Nursing Resource Center
www.digestive.niddk.nih.gov	PsycInfo
www.epilepsyfoundation.org	PsycArticles
www.fda.gov	PubMed

(Continues)

TABLE 4-6 (Continued)

Websites	Databases
www.healthfinder.gov	Science Direct
www.lungusa.org	UpToDate
www.mayoclinic.com	Wiley Online Library
www.medlineplus.gov	
www.medscape.com	
www.ncsbn.org	
www.nhlbi.nih.gov	
www.nia.nih.gov	
www.ngc.gov	
www.nih.gov	
www.nursingworld.org	

© Cengage Learning 2014

Evaluation of Information Found on the Internet

Traveling through the Internet, one must always evaluate the information that is found. A simple mnemonic, "Are you PLEASED with the site?" is very helpful (Nicoll, 2003). (See Table 4-7.)

Nurses have always had to use decision-making and critical-thinking skills in everyday practice. The exponential growth of health information and technology is a double-edged sword in practice today. There is so much information available, discerning what is reputable and the best available evidence requires practice and a judicious eye. Keeping up with health technology and advances is now an integral part of nursing practice, much like a stethoscope, and is required in any place you will practice in your career.

CASE STUDY **4-3**

A patient has been told that her baby may have Ebstein's anomaly, a rare genetic disorder causing cardiac defects. The mother has never heard of this and neither have you, the nurse.

How will you find reliable information to give to the mother?

How will you help her navigate information on the Internet to stay away from unreliable sources?

How will you share this information with your colleagues?

TABLE 4-7
Website Evaluation: Ask Yourself, "Am I PLEASED with the Site?"

Purpose
Links
Editorial (site content)
Author
Site navigation
Ethical disclosure
Date site last updated

Source: Compiled with information from Health on the Net Foundation. HONcode Site Evaluation form. (2009). Available at http://www.hon.ch/cgi-bin/HONcode/Inscription/site_evaluation.pl?language=en&userCategory=individuals (accessed 4-16-09)

KEY CONCEPTS

- In the decision-making process, there are five levels.
- Critical thinking involves examining problems or situations from every viewpoint. Use of the universal intellectual standards will improve a nurse's critical thinking.
- Practicing reflective thinking, intuitive thinking, and problem solving helps individuals become better critical thinkers.
- Decision-making tools are helpful when the nurse needs to separate multiple factors surrounding a situation during the decision-making process.
- Nursing informatics focuses on nursing data, information, and knowledge and manages this information, including the communication of it, within the broader context of health informatics.
- The electronic health record is an integral part of the health care documentation process.
- Information literacy is necessary for nurses searching for evidence to provide care reflecting current evidence-based practice.
- There are situations in which the nurse makes an individual decision. Other situations call for group decision making.

KEY TERMS

consensus
critical thinking
decision making
intuitive thinking
nursing informatics
problem solving
reflective thinking

REVIEW QUESTIONS

1. A new nurse is trying to set her goals for the next five years. She plans to eventually become an acute care nurse practitioner in the ICU setting. She knows she needs to become more experienced, obtain appropriate certification, go back to school, and take the practitioner exam. She would like to see a visual of the time it will take her to realistically accomplish those goals. She should use which of the following?
   A. Decision tree
   B. Gantt chart
   C. Decision grid
   D. Problem-solving process
2. A task force designed to examine solutions for low patient satisfaction in an emergency department has decided to write their ideas down, present their ideas to the taskforce, discuss the ideas, and then privately vote on the ideas. This is an example of which group process?
   A. Consensus building
   B. Delphi technique
   C. Problem-solving process
   D. Nominal group technique

3. A nurse manager decides to form a task force to identify reasons and solutions for patient dissatisfaction on your unit. What are the advantages of forming this task force? Select all that apply.

A. The decisions will be made more quickly.
B. High-quality decision making is possible due to more solutions being generated.
C. Acceptance of decisions is more likely.
D. There is access to a larger resource base.
E. Conflict during the decision-making process is less likely.
F. Ownership of the solution will be promoted.

4. A nurse needs to assist a patient in walking down the hall twice daily as part of the patient's postoperative activities. It is the middle of the afternoon, and the patient is asleep. The nurse would like to allow the patient to sleep because the patient was awake a majority of the night. However, if the nurse does not ambulate the patient now, it is possible that the rest of the nurse's afternoon activities will prevent her from returning to the patient to ambulate before the end of her shift. The nurse must decide whether to ambulate the patient now. What is the next step of the decision-making process?

A. Determine the outcome or goal that is desired.
B. Identify alternatives and determine benefits and consequences of each.
C. Make the decision.
D. Evaluate the decision.

5. A newly licensed RN is hired in an intensive care setting. The preceptor wants the nurse to become more proficient in caring for ventilated patients. There are four experiences available that could increase these skills. Which is the best choice to improve ventilator skills?

A. Read the intranet policy on ventilators.
B. Go into an empty patient room that has a ventilator in the room.
C. Visit the simulation lab with a mechanically intubated patient simulator.
D. Care for a patient on a ventilator who is diagnosed with adult respiratory distress syndrome.

6. An RN with four months of experience is trying to improve decision-making skills. Which response by the nurse would indicate understanding of decision-making skills of new nurses?

A. "I should use my intuition to guide my practice."
B. "Memorizing care protocols will help me with decisions."
C. "I should rely on what I learned in school."
D. "Better decision making will come with time and I shouldn't really worry about it now."

7. A nurse is reviewing helpful decision-making ideas. Which decision-making tips are helpful for the nurse? Select all that apply.

A. Procrastination is helpful.
B. Draw on past experiences.
C. Make decisions based on emotions.
D. Consider all the possible outcomes.
E. Identify why the decision needs to be made.
F. Do not rely on your ability to make a decision.

8. A nurse manager has a group of three nurses who do not communicate with each other and do not act as team members. The manager fears this lack of teamwork and good communication could negatively impact patient outcomes. The manager thinks of four possible ways to improve team work and communication. Which is the best option?
   A. Change the schedule so they do not work together.
   B. Reprimand them individually and document that in their employee files.
   C. Explore their feelings as a group and allow them to vent their feelings.
   D. Schedule the group for a patient demise simulation scenario and have them work together for a positive patient outcome.

9. Which procedure by the nurse would be in accordance with the National Patient Safety Goals to reduce the likelihood of patient harm?
   A. Use a one-person verification process.
   B. Implement a surveillance program to evaluate lunchtime activities.
   C. Implement evidence-based practices to prevent health care–associated infections.
   D. Use nursing judgment when deciding to insert urinary catheters in patients with mobility issues.

10. Nurses document in the electronic health record (EHR). Which statements are true regarding the EHR? Select all that apply.
   A. The EHR verifies the accuracy of charting.
   B. Quality measures are more easily tracked.
   C. The documentation process is streamlined.
   D. The flow of information is facilitated.
   E. The EHR is a type of technology in which nurses need proficiency in order to document care.
   F. Nurses' narrative notes to explain events are not required anymore.

REVIEW ACTIVITIES

1. You are taking the NCLEX in 10 weeks and need to prepare. Draw a PERT diagram to depict the sequence of tasks necessary for the successful completion of the NCLEX.
2. The education forms are not being filled out correctly for new admissions in your medical-surgical unit. Decide on your own the best action to take in this situation. Then, get into a group and decide on the best action to take. Compare the differences between individual and group decision making. What did you learn?
3. Identify a problem that you have been considering. Using the decision-making grid below, rate the alternative solutions to the problem on a scale of 1 to 3 on the elements of cost, quality, importance, location, and any other elements that are important to you. Did this exercise help you to clarify your thinking?

	Cost	Quality	Importance	Location	Other
Alternative A					
Alternative B					
Alternative C					

4. You have been asked to locate the latest evidence on pressure ulcer prevention. Where will you start? How will you know the information is reliable and the latest?

EXPLORING THE WEB

- Review this site for extra information on intuitive thinking: *http://www.typelogic.com*
- The Unified Medical Language System is developed to compensate for differences in concepts in several biomedical terminologies: *http://www.nlm.nih.gov/research/umls*
- Note the universal intellectual standards at the Foundation for Critical Thinking: *http://www.critical thinking.org*
- Visit this critical-thinking site: *http://www.insightassessment.com*
- Review this site on applying artificial intelligence to clinical situations: *http://www.medg.lcs.mit.edu*

REFERENCES

Benner, P., Hughes, R. G., & Sutphen, M. (2008).†† Clinical reasoning, decision making, and action: Thinking critically and clinically. In R. G. Hughes (Ed.),† *Patient safety and quality: An evidence-based handbook† for nurses.* AHRQ† Publication No. 08-0043. Rockville, MD: Agency for Healthcare Research† and Quality.

Benner, P., Tanner, C., & Chelsa, C. (2009). *Expertise in nursing practice: Caring, clinical judgment, and ethics,* (2nd ed.). New York, NY: Springer.

Centers for Medicare and Medicaid Services (CMS). (2010). Meaningful use. Retrieved October 29, 2011, from https://www.cms.gov/EHRIncentivePrograms/30_Meaningful_Use

Comsti, T. (2011). Peer-to-peer health care: Fox shows how the Internet is changing health care. *NIH Record., 62*(19). Retrieved September 20, 2011, from http://nihrecord.od.nih.gov/newsletters/2011/09_16_2011/story2.htm

Day, L., & Smith, E. L. (2007). Website evaluation exercises. Retrieved October 11, 2011, from http://www.qsen.org/teachingstrategy.php?id=40

DeLaune, S., & Ladner, P. (2011). *Fundamentals of nursing: Standards and practice* (4th ed.). Clifton Park, NY: Delmar Cengage Learning.

Delbecq, A. L., Gustafson, A. C., & Van de Ven, A. H. (1971). A group process model for problem identification and program planning. *Journal of Applied Behavioral Science, VII,* 466–491.

Delbecq, A. L., Van de Ven, A. H., & Gustafson, D. H. (1975). *Group techniques for program planners.* Glenview, IL: Scott Foresman and Company.

Durham, C. F., & Alden, K. R. (2008).†† Enhancing patient safety in nursing education through patient† simulation. In R. G. Hughes (Ed.),† *Patient safety and quality: An evidence-based handbook† for nurses.* AHRQ† Publication No. 08-0043. Rockville, MD: Agency for Healthcare Research† and Quality.

Fineout-Overholt, E., Mazurek Melynk, B., Stillwell, S. B., & Williamson, K. M. (2010, March). Evidence-Based practice step by step: Implementing an evidence-based practice change. *American Journal of Nursing, 111*(3), 54–60.

Gardner, P. (2003). *Nursing process in action.* Clifton Park, NY: Delmar Cengage Learning.

Healthcare Information and Management Systems Society (HIMSS). (2008). Electronic health records: A global perspective. *The Healthcare Information and Management Systems Society.* Retrieved September 27, 2011, from http://himss.org/content/files/200808_EHR GlobalPerspective_whitepaper.pdf?src=winews2009114

Health on the Net Foundation. (2009). HONcode site evaluation form. Accessed April 16, 2009, at http://www .hon.ch/cgi-bin/HONcode/Inscription/site_evaluation .pl?language=en& user Category=individuals.

Henneman, E. A., Cunningham, H., Roche, J. P., & Curnin, M. E. (2007). Human patient simulation: Teaching students to provide safe care. *Nurse Educator, 32*(5), 212–217.

History Learning Site. (2011). Martin Luther King. Retrieved October 11, 2011, from http://www .historylearningsite.co.uk/mlk1.htm

Joint Commission. (2011). National patient safety goals. Retrieved October 31, 2011, from http://www .jointcomission.org.

Jones, J., & Nicoll, L. H. (2012). Nursing and health care informatics. In P. Kelly (Ed.), *Nursing leadership and management,* (3rd ed.). Clifton Park, NY: Delmar Cengage Learning.

Jones, R. A. P., & Beck, S. E. (1996). *Decision making in nursing.* Clifton Park, NY: Delmar Cengage Learning.

Keenan, G. M., Yakel, E., & Tschannen, D. (2008). In R. G. Hughes (Ed.),† *Patient safety and quality: An evidence-based handbook† for nurses.* AHRQ† Publication No. 08-0043. Rockville, MD: Agency for Healthcare Research† and Quality.

Kelley, T. F., Brandon, D. H., & Docherty, S. L. (2011). Electronic nursing documentation as a strategy to improve quality of patient care. *Journal of Nursing Scholarship, 43,*† 154–162. doi:† 10.1111/j.1547-5069.2011.01397.x

Kohn L. T., Corrigan, J. M., Donaldson, M. S. (Eds.). (2000). *To err is human: Building a safer health system.* A report of the Committee on Quality of Health Care in America, Institute of Medicine. Washington, DC: National Academies Press.

Lipowicz, A. (2011). VA wants help modernizing health care records system. *Washington Technology.* Retrieved September 27, 2011, from http://washingtontechnology.com/articles/2011/01/28/va-looking-for-help-to-set-up-governance-for-open-source-vista.aspx

Little-Stoetzel, S., & Fane, B. K. (2012). Decision making and critical thinking. In P. Kelly (Ed.), *Nursing leadership and management,* (3rd ed.) (pp. 526–543). Clifton Park, NY: Delmar Cengage Learning.

Merriam Websterí's Online Dictionary. (2011). Consensus. Retrieved September 22, 2011, from http://www.merriam-webster.com/dictionary/consensus

National Priority Partnership. (2010). Input to the secretary of health and human services on priorities for the 2011 national quality strategy. National Quality Forum, Washington, DC. Retrieved October 31, 2011, from http://www.nationalprioritiespartnership.org

National Quality Forum. (2011). About us. Retrieved October 31, 2011, from http://www.qualityforum.org/About_NQF/About_NQF.aspx

Nicoll, L. H. (2003). Nursing and health care informatics. In P. L. Kelly-Heidenthal (Ed.), *Nursing leadership & management.* Clifton Park, NY: Delmar Cengage Learning.

Paul, R. (1992). *Critical thinking: What every person needs to survive in a rapidly changing world.* Santa Rosa, CA: Foundation for Critical Thinking.

Paul, R., & Elder, L. (1996). Foundation for critical thinking. Retrieved from http://www.criticalthinking.org

Pesut, D. J., & Herman, J. (1999). *Clinical reasoning: The art & science of critical & creative thinking.* Clifton Park, NY: Delmar Cengage Learning.

Pretz, J. E., & Folse, V. N. (2011). Nursing experience and preference for intuition in decision making. *Journal of Clinical Nursing, 20,*† 2878–2889. doi:† 10.1111/j.1365-2702.2011.03705.x

Technology Informatics Guiding Educational Reform (TIGER). (2009). Collaborating to integrate evidence and informatics into nursing practice and education. Retrieved October 31, 2009, from http://www.tigersummit.com/9_Collaboratives.html

Vroom, V. H., & Yetton, P. (1973). *Leadership and decision making.* Pittsburgh, PA: University of Pittsburgh Press.

Yao, B. H. (2010). The dos and don'ts of successful decision making. *Ezine@rticles.* Retrieved September 29, 2011, from http://ezinearticles.com/?The-dos-and-donts-of-successful-decision-making&id=4873870

SUGGESTED READINGS

Anderson, G. L., & Tredway, C. A. (2009). Transforming the nursing curriculum to promote critical thinking online. *Journal of Nursing Education, 48*(2), 111–115.

Artinian, N. T. (2007, January–February). Telehealth as a tool for enhancing care for patients with cardiovascular disease. *Journal of Cardiovascular Nursing, 22*(1), 25–31.

Bittner, N. P., & Gravlin, G. (2009). Critical thinking, delegation, and missed care in nursing practice. *Journal of Nursing Administration, 39*(3), 142–146.

Bowles, K. H., & Baugh, A. C. (2007, January–February). Applying research evidence to optimize telehomecare. *Journal of Cardiovascular Nursing, 22*(1), 5–15.

Cholewka, P. A., & Mohr, B. (2009). Enhancing nursing informatics competencies and critical-thinking skills using wireless clinical simulation laboratories. *Studies in Health Technology and Informatics, 146,* 561–563.

Demiris, G. (2007). Interdisciplinary innovations in biomedical and health informatics graduate education. *Methods in Infectious Medicine, 46*(1), 63–66.

Evans, C. (2005). Clinical decision-making theories: Patient assessment in autonomy and extended roles. *Emergency Nurse, 13*(5), 16–20.

Hernandez, C. A. (2009). Student articulation of a nursing philosophical statement: An assignment to enhance critical-thinking skills and promote learning. *Journal of Nursing Education, 48*(6), 343–349.

Lyons, E. M. (2008). Examining the effects of problem-based learning and NCLEX-RN scores on the critical-thinking skills of associate-degree nursing students in a southeastern community college. *International Journal of Nursing Education Scholarship, 5*(21). (Epub 2008, June 5).

McMullen, M. A., & McMullen, W. F. (2009). Examining patterns of change in the critical-thinking skills of graduate nursing students. *Journal of Nursing Education, 48*(6), 310–318.

Pickett, J. (2009). Critical thinking a necessary factor in nursing workload. *American Journal of Critical Care, 18*(2), 101.

Zurmehly, J. (2008). The relationship of educational preparation, autonomy, and critical thinking to nursing job satisfaction. *Journal of Continuing Education in Nursing, 39*(10), 453–460.

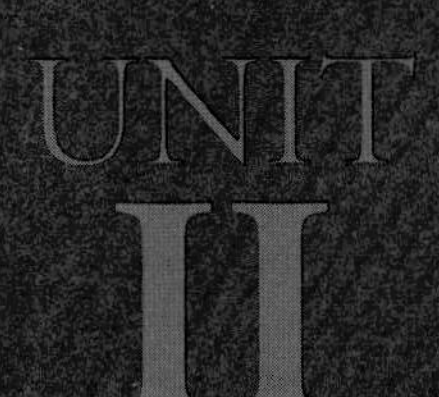

LEADERSHIP AND MANAGEMENT OF THE INTER-PROFESSIONAL TEAM

CHAPTER 5

Inter-Professional Teamwork and Collaboration

EDNA HARDER MATTSON, RN, BN, BA(CRS), MDE, CTSN, CAE; KARIN POLIFKO-HARRIS, RN, PHD, CNAA; CRISAMAR J. ANUNCIADO, RN, MSN, FNP-BC; JACKLYN RUTHMAN, RN, PHD; AND DEBORAH ERICKSON, RN, PHD

Teamwork is the ability to work together toward a common vision, the ability to direct individual accomplishment toward organizational objectives. It is the fuel that allows common people to attain uncommon results.

–ANDREW CARNEGIE, 1984

OBJECTIVES

Upon completion of this chapter, the reader should be able to:

1. Identify teamwork and collaboration within a health care system.
2. Discuss TeamSTEPPS, Crew Resource Management, and horizontal and lateral violence.
3. Review the Health Insurance Portability and Accountability Act (HIPAA).
4. Review the stages of group process and working with inter-professional health care team members.
5. Describe the benefits of delivering patient-centered care and considering the patient and family as partners on the inter-professional team.
6. Discuss teamwork and collaboration as an extension of organizational performance

As a new nurse, you are making the day's assignments for a 34-bed medical-surgical unit. Working with you today will be another two registered nurses, two licensed practical nurses, and one nursing assistant. You graduated only a year ago and you were recently promoted to the role of charge nurse. Today, one of the licensed practical nurses and the nursing assistant are challenging your patient care assignments, saying you do not have enough experience to make a fair assignment. They are trying to get the two registered nurses *to* side with them. It appears that the two registered nurses often work together, as do the two licensed practical nurses. You know you made the best assignments given the staff available, yet you are wondering if there is a better solution.

What would be the best way to address the assignment concerns of the nursing staff?

What factors did you consider in making the assignments?

How would you engage the staff in seeking their input for making staff assignments?

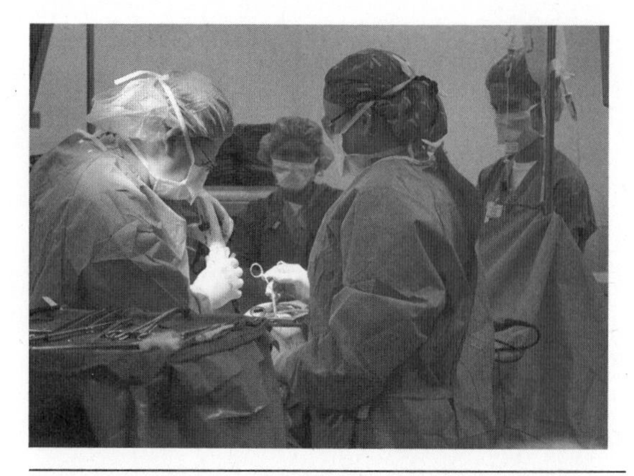

Source: Courtesy of Advocate Good Shepherd Hospital, Barrington, Illinois

In today's health care environment, great demands are placed on each health care professional to provide the best quality of care efficiently, safely, and cost-effectively to optimize patient care outcomes. Many nursing leaders and managers encourage reflection on achievement of standards of quality patient care by nurses. Many health care providers recognize that effective inter-professional teamwork and collaboration are needed to create a safe patient care environment. Inter-professional teamwork and collaboration among staff nurses and other disciplines in the health care setting are so critical to optimizing patient care safety and outcomes that they are a priority for most health care administrators, directors, and managers. This chapter discusses teamwork and collaboration within a health care system and discusses TeamSTEPPS, Crew Resource Management, and horizontal and lateral violence. It reviews the Health Insurance Portability and Accountability Act (HIPAA) and reviews the stages of group process and working with inter-professional health care team members. The chapter describes the benefits of delivering patient-centered care and considering the patient and family as partners on the inter-professional team. Finally, the chapter discusses teamwork and collaboration as an extension of organizational performance.

TEAMWORK AND COLLABORATION

The Quality and Safety Education for Nurses (QSEN) initiative, funded by the Robert Wood Johnson Foundation to address nursing competency concerns of the Institute of Medicine (2004), defined teamwork and collaboration as functioning "effectively within nursing and inter-professional teams, fostering open communication, mutual respect, and shared decision making to achieve quality patient care" (QSEN, 2011). Teamwork and collaboration celebrate patient-centered care, which "recognizes the patient or designee as the source of control and full partner in providing compassionate care based on respect for the patient's preferences, values, and needs" (QSEN, 2011). A study conducted by Kalisch & Lee (2011) found that the ability to provide quality and safe care is associated with teamwork, which in turn requires adequate staffing.

The move to interdisciplinary or inter-professional teams in the provision of quality patient care begins with health care team attitudinal changes. Embracing the values of caring and collaborative patient care, including the patient and family as significant partners, is essential for all stakeholders (QSEN, 2011).

Verma, Paterson, and Medves state that changing the culture in academic health sciences begins with the development and evaluation of an interdisciplinary curriculum at the undergraduate level (2006). The governing bodies of educational institutions, chief executive officers, and related senior managers acknowledge that interdisciplinary practice is essential in meeting the complexity of health care needs (per Refs Governance Institute, 2009). In addition, the approach to interdisciplinary education at the undergraduate and graduate levels must be reinforced throughout the lifespan of health care providers to maintain effective clinicians and expert team members (Weaver, Rosen, Salas, Baum, & King, 2010). Inter-professional teamwork and collaboration can be reinforced by the development of TeamSTEPPS as a structured program to analyze the problems of ineffective health care teams and develop strategies to improve safety within the organization (Agency for Healthcare Research and Quality, 2012).

The Quality and Safety Education for Nurses website, www.qsen.org, (QSEN, 2011) identifies self-awareness of one's own strengths, limitations, and values in functioning as a member of a team as the initial competency in developing the skill to function within a team. This self-awareness must be followed with a plan for self-development in inter-professional teamwork and collaboration and must begin with treating each team member with dignity and respect. Health care team members must understand and respect the scope of practice and roles of all health care team members. "Communication practices that minimize risk associated with (shift report) handoffs among providers and across transition in care" (Preheim, Armstrong, & Barton, 2009, p. 694) must be utilized. Nurses must also acknowledge their own potential to contribute to effective team functioning (Preheim, Armstrong, & Barton, 2009).

TeamSTEPPS

TeamSTEPPS is an evidence based teamwork system designed for health care professionals to improve safety concerns within organizations. TeamSTEPPS, available at, http://teamstepps.ahrq.gov/, was developed by the Department of Defense's Patient Safety Program in collaboration with the Agency for Healthcare Research and Quality. The three phases of TeamSTEPPS are designed at creating and sustaining a culture of safety. The three phases are using a pretraining assessment to determine the readiness of the site to participate, using onsite trainers and health care staff, and having an implementation and sustainable plan.

TeamSTEPPS focuses on skills and actions that improve teamwork and collaboration in reducing and preventing errors in patient care (Rabinovitch, Johnson, Mazzapica & O'Leary 2010). The TeamSTEPPS logo at, http://teamstepps.ahrq.gov/teamsteppslogo.htm, identifies important concepts related to trainable teamwork skills. These are leadership, communication, situation monitoring, and mutual support. If a team has tools and strategies, it can leverage to build competency in each of those skills. Note that teamwork is an essential component of practice on a 24/7 basis in health care; however increased research is required to fully understand the processes and effectiveness of teams (Kalisch & Lee, 2009).

Setting of Care: Primary, Secondary, and Tertiary Care

Factors to be considered in effective teamwork and collaboration include the nature of the services, such as primary, secondary, and tertiary care, the availability and characteristics of the resources, and changes in availability of the resources. Primary health care includes health promotion and education, early detection of disease, preventive care, and environmental protection (World Health Organization, 2011). The World Health Organization describes primary health as reducing social disparities and focusing on patient needs and expectations, public policy reforms, and leadership reforms. Many countries recognize that primary health services involving an inter-professional approach are vital in improving the health care of its citizens. Secondary care focuses on diagnosis and treatment in acute and emergency care settings, and tertiary care focuses on long-term, rehabilitation, and palliative care. Direct and indirect communication practices among the providers of primary, secondary, and tertiary care services are essential in improving care for patients (Farup, Blix, Førre, Johnson, Lange, Johannessen & Petersen (2011).

Communication Process

Communication is an interactive process that occurs when a person (the sender) sends a verbal or nonverbal message to another person (the receiver) and receives

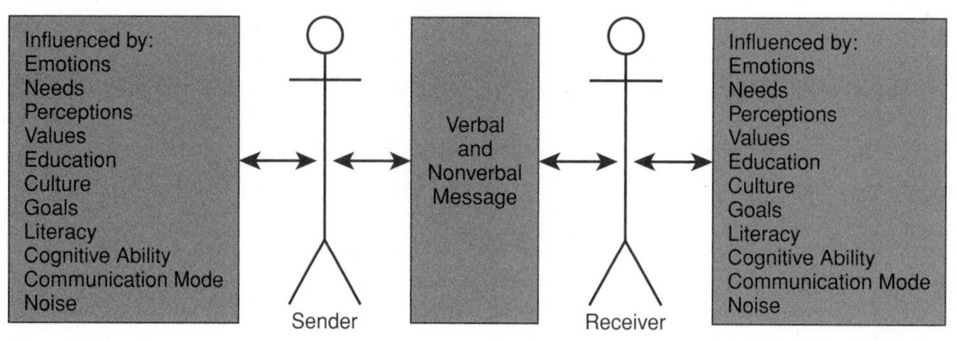

FIGURE 5-1

Communication process.

© Cengage learning 2014

feedback. The communication process is influenced by emotions, needs, perceptions, values, education, culture, goals, literacy, cognitive ability, the communication mode, and noise (Figure 5-1). Communication in health care is used to coordinate patient care, and nowhere more so than communicating changes in patient conditions to other team members or during care handoffs within a specific disciplinary team (Welsh, Flanagan, & Ebright, 2010).

Staff communication and coordination are also relevant to the health care organization's ability to comply with the requirements of accrediting bodies. For example, both the Joint Commission (JC, 2011) and the National Committee on Quality Assurance (NCQA , 2011), two leading accrediting bodies in the health care industry, have adopted accreditation standards that address the need for good coordination among professional groups, patient care units, and service components within health care organizations.

Several studies of ICUs indicate that effective communication and coordination among clinical staff result in more efficient and better quality of care (Knaus, Draper, Wagner, & Zimmerman, 1986; Baggs, Ryan, Phelps, Richeson, & Johnson, 1992; Shortell et al., 1994; Young et al., 1997; Young et al., 1998). Additionally, research suggests that ineffective coordination and communication among hospital staff contribute substantially to adverse events. For example, one study of the care of 1,047 patients in a large, tertiary care hospital found that approximately 15 percent of the 480 adverse events identified (e.g., failure to order indicated tests and misplaced test results), had causes related to the interaction of staff, such as the failure of a consultant team to communicate adequately with the requesting team (Andrews et al., 1997).

Electronic Communication

Communication is shifting to an electronic mode, with computer technology playing an increasingly dominant role. Health care providers are using a variety of technologies, including telephones, voice mail, personal data assistants, iPhones, BlackBerry, fax, e-mail, and video conferencing. These methods require careful communication. For example, e-mail now allows almost instantaneous communication around the world, but it also accommodates individual preferences with respect to the timing of the response. This allows a person to send a message early in the day and allows the team members the opportunity to respond as their schedules permit. Using e-mail may save a patient and caregiver from travel or loss of work. However, using e-mail requires that nurses acting in a caregiver role have sharp assessment skills and good writing skills. The speed with which exchanges can now be made using technology has reduced acceptable response times. Therefore, the first tip when communicating using technology is that it is important that both parties have an understanding about the circumstances under which different modes of communication will be used. Although one practitioner who is "connected" may be comfortable receiving urgent patient information such as an elevated potassium level electronically (perhaps by e-mail), most

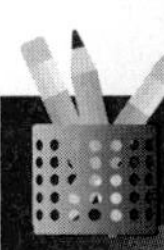

CASE STUDY 5-1

Go to http://teamstepps.ahrq.gov/. Read about TeamSTEPPS, which is an evidence-based teamwork system to improve communication and teamwork skills among health care professionals. TeamSTEPPS provides higher quality, safer patient care by producing highly effective health care teams that optimize the use of information, people, and resources to achieve the best clinical outcomes for patients; increasing team awareness and clarifying team roles and responsibilities; resolving conflicts and improving information sharing; and eliminating barriers to quality and safety.

TeamSTEPPS has a three-phased process aimed at creating and sustaining a culture of safety in an organization. Do you think TeamSTEPPS has the potential to improve patient care? Are clinicians using TeamSTEPPS in your clinical area?

practitioners would expect a telephone call if the data being shared is potentially life threatening.

Practitioners may be satisfied to receive a fax if the data is not urgent. Often, organizations have policies that guide under what circumstances a particular mode of communication is used, so be sure to understand your institution's policy for communicating urgent information.

Another tip is to respond in a timely manner. Timeliness is defined by what information is being shared and the route being used. A fax delivered to a practitioner's office over the weekend will likely not generate a reply before Monday. E-mail, in general, provides great immediacy, but the telephone remains the primary tool for communicating urgent information. Tips for communicating by e-mail include the following:

- NO CAPITAL LETTERS—this looks like you are shouting.
- Be brief and reply sparingly, as appropriate.
- Use clear subject lines.
- Cool off before responding to an angry message. Answer tomorrow.
- Forward e-mail messages from others only with their permission.
- Forward jokes selectively, if ever.
- Use good judgment; e-mail may not be private.

Keep in mind that accurate spelling, correct grammar, and organization of thought assume greater importance in the absence of verbal and nonverbal cues that are given in face-to-face encounters. Always proofread correspondences prior to sending them. Imagine yourself as the recipient of the document. Look for complete sentences, logical development of thought and reasoning, accuracy, and appropriate use of grammar, punctuation, and capitalization.

Using Social Media in Health care Organizations

The use of social media has become a current vehicle for efficient communication in the workplace. Educational institutions and professional organizations are no exception. Facebook began as a media for the meeting of college students (DeSilets, 2009). Electronic mail is currently under scrutiny in relation to the widespread use of e-mail in organizations, monitoring communication techniques, and concerns of the organizations' legal right to monitor, and the employees' expectations of privacy (Snyder, 2010). An employee's communication on social media must respect the privacy of all. Exercising good judgement is essential in posting information and nursing leaders must be diligent about warning the staff about violating their confidentiality agreement with the employer (Scott & Troutman, 2009). Five California nurses were recently fired after allegedly discussing patients on Facebook (Fink, 2010).

Health Insurance Portability and Accountability Act (HIPAA)

The U.S. Department of Health and Human Services (HHS) issued the Privacy Rule to implement the requirements of the Health Insurance Portability and Accountability Act of 1996 (HIPAA). The Privacy Rule standards address the use and disclosure of individuals' health information by organizations subject to the Privacy Rule as well as standards for individuals' privacy rights to understand and control how their health information is used. Within HHS, the Office for Civil Rights (OCR) has responsibility for implementing and enforcing the Privacy Rule with respect to voluntary compliance activities and money penalties.

A major goal of the Privacy Rule is to ensure that individuals' health information is properly protected while allowing for the flow of health information needed to provide and promote high-quality health care and the protection of the public's health and well-being. The Privacy Rule introduced new standards for protecting the privacy of individuals' identifiable health information. There are 18 personal health identifiers. This law may also apply to health information that is shared for research purposes (http://www.hhs.gov/ocr/privacy/index.html) (Table 5-1).

Patients and Families as Active Participants

Recognizing patients and families as active participants in the health care system is essential. The Obama Administration has launched the Partnership for Patients: Better Care, Lower Costs, a new public-private partnership that will help improve the quality, safety, and affordability of health care for all Americans. The Partnership for Patients brings together leaders of major hospitals, employers, physicians, nurses, and patient advocates along with state and federal governments in a shared effort to make hospital care safer, more reliable, and less costly. The two goals of this new partnership are to keep patients from getting injured or sicker and help patients heal without complications. It is hoped that by the end of 2013, preventable hospital-acquired conditions would decrease by 40 percent compared to 2010. Achieving this goal would mean approximately 1.8 million fewer injuries to patients with more than 60,000 lives saved over three years.

Nurses play a vital role in including patients and families on teams, listening to their concerns, and incorporating patients' and families' input into the unit and the health care system (Comp, 2011). Haines and Warren (2011) highlight the role of nurses in encouraging clinical leaders to engage their teams and to implement and embed the changes of partnering with patients and family members in nursing practice. All members of the health care team including "clinical and nonclinical colleagues should be encouraged to engage in quality assurance, education, and dissemination of good practice" (p. 23). The involvement of patients and family members can provide

TABLE 5-1
Elements that are Considered Patient Identifiers Under the Health Insurance Portability and Accountability Act of 1996 (HIPAA)

- Names
- All geographic subdivisions smaller than a state, including street address, city, county, precinct, ZIP code
- All elements of dates (except year) for dates directly related to an individual, including birth date, admission date, discharge date, date of death; all ages over 89
- Telephone numbers
- Fax numbers
- E-mail addresses
- Social Security numbers
- Medical record numbers
- Health plan beneficiary numbers
- Account numbers
- Certificate/license numbers
- Vehicle identifiers and serial numbers
- Device identifiers and serial numbers
- Web universal resource locators (URLs)
- Internet Protocol (IP) address numbers
- Biometric identifiers, including fingerprints and voiceprints
- Full-face photographic images and any comparable images
- Any other unique identifying number, characteristic, or code unless otherwise permitted

Source: Compiled with information from U.S. Department of Health and Human Services. (2003). *Protecting personal health information in research: Understanding the HIPAA privacy rule.* NIH Publication Number 03-5388.

guidance for staff development, education, and sharing of best practices within the unit and the organization (Bryan, 2009).

STAGES OF GROUP PROCESS

The World Health Organization (WHO, 2007) defines a team as "two or more people working interdependently towards a common goal." Getting a group of people together does not make a team. As mentioned earlier, teamwork and collaboration to function effectively within nursing and inter-professional teams, fostering open communication, mutual respect, and shared decision making to achieve quality patient care is part of being a team (QSEN, 2012). A team develops products that are the result of the team's collective effort and involves collaboration. All teams go through predictable phases of collaboration and group development group development as they evolve from an immature stage to a mature stage. It is critical to note that not all teams reach maturity, for a variety of reasons: perhaps there is ineffective leadership, problematic members, unclear goals and communication, or lack of focus or energy. Some teams may become fully functional and mature quickly, bypassing a stage or two along the way. It is typical for high-functioning teams whose members are trusting of one another to be able to make decisions quickly and accurately; it may take longer for other teams, whose members need to get to know and trust one another, before the actual work of the team can take place.

Tuckman and Jensen (1977) identified five stages that a group normally progresses through as it develops. These stages are known as **group process** and consist of: Forming, Storming, Norming, Performing, and Adjourning (Table 5-2).

The first stage of the team process is the Forming stage. This stage occurs when the group is created and meets as a team for the first time. The team members come to the meeting with zest and a sense of curiosity, adventure, and even apprehension as they orient themselves to each other and get to know each other through personal interaction and perhaps team-building activities. With the help of the team leader or facilitator, they will explore the purpose and goals of the team, what contribution they can bring to the table, and set boundaries for the teamwork.

The second stage of the team process is the Storming stage. As the group relaxes and becomes more comfortable, interpersonal issues or opposing opinions

TABLE 5-2
Tuckman and Jensen's Stages of Group Process

Stages	Description
Forming	***Relationship development:*** Team orientation, identification of role expectations, beginning team interactions, explorations, and boundary setting occurs.
Storming	***Interpersonal interaction and reaction:*** Dealing with tension and conflict or confrontation may occur.
Norming	***Effective cooperation and collaboration:*** Personal opinions are expressed and resolution of conflict with formation of solidified goals and increased group cohesiveness occurs.
Performing	***Group maturity and stable relationships:*** Team roles become more functional and flexible. Structural issues are resolved leading to supportive task performance through group-directed collaboration and resources sharing.
Adjourning	***Termination and consolidation:*** Team goals and activities are met leading to closure, evaluation, and outcomes review. This may also lead to reforming when the need for improvement or further goal development is identified.

Source: Compiled with information from Tuckman, B. W., & Jensen, M. A. C. (1977). Stages of Small Group Development Revisited. *Group and Organizational Studies, 2*(4), 419–427; Hall, P., & Weaver, L. (2001). Interdisciplinary Education and Teamwork: A Long and Winding Road. *Medical Education, 35*, 867–875; Polifko-Harris, K. (2003). Effective Team Building. In P. L. Kelly, (Ed.). *Nursing Leadership & Management.* (2nd ed.). Clifton Park, NY: Delmar Cengage Learning.

may arise that may cause conflict between members of the team and with the team leader. This may cause feelings of uneasiness in the group. It is important at this stage to understand that conflict is a healthy and natural process of team development. When members of the team come from various disciplines and specialties, they are likely to approach an issue from several completely different standpoints. These differences need to be openly confronted and addressed so that effective resolution of the issue may occur in a timely manner. Real teams do not emerge unless individuals on them take risks involving conflict, trust, interdependence, and hard work (Katzenbach & Smith, 2003).

The third stage is called Norming. After resistance is overcome in the Storming stage, a feeling of group cohesion develops. Team members master the ability to resolve conflict. Although complete resolution and agreement may not be attained at all times, team members learn to respect differences of opinion and may work together through these obstacles to achieve team goals. Communication of ideas, opinions, and information occurs through effective cooperation among the team members. Overcoming barriers to performance is how groups become teams (Katzenbach & Smith, 2003).

The fourth stage of the team development process is the Performing stage. In this stage, group cohesion, collaboration, and solidarity are evident. Personal opinions are set aside to achieve group goals. Team members openly communicate, know each other's roles and responsibilities, take risks, and trust or rely on each other to complete assigned tasks. The group reaches maturity at this stage. One of the biggest strengths of this stage is the emphasis on maintaining and improving interpersonal relationships within the team as each member functions within the whole. Kenneth Blanchard, one of the authors of *The One Minute Manager* (1981), sums it up with his comment "None of us is as smart as all of us."

The fifth and final stage of team process development is the Adjourning stage. Termination and consolidation occur in this stage. When the team has achieved its goals and assigned tasks, the team closure process begins. The team reviews its activities and evaluates its progress and outcomes by answering the questions: Were the team goals sufficiently met? Was there anything that could have been done differently?

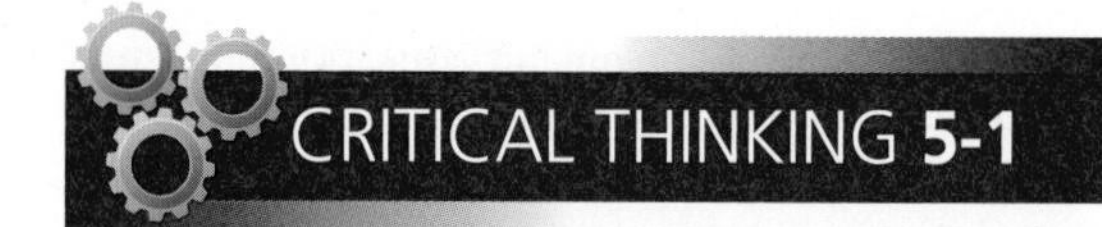

You are having a coffee break with another nurse who mentions a problem she is having with care delivery. The nurse is not sure how to solve it. You want to be helpful and supportive and yet avoid giving advice. Ask the nurse if she can describe the problem fully for you. Do not interrupt. Then, ask the nurse some questions about the problem, and seek clarification until you are clear on the problem and the nurse has fully described it. Do not give advice. Use your communication skills, such as attending, clarifying, and responding, and ask the nurse such things as, "Tell me more about that," "What did you think about it?," and so forth, until you are both clear on the issue. At the end of this process, you can just finish by relaxing for the rest of your break or you can ask the nurse, "Do you want advice about your problem?"

Many times, this process will help the nurse solve the problem by himself or herself. If the nurse does want advice, you can give some suggestions if you are comfortable doing so. Do you think this process can strengthen people's ability to find answers to their problems? Do you think this process would be helpful to you in working with others on the unit? Do you think this approach honors people's integrity and ability to solve their own problems?

Source: Adapted from Parsons, M.(2003). Personal communication.

The team leader summarizes the group's accomplishments and the role played by each member in achieving its goals. It is important to provide closure or feedback regarding the team process to leave each team member with a sense of accomplishment. This is particularly relevant within a health care team.

COMMON TEAM MEMBER ROLES

In any team, there are bound to be both participants who are helpful and those who are not helpful in their behaviors. Sometimes the behaviors are unconsciously acted out. At other times, a team member is quite clear and focused about the role he or she is playing, such as the role of the aggressor. In any case, it is imperative that the astute team leader be aware of everyone's roles and use excellent communication skills to facilitate the group process.

Common member roles in groups fit into three categories: group task roles, group maintenance roles, and self-oriented roles. Note that successful teams include both group leader roles and group follower roles.

Group task roles help a group develop and accomplish its goals. Among these roles are the following:

- Initiator-contributor: Proposes goals, suggests ways of approaching tasks, and recommends procedures for approaching a problem or task
- Information seeker: Asks for information, viewpoints, and suggestions about the problem or task
- Information giver: Offers information, viewpoints, and suggestions about the problem or task
- Coordinator: Clarifies and synthesizes various ideas in an effort to tie together the work of the members
- Orienter: Summarizes, points to departures from goals, and raises questions about the discussion direction
- Energizer: Stimulates the group to higher levels and better quality of work

Group maintenance roles do not directly address a task itself, but instead help foster group unity, positive interpersonal relations among group members, and development of the ability of members to work effectively together. Group maintenance roles include the following:

- Encourager: Expresses warmth and friendliness toward group members, encourages them, and acknowledges their contributions
- Harmonizer: Mediates disagreements between members and attempts to help reconcile differences
- Gatekeeper: Tries to keep lines of communication open and promotes the participation of all members
- Standard setter: Suggests standards for ways in which the group will operate and checks whether members are satisfied with the functioning of the group
- Group observer: Watches the internal operations of the group and provides feedback about how participants are doing and how they might be able to function better
- Follower: Goes along with the group and is friendly but relatively passive

Self-oriented roles are related to the personal needs of group members and often negatively influence the effectiveness of a group. These roles include the following:

- Aggressor: Deflates the contributions of others by attacking their ideas, ridiculing their feelings, and displaying excessive competitiveness
- Blocker: Tends to be negative, stubborn, and resistive of new ideas—sometimes in order to force the group to readdress a viewpoint that it has already dealt with
- Recognition seeker: Seeks attention, boasts about accomplishments and capabilities, and works to prevent being placed in an inferior position in the group
- Dominator: Tries to assert control and manipulates the group or certain group members by using methods such as flattering, giving orders, or interrupting others (Bartol & Martin, 1998)

Types of Teams

The purpose of health care teams is to meet patient care needs. Teams may be discipline specific with similar backgrounds and abilities such as a nursing policy and procedure team. Other teams may be developed with inter-professional members who have a variety of skills and talents and provide different perspectives and ideas on how to solve problems. Everyone on an inter-professional team is trained in a specialty and looks at health care delivery with a different focus, for example, as nurses, physicians, social workers, dieticians, or case managers. Having so many inter-professional viewpoints can be difficult, especially if a single decision is needed and everyone has different opinions. This presents challenges for effective teamwork that "can only be fully understood from experiencing them in the clinical setting" (Anderson & Thorpe, 2010, p. 20). Nursing leaders should encourage experiential learning by nursing students and staff by involving them with interdisciplinary groups in multiple settings such as families, schools, and communities (Selle, Salamon, Boarman, & Sauer, 2008).

To get the work of an organization completed, multiple formal and informal teams may develop. Formal teams may include a temporary ad hoc team that meets to accomplish a specific purpose, such as preparing for accreditation by the Joint Commission, or a permanent standing team that meets regularly to accomplish organizational objectives, such as the Intensive Care Committee.

Informal teams may also evolve in organizations. The importance of informal workgroup structure and group processes has been recognized for many years (Shortell & Kaluzny, 2006). The Hawthorne experiments firmly established the proposition that an individual's performance is determined in large part by informal relationship patterns that emerge within workgroups (Roethlisberger & Dickson, 1939). The workgroup has an impact on individual behaviors and attitudes because it controls so many of the stimuli to which the individual is exposed in performing organizational tasks (Hasenfeld, 1983).

Informal groups are not directly established or sanctioned by the organization, but often form naturally by individuals in a service organization to fill a personal or social interest or need. Shortell and Kaluzny (2006) identify a number of circumstances under which informal groups can have a negative impact on an organization. Groups may become overly exclusionary and this leads to interpersonal conflict. Informal groups can also become so powerful that they undermine the formal authority structure of the organization. Informal groups can assume a change agent role. Informal groups are often responsible for facilitating improvements in working conditions. Such informal groups sometimes evolve into formal groups. Informal groups may also emerge to deal with a particular organizational problem or to work toward changes in organizational policies and procedures. In sum, informal groups play a unique role in organizations. These roles may be positive or negative.

A team may also be advisory, such as a team that meets to discuss concerns of the professional nursing staff and then reports back to the chief nurse executive for decision making, or the team may be self-directed and make decisions on its own. Whatever the type, formal or informal, all teams must effectively communicate to achieve their objectives.

GREAT TEAM GUIDELINES

Great teams do not just happen; there is behind-the-scenes planning, preparation, and forward thinking before anyone works together. Theories of effective teams have been discussed in the literature for several decades by Lewin (1951), McGregor (1960), Argyris (1964), Burns (1978), Bennis (1989), and Senge (1990). What are the guidelines for encouraging great teams? A great team accomplishes what it sets out to do, with everyone on the team participating to achieve the desired outcomes. Effective teamwork is achieved when there is synergy. Mark Twain defines synergy as "the bonus that is achieved when things work together harmoniously." Steven Covey maintains that synergy means that the whole is greater than the sum of its parts (1989). The American Association of Critical Care Nurses has a Synergy Model of Professional Caring & Ethical Practice that guides the nurse and results in synergy, where the needs and characteristics of a patient, clinical unit, or system are matched with a nurse's competencies (Hardin & Kaplan, 2005). Effective nurses and teams achieve synergy. They develop the ingredients for creating a winning team where people with different ideas, backgrounds, and beliefs work together synergistically and harmoniously.

First and foremost, these winning teams must have a clearly stated purpose: What are the goals? What are the objectives? What does the leader see the team accomplishing? Are any budget requirements, decision-making ability, and lines of authority for the team spelled out? An effective team keeps the larger organization's goals in mind as it progresses; otherwise, its goals will be inconsistent with those of the parent organization.

Second is an assessment of the team's composition: What are the team members' personal strengths and weaknesses? How do the team members see themselves as individuals? Do they see themselves as part of a cohesive team? Are the contributions of all team members valued? Are all team members' opinions respected? Does the team have a plan to avoid groupthink? Are any additional members with special expertise needed? What are the roles of each team member?

Third is the communication link. Are effective communication patterns in place? Is there a need to improve communication, either in written or verbal format? Does the team work well together and is communication open, with minimal hidden agendas of the members? Can the truth be told in a compassionate and sympathetic manner in order to reach a difficult decision?

Active participation by all team members is a critical fourth item. Does everyone have a designated responsibility? Do people listen to one another? Is "we versus they" thinking discouraged? Are all team members involved in shaping plans and decisions? Are they all carrying their weight on the team, or are some members not doing their part? What are the relationships of the team members? Is there mutual trust and respect for members and their decisions, however unpopular? Are there political turf issues that must be resolved before proceeding? The climate of the team should be relaxed but supportive.

Is there a clear plan as to how to proceed? Is there a way to acknowledge team accomplishments and positive change? This fifth element leads to an action plan that everyone agrees with early on, and one that is revisited at certain designated times. Feedback by team members and others affected by the team's decisions is necessary to keep focus.

The sixth guideline is actually ongoing, in that assessment and evaluation are continuous throughout the team's history. Outcomes have to be consistent and related to the expectations of the organization. Creativity is also encouraged at the team level; perhaps a member has an idea to solve a problem that no one has ever tried. In a supportive environment, pros and cons of all reasonable ideas should be freely discussed. A team needs to periodically evaluate its progress. See Table 5-3.

TABLE 5-3
Team Evaluation Checklist

	YES	NO
1. Is the environment/climate conducive to team building?	____	____
2. Do the team members have mutual respect for and trust in one another?	____	____
3. Are the team members honest with one another?	____	____
4. Does everyone actively participate in the team's decision making and problem solving?	____	____
5. Are the purpose, goals, and objectives of the team obvious to all participants?	____	____
6. Are the goals met?	____	____
7. Are creativity and mutual support of new ideas encouraged by all team members?	____	____
8. Does the team work to avoid groupthink?	____	____
9. Is the team productive, and does it see actual progress toward goal attainment?	____	____
10. Does the team begin and end its meetings on time?	____	____
11. Does the team leader provide vision and energy to the team?	____	____
12. Do any persons on the team serve in the common team member roles of group task role, group maintenance role, or self-oriented role, as identified earlier in this chapter?	____	____

Source: Compiled with information from Polifko-Harris, K. (2003). Effective team building. In P. L. Kelly, *Nursing Leadership and Management.* (2nd ed.). Clifton Park, NY: Delmar Cengage Learning.

TEAMWORK ON A PATIENT CARE UNIT

The role of the nurse is multifaceted. Depending on the scenario, a nurse may work directly or indirectly with a wide variety of staff on the health care team. A registered nurse (RN) is directly responsible for the care of the patient, but that care encompasses ensuring that the nursing and medical practitioner's orders are carried out and that nursing assistive personnel document the intakes and outputs accurately for the shift. The RN ensures that the licensed practical nurse completes the ordered treatments; that discharge planning is coordinated with the social worker, the case manager, the pharmacist, and the administration; that the family understands how to dress the patient's wound; and, finally, that the patient understands the discharge instructions. The role of the RN team leader incorporates the entire spectrum of care provided to the patient and family by a wide variety of people. The effective nurse will possess excellent

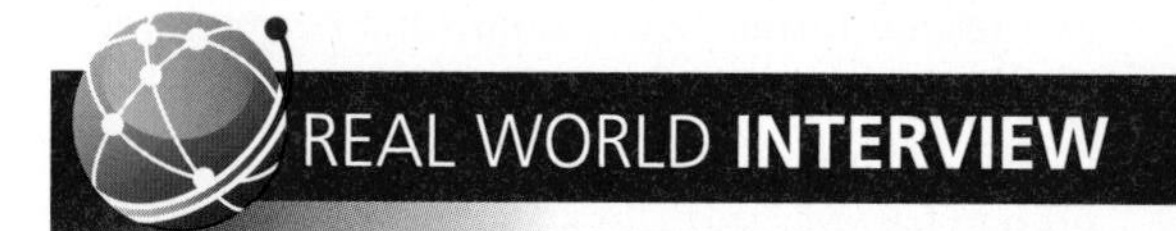

An elderly nonverbal patient with a history of schizophrenia was admitted to our surgical unit for dehydration. She was in need of total care, especially with respect to hygiene, which had been neglected. She was dependent on staff to turn and position her. Her level of awareness suggested she was unable to use a call light for help.

This patient challenged staff for a variety of reasons. First, due to multiple other health problems, she was not a candidate for surgery. This placed her among the patients who don't really "fit" the surgical unit where she was admitted. Nonetheless, my goal was to advocate for comfort care with her physician while also encouraging subordinates to provide quality care even though the goal was not for cure with this particular patient. The patient's inability to communicate verbally added to the challenge. It was unclear how aware the patient was of the care she was receiving. Her nonverbal status blocked her ability to dialogue. This caused us to rely on nonverbal cues. Respect for patients with or without their verbal feedback is essential. The CNA and I tackled the needed bed bath together. Teamwork kept the focus on the goal for the patient, which was to optimize comfort and maintain skin integrity. It allowed me to complete a thorough assessment and to model desired communication with the patient, whom I addressed by name. I inquired whether she was in pain, to which she responded with twisting motions. I continued the one-way conversation, attempting to clarify what her nonverbal responses meant. She pointed to her shoulder, so we repositioned her and she settled down, resting quietly. As is often the case, the CNA willingly returned to reposition the patient with confidence the remainder of the shift. The patient's inability to verbalize needs was perceived as less of a barrier once we were successful in overcoming it together.

I find that CNAs will often volunteer to complete entire tasks they feel capable of performing independently. They also need to be assured that they will not be expected to handle clinical situations for which they do not feel qualified. This mutual respect for each other is essential to an ongoing working relationship. They honor my standard of care and will often complete tasks, going above and beyond what I ask. For example, later in the afternoon, the CNA returned to the patient and washed and braided her hair. Since this same patient would not likely use the call light, I also explained our goal to the high school student volunteer and I asked her to check the patient's position whenever she went by the room. I instructed her to let me know if the patient appeared uncomfortable, assuring her that I would reposition the patient as needed. The student expressed that she thought it was cool how nurses communicate with patients who can't talk. I believe through effective communication our team achieved the goal of optimizing this patient's comfort in spite of many potential barriers.

LARI SUMMA, RN, BSN
Team Leader
Peoria, Illinois

communication skills, both written and verbal; be sensitive of others' cultural and value differences; be aware of others' abilities; and show genuine interest in the team members.

Status Differences

Status is the measure of worth conferred on an individual by a group. Status differences are seen throughout organizations and serve some useful purposes (Shortell & Kaluzny, 2006). Differences in status motivate people, provide them with a means of identification, and may be a force for stability in the organization (Scott, 1967).

Status differences have a profound effect on the functioning of teams. Research findings are fairly consistent in showing that high-status members initiate communication more often, are provided more opportunities to participate, and have more influence over the decision-making process (Owens, Mannic, & Neale, 1998). Thus, an individual from a lower-status professional group may be intimidated or ignored by higher-status team members. The group, as a result, may not benefit from this person's expertise. This situation is very likely in health care, where status differences among the professions are well entrenched (Topping, Norton, & Scafidi, 2003). Often, multidisciplinary teams are idealistically expected to operate as a company of equals, yet the reality of the situation makes this difficult (Shortell & Kaluzny, 2006). In a study of end-stage renal disease teams in which the equal participation ideology was accepted by most team participants, it was clear that the medical practitioners, who were perceived as having higher professional status than other groups, had greater involvement in the actual decision-making process (Deber & Leatt, 1986). The mismatch between expectations and reality made many team members, particularly staff nurses, feel a sense of role deprivation, with accompanying implications for morale and job satisfaction. This problem is exacerbated in teams characterized by gender diversity. In one study, men were more likely to want to exit teams that were female-dominated for those that were male-dominated or homogenous. Men have historically been perceived as having higher status in managerial roles in organizations, thereby affecting the men's satisfaction with the team (Chatman & O'Reilly, 2004). Status differences may significantly impact patient outcomes. According to the recent report *Keeping Patients Safe: Transforming the Work Environment of Nurses,* "counterproductive hierarchical communication patterns that derive from status differences" are partly responsible for many medical errors (Institute of Medicine, 2003, p. 361). Further, a review of medical malpractice cases from across the country found that medical practitioners, perceived by some as the higher-status members of the team, often ignored important information communicated by nurses, perceived by some as the lower-status members of the team. Nurses in turn were found to withhold relevant information for diagnosis and treatment from medical practitioners (Schmitt, 2001). Lately, changes in the status-conscious environment have prompted more attention to interdisciplinary service learning (Dacey, Murphy, Anderson, & McCloskey, 2010). Technological and pharmaceutical advances have demanded an inter-professional approach to promoting safe and competent care. Dacey and others (2010) illustrated the benefit of inter-professional service learning with pharmacy students where "pharmacy students had the most knowledge about drug therapy for cardiovascular disease" (p. 698). Changes in collaborative practice are underway, for example, the 2005 publication of the *Journal of Interprofessional Care.* Subsequent publications are addressing inter-professional practice more, but the number of articles authored by nurses is limited in comparison to other disciplines.

Crew Resource Management

Safe, competent, high-quality patient care, like other technically complex and high-risk fields, is an interdependent process carried out by teams of individuals with advanced technical training who have varying roles and decision-making responsibilities (Shea-Lewis, 2009). While technical training assures proficiency in specific tasks, it does not address the potential for errors created by communication and decision making in dynamic environments. Experts in aviation have developed safety training focused on effective team management, known as Crew Resource Management (CRM). Over the past 20 years, lessons from aviation's approach to team training have been applied to medicine, notably in surgical care (McGreevy et al., 2006) with modifications to support health care organization (Barach, 2007).

Modeling CRM practices is also recommended for adoption in obstetrical care (Neilsen & Mann, 2008). CRM training encompasses a wide range of knowledge, skills, and attitudes including communication, assertiveness, situational awareness, problem solving, decision making, and teamwork. Initiatives are underway to integrate team training into undergraduate and postgraduate education (Weaver et al., 2010).

Assertiveness is the willingness to actively participate, state, and maintain a position until convinced by the facts that other options are better. It requires initiative and the courage to act. Assertiveness differs from passive behavior which is often submissive to avoid conflict, and demonstrates a lack of initiative. Assertiveness also differs from aggressive behavior which can be dominating, hostile, belligerent, and argumentative. Situational awareness refers to the degree of accuracy by which one's perception of his or her current environment mirrors reality. Factors that reduce situational awareness include insufficient communication, fatigue and stress, task overload, task underload, group mindset, "press on regardless" philosophy, and degraded operating conditions.

CRM fosters a climate or culture where the freedom to respectfully question authority is encouraged. However, the primary goal of CRM is not enhanced communication, but enhanced situational awareness. CRM recognizes that a discrepancy between what is happening and what should be happening is often the first indicator that an error is occurring. This is a delicate area for many organizations, especially ones with traditional hierarchies like health care. Appropriate communication techniques must be taught to all nursing and medical practitioners so they understand that the questioning of authority need not be threatening, and so that all understand the correct way to question orders. A significant practice of CRM is identified as the sterile cockpit rule in depicting the need for improving the knowledge of each crew member's role at every stage of the flight, so that they can be sensitive to the other's workload level. West, et al. (2012) applied the sterile cockpit rule to the workload of nursing assistants in which all staff provided support for the nursing assistants' uninterrupted contribution to the care of patients.

The Foundation for Firefighter Health and Safety (2002) developed a five-step assertive statement process that encompasses inquiry and advocacy steps. The five steps are:

- Opening or attention getter—Address the individual as, for example, "Dr. Karen" or "Michelle," or whatever name or title will get the person's attention.
- State your concern—State what you see in a direct manner. "Mr. Jones has a pulse of 160."
- State the problem as you see it—"Mr. Jones is going into ventricular tachycardia."
- State a solution—"Mr. Jones needs an anti-arrhythmic medication."
- Obtain agreement (or buy-in)—"Do you want to order an antiarrhythmic medication?"

The five steps are difficult but important skills to master, and they require a change in interpersonal dynamics and organizational culture.

Communicating with Supervisors

Communicating with a supervisor about team problems can be intimidating, especially for a new nurse. It is important to communicate with your boss in order to develop a good working relationship (Gabarro & Kotter, 1993). See Table 5-4. Note that observing professional courtesy is an important first step. Alert your supervisor to any problems immediately, follow the policy and procedure of your agency, and, if it is not an emergency, request an appointment to discuss a problem further. This demonstrates respect and allows for the conversation to occur at an appropriate time and place. Be prepared to state the concern clearly and accurately. Provide supporting evidence. State a willingness to cooperate in finding a solution and then match behaviors to words. Persist in the pursuit of a solution.

Communicating with Coworkers

Nurses depend on their coworkers in many ways to collectively provide quality patient care. Nowhere is this more important than in the acute care setting where nursing services are nonstop around the clock. Handoff transfer of information about patient care from nurse to nurse is one of the most important and frequent communications between coworkers.

TABLE 5-4
How to Improve Your Ability to Work With Your Boss

Know your boss's:
- Goals and objectives
- Pressures
- Strengths, weaknesses, and blind spots
- Working style

Understand your own:
- Objectives
- Pressures
- Strengths, weaknesses, and blind spots
- Working style
- Predisposition toward dependence on authority figures

Develop a relationship that:
- Meets both your objectives and styles
- Keeps your boss informed
- Is based on dependability and honesty
- Selectively uses your boss's time and resources

Source: Adapted from Gabarro, J, & Kotter, J. P. (1993, May–June). Managing your boss. *Harvard Business Review,* 150–157.

Accurate handoffs are crucial to achieving quality patient care.

The Golden Rule

An excellent guide for communicating with coworkers is the golden rule: "Do unto others as you would have them do unto you." As a nurse who will be responsible for overseeing others' work, a valuable perspective for you to maintain is that all members of the team are important to successfully realize quality patient care. Offering positive feedback such as, "I appreciate the way you interacted with Mr. T. to get him to ambulate twice this shift," goes a long way toward team building, and it improves coworkers' sense of worth. Nurses also have an opportunity to act as teachers to coworkers. Often in a hospital setting, nurses teach by example. Demonstrating the desired behavior allows the coworker to copy the behavior. It is important to allow time for return demonstrations to evaluate whether the coworker has learned the intended skill. For example, as the nurse, you may demonstrate how to position a patient with special needs, encouraging the coworker to assist and ask questions. The next time repositioning is indicated, accompany the coworker and observe his or her ability to successfully complete the task. Offer constructive feedback. Be patient. Remember your own learning curve when mastering new skills and behaviors and allow those you supervise the opportunity to grow. Be open to the possibility that coworkers, particularly those with experience, may have a few pearls of wisdom to share with you as well.

Communicating with Other Nursing and Medical Practitioners

Sometimes new graduates are intimidated by other nursing and medical practitioners they work with. Cardillo (2001) gives several tips on working with

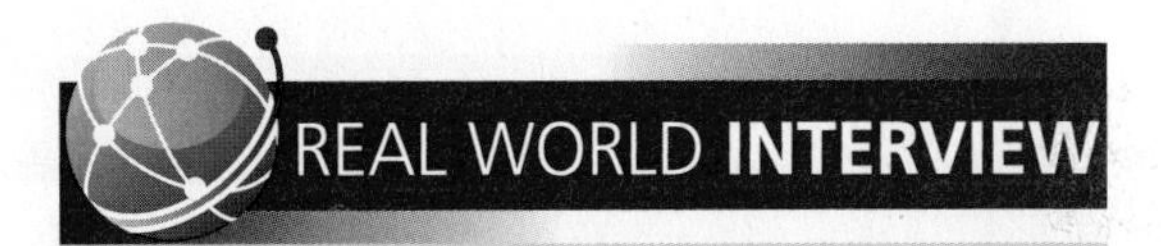

As an emergency medicine physician, I am frequently interfacing with nurses during life-threatening medical scenarios. Whether it is an acute myocardial infarction or respiratory failure or even a very sick child, the dialogue is standard. There is a set tone of urgency on both our parts, and we get straight to work with little discussion. I think when we work as a team, we are like a well-oiled machine. The nurse anticipates my needs and I hers or his, and we follow our protocols. The absolute focus is on the patient and getting him or her out of immediate danger. That is what the emergency department does best. We "stabilize" the patient's acute life-threatening event. The rapport between MD and RN is built from an understanding of mutual competency. I know my nurses in the ED and they know me. I could not save lives day in and day out without the teamwork mentality.

ELIZABETH HORVATH, D.O.
Crystal Lake, Illinois

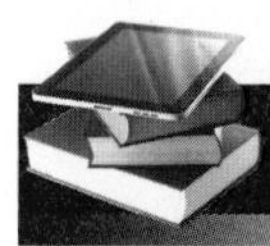

EVIDENCE FROM THE **LITERATURE**

Citation: Miller, K., Riley, W., & Davis, S. (2009). Identifying key nursing and team behaviours to achieve high reliability. *Journal of Nursing Management, 17*, 247–255.

Discussion: The aim of this study was to identify key nursing and interdisciplinary team behaviors that promote high reliability during critical events. Technical and team competence are necessary to achieve high reliability in interdisciplinary teams to ensure optimum patient care safety. Technical competence is generally guaranteed because of professional training, licensure, and practice standards. During critical events, team competence is difficult to observe, measure, and evaluate in interdisciplinary teams. Markers of team competence include having clear situational awareness; using the Situation, Background, Assessment, Recommendation, and Response (SBARR) method of communication (Table 5-5); using closed-loop communication, that is, repeating back information when one team member makes a request of another team member; and having a shared mental model of requirements, procedures, and role responsibilities of the team. These markers of team competence, which are necessary for nurses to contribute to highly reliable interdisciplinary teams, are not consistently observed during critical events. This constitutes a breach in defensive barriers for ensuring patient safety.

Implications for Nursing: Nurses make an important contribution to ensuring effective technical and team competence through appropriate and timely transfer of information during critical events. Nurses need to identify important clinical and environmental cues and act to ensure that the team progresses along the optimal course for patient safety.

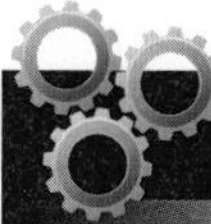

CRITICAL THINKING **5-2**

Teamwork on a patient care unit—Day shift routine

Throughout the day shift, nursing and unit staff communicate and work together to deliver quality patient care.

7:00 AM	Day shift takes handoff shift report from night shift
7:15 AM	Charge nurse reviews patient care assignments with all nurses and unit staff; goals and priorities are set
7:20 AM	Patient assessment, vital sign assessment, lab work, intravenous (IV) assessment, etc.
7:30 AM	Breakfast served
7:45 AM	A.M. care begins
8:00 AM	Medications given, practitioners make rounds, patients sent for diagnostic tests, nursing care standards followed, documentation begun, hourly regular patient rounds and team planning with other disciplines, medications given, etc.
11:30 AM	Vital sign assessment
12:00 PM	Lunch served, medications given
2:00 PM	Intake and output reports completed; documentation completed
3:00 PM	Hand off shift report from day shift to evening shift

How does teamwork get patient care completed? Does patient care on your clinical unit follow a similar time sequence as this routine above?

other practitioners. She suggests that it is useful to establish rapport and introduce yourself to the other practitioners you work with. Do this early in your working relationships and do not be intimidated. You and the other practitioners are all on the health care team to meet the patient's goals. At least one study has indicated that when nurses and physicians work together, patient death rates or readmission rates decrease (Baggs & Ryan, 1990). Both you and the other health care practitioners are important to your patient's welfare. Use the Situation, Background, Assessment, Recommendation, Response (SBARR) method to organize and clarify calls to other practitioners.

Cardillo (2001) also suggests that nurses be assertive. Do not call another practitioner or doctor and say, "I'm sorry to bother you." You are not bothering her. That is her job and you are doing your job by calling her. If you do not understand something, ask questions. Many practitioners and physicians love to teach. Be honest and up front. Tell the practitioner if something is new to you.

Show respect and consideration for the practitioner you work with, but do not be a doormat. Give due respect and expect the same from him or her. Present information in a straightforward manner, clearly delineating the problem and supporting it with pertinent evidence. This is especially important when reporting changes in patient conditions. Nurses are responsible for knowing classic symptoms of conditions, orally apprising the physician of changes, and recording all observations in the chart

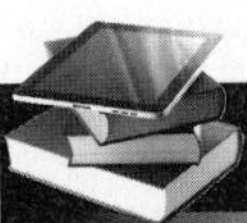

EVIDENCE FROM THE **LITERATURE**

Citation: Haig, K. M., Sutton, S., & Whittington, J. (2006). The SBARR technique: Improves communication, enhances patient safety. *Joint Commission's Perspectives on Patient Safety, 5*(2), 1–2.

Discussion: Communication failures are the root cause of nearly two-thirds of sentinel events in hospitals. This is due, in part, because nursing and medical practitioners are trained to communicate differently. The SBARR technique (Situation, Background, Assessment, Recommendation, Response) is designed to improve communication among health care personnel and improve patient safety.

- *Situation:* What is going on with the patient? Identify self, unit, patient, room number. Briefly state the problem, when it started, and its severity.
- *Background:* Provide background information related to the situation, as needed. Be aware of patient's admitting diagnosis, date of admission, current medications, allergies, IV fluids, most recent vital signs, lab results with date and time each was performed, other clinical information, and patient code status. The practitioner may ask you for these when you call.
- *Assessment:* What is your assessment? Do you think the patient's condition is deteriorating? Do you think the patient needs medication?
- *Recommendation:* What is your recommendation or what do you want? Know what you want from the practitioner before you call. Don't hang up without communicating this to the practitioner and assuring that your patient's needs are met—e.g., patient needs to be admitted, patient needs to be seen, order needs to be changed, or medication needs to be added.
- *Response:* Document response of practitioner and any further actions you take to meet patient needs.

Implications for Practice: Nursing and medical practitioners who use the SBARR technique will improve their communications. Patients will be the beneficiaries.

(Sanchez-Sweatman, 1996). If the other practitioner is out of line, you might say, "I don't appreciate being spoken to in that way," or "I would appreciate being spoken to in a civil tone of voice and I promise to do the same with you," or something similar. It is helpful to alert your nursing manager if a practitioner's behavior is inappropriate. Leadership support is essential to elimination of this problem.

Calfee (1998) offers suggestions for handling telephone miscommunications. For example, if a physician hangs up, document that the call was terminated and fill out an incident report. If, for example, the physician gives an inappropriate answer or gives no orders for a patient complaint of pain, document the call, the information relayed, and the fact that no orders were given. In addition, document any other steps such as notifying the supervisor that were taken to resolve the problem.

Cardillo (2001) also suggests that nurses seek clarification from the practitioner if an order is unclear. If an order is inappropriate or incorrect, rather than saying, "This order does not seem appropriate for this patient," which would likely put the practitioner on the defensive, try, "Teach me something, Dr. Jones; I've never seen a dose of Lopressor that high. Can you explain the therapeutic dynamics to me?" or "Dr. Smith, I can't figure out why you ordered a brain scan on this patient. Can you help me out here?" This approach often results in the practitioner either reevaluating an order or changing it. If the practitioner does not change an order that you think is inappropriate or you cannot reach the practitioner, let your supervisor know and follow the chain of command guidelines of the agency where you work. Patient safety must always be safeguarded.

Communicating with Patients and Families

Communication with patients and families is optimized by many skills, including touch. Nurses routinely use touch as a way to communicate caring and concern. Occasionally, language barriers will limit communication to the nonverbal mode. For instance, a stroke patient who cannot process words can still interpret a gentle hand on his or her shoulder.

Communication requires an openness and honesty with concurrent respect for patients and families. In addition, it is important to honor and protect patients' privacy with the nurse's actions and words.

Mentoring

Mentoring is a one-on-one relationship between an expert nurse preceptor and a novice nurse that focuses on professional aspects of nursing and is mutually beneficial. The optimal novice nurse is hardworking, willing to learn, and anxious to succeed. Good communication between the preceptor and the novice helps the novice nurse develop expert status and career direction. The preceptor's wisdom is typically shared through listening, affirming, counseling, encouraging, and seeking input from the novice. Sharing the same work schedule helps the preceptor and novice share information and provides opportunities for the novice to shadow the preceptor. The preceptor can also anticipate added challenges that will likely occur with the novice's increasing responsibilities. Nursing leaders should develop mentorship models to improve the new nursing graduate's direct care, decision making, and collaborative skills (Komaratat & Oumtanee, 2009). Role-playing, based on an evolving real-world case scenario in which the expert preceptor nurse guides the novice to practice the response to new and sometimes challenging situations, is a safe learning strategy. Giving end-of-shift handoff reports followed by feedback from nursing and medical practitioners allows novice nurses to critically reflect on the value of their communication with other care providers (Skaalvik, Normann, & Henriksen, 2010).

Responsibility of Nursing Leaders

Nursing leaders have a responsibility to ensure that developing the knowledge, skills, and attitudes of teamwork and collaboration empower nurses as team members rather than disempowering them (Cusack & Smith, 2010). The timeless adage "actions speak louder than words" is relevant in providing consistent safe and competent care. Nursing leaders must model

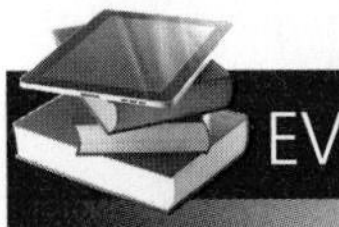

EVIDENCE FROM THE **LITERATURE**

Citation: Longo, J., and Sherman, R.O. (2007, March). Leveling horizontal violence. *Nursing Management, 38(3), 38* 34–37.

Discussion: Horizontal violence has been described as an expression of oppressed group behavior evolving from feelings of low self-esteem and lack of respect from others. Despite recent research that indicates a significant improvement in RNs' perceptions of satisfaction with their careers and work environments, the majority of nurses still disagree when asked if nursing is a good career for people who want respect in their jobs. Nurses may have been described as an oppressed group because the nursing profession is primarily female and has existed under a historically patriarchal system headed by male physicians, administrators, and marginalized nurse managers.

Horizontal violence between nurses is an act of aggression perpetrated by one colleague toward another colleague. Although horizontal violence usually consists of verbal or emotional abuse, it can also include physical abuse and may be subtle or overt. Acts of horizontal violence can include talking behind one's back, belittling or criticizing a colleague in front of others, blocking information or a chance for promotion, and isolating or freezing a colleague out of group activities. Repeated acts of horizontal violence against another are often referred to as "workplace bullying."

Common behaviors characterized as horizontal violence include:

- Nonverbal behaviors such as the raising of eyebrows or making faces in response to comments from the victim
- Verbal remarks that could be characterized as being snide, or abrupt responses to questions raised by the victim
- Activities that undermine the victim's ability to perform professionally, including either refusing or not being available to give assistance
- The withholding of information about a practice or patient that will undermine a victim's ability to perform professionally
- Acts of sabotage that deliberately set victims up for negative situations in their work environment
- Group infighting and establishing of cliques designed to exclude some staff members
- Scapegoating or attributing all that goes wrong in a situation to one individual
- Failure to resolve conflicts directly with the individual involved, choosing instead to complain to others about an individual's behavior
- Failure to respect the privacy of others
- Broken confidences

Implications for Nursing: Nurses can work to recognize horizontal violence or workforce bullying in the profession. As these behaviors are recognized, they can be eliminated.

a collaborative approach in embracing interdisciplinary, evidence-based practice involving patient and family as members of the interdisciplinary team (Newhouse & Spring, 2010). Supporting nurses in identifying and delivering nursing care that is respectful of colleagues and patients is essential in the role of nursing leaders (Burhans & Alligood, 2010).

ORGANIZATIONAL COMMUNICATION

Avenues of communication are often defined by an organization's formal structure. The formal structure establishes who is in charge and identifies how different levels of personnel and various departments relate within the organization. Some of these relationships are typically depicted by an organizational chart. When the chief executive officer of an organization announces that the company will adopt a new policy that all employees will follow, that is downward communication. The message starts at the top and is usually disseminated by levels through the chain of communication. Upward communication is the opposite of downward communication. The message originates at some level below the top of the organization and moves upward. For example, when a nurse recommends a more efficient approach to organizing care to his nurse manager, who takes the recommendation to her superior, who uses the recommendation to develop a new policy—that is upward communication.

Besides the upward and downward chain network of communication, other common networks of communication have been identified, for example, a Y network, a wheel network, a circle network, and an all-channel network of communication (Longest, Rakich, & Darr, 2000). A Y pattern of communication would be two people reporting to another person who reports to others. An example is two staff nurses who report to the nursing unit director, who reports to the vice president for nursing, who reports to the president.

A wheel network of communication looks like an X in a wheel and could be a situation in which four nurses report to one nurse manager. There is no interaction among the four nurses, and all communications are channeled through the nurse manager at the center of the wheel. This wheel network is rare in health care organizations. Even though this type of wheel network communication is not used routinely, it may be used in circumstances in which urgency or secrecy is required. For example, the president of an organization who has an emergency might communicate with the vice presidents in a wheel network because time does not permit using other modes.

A circle network of communication allows communicators in the network to communicate directly only with two others, next to them in the circle. Because each communicates with another communicator in the circle network, the effect is that everyone communicates with someone, and there is no central authority or leader.

Finally, an all-channel network of communication is a circle network, except that all communicators may interact with every other communicator in the network, not just the communicator next to them (Longest, Rakich, & Darr, 2000).

Communication networks vary along several dimensions. The most appropriate network depends upon the situation in which it is used. The wheel and all-channel networks tend to be fast and accurate compared with the chain and Y-pattern networks. The chain and Y-pattern networks promote clear-cut lines of authority and responsibility but may slow communications. The circle and all-channel networks enhance morale among those in the networks better than other patterns. Nurses must construct communication networks to fit the various communication situations they face. Note that e-mail has had the effect of flattening some organizational communications to sometimes allow more direct access between levels that were formerly controlled through middle managers.

A final avenue worth mentioning, which is not a formal avenue, is the grapevine. The **grapevine** is an informal avenue in which rumors circulate. It ignores the formal chain of command. The major benefit of the grapevine is the speed with which information is spread, but its major drawback is that it often lacks accuracy. For example, nurses who inform an oncoming shift about a rumor that layoffs or mandatory overtime is imminent in the absence of any information from hospital administration are participating in grapevine communication.

OVERCOMING COMMUNICATION BARRIERS

Despite the best intentions and efforts, communication barriers may occur; however, these incidences can be minimized. DuBrin (2000) has identified nine strategies and tactics for overcoming communication barriers. See Table 5-5. In addition to these strategies, it is helpful to use stress management techniques to avoid communication barriers.

Horizontal or Lateral Violence

Horizontal or lateral violence is hostile and aggressive behavior by an individual or group members toward another member or groups of members of the larger group. It is generally nonphysical, but may involve shoving, hitting, or throwing objects, or other overt and covert behaviors of hostility. It includes all acts of unkindness, discourtesy, sabotage, divisiveness, infighting, bullying, lack of cohesiveness, scapegoating, and criticism. Horizontal or lateral violence is behavior associated with oppressed groups and can occur in any arena where there are unequal power relations, and one group's self-expression and autonomy are controlled by forces with greater prestige, power, and status than themselves. It is generally psychologically, emotionally, and spiritually damaging behavior and can have devastating long-term effects on the recipients.

Horizontal or lateral violence may also be demonstrated by an individual or a group in response to unhealthy organizational factors that must be

TABLE 5-5
Overcoming Communication Barriers

Concept	Application
Understand the receiver	Ask yourself, "What is in it for the other person?" Work to develop an understanding of the other person's needs.
Communicate assertively	Be direct. Use "I" statements; e.g., "I want you to . . ." Explain ideas clearly and with feeling. Repeat important messages. Use various communication channels; e.g., written, e-mail, and verbal.
Use two-way communication	Ask questions. Communicate face to face.
Unite with a common vocabulary	Define the meaning of important terms, such as "high quality," so all understand their meaning.
Elicit verbal and nonverbal feedback	Request and offer verbal feedback often. Document important agreements. Observe nonverbal feedback.
Enhance listening skills	Pay attention to what is said, what is not said, and nonverbal signals. Continue listening carefully even when you do not like the message. Give summary reflections to ensure understanding; e.g., "You say you were late giving medication because the pharmacy did not deliver meds on time." Engage in concluding discussions; e.g., "Has your unit been late with medications due to problems with pharmacy deliveries before?" Ask questions to explore problems. Paraphrase the speaker's words to decrease miscommunication, rather than blurting out questions as soon as the other person finishes speaking.
Be sensitive to cultural differences	Know that cultural communication barriers exist. Show respect for all workers. Minimize use of jargon specific to your culture. Be sensitive to cultural etiquette; e.g., use of first names, eye contact, hand gestures, personal appearance.

(Continues)

TABLE 5-5 (Continued)

Be sensitive to gender differences	Be aware that men and women may have some differences in communication style; e.g., men may call attention to their accomplishments and women tend to be more conciliatory when facing differences. Know that male-female stereotypes often do not fit the person you are working with. Avoid barriers by knowing differences exist, and do not take things personally. Males can improve communication by showing more empathy, and females by becoming more direct.
Engage in metacommunication	Communicate about your communication to resolve a problem; e.g., "I'm trying to get through to you, but either you don't react to me or you get angry. What can I do to improve our communication?"

Source: Compiled with information from DuBrin, A. J. (2000). *The active manager.* London, England: South-Western College Publishing.

identified and eliminated or the behavior will continue or increase. Horizontal or lateral violence differs from a simple conflict that can be readily resolved in that it is demonstrated more frequently and lasts for a longer period of time. Lutgen-Sandvik, Tracy, and Alberts (2007) describe workplace bullying in which the individual "experiences at least two negative acts, weekly or more often, for six or more months in situations where targets find it difficult to defend against or stop the abuse" (p. 841).

Acknowledging horizontal or lateral violence early is an initial step in addressing it. However, addressing it with the goal of eliminating unhealthy organizational factors is more challenging. Organizational factors contributing to horizontal or lateral violence may include organizational volatility, leadership styles, the organizational hierarchy, and oppressed group behavior (Johnson, 2009). It is important to develop an organizational culture that provides a safe place to practice and to develop policies that clearly articulate how horizontal or lateral violence will be identified, addressed, and stopped.

Avoiding Groupthink

Effective leaders work to avoid groupthink. Groupthink is defined as "the tendency to have the same opinion as the other members of the group as a way to avoid conflict, reduce interpersonal pressure, or maintain an illusion of unity and cohesion" (Wienclaw, 2010, p. 5). Groupthink occurs when maintaining the pleasant atmosphere of the team becomes more important to members than reaching a good decision (Shortell & Kaluzny, 2006). There is a reduced willingness to disagree and challenge others' views in groupthink. Some or all of the following symptoms may indicate the presence of groupthink (Janis, 1972):

- *The illusion of invulnerability:* Team members may reassure themselves about obvious dangers and become overly optimistic and willing to take extraordinary risks.
- *Collective rationalization:* Teams may overlook blind spots in their plans. When confronted with conflicting information, the team may spend considerable time and energy refuting the information and rationalizing a decision.
- *Belief in the inherent morality of the team:* Highly cohesive teams may develop a sense of self-righteousness about their role that makes them insensitive to the consequences of decisions.
- *Stereotyping others:* Victims of groupthink hold biased, highly negative views of competing teams. They assume that they are unable to negotiate with other teams, and rule out compromise.

- *Pressures to conform:* Group members face severe pressures to conform to team norms and to team decisions. Dissent is considered abnormal and may lead to formal or informal punishment.
- *The use of mind guards:* Mind guards are used by members who withhold or discount dissonant information that interferes with the team's current view of a problem.
- *Self-censorship:* Teams subject to groupthink pressure members to remain silent about possible misgivings and to minimize self-doubts about a decision.
- *Illusion of unanimity:* A sense of unanimity emerges when members assume that silence and lack of protest signify agreement and consensus.

Shortell and Kaluzny (2006) state that the consequences of groupthink are that teams may limit themselves, often prematurely, to one possible solution and fail to conduct a comprehensive analysis of a problem. When groupthink is well entrenched, members may fail to review their decisions in light of new information or changing events. Teams may also fail to consult adequately with experts within or outside the organization, and fail to develop contingency plans in the event that the decision turns out to be wrong.

Team leaders can help avoid groupthink. First, leaders can encourage members to critically evaluate proposals and solutions. When a leader is particularly powerful and influential, yet still wants to get unbiased views from team members, the leader may refrain from stating his or her own position until later in the decision-making process. Another strategy is to assign the same problem to two separate work teams. Most importantly, groupthink can be avoided by proactively engaging in a process of critical appraisal of ideas and solutions, and by understanding the warning signs of groupthink (Shortell & Kaluzny, 2006).

CRITICAL THINKING 5-3

The Luck Factor, published in 2004, authored by R. Wiseman, discusses research that illustrates luck as something that can be learned if one pays attention to four principles:

- Lucky people create, notice, and act on the chance opportunities in their lives.
- Lucky people make successful decisions by using their intuitions and gut feelings.
- Lucky people's expectations about the future help them fulfill their dreams and ambitions.
- Lucky people are able to transform their bad luck into good fortune.

Do you agree with Wiseman's findings? Can you use "luck" as well as careful planning to improve your nursing career? Your life? Discuss.

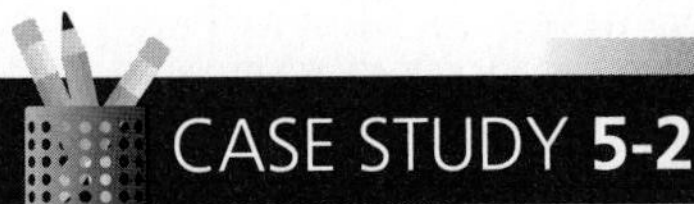

CASE STUDY 5-2

You volunteer to serve on a task force exploring the high incidence of patient falls in your department. The task force has been meeting for almost a year without making much progress. Your first meeting is scheduled in two weeks' time and is scheduled to last one hour.

What actions may be helpful in preparing to serve on the task force?

At the first meeting you attend, you observe that the meeting lacks focus with several members using the time to voice their complaints about nursing leadership, ranging from lack of support to hostile communication behaviors. Shortly before the meeting ends, one of the members confronts you about what you think of the meeting and asks you for your opinion on the number of falls. How would you respond?

KEY CONCEPTS

- ✦ Teams consist of people who collaborate and come together for a common purpose and who need each other's contributions to achieve the overall goal.
- ✦ Horizontal and lateral violence (workforce bullying) interferes with safe patient care.

- The Health Insurance Portability and Accountability Act (HIPAA) protects patient privacy.
- There are various stages of group process.
- Working with inter-professional health care team members can improve patient-centered care, along with quality and safety.
- The patient and family are partners with the inter-professional health care team.
- Teamwork and collaboration are an extension of organizational performance.
- Crew Resource Management (CRM) and TeamSTEPPS are methods for improving team performance and communication.
- Team members perform various roles, which may ultimately enhance or hinder the team's progress toward goal attainment.
- Great teams have clearly stated purposes, goals, effective communication, an action plan, and continuously evaluate their progress toward outcomes.
- Clear team communication is essential to achieving organizational goals.
- Groupthink must be avoided to ensure effective team functioning.

KEY TERMS

communication
grapevine
group process

REVIEW QUESTIONS

1. Based on the Tuckman and Jensen Team Process, what stage of team development consists of team members working harmoniously together, engaging in open communication, taking risks, and trusting each other to complete assigned tasks?
   A. Forming
   B. Storming
   C. Norming
   D. Performing
2. Which of the following is NOT a characteristic of groupthink?
   A. Use of mind guards
   B. Illusion of unanimity
   C. Free discussion of ideas
   D. Pressure to conform
3. Which of the following showed that an individual's performance is often determined in large part by the workgroup?
   A. Kaluzny study
   B. Dickson research
   C. Carnegie study
   D. Hawthorne experiments
4. All but which of the following are steps to improve communication using the SBARR technique?
   A. Share the situation.
   B. Provide background information.
   C. Ensure patient safety.
   D. Ask for a recommendation from the practitioner.

5. You are aware that two nursing staff are speaking negatively about the assignment you have made for the upcoming shift. How should you address it initially?
   A. Discuss the situation with the human resources personnel in your hospital.
   B. Explore concerns about the staff assignment with the two staff members.
   C. Accuse the staff members of insubordination and report it to the manager.
   D. Ask a nursing leader from another unit to review your assignment.

6. What behavior could the health care team borrow from the aviation industry and use during emergency situations?
   A. Foster a climate where the freedom to respectfully question authority is encouraged.
   B. Gain familiarity with the organizational chart and reporting relationships.
   C. Interpret the vision of the organization as a member of the health care industry.
   D. Explore everyone's opinion before taking action.

7. Which of the following are elements of Crew Resource Management? Select all that apply.
   A. Teamwork
   B. Assertiveness
   C. Communication
   D. Problem solving
   E. Brainstorming
   F. Situational awareness

8. Which of the following are group maintenance roles that foster group unity, positive interpersonal relationships among group members, and development of the ability of members to work effectively together? Select all that apply.
   A. Challenger
   B. Equalizer
   C. Harmonizer
   D. Gatekeeper
   E. Group observer
   F. Standard setter

9. Which of the following are group task roles that help a group develop and accomplish its goals? Select all that apply.
   A. Orienter
   B. Energizer
   C. Harmonizer
   D. Information giver
   E. Gatekeeper
   F. Information seeker

10. Which of the following are considered patient identifiers under HIPAA legislation? Select all that apply.
   A. Fax number
   B. Fingerprints
   C. E-mail address
   D. Phone number
   E. Vehicle serial number
   F. Health plan beneficiary number

REVIEW ACTIVITIES

1. You are a nurse on a 38-bed medical-surgical unit. In light of some vacancies, the nurse manager has hired a licensed practical nurse to fill a position in which only registered nurses had worked before.
   - What are some things you can do to assist the new person in becoming a member of your team?
   - Would nursing assignments change with the addition of the new practical nurse?
2. On the unit on which you work as a registered nurse, the team is quite inter-professional in nature: you directly work with licensed practical nurses, nursing assistive personnel, a secretary, one housekeeper, one respiratory therapist, one case manager, and one clinical nurse specialist.
   - What are some of the advantages of working with inter-professional teams?
   - What are some of the challenges of working with inter-professional teams?
   - How does one best communicate with an inter-professional team?

EXPLORING THE WEB

- Agency for Healthcare Research and Quality: *http://www.ahrq.gov*
- Quality & Safety Education for Nurses: *http://www.qsen.org*
- Institute of Medicine (IOM): *http://www.iom.edu*
- National Academy of Sciences: *http://www.nap.edu*
- The Institute for Patient- and Family-Centered Care: *http://www.ipfcc.org*
- World Health Organization: *http://www.who.int/en*

REFERENCES

Agency for Healthcare Research and Quality. (2012). TeamSTEPPS: National implementation. Retrieved September 1, 2012, from http://teamstepps.ahrq.gov/about-2cl_3.htm

Anderson, E. S., & Thorpe, L. (2010). Learning together in practice: An interprofessional education programme to appreciate teamwork. *The Clinical Teacher, 7*(1), 19–25.

Andrews, L. B., Stocking, C. T., Krizek, T., Gottlieb, L., Krizek, C., Vargish, T., et al. (1997, February). An alternative strategy for studying adverse events in medical care. *Lancet, 349*, 309–313.

Argyris, C. (1964). *Integrating the individual and the organization*. New York, NY: Wiley.

Baggs, J. G., & Ryan, S. A. (1990). ICU nurse-physician collaboration and nursing satisfaction. *Nursing Economics, 8*(6), 386–392.

Baggs, J. G., Ryan, S. A., Phelps, C. E., Richeson, J. F., & Johnson, J. E. (1992). The association between interdisciplinary collaboration and patient outcomes in a medical intensive care unit. *Heart and Lung: Journal of Critical Care, 21*(1), 18–24.

Barach, P. (2007). A team-based risk modification programme to make health care safer. *Theoretical Issues in Ergonomic Science, 8*(5), 481–494.

Bartol, K. M., & Martin, D. C. (1998). *Management*, (3rd ed.). Boston, MA: McGraw-Hill.

Bennis, W. (1989). *Why leaders can't lead*. San Francisco, CA: Jossey-Bass.

Blanchard, K. H., & Johnson, S. (1981). *The one-minute manager*. New York, NY: Partnership and Candle Communications Corporation.

Bryan, J. (2009). Engaging clients, families, and communities as partners in mental health. *Journal of Counseling & Development, 87*(4), 507–512.

Burhans, L. M., & Alligood, M. R. (2010). Quality nursing care in the words of nurses. *Journal of Advanced Nursing, 66*(8), 1689–1697.

Burns, J. M. (1978). *Leadership*. New York, NY: Harper & Row.

Calfee, B. E. (1998). Making calls to the physician. *Nursing, 98*, 10, 17.

Cardillo, D. W. (2001). *Your first year as a nurse*. Roseville, CA: Prima.

Chatman, J., & O'Reilly, C. (2004). Asymmetric effects of work group demographics on men's and women's responses to work group composition. *Academy of Management Journal, 47*(2), 193–208.

Comp, D. (2011). Improving parent satisfaction by sharing the inpatient daily plan of care: An evidence review with implications for practice and research. *Pediatric Nursing, 37*(5), 237–242.

Covey, S. (1989). *The 7 habits of highly effective people.* New York, NY: Fireside.

Cusack, L., & Smith, M. (2010). Power inequalities in the assessment of nursing competency within the workplace: Implications for nursing management. *The Journal of Continuing Education in Nursing, 41*(9), 408–412.

Dacey, M., Murphy, J. I., Anderson, D. C., & McCloskey, W. W. (2010). An interprofessional service-learning course: Uniting students across educational levels and promoting patient-centered care. *Journal of Nursing Education, 49*(2), 696–699.

Deber, R. B. & Leatt, P. (1986). The multidisciplinary renal team: Who makes the decisions? *Health Matrix, 4*(3), 3–9.

DuBrin, A. J. (2000). *The active manager.* London, England: South-Western College Publishing.

Farup, P. G., Blix, I., Førre, Johnson, G., Lange, O., Johannessen & Petersen, H. (2011). What causes treatment failure - the patient, primary care, secondary care or inadequate interaction in the health services. *BMC Health ServicesResearch*, 11:111. Retrieved October 31, 2012 from http://www.ncbi.nlm.nih.gov/pubmed/21599926

Finest quotes retrieved october 31, 2012 from http://www.finestquotes.com/select_quote-category-Team%20Work-page-0.htm

Fink, J. (2010). Five nurses fired for Facebook postings. Retrieved January 17, 2012, from http://scrubsmag.com/five-nurses-fired-for-facebook-postings/

Foundation for Firefighter Health and Safety. (2002) Crew Resource Management. Retrieved October 31, 2012 from http://www.iaff.org/06news/NearMissKit/6.%20Crew%20Resource%20Management/CRM.pdf

Gabarro, J., & Kotter, J. P. (1993, May–June). Managing your boss. *Harvard Business Review*, 150–157.

Gardner, S. F., Chamberlin, G. D., Heestand, D. E., & Stowe, C. D. (2002). Interdisciplinary didactic instruction at academic health centers in the United States: attitudes and barriers. *Advances in Health Sciences Education 7*(3): 179–190.

Governance Institute. (2009). Leadership in healthcare organizations: A guide to Joint Commission standards. Retrieved September 1, 2012, from http://www.jointcommission.org/Library/publications

Haig, K. M., Sutton, S., & Whittington, J. (2006). The SBARR technique: Improves communication, enhances patient safety. *Joint Commission's Perspectives on Patient Safety, 5*(2), 1–2.

Haines, S., & Warren, T. (2011). Staff and patient involvement in benchmarking to improve care. *Nursing Management, 18*(2), 22–25.

Hall, P., & Weaver, L. (2001). Interdisciplinary education and teamwork: A long and winding road. *Medical Education, 35*, 867–875.

Hardin, S. R., & Kaplan, R. (2005). *Synergy for clinical excellence: American Association of Critical Care Nurses.* Boston, MA: Jones & Bartlett.

Hasenfeld, Y. (1983). *Human service organizations.* Englewood Cliffs, NJ: Prentice Hall.

Institute of Medicine (IOM). (2003). *Keeping patients safe: Transforming the work environment of nurses.* Washington, DC: The National Academies Press

Institute of Medicine (IOM). (2004). *Keeping patients safe: Transforming the work environment of nurses.* Washington, DC: The National Academies Press.

Janis, L. (1972). *Victims of groupthink.* Boston, MA: Houghton-Mifflin.

Johnson, S. L. (2009). International perspectives on workplace bullying among nurses: A review. *International Nursing Review, 56*(1), 34–40.

Joint Commission. (2011). Inspiring health care excellence. Retrieved September 1, 2012, from http://www.jointcommission.org

Kalisch, B. J., & Lee, K. H. (2011). Nurse staffing levels and teamwork: A cross-sectional study of seven patient care units in acute care hospitals. *Journal of Nursing Scholarship, 43*(1), 82–88.

Katzenbach, J. R., & Smith, D. K. (2003). *The wisdom of teams: Creating the high-performance organization.* New York, NY: Harper Collins Publishers.

Knaus, W. A., Draper, E. A., Wagner, D. P., & Zimmerman, J. E. (1986). An evaluation of outcome from intensive care in major medical centers. *Annals of Internal Medicine, 104*(3), 410–418.

Komaratat, S., & Oumtanee, A. (2009). Using a mentorship model to prepare newly graduated nurses for competency. *The Journal of Continuing Education in Nursing, 40*(10), 475–480.

Lewin, K. (1951). *Field theory in social sciences.* New York, NY: Harper & Row.

Longest, B. B., Jr., Rakich, J. S., & Darr, K. (2000). *Managing health services organizations and systems* (4th ed.). Baltimore, MD: Health Professions Press.

Longo, J., & Sherman, R. O. (2007). Leveling horizontal violence. *Nursing Management, 38*(3), 34–37, 50–51.

Lutgen-Sandvik, P., Tracy, S. J., & Alberts, J. K. (2007). Burned in bullying in American workplace: Prevalence, perception, degree and impact. *Journal of Management Studies, 44*(6), 837–862.

McGreevy, J., Otten, T., Poggi, M., Robinson, C., Castaneda, D., & Wade, P. (2006). The challenge of changing roles and improving surgical care now: Crew resource management. *American Surgeon, 72*(110), 1082–1087.

McGregor, D. (1960). *The human side of enterprise.* New York, NY: McGraw-Hill.

Miller, K., Riley, W., & Davis, S. (2009). Identifying key nursing and team behaviours to achieve high reliability. *Journal of Nursing Management, 17,* 247–255.

National Committee on Quality Assurance (NCQA). (2011). The healthcare effectiveness data and information. Retrieved September 1, 2012, from http://web.ncqa.org

Neilsen, P., & Mann, S. (2008). Team function in obstetrics to reduce errors and improve outcomes. *Obstetrics and Gynecology Clinics in North America, 35*(1), 81–95.

Newhouse, R. P., & Spring, B. (2010). Interdisciplinary evidence-based practice: Moving from silos to synergy. *Nursing Outlook, 2010*(6), 309–317.

NHS Institute for Innovation and Improvement. (2008). Quality and service improvement tools. Retrieved September 1, 2012, from http://www.institute.nhs.uk?quality_and_service_improvment_tools/quality_and_service

Owens, D. A., Mannic, E. A., & Neale, M. A. (1998). Strategic formation of groups: Issues in task performance and team member selection. In D. H. Gruenfeld (Ed.), *Research on managing groups and teams* (pp. 149–165). Stamford, CT: MAI Press.

Polifko-Harris, K. (2003). Effective team building. In P. L. Kelly (Ed.), *Nursing leadership & management* (2nd ed.). Clifton Park, NY: Delmar Cengage Learning.

Preheim, G. J., Armstrong, G. E., & Barton, A. J. (2009). The new fundamentals in nursing: Introducing beginning quality and safety education for nurses' competencies. *Journal of Nursing Education, 48*(2), 694–697.

Quality & Safety Education for Nurses (QSEN). (2012). Teamwork and collaboration. Retrieved September 1, 2012,from http://www.qsen.org/definition.php?id=2

Roethlisberger, F. J., & Dickson, W. J. (1939). *Management and the worker.* Cambridge, MA: Harvard University Press.

Sanchez-Sweatman, L. (1996, September.). Communicating with physicians. *The Canadian Nurse, 92*(8), 49–50.

Schmitt, M. H. (2001). Collaboration improves the quality of care: Methodological challenges and evidence from U.S. health care research. *Journal of Interprofessional Care, 15*(1), 47–66.

Scott, D., & Troutman, A. K. (2009). Facebook firings show privacy concerns with social networking sites: Remind staff about slippery slope with online postings. *Healthcare Risk Management, 31*(5), 50–52.

Scott, W. G. (1967). *Organization theory.* Homewood, IL: Irwin.

Selle, K. M., Salamon, K., Boarman, R., & Sauer, J. (2008). Providing interprofessional learning through interdisciplinary collaboration: The role of "modelling". *Journal of Interprofessional Care, 22*(1), 85–92.

Senge, P. M. (1990). *The fifth discipline.* New York, NY: Doubleday Books.

Shea-Lewis, A. (2009). Teamwork: Crew resource management in a community hospital. *Journal of Healthcare Quality, 31*(5), 14–18.

Shortell, S. M., & Kaluzny, A.D. (2006). *Health care management* (5th ed.). Clifton Park, NY: Delmar Cengage Learning.

Shortell, S. M., Zimmerman, J. E., Rousseau, D. M., Gillies, R. R., Wagner, D. P., Draper, E. A., et al. (1994). The performance of intensive care units: Does good management make a difference? *Medical Care, 32*(5), 508–525.

Skaalvik, M. W., Normann, H. K., & Henriksen, N. (2010). To what extent does the oral shift report stimulate learning among nursing students? A qualitative study. *Journal of Clinical Nursing, 19*(15/16), 2300–2308.

Topping, S., Norton, T., & diScafi, B. (2003). Coordination of services: The use of multidisciplinary, interagency teams. In S. Dopson & A. L. Mark (Eds.), *Leading health care organizations* (pp. 100–112). New York: Palgrave Macmillan.

Tuckman, B. W. & Jensen, M. A. C. (1977). Stages of small group development revisited. *Group and Organizational Studies, 2*(4), 419–427.

U.S. Department of Health and Human Services HHS. (2003). Protecting personal health information research: Understanding the HIPAA privacy rule. NIH Publication Number 03–5388.

U.S. Department of Health & Human Services. (2012). The Health Insurance Portability and Accountability Act of 1996 (HIPAA) Privacy and Security Rules. Retrieved October 31, 2012 from http://www.hhs.gov/ocr/privacy/index.html

Verma, S., Paterson, M., & Medves, J. (2006). Core competencies for health care professionals: What medicine, nursing, occupational therapy, and physiotherapy share. *Journal of Allied Health, 35*(2), 109–115.

Weaver, S. J., Rosen, M. A., Salas, E., Baum, K. D., & King, H. B. (2010). Integrating the science of team training: Guidelines for continuing education. *The Journal of Continuing Education in the Health Professions, 30*(4), 208–220.

Welsh, C. A., Flanagan, M. E., Ebright, P. (2010). Barriers and facilitators to nursing handoffs: Recommendations for redesign. *Nursing Outlook, 58*(3), 148–154.

West, P., Sculli, G., Fore, A. , Okam, N., Dunlap, C., Neily, J., & Mills, P. et al. (2012). Improving patient safety and optimizing nursing teamwork using crew management techniques. *The Journal of Nursing Administration, 42*(1), 15–20.

Wienclaw, R. A. (2010). *Conflict management, Research Starters Academic Topic Overviews: EBSCO Research Starter.* Ipswich, Massachusetts EBSCO Publishing.

Wiseman, R. (2004). *The luck factor*. London, England, UK: Random House.

World Health Organization (WHO). (2007). Team building. Retrieved September 1, 2012, from http://www.who.int/cancer/modules/Team%20building.pdf

World Health Organization (WHO). (2011). Health topics: Primary health care. Retrieved September 1, 2012, from http://www.who.int/topics/primary_health_care/en

Young, G. J., Charns, M. P., Daley, J., Forbes, M. G., Henderson, W., & Khuri, S. F. (1997). Best practices for managing surgical services: The role of coordination. *Health Care Management Review, 22*(4), 72–81.

Young, G. J., Charns, M. P., Desai, K., Khuri, S. F., Forbes, M. G., Henderson, W., et al. (1998). Patterns of coordination and surgical outcomes: A study of surgical services. *Health Services Research, 33*(5).

Youngwerth, J. & Twaddle, M. (2011). Cultures of interdisciplinary teams: How to foster good dynamics. *Journal of Palliative Medicine, 14*(5), 650–654.

SUGGESTED READINGS

Angood, P., Dingman, J., Foley, M. E., Ford, D., Martins, B., O'Regan, P., et al. (2010). Patient and family involvement in contemporary health care. *Journal of Patient Safety, 6*(1), 38–42.

Baker, S. J. (2010). Bedside shift report improves patient safety and nurse accountability. *Journal of Emergency Nursing, 36*(4), 355–358.

Beswick, S., Hill, P., & Anderson, M. A. (2010). Comparison of nurse workload approaches. *Journal of Nursing Management, 18*(5), 592–598.

Carter, K. F., & Burnette, H. D. (2011). Creating patient-nurse synergy on a medical-surgical unit. *MEDSURG Nursing, 20*(5), 249–254.

Clark, R. C., & Allison-Jones, L. (2011). Investing in human capital: An academic-service partnership to address the nursing shortage. *Nursing Education Perspectives, 32*(1), 18–21.

Conway, J. (2008). Patients and families: Powerful new partners for healthcare and caregivers. *Healthcare Executive, 23*(1), 60–62.

Joint Commission. (2005). The SBARR technique: Improves communication, enhances patient safety. *Joint Commission's Perspectives on Patient Safety, 5*(2), 1–2.

Peck, N. C., Kleiner, K. H., & Kleiner, B. H. (2011). Managing generational diversity in the hospital setting. *Cultural & Religion Review Journal.,* (1), 54–68.

Reid, R., Allstaff, K., & Bruce, D. (2009). An educated workforce which works collaboratively. Deriving best-evidence operating principles for interprofessional learning in Tayside: A qualitative study. *Journal of Interprofessional Care, 23*(5), 534–538.

Smith, M. K. (2005). Bruce W. Tuckman—forming, storming, norming, and performing in groups. *Encyclopedia of Informal Education*. Retrieved November 3, 2011, from http://www.infed.org/thinkers/tuckman.htm

Tevington, P. (2011). Mandatory nurse–patient ratios. *MEDSURG Nursing, 20*(5), 265–268.

Thomas, M. B., Benbow, D. A., & Ayers, V. D. (2010). Continued competency and board regulation: One state expands options. *The Journal of Continuing Education in Nursing, 41*(11), 524–528.

Yarbrough, S., & Klotz, L. (2007). Incorporating cultural issues in education for ethical practice. *Nursing Ethics, 14*(4), 492–502.

CHAPTER 6

Change, Innovation, and Conflict

CAROLYN A. CHRISTIE-McAULIFFE, RN, PHD, FNP; KRISTINE E. PEFENDT, RN, MSN; AND MARGARET ANDERSON, RN, EDD

Never doubt that a small group of thoughtful, committed citizens can change the world; indeed, it's the only thing that ever has.

–MARGARET MEAD, 2002

OBJECTIVES

Upon completion of this chapter, the reader should be able to:

1. Discuss traditional theories of change.
2. Discuss chaos theory and the concept of the learning organization.
3. Review the concept of innovation.
4. Discuss the concept of conflict.
5. Review conflict management.

Lakeisha is a new graduate. She is in her fifth week of orientation with her preceptor, Denise, and has been doing fairly well. Recently, Lakeisha disagreed privately with Denise about how to do a patient care procedure. While Lakeisha was careful to disagree in a professional manner, Denise has been acting irritated with her ever since the discussion. How can Lakeisha deal with this conflict with Denise? Is conflict ever useful?

This chapter is designed to introduce the concepts of change, innovation, chaos, organizational learning, and conflict. The ability to change and be innovative is useful both in life and in health care situations. The ability to manage any conflict that may ensue from change and innovation requires that the nurse gain understanding of these concepts.

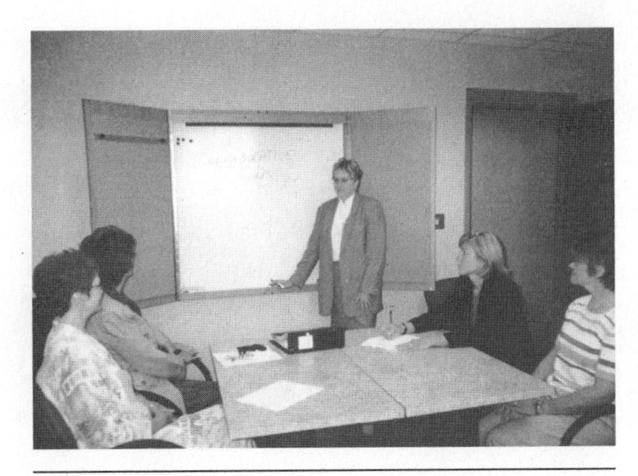

© Cengage Learning 2014

CHANGE

Change can be defined as "the act or process of substitution, alteration, or variation" (Webster's New World Dictionary, 2000, p. 245). The outcome may be the same, but the actions performed to get to the outcome may be different.

There are many types of change—personal, professional, and organizational. For example, a change to new patient admission forms may necessitate a different method of assessing the patient or change the number of people involved in the admission process. Rather than one registered nurse conducting the entire admission process, the process may be broken down so that individuals with different skill levels conduct parts of the process utilizing collaboration and teamwork. The goal of the change is still the admission of the patient to a unit; how it is done may be different. Adoption of the new admission form may involve personal, professional, and organizational changes. See Table 6-1.

Individual persons, professionals, and organizations that adapt successfully to change are more likely to survive in a competitive health care environment.

Traditional Change Theories

The change theories illustrated here are Lewin's Force-Field Model (1951), Lippitt's Phases of Change (1958), Havelock's Six-Step Change Model (1973), and Rogers's Diffusion of Innovations Theory (1995). These are classic change theories. See Table 6-2.

Lewin's model has three simple steps: unfreezing, moving to a new level, and refreezing.

TABLE 6-1
Types of Voluntary and Involuntary Change

Personal	A change made in one's life, often for self-improvement.
Professional	A change in one's career, such as obtaining additional academic credentials or being promoted to a new work position.
Organizational	A change in an organization to achieve organizational goals.

© Cengage Learning 2014

TABLE 6-2
Traditional Change Theories

Theorist and Year	Lewin (1951)	Lippitt (1958)	Havelock (1973)	Rogers (1995)
Title of Model	Force-Field Model	Seven Phases of Change	Six-Step Change Model	Diffusion of Innovations Theory
Steps in Model	1. Unfreeze.	1. Diagnose problem.	1. Build relationship.	1. Awareness.
	2. Move.	2. Assess motivation and capacity for change.	2. Diagnose problem.	2. Interest.
	3. Refreeze.	3. Assess change agent's motivation and resources.	3. Acquire resources.	3. Evaluation.
		4. Select progressive change objective.	4. Choose solution.	4. Trial.
		5. Choose appropriate role of change agent.	5. Gain acceptance.	5. Adoption.
		6. Maintain change.	6. Stabilize and self-renew.	
		7. Terminate helping relationship.		

Sources: Compiled with information from Lewin, K. (1951). *Field History in Social Science.* New York, NY: Harper & Row; Lippitt, R., et al. (1958). *The Dynamics of Planned Change.* New York, NY: Harcourt Brace; Havelock, R. G. (1973). *The Change Agent's Guide to Innovation in Education.* Englewood Cliffs, NJ: Educational Technology; Rogers, E. M. (1995). *Diffusion of Innovations* (4th ed.). New York, NY: Free Press.

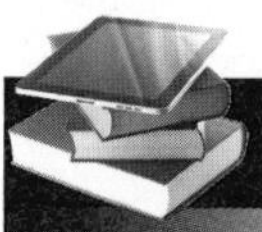

EVIDENCE FROM THE **LITERATURE**

Citation: Brookes, J. (2011). Engaging staff in the change process. *Nursing Management, 18*(5), 16–19.

Discussion: Brookes discovered first-hand the consequence of autocratic leadership and problem-focused management. As a new manager to a pediatric acute care floor, she found a myriad of problems including low morale, ineffective recruitment and/or retention of nurses, as well as high absenteeism and many medication errors. Rather than utilize traditional change management strategies, Brookes decided to engage in a creative process based on "appreciative inquiry" and participatory management. Brookes found the process to be particularly positive, articulating with staff a clear vision for improving strengths and positively addressing problems. The end result was radical and lasting positive change with improved recruitment and retention and a simultaneous decrease in medication and other care-related errors.

Implications for Practice: Brookes's article supports the idea that any nurse can facilitate and support positive change and transformation whether he or she is the formal leader or a follower. In this case, the nursing staff can be given as much credit as Brookes herself for positively addressing the needed change for this pediatric unit.

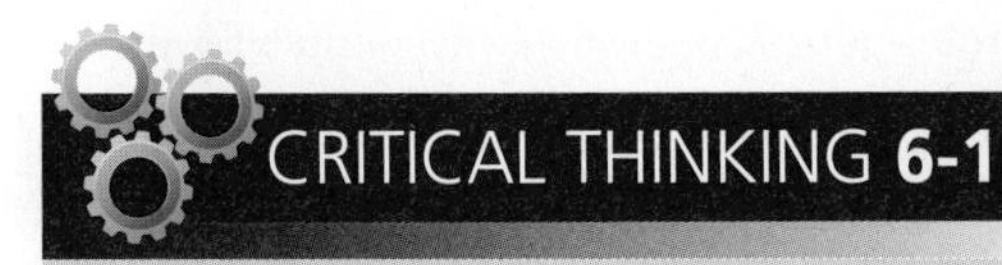

LaTonya works the night shift on her unit. She is concerned that the medication carts stock high dosages of intravenous potassium chloride. LaTonya knows that high dosages of this medication are lethal. She believes that this medication should be made up by the pharmacy only on an "as needed" basis in response to a specific patient's needs. How can LaTonya work as a change agent, unfreeze the current situation, and move to a new way of preparing this medication? How can she then refreeze this needed change?

The theories described in Table 6-2 are linear in nature, meaning they more or less proceed in an orderly manner from one step to the next; for example, from unfreezing to moving to a new level to refreezing. Unfortunately, change is not often this simple and often requires more personal, professional, and organizational adjustment.

Unfreezing means that the current or old way of doing something is thawed or open for change. People begin to be aware of the need for doing things differently, that change is needed for a specific reason. This change can be easy for some people and difficult for others. In the next step, moving to a new level, change is implemented. In the third step, refreezing occurs. This means that the new way of doing things is incorporated into the routines or habits of the affected people. Although these steps sound simple, the process of change is more complicated than it initially appears.

Emerging Change Theories

Two other emerging theories of change are also useful in understanding health care organizations. These theories are *chaos theory* and *learning organization theory.*

Chaos Theory

Chaos theory hypothesizes that chaos actually has an order. That is, although the potential for chaos appears to be random at first glance, further investigation reveals some order to the chaos. Health care organizations have repeatedly experienced chaos during the past 20 years. Chaos theory would say that this is normal. Most organizations go through periods of rapid change and innovation and then stabilize before chaos erupts again. Even though each chaotic occurrence is similar to the one that occurred before, each is different. The political, scientific, and behavioral components of the organization are different from before, so the chaos looks different. Order emerges through fluctuation and chaos. Thus, the potential for chaos means that nurses and the organization must be able to organize and implement change quickly and forcefully. There is little time for orderly linear change.

Learning Organization Theory

Peter Senge (1990) first described **learning organization theory**. Learning organizations are based on five learning disciplines and demonstrate responsiveness and flexibility. Senge believes that because organizations are open systems, they could best respond to unpredictable changes in the environment by using a learning approach in their interactions and inter-professional workings with one another. The whole cannot function well without a part, regardless of how small that part may seem. An example in health care is that the billing department cannot submit an accurate bill to the insurance company without the cooperation of the nursing staff. If the patient is not charged appropriately by nursing for items used in his or her care, then the billing department cannot prepare an accurate inventory. Then, the organization cannot be paid for the actual services and supplies used. The learning organization understands these interrelationships and responds quickly to improve relationships. This may be through dialogue and teamwork and problem solving. All parties must understand what is at stake for cooperation and working together to occur. Senge, Kleiner, Roberts, Ross, and Smith (1994) emphasize that the core of the learning organization is based on five "learning disciplines"—lifelong programs of study and practice.

- Personal Mastery. Learning to expand our personal capacity to create the results we most desire, creating an organizational environment that encourages all members of the team to develop themselves toward the goals and purposes they choose.
- Mental Models. Reflecting on, continually clarifying, and improving our internal pictures of the world, and seeing how this vision shapes our actions and decisions.
- Shared Vision. Building a sense of commitment in a group by developing shared images of the future we seek to create, and developing the principles and guiding practices by which we hope to get there.
- Team Learning. Encouraging teamwork and conversational and collective thinking skills, so groups of people can reliably develop intelligence and ability greater than the sum of individual members' talents.
- Systems Thinking. A way of thinking about and understanding the forces and interprofessional relationships that shape the behavior of systems. *Systems thinking* highlights the fact that change in one area will affect other areas of the system. This discipline helps us to see how we can act more in tune with the larger processes of the natural and economic world.

In organizations, Senge believes the individuals who contribute most to the enterprise are the ones who are committed to the practice of these five learning disciplines. People using these principles are: expanding their own capacity to improve and master their environment; clarifying and sharing their vision of the world and the future they hope to create; building team learning; and understanding the behavior of the systems they are helping to develop.

Change Promotion

Bennis, Benne, and Chin (1969) identified three strategies to promote change in groups or organizations. Different strategies work in different situations. The power or authority of the change agent has an impact on the strategy selected. See Table 6-3. The **change agent** is one who is responsible for implementation of a change project. This person may be from within or outside an organization. Most change agents use a variety of approaches to promote successful change. See Table 6-4.

Registered nurses providing care in an interprofessional environment continuously function from a fluctuating perspective of being a leader in some cases and a follower in others. In either situation, supporting the process of positive change becomes a necessary responsibility of every nurse. In that sense, anyone can be an agent of change.

Response to Change

Lewin (1951) identified forces that were supportive of, as well as barriers to, change. He called these "driving" and "restraining" forces. If the restraining forces outweigh the driving forces, then the change must be abandoned because it cannot succeed. Driving and restraining forces include political issues, technology issues, cost and structural issues, and people issues. The political issues include the power groups in favor of or against the proposed change. This may include practitioners, administrators, civic and community groups, or state or federal regulators. The technology or informatics issues include whether to update old equipment, computer systems, implementing bar code scanning, or methods of accounting for supply use. Structural issues include the costs, desirability, and feasibility of remodeling or building new construction for the change project. People issues include the commitment of the interprofessional staff, their

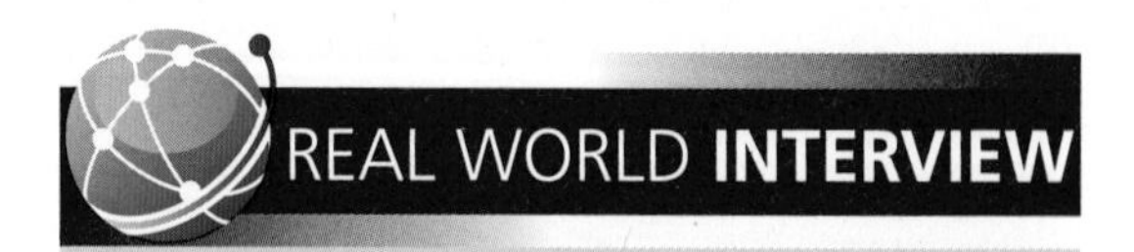

One of the things I have learned about change is that fear of the change is worse than the change itself. Now I concentrate on assisting my staff to focus on the reasons the change is necessary, and involving them in the process of finding solutions to the problem.

JOY CHURCHILL, RN
Team Leader
Highland Heights, Kentucky

TABLE 6-3
Strategies for Change

Strategy	Description	Example
Power-coercive Approach	Used when resistance is expected but change acceptance is not important to the power group. Uses power, control, authority, and threat of job loss to gain compliance with change—"Do it or get out."	Student must achieve a passing grade in a class project to complete the course requirements satisfactorily.
Normative-reeducative Approach	Uses the individual's need to have satisfactory relationships in the workplace as a method of inducing support for change. Focuses on the relationship needs of workers and stresses "going along with the majority."	A new RN who is working 8-hour shifts is encouraged by the other unit staff to embrace a new unit plan for 12-hour staffing.
Rational-empirical Approach	Uses knowledge to encourage change. Once workers understand the merits of change for the organization or understand the meaning of the change to them as individuals and the organization as a whole, they will change. Stresses training and communication. Used when little resistance is anticipated.	Staff are educated regarding the scientific merits of a needed change.

© Cengage Learning 2014

level of education and training, and their interest in the project. The most common people issue is fear of job loss or fear of not being valued. It bears repeating that if the restraining forces outweigh the driving forces, then the change will not succeed, and it should be abandoned or rethought. See Figure 6-1.

Several factors affect staff response to change. The first is trust. Staff must trust that each member is doing the right thing and that each is capable of producing successful change. In addition to capability, predictability is important. Another factor is the individual's ability to cope with change. Silber (1993) points out four factors that affect an individual's ability to cope with change:

1. Flexibility for change; that is, the ability to adapt to change.
2. Evaluation of the immediate situation; that is, if the current situation is unacceptable, then change will be more welcome.
3. Anticipated consequences of change; that is, the impact change will have on one's current job.
4. Individual's stake, or what the individual has to win or lose, in the change; that is, the more individuals perceive they have to lose, the more resistance they will offer.

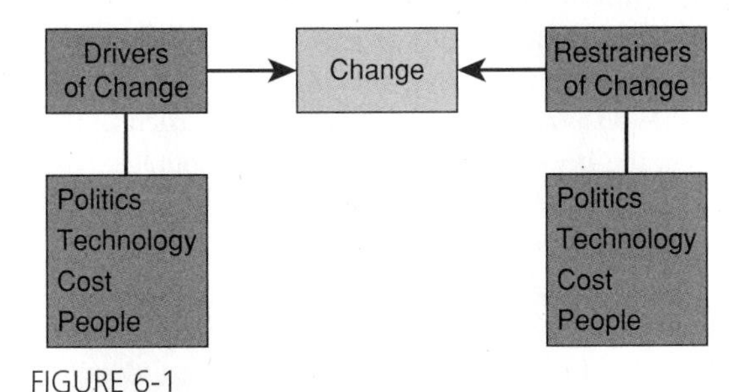

FIGURE 6-1

Forces driving and restraining change.

© Cengage Learning 2014

Bushy (1992) has identified six behavioral responses to planned change. See Table 6-5.

Regardless of the importance and necessity of change, the human response is very important and

TABLE 6-4
Change Agent Approaches

1. Begin by articulating the vision clearly and concisely. Use the same words over and over. Constantly remind people of the vision.
2. Map out a tentative timeline and the steps of the project. Have a good idea of how the project should go.
3. Plant seeds or mention some ideas or thoughts to key individuals from the first step through the evaluation step so that some notion of what is expected is always under consideration.
4. Make sure the committee is heavily loaded with those who will be affected by the change, and other experts as needed. Select a variety of people. For example, an innovator, someone from the late majority group, a laggard, and a rejector (Table 6-5) are probably good to include. These people provide insight into what others are thinking.
5. Set up consistent meeting dates and keep them. Have an agenda and constantly check the timeline for target activities.
6. Give regular updates and progress reports, both verbally and in writing, to the executives of the organization and those affected by the change. If the change agent does not do this, someone on the project team will, and the change agent wants to control the messages.
7. Check out rumors of conflict and confront conflict head-on. Do not back away from conflict or ignore it.
8. Maintain a positive attitude and do not get discouraged.
9. Stay alert to political forces, both for and against the project. Get consensus on important issues as the project goes along, especially if policy, financial, or philosophical issues are involved. Obtain consensus quickly from both executives and staff on major issues or potential barriers to the project.
10. Know the formal and informal leaders. Create a relationship with them. Consult them often.
11. Have self-confidence and trust in oneself and one's team. This will overcome a lot of obstacles.

Source: Compiled with information from Lancaster, J. (1999). *Nursing Issues in Leading and Managing Change.* St. Louis, MO: Mosby.

cannot be dismissed. So often, in one's zeal to respond to a need, the change agent forgets that the human side of change must be dealt with. People have a right to their feelings and a right to express them. The important point is that the change agent works with people's responses and helps them move on to the goal of implementing the change.

INNOVATION

Innovation can be defined as the process of creating new services or products. Shortell & Kaluzny (2006) state that "change" and "innovation" are different. "Change" is a generic concept that refers to any modification. "Innovation" is more restricted to new modifications in ideas or practices. Porter-O'Grady and Malloch (2011), authors of *Quantum Leadership: Advancing Innovation, Transforming Health Care*, discuss the role of leadership within nursing and health care relative to sustainability and success. They outline key factors needed of leaders to create a "healing environment" for both health care professionals as well as their patients. In particular, they stress the need for including creativity, courage, emotional competence, and transformative leadership in all levels of management and care.

An example of innovation in health care has been applied to the problem of medication errors. Injuries and death from medication errors have been identified by internal and external groups, creating pressure for change in performance and the promotion of safety.

TABLE 6-5
Responses to Change

1. Innovators: Change embracers. Enjoy the challenge of change and often lead change.
2. Early adopters: Open and receptive to change, but not obsessed with it.
3. Early majority: Enjoy and prefer the status quo, but do not want to be left behind. They adopt change before the average person.
4. Late majority: Often known as the followers. They adopt change after expressing negative feelings and are often skeptics.
5. Laggards: Last group to adopt a change. They prefer tradition and stability to innovation. They are somewhat suspicious of change.
6. Rejectors: Openly oppose and reject change. They may be surreptitious or covert in their opposition. They may hinder the change process to the point of sabotage.

© Cengage Learning 2014

Once the medication performance gap was recognized and identified by interprofessional health care groups, nursing and medical practitioners, working in collaboration with pharmacists and other team members, they were able to analyze why medication errors were occurring. Rather than blaming the person who administered the medication, an innovative "systems" approach revealed why the errors were occurring. Systems errors included illegible handwriting, unfamiliar medications, dosage calculation errors, food and drug interactions, and lack of documentation of patient allergic reactions.

By applying an innovative systems approach to problem solving, new safety structures and health care processes were implemented and institutionalized. Health care structures and processes were developed using informatics to include a computerized, medication-order entry system, and all personnel were educated in the system. This system changed the process of how health care orders were written. Handwritten orders that were prone to interpretation errors were replaced by clear, concise, computer-generated orders. Informatics incorporated multiple checks and balances into the computer system to document allergies, health care conditions, and current height and weight to assist in appropriate medication ordering and dosing. Nurses and dietitians reviewed the computerized patient information profiles for possible food and drug allergies and interactions. Pharmacists reviewed orders using this computer system before dispensing medications to analyze whether the medication dosage was indeed correct, based on the patient's height and weight. Nurses review computer-generated medication administration records (MARs). Barcoding systems are now used to ensure that the right drug is being administered to the right patient at the right time. Centralized computerized charting for nurses and other health care providers now aids in the accurate and timely flow of information. Patient histories and current lab results can be accessed and assessed quickly. Nurses access a database from their portable computers. This use of technology speeds the flow of information to the medical or nursing practitioner and back to the nurse caring for the patient. By improving the flow of essential information, patient safety is enhanced. Hopefully, ongoing evaluation of these innovative measures will indicate that medication errors are occurring less frequently and that patient outcomes are improving.

A poignant example of innovation within the context of quality of care and patient safety is the Quality and Safety Education for Nurses (QSEN) project that evolved from several studies and initiatives by organizations such as the Institute of Medicine (IOM), the American Association of Colleges of Nursing (AACN), the National League for Nurses (NLN), and the Robert Wood Johnson Foundation. The QSEN project aimed to "meet the challenge of preparing future nurses who will have the knowledge, skills, and attitudes necessary to continuously improve the quality and safety of the health care systems within which they work" (QSEN, 2011, p.1). Within this goal, QSEN stipulates six core competencies that nurses should demonstrate with knowledge, skill, and attitude: patient-centered care, teamwork and collaboration, evidenced-based practice, quality improvement, safety, and informatics. An especially exciting opportunity offered by QSEN is the Student Innovator Award that rewards nursing students' suggestions for change projects aimed at improving an aspect of the quality and/or safety of patient care. Within a two-year time span of the award's inception, 221 graduate nurses who were exposed to the creative and critical thinking skills of the Institute for Healthcare Improvement's Transforming Care at the Bedside (TCAB) proposed, conducted, and evaluated over 91 projects (QSEN, 2011).

CONFLICT

An important part of the change process is the ability to resolve conflict. **Conflict** is a disagreement about something of importance to the people involved. Conflict resolution skills are leadership and management tools that all registered nurses should have in their repertoire. Conflict itself is not bad. Conflict can be healthy. It, like change, allows for creativity, innovation, new ideas, and new ways of doing things. It allows for the healthy discussion of different views and values and adds an important dimension to the provision of quality patient care. Without some conflict, groups or work teams tend to become stagnant and routinized. Nothing new is allowed to penetrate the "way we have always done it" mentality. Conflict can be stimulated by such things as changing material resources, quality improvement initiatives, invasion of personal space, safety or security issues, cultural differences, scarce nursing resources, increased workload, group competition, and various nursing demands and responsibilities.

The Conflict Process

In 1975, Filley suggested a process for conflict resolution that is widely accepted. In this process, there are five stages of conflict:

1. Antecedent conditions
2. Perceived and/or felt conflict
3. Manifest behavior
4. Conflict resolution or suppression
5. Resolution aftermath

In Filley's model, conflict and conflict resolution follow a specific course. The process begins with specific preexisting conditions called "antecedent conditions." As the situation develops, conflict is perceived or felt by the involved parties. This triggers a response or manifest behavior. The conflict is either resolved or suppressed, leading to the development of new feelings and attitudes that may create new conflicts. Conflict resolution is vital in change. The antecedent conditions that Filley suggests may or may not be the cause of the conflict, but they certainly move the disagreement to the conflict level. The sources of these conditions include disagreement about goals, values, or resource utilization. Other issues may also serve as antecedent conditions such as the dependency of one group on another. For instance, the nursing department is dependent on the pharmacy department to provide drugs for the nursing unit in a timely fashion. The goals and priorities of pharmacy and nursing may be different at the time the nurse requests the drugs, and so a source of disagreement arises. If the circumstances for disagreement continue, a conflict will develop.

Methods of Conflict Management

There are essentially seven methods of conflict management. These methods dictate the outcomes of the conflict process. Although some methods are more desirable or produce more successful outcomes than others, there may be a place in conflict management for all the methods, depending on the nature of the conflict and the desired outcomes. Table 6-6 is a summary of these methods, highlighting some of their advantages and disadvantages.

Negotiation in Conflict Management

According to Lewicki, Hiam, and Olander (1996), there are five basic approaches to negotiating in conflict management: collaborative (win-win), competitive (win at all costs), avoiding (lose-lose), accommodating (lose to win), and compromise

TABLE 6-6
Summary of Conflict Management Methods

Conflict Management Method	Advantages	Disadvantages
Accommodating—smoothing or cooperating; one side gives in to the other side	One side is more concerned with an issue than the other side; stakes not high enough for one side and that side is willing to give in	One side holds more power and can force the other side to give in; the importance of the stakes are not as apparent to one side
Avoiding—ignoring the conflict	Does not make a big deal out of nothing; conflict may be minor in comparison to other priorities; allows tempers to cool	Conflict can become bigger than anticipated; source of conflict might be more important to one person or group than others
Collaborating—both sides work together to develop optimal outcomes	Best solution for the conflict and encompasses all important goals to each side	Takes a lot of time; requires commitment to success
Competing—the two or three sides are forced to compete for the goal	Produces a winner; good when time is short and stakes are high	Produces a loser; may leave anger and resentment on losing side
Compromising—each side gives up something and gains something	No one should win or lose, but both should gain something; good for disagreements between individuals	May cause a return to the conflict if what is given up becomes more important than the original goal
Confronting—immediate and obvious movement to stop conflict at the very start	Does not allow conflict to take root; very powerful	May leave impression that conflict is not tolerated; may make something big out of nothing
Negotiating—high-level discussion that seeks agreement, but not necessarily consensus	Stakes are very high and solution is rather permanent; often involves powerful groups	Agreements are permanent, even though each side has gains and losses

© Cengage Learning 2014

(split the difference). These five approaches to negotiation are influenced by the importance of maintaining the relationships relative to the importance of achieving one's desired outcomes (Figure 6-2). Note that as the relationship's and the outcome's value increase, the amount of collaboration increases.

Strategies to Facilitate Conflict Management

Open, honest, clear communication is the key to successful conflict management. The nurse manager/leader and all parties to the conflict must agree to communicate with one another openly and honestly. Courtesy and active listening are encouraged.

The Quality and Safety Education for Nurses (QSEN) site (www.qsen.org) provides relevant and helpful resources to nurse educators as well as nurses for each of the six competencies, including many strategies for improved communication as it impacts all aspects of nursing functions. However, effective communication is most critical to collaboration and teamwork. Within the resources provided, two teaching strategies have been provided that help address the need for standardized communications across

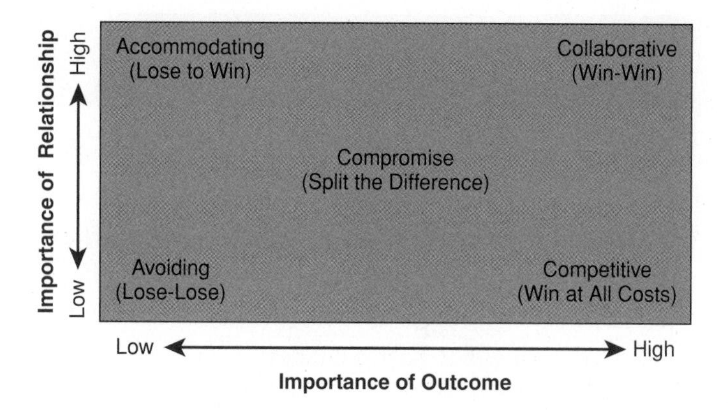

FIGURE 6-2

Negotiation strategies.
© Cengage Learning 2014

disciplines in order to provide seamless patient care. The first strategy, called Situation, Background, Assessment, Recommendation, and Response (SBARR), is a method of improving communication particularly in situations needing quick, concise interchange. The second strategy, 60-Second Situational Assessment, is a tool for developing both assessment skills and awareness of observable data. Both tools can be used for clinical as well as organizational situations requiring clear and effective communication.

In addition to maximizing communication skills, the setting for the discussions for conflict management should be private, relaxed, and comfortable. If possible, external interruptions from phones, pagers, overhead speakers, and personnel should be avoided or kept to a minimum. The setting should be on neutral territory so that no one feels overpowered. The ground rules (e.g., not interrupting, who should go first, time limits) should be agreed upon in the beginning. Adherence to ground rules should be expected.

In the conflict management process, it is expected that both sides in the conflict will comply with the results. If one party cannot agree to comply with the decisions or outcomes, there is no point to the process.

REAL WORLD INTERVIEW

Change is all about growing and developing, but the change agent or nurse manager has to be honest and truthful. Once he or she lies to us, then trust is destroyed and the change will surely fail. It's okay to not have the answer or not to be able to give the answer, but don't lie about it.

CARON MARTIN, RN
Staff Nurse
Highland Heights, Kentucky

Conflict Management, Change, and Innovation

Conflict management is an important part of the change and innovation process. Change and innovation can often threaten individuals and groups, making conflict an inevitable part of the process. It is important to keep in mind that some conflicts resolve themselves, so the change agent should not be too quick to jump into an intervention mode.

A guide for assessing conflict is identified in Figure 6-3. Figure 6-4 provides a guide for assessment of the level of conflict. If the level of conflict is too high, the nurse manager must apply conflict management strategies. Change, innovation, and conflict are all positive processes that promote growth. Leaders, managers, and staff should be encouraged to embrace

Interpersonal or intergroup?

1. **Who?**
   - Who are the primary individuals or groups involved? Characteristics (values; feelings; needs; perceptions; goals; hostility; strengths, past history of constructive conflict management; self-awareness)?
   - Who, if anyone, are the individuals or groups that have an indirect investment in the result of the conflict?
   - Who, if anyone, is assisting the parties to manage the conflict constructively?
   - What is the history of the individuals' or groups' involvement in the conflict?
   - What is the past and present interpersonal relationship between the parties involved in the conflict?
   - How is power distributed among the parties?
   - What are the major sources of power used?
   - Does the potential for coalition exist among the parties?
   - What is the nature of the current leadership affecting the conflicting parties?
2. **What?**
   - What is (are) the issues(s) in the conflict?
   - Are the issues based on facts? Based on values? Based on interests in resources?
   - Are the issues realistic?
   - What is the dominant issue in the conflict?
   - What are the goals of each conflicting party?
   - Is the current conflict functional? Dysfunctional?
   - What conflict management strategies, if any, have been used to manage the conflict to date?
   - What alternatives in managing the conflict exist?
   - What are you doing to keep the conflict going?
   - Is there a lack of stimulating work?
3. **How?**
   - What is the origin of the conflict? Sources? Precipitating events?
   - What are the major events in the evolution of the conflict?
   - How have the issues emerged? Been transformed? Proliferated?
   - What polarizations and coalitions have occurred?
   - How have parties tried to damage each other? What stereotyping exists?
4. **When/Where?**
   - When did the conflict originate?
   - Where is the conflict taking place?
   - What are the characteristics of the setting within which the conflict is occurring?
   - What are the geographic boundaries? Political structures? Decision-making patterns? Communication networks? Subsystem boundaries?
   - What environmental factors exist that influence the development of functional versus dysfunctional conflict?
   - What resource persons are available to assist in constructive conflict management?

Functional or dysfunctional?	**YES**	**NO**
Does the conflict support the goals of the organization?	[ ]	[ ]
Does the conflict contribute to the overall goals of the organization?	[ ]	[ ]
Does the conflict stimulate improved job performance?	[ ]	[ ]
Does the conflict increase productivity among work group members?	[ ]	[ ]
Does the conflict stimulate creativity and innovation?	[ ]	[ ]
Does the conflict bring about constructive change?	[ ]	[ ]
Does the conflict contribute to the survival of the organization?	[ ]	[ ]
Does the conflict improve initiative?	[ ]	[ ]
Does job satisfaction remain high?	[ ]	[ ]
Does the conflict improve the morale of the work group?	[ ]	[ ]

A yes response to the majority of the questions indicates that the conflict is probably functional. If the majority of responses are no, then the conflict is most likely a dysfunctional conflict.

FIGURE 6-3.

Guide for the assessment of conflict.

(*Source:* From MacFarland, G., Leonard, H., & Morris, M. (1984). *Nursing Leadership and Management: Contemporary Strategies.* Clifton Park, NY: Delmar Cengage Learning.)

Is conflict too low?	YES	NO
Is the work group consistently satisfied with the status quo?	[ ]	[ ]
Are no or few opposing views expressed by work-group members?	[ ]	[ ]
Is little concern expressed about doing things better?	[ ]	[ ]
Is little or no concern expressed about improving inadequacies?	[ ]	[ ]
Are the decisions made by the work group generally of low quality?	[ ]	[ ]
Are no or few innovative solutions or ideas expressed?	[ ]	[ ]
Are many work-group members "yes-men"?	[ ]	[ ]
Are workgroup members reluctant to express ignorance or uncertainties?	[ ]	[ ]
Does the nurse manager seek to maintain peace and group cooperation regardless of whether this is the correct intervention?	[ ]	[ ]
Do the workgroup members demonstrate an extremely high level of resistance to change?	[ ]	[ ]
Does the nurse manager base the distribution of rewards on "popularity" as opposed to competence and high job performance?	[ ]	[ ]
Is the nurse manager excessively concerned about not hurting the feelings of the nursing staff?	[ ]	[ ]
Is the nurse manager excessively concerned with obtaining a consensus of opinion and reaching a compromise when decisions must be made?	[ ]	[ ]

A yes response to the majority of these questions can be indicative of a too-low conflict level in a work group.

Is conflict too high?	YES	NO
Is there an upward and onward spiraling escalation of the conflict?	[ ]	[ ]
Are the conflicting parties stimulating the escalation of conflict without considering the consequences?	[ ]	[ ]
Is there a shift away from conciliation, minimizing differences, and enhancing goodwill?	[ ]	[ ]
Are the issues involved in the conflict being increasingly elaborated and expanded?	[ ]	[ ]
Are false issues being generated?	[ ]	[ ]
Are the issues vague or unclear?	[ ]	[ ]
Is job dissatisfaction increasing among workgroup members?	[ ]	[ ]
Is the workgroup productivity being adversely affected?	[ ]	[ ]
Is the energy being directed to activities that do not contribute to the achievement of organizational goals (e.g., destroying opposing party)?	[ ]	[ ]
Is the morale of the nursing staff being adversely affected?	[ ]	[ ]
Are extra parties getting dragged into the conflict?	[ ]	[ ]
Is a great deal of reliance on overt power manipulation noted (threats, coercion, deception)?	[ ]	[ ]
Is there a great deal of imbalance in power noted among the parties?	[ ]	[ ]
Do the individuals or groups involved in the conflict express dissatisfaction about the course of the conflict and feel that they are losing something?	[ ]	[ ]
Is absenteeism increasing among staff?	[ ]	[ ]
Is there a high rate of turnover among personnel?	[ ]	[ ]
Is communication dysfunctional, not open, mistrustful, and/or restrictive?	[ ]	[ ]
Is the focus being placed on nonconflict relevant to sensitive areas of the other party?	[ ]	[ ]

A yes response to the majority of these questions can be indicative of a conflict level in a work group that is too high.

FIGURE 6-4

Guide for the assessment of level of conflict.

(*Source:* From MacFarland, G., Leonard, H., & Morris, M. (1984). *Nursing Leadership and Management: Contemporary Strategies.* Clifton Park, NY: Delmar Cengage Learning.)

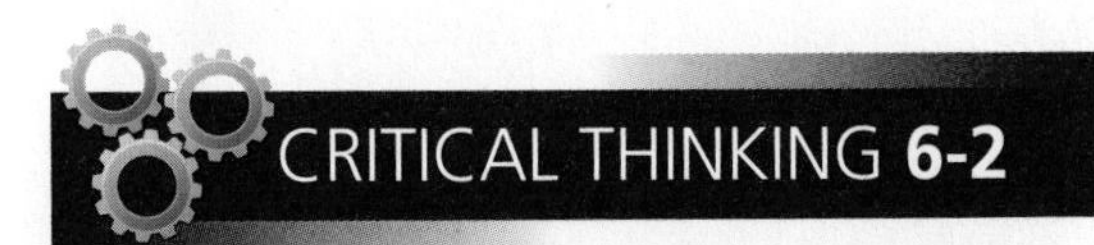

CRITICAL THINKING 6-2

Review Table 6-6, Summary of Conflict Management Methods. Think about a recent personal or professional time when you disagreed with someone. Which conflict management technique did you use? Did it help you achieve your goal?

all three processes and explore them as opportunities for personal and professional growth. Establishing trust and effective communication as well as embracing values and vision of an organization allow today's nurse the ability to function as an agent of change, innovation, and transformation (Porter-O'Grady & Malloch, 2011; Curtin, 2011).

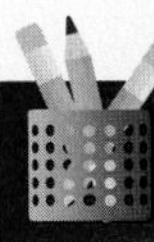

CASE STUDY 6-1

James's staff was about three weeks into the latest change in care delivery when one of the staff nurses, Linda, returned from maternity leave. Linda tends to be negative about change, but she has terrific clinical skills and has often served as a preceptor for new staff. James knew that if Linda could avoid her tendency toward the negative, then not too much would happen to get the change off course. Linda's first words to James were, "Whose brilliant idea is this? I do not want to work with Kathy. She is an idiot." James smiled and said, "Welcome back, Linda. We have missed you. How's the baby? Any pictures?" What do you think James should do to help Linda adjust to the change? Should James explore Linda's feelings about Kathy? Which is more stressful for Linda, the change or working with Kathy? Should James have done something to prepare Linda for this change in her assignment to work with Kathy?

KEY CONCEPTS

- Change is defined as making something different from what it was.
- Major change theorists include Lewin, Lippitt, Havelock, and Rogers.
- Senge's model of five disciplines describes the learning organization.
- The change agent is an important part of the change process. The change agent can facilitate and support organizational transformation as a follower and/or as a leader.
- Chaos theory says that most organizations go through periods of rapid change and innovation and then stabilize before chaos erupts again.
- Innovation is the process of creating new services or products.
- Conflict is a normal part of any change project and is often healthy and positive.
- Conflict can move the change process along if it is handled well. Conflict can stop the change process if it is handled poorly or allowed to get out of control.
- The techniques for conflict management include avoiding, accommodating, compromising, competing, negotiating, confronting, and collaborating.

KEY TERMS

change
change agent
conflict
innovation
learning organization theory

REVIEW QUESTIONS

1. A nurse is having a conflict with a nurse's aide because she feels that the nurse's aide is rude to patients. While trying to figure out the way to fix this conflict, which conflict management technique should the nurse employ?
   A. Avoiding
   B. Competing
   C. Negotiating
   D. Collaborating
2. As a new nurse, you notice there is one nurse on the unit who seems to help positive change come about and who seems to help the other nurses resolve their differences. Which characteristics listed apply to this person? Select all that apply.
   A. Secretive
   B. Trustworthy
   C. Good communicator
   D. Avoiding
   E. Dictatorial
   F. Effective listener
   G. Loud and rude
3. A nurse is overheard saying, "I'm so sick of change; everyday I have to learn something new. Why can't we leave things the way they were?" Which reply by the nurse manager explaining why change is necessary is most correct?
   A. "We have to maintain the status quo."
   B. "Changes are implemented to improve quality and safety."
   C. "We change things to encourage staff turnover."
   D. "Change makes us look like we are using cutting-edge technology."
4. Nurses are discussing who proposed the original change theory. One nurse states, "I remember! It was _______________ (fill in the blank) that first proposed original change theory."
   A. Rogers
   B. Havelock
   C. Lewin
   D. Lippitt
5. There are many forms of communication in the medical center in which you work including word of mouth, staff-meeting minutes, unit director memos, and the medical center newsletter. Which method of communication would be considered unreliable about news of future layoffs in nursing?
   A. Word of mouth
   B. Staff-meeting minutes
   C. Unit director memos
   D. Medical center newsletter
6. The health care environment can be described as chaotic. What are the global reasons for this chaos? Select all that apply.
   A. Innovations
   B. Emerging evidence
   C. Social changes
   D. Staffing
   E. Introduction of more technology
   F. Changes in nursing education

7. Elements of leadership that best facilitate a "healing environment" for both patients and health care professionals are many. Which elements facilitate a healing environment? Select all that apply.
   A. Creativity
   B. Courage
   C. Emotional competence
   D. Corporate greed
   E. Transformative leadership
   F. Sense of entitlement

8. A discussion regarding conflict occurs in the nursing break room. Many statements are made. Which statements related to conflict are correct? Select all that apply.
   A. Conflict can lead to positive change.
   B. Conflict can allow for creativity and innovation.
   C. Conflict requires conflict-resolution skills.
   D. Without conflict, groups can improve.
   E. Conflict can be a part of change.
   F. Conflict should be avoided if groups are to function smoothly.

9. Quality and safety are integral to providing care to patients in the hospital setting. Which are examples of innovations improving patient safety? Select all that apply.
   A. Phone-in dietary requests 24 hours a day
   B. Lift teams
   C. Barcode medication administration
   D. Electronic order entry
   E. Standardized uniforms for nurses
   F. Bed alarms

10. The new nurse notes that when the six-week schedule was published, many of the staff, including the new nurse, were very angry about their schedules. Which conflict resolution technique will be most effective for arriving at a solution for the unit?
    A. Avoiding
    B. Competing
    C. Negotiating
    D. Collaborating

REVIEW ACTIVITIES

1. Select a change project that you have experienced in a clinical situation and discuss with your classmates how the change agent maintained momentum for the project. What approaches did the change agent use?
2. Discuss with a nurse manager how she determines whether a conflict is occurring and what steps she takes to manage it. Share the information with your classmates.
3. Visit the QSEN website and explore the Quality/Safety Competencies section. Review the discussions for each of the six core competencies in order to consider where you see yourself relative to the knowledge, skill, and attitude of each.

EXPLORING THE WEB

Look up the *Journal of Conflict Resolution* and describe its purpose. Would this journal be useful to the new nurse manager? A new nurse? Anyone else in health care?

http://www.jcr.sagepub.com

Explore the following websites to learn more about change, conflict management, and innovation:

- International Association for Conflict Management: *http://www.iacm-conflict.org*
- National League for Nursing: *http://www.nln.org*
  Click on *Position Statement* and *Innovation in Nursing Education.*
- American Nurses Credentialing Center: *http://www.nursecredentialing.org*
  Click on the Magnet Prize Program.

REFERENCES

Agnes, M. & Guralnik, B. D. (2000). *Webster's new world collegiate dictionary* (4th ed.). Foster City, CA: IDG Books Worldwide Inc.

Bennis, W., Benne, K., & Chin, R. (Eds.). (1969). *The planning of change* (2nd ed.). New York, NY: Holt, Rinehart, Winston.

Brookes, J. (2011). Engaging staff in the change process. *Nursing Management, 18*, 16–19.

Bushy, A. (1992). Managing change: Strategies for continuing education. *The Journal of Continuing Education in Nursing, 23,*197–200.

Curtin, L. (2011) Quantum leadership: Succeeding in interesting times. *Nurse Leader, 9*(1), 38–38.

Filley, A. C. (1975). *Interpersonal conflict resolution.* Glenview, IL: Scott Foresman.

Havelock, R. G. (1973). *The change agent's guide to innovation in education.* Englewood Cliffs, NJ: Educational Technology.

Lancaster, J. (1999). *Nursing issues in leading and managing change.* St. Louis, MO: Mosby.

Lewicki, R. J., Hiam, A., & Olander, K. W. (1996). *Think before you speak.* New York, NY: John Wiley & Sons.

Lewin, K. (1951). *Field theory in social science.* New York, NY: Harper & Row.

Lippitt, R., Watson, J., & Westley, B. (1958). *The dynamics of planned change.* New York, NY: Harcourt, Brace.

MacFarland, G., Leonard, H., & Morris, M. (1984). *Nursing leadership and management: Contemporary strategies.* Clifton Park, NY: Delmar Cengage Learning.

Margaret Mead. (n.d.). BrainyQuote.com. Retrieved October 27, 2012, from http://www.brainyquote.com/quotes/quotes/m/margaretme100502.html

Porter-O'Grady, P., & Malloch, K. (2011). *Quantum leadership: Advancing innovation, transforming health care* (3rd ed.). Sudbury, MA: Jones & Bartlett Learning.

Quality & Safety Education for Nurses (QSEN). (2011). Retrieved September 1, 2012, from http://www.qsen.org

Rogers, E. M. (1995). *Diffusion of innovations* (4th ed.). New York, NY: Free Press.

Senge, P. M. (1990). *The fifth discipline: The art and practice of the learning organization.* New York, NY: Doubleday.

Senge, P., Kleiner, A., Roberts C., Ross, R. B., & Smith, B. (1994). *The fifth discipline fieldbook.* New York, NY: Doubleday.

Shortell, S. M., & Kaluzny, A. D. (2006). *Health care management* (5th ed.). Clifton Park, NY: Delmar Cengage Learning.

Silber, M. B. (1993, September). The "C"s in excellence: Choice and change. *Nursing Management, 24*(9), 60–62.

SUGGESTED READINGS

Begun, J., Zimmerman, B., & Dooley, K. (2006). Health care organizations as complex adaptive systems. Retrieved September 8, 2006, from http://www.change-ability.ca/ComplexAda ptive.pdf

Bolman, L. G., & Deal, T. E. (2008). *Reframing organizations: Artistry, choice, and leadership* (4th ed.). San Francisco, CA: Jossey-Bass.

Bushy, A., & Kamphius, J. (1993, March). Response to innovation: Behavioral patterns. *Nursing Management, 24*(3), 62–64.

Clifton, D. O., Anderson, E., & Schreiner, L. A. (2006). *Strengths quest: Discover and develop your strengths in academics, career, and beyond.* New York, NY: Gallup Press.

Gleick, J. (1987). *Chaos: Making a new science.* New York, NY: Viking.

Kotter, J. P. (1996). *Leading change.* Boston, MA: Harvard Business School Press.

MacGuire, J. M. (2006, January). Putting nursing research findings into practice: Research utilization as an aspect of the management of change. *Journal of Advanced Nursing, 53*(1), 65–71.

Marquis, B. L., & Huston, C. J. (2006). *Leadership roles and management functions in nursing: Theory applied* (5th ed.). Philadelphia, PA: Lippincott.

McCartney, P. (2006, November–December). The International Council of Nurses innovations database. *American Journal of Maternal/Child Nursing, 31*(6), 389.

National Council of State Boards of Nursing. (2010). *Professional boundaries: A nurse's guide to the importance of appropriate professional boundaries.* Retrieved September 26, 2012, from https://www.ncsbn.org/Professional Boundaries_Complete.pdf

Senge, P., Flowers, B. S., & Scharmer, C. O. (2005). *Presence: An exploration of profound change in people, organizations, and society.* New York, NY: Doubleday.

Shortell, S., & Kaluzny, A. D. (2000). *Health care management: Organization design and behavior* (4th ed.). Clifton Park, NY: Delmar Cengage Learning.

Thomas, L. M., Reynolds, T., & O'Brien, L. (2006, September). Innovation and change: Shaping district nursing services to meet the needs of primary health care. *Journal of Nursing Management, 74*(6), 447–454.

Waldrop, M. M. (1992). *Complexity: The emerging science at the edge of order and chaos.* New York, NY: Simon & Schuster.

Waterman, T., & Peters, R. H. (1982). *In search of excellence.* Cambridge, MA: Harper Collins.

Whitehead, D. K., Weiss, S. A., & Tappen, R. M. (2010). *Essentials of nursing leadership and management.* (5th ed.) Philadelphia, PA., F.A. Davis..

CHAPTER 7

Power and Politics

PATRICIA M. SCHOON, RN, MPH, PHN;
TERRY W. MILLER, RN, PHD;
PATSY MALONEY, RN-BC, MSN, MA, EDD, NEA-BC;
RICHARD J. MALONEY, BS, MA, EDD, MAHRM;
AND JANICE TAZBIR, RN, MS, CS, CCRN

Be the change you want to see in the world.

–MAHATMA GANDHI 1869–1948

OBJECTIVES

Upon completion of this chapter, the reader should be able to:

1. Describe power, sources of power, and how to use personal and professional power to improve the well-being of patients, nurses, and the health care system.
2. Discuss how the nurse can be an advocate in providing for patient safety and improving patient care.
3. Discuss the role of the American Nurses Association as an advocate for nurses and a force for change in the health care system.
4. Understand the purpose and process of collective bargaining by professional nursing organizations and unions.
5. Describe how to use the political process to advocate for change in the health care system.
6. Describe how to use collective social action and the media to influence the public, health care consumers, stakeholders, and elected officials in advocating for improve-

Nurse Pat, a new graduate who just finished orientation, is working with a patient for whom a surgical consult has been written. The unit clerk and a long-time nurse on the unit remark that Dr. Killian, the practitioner doing the surgical consultation, should be named "Dr. Killjoy" because she humiliates new nurses to try to put them in their place. Based on previous reports by other nurses on the unit, Pat knows Dr. Killian has the reputation of being demeaning and inappropriately demanding when interacting with new nurses. Two hours later, Dr. Killian appears on the unit and asks to see the nurse who did the surgical admission sheet.

What type of power does Dr. Killian illustrate?

How could Pat increase his power to improve his approach to Dr. Killian?

We CAN
Improve Patient Care
We CAN
Heal Health Care

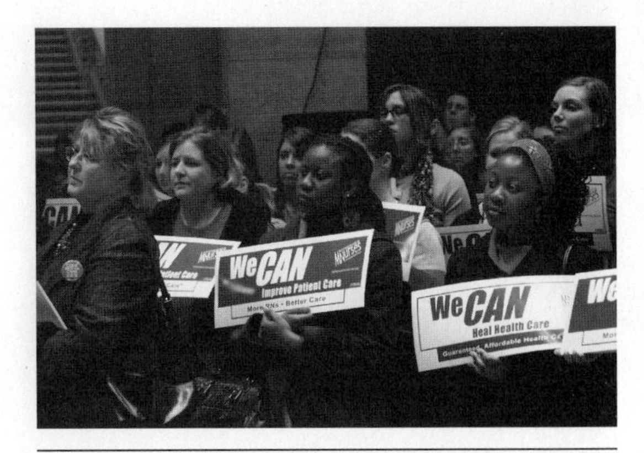

Source: Photo used by permission of Minnesota Nurses Association, © 2009. MNA Capitol Rally for Safe Statting.

Nurses advocate for their patients because they care (Curtin, 1979; Falk-Rafael, 2005). They advocate for patient safety, autonomy, well-being, and equity in health care access and services (Bu & Jezewski, 2006). In order to advocate effectively, nurses need to be empowered and know how to use their personal and professional power to create positive change both individually and collectively. When nurses are licensed as registered nurses, they enter into a professional contract with society to promote and protect the health of their patients and their community. Nursing may begin at the bedside but it does not end there.

Effective nurses are powerful. They show objectivity, creativity, and knowledge throughout their practice and regardless of their work setting. They exert power by understanding the concept of power from multiple perspectives and by using this understanding to change and improve care. This chapter discusses power, sources of power, how nurses can use power, politics, collective social action, and collective bargaining to advocate for the health of their patients and community, their profession, and an improved health care system. It also discusses how to use media and the political process to advocate for change in the health care system.

POWER

Nurses use their power in a moral and ethical manner when they use their power to empower others. **Power** is described as having control over others and the ability to influence and shape the behaviors of others (Zelek & Phillips, 2003). Power is used to create, acquire, and use resources to achieve one's goals. Nurses as independent practitioners need to be able to act independently in order to use their power (Manojlovich, 2007). Nursing power and professionalism are interrelated; when nurses have power, they can control the practice of nursing and function independently (Rutty, 1998). If nurses do not utilize their power to control nursing practice, others will do so. Each of us has an individual power base best described as a three-legged stool. The "seat" of power is supported by one's personal, professional, and **organizational power**. Nurses need to become skilled in using all legs of their power base if they are going to advocate effectively. The components of the nursing power base and empowerment strategies are found in Table 7-1. Conversely, power has been used for personal gain to the detriment of others. Orientation to personal gain and power as a bad thing (and therefore something to be avoided) is reflected in a quotation from Lord Acton (Seldes, 1985, p. 234): "Power tends to corrupt, and absolute power corrupts absolutely." People having this belief tend to believe that those wielding or afforded power ultimately should not have power because of their potential to misuse it, that people desiring power should not be trusted because their

TABLE 7-1
A Framework for Becoming Empowered and Empowering Others

Definition	Components	Empowerment Strategies
Personal power is the power you acquire and exercise through your informal and formal roles in your family and community.	◆ Personal roles: family and friends ◆ Community roles: neighborhood, volunteer, elected official; culture and ethnic ties ◆ Organizational membership: religious, political, other	◆ Become involved as a citizen in an issue you are passionate about. ◆ Get to know your neighbors and community. ◆ Identify yourself to family, friends, neighbors, community members, and stakeholders as a professional who is committed to improving the health of the community. ◆ Participate in community or organizational meetings. Share your knowledge about health care. ◆ Form linkages and networks between different groups and organizations that share common beliefs and goals. ◆ Know your elected and appointed officials.
Professional power is the power you acquire and exercise through your formal role as a professional nurse.	◆ Legitimacy through licensure ◆ Social contract with public ◆ Professional expertise and competencies ◆ Membership in professional organizations ◆ Professional networks	◆ Find a professional and career mentor. ◆ Join a professional nursing organization. ◆ Attend conferences and meetings. ◆ Continue your education through continuing education, certification, and formal higher education. ◆ Strive to provide evidence-based care. ◆ Develop strategies for monitoring quality and safety of care. ◆ Role model professional nursing practice. ◆ Become a mentor for novice nurses.
Organizational power is the power you acquire and exercise through your formal and informal roles in your workplace and the health care system.	◆ Position and job description ◆ Organizational communication ◆ Coordination of care ◆ Dispersed power of nursing throughout organization and society	◆ Become involved in the work of the organization beyond patient care. ◆ Become a member of a practice committee. ◆ Collaborate with other disciplines, management, and administration. ◆ Join an interdisciplinary group whose goal is improvement in patient care or population health. ◆ Work with a consumer group to improve health care in your community. ◆ Be politically active at the local level. Be Glocal: think global, act local. At some point you may wish to become involved at the state and national levels.

© Cengage Learning 2014

motivation for acquiring power is inherently wrong—they want power for personal gain at any cost.

The other point of view, that power is a good thing, that is, a force that is used for good purposes, is reflected in Gracian's (1892, p. 172) saying: "The sole advantage of power is that you can do more good." Nurses, in general, are likely to see power as a positive thing and are more inclined to use this positive power to help others.

Sources of Power

Most researchers agree that the **sources of power** are diverse and vary from one situation to another. They also agree that these sources of power are a combination of conscious and unconscious factors that allow an individual to influence others to do as the individual wants (Fisher & Koch, 1996). Articles and textbooks about nursing administration, educational leadership, and organizational management commonly include references to the work of Hersey, Blanchard, and Natemeyer (1979), an expansion of the power typology originally developed by French and Raven in 1959. The typology helps nurses understand how different people perceive power and subsequently relate to others in the work setting and in attempts to achieve their goals. Power is described as having a basis in expertise, legitimacy, reference (charisma), reward and coercion, or connection. More recently, another power source—information—has been added to the typology (Wells, 1998). Generally speaking, nurses exert influence derived from one or a combination of these power sources. See Table 7-2.

TABLE 7-2
Sources and Examples of Power

Type	Source	Examples for Nursing
Expert	Power derived from the knowledge and skills nurses possess. The more proficiency the nurse has, the more the nurse is received as an expert.	Communicating information from current evidence-based journals and bringing expert knowledge to patient care.
Legitimate	Power derived from an academic degree, licensure, certification, experience in the role, and job title in the organization.	Wearing or displaying symbols of professional standing, including license and certification.
Referent	Power based on the trust and respect that people feel for an individual, group, or organization with which one is associated.	Gaining power by affiliating with nurses and others who have power in the organization.
Reward	Power that comes from the ability to reward others to influence them to change their behavior.	Using a hospital award to alter other's behavior.
Coercive	Power that comes from the ability to punish others to influence them to change their behavior.	Using the hospital disciplinary evaluation system to alter another's behavior.
Connection	Power that comes from personal and professional relationships that enhance one's resources and the capacity for learning and information sharing.	Developing good working relationships and mentoring with the boss and other powerful people.
Information	Power based on information that someone can provide to the group.	Sharing useful knowledge gleaned from the Internet and other sources with coworkers.

Source: Developed with information from Hersey, P., Blanchard, K., & Natemeyer, W. (1979). Situational leadership, perception and impact of power. *Group and Organizational Studies, 4*; French, J. P. R., Jr., & Raven, B. (1959). The bases of social power, in D. Cartwright and A. Zander (Eds.), *Group Dynamics*. New York, NY: Harper and Row; and Wells, S. (1998). *Choosing the future: The power of strategic thinking.* Boston , MA: Butterworth-Heinemann.

Effective nurses use these sources of power and combine reference (charismatic) power and expert power from a legitimate power base, adding carefully measured portions of reward power and little or preferably no coercive power (Fisher & Koch, 1996). These leaders gather and use information in new and creative ways. When nurses act powerfully as advocates for patients and their families and are recognized by others as powerful, they demonstrate eight components of powerful professional practice (Ponte et al., 2007). See Table 7-3.

Nurses who work within health care institutions are empowered in three ways: psychologically, relationally, and structurally (Manojlovich, 2007). Psychological power is a combination of personal motivation that is facilitated by an empowering work culture. Relational empowerment occurs when nurses foster and nurture others resulting in mutual empowerment. Structural empowerment occurs when the organization provides opportunities for career enhancement and advancement, as well as support and resources for professional nursing responsibilities. Empowered nurses have higher levels of job satisfaction, provide better patient-centered care, and have better patient outcomes (Manojlovich, 2007).

TABLE 7-3
Components of Powerful Professional Nursing Practice in Nursing Leaders

Nurse Leaders who are identified as powerful demonstrate:

1. Unique nursing role in provision of patient-centered and family care.
2. Commitment to continuous learning and evidence-based practice.
3. Professional nursing behaviors and the critical nature of presence.
4. Collaboration with nurses and interdisciplinary team.
5. Ability to influence decisions and resource allocation.
6. Actions that are inspirational and compassionate.
7. Ability to facilitate nurses' voices being heard and to mentor novice nurses.
8. Ability to evaluate the power of nursing and the nursing department by assessing the organization's mission and values and its commitment to enhancing power of diverse perspectives.

Source: Modified from Ponte, Glazer, Dan, McCollum, Gross, Tyrrell, Branowicki, Noga, Winfrey, Cooley, Saint-Eloi, Hays, Nicolas, & Washington, et al. 2007.

Use of Power

Nursing involvement in power and politics includes using power to improve the position of patients and nurses. Nurses use their power with colleagues, administrators, and subordinates. Nurses can also use power in the legal system, their professional nursing organizations, and the media to work to improve care. Nurses must grow in their ability to work with all of these groups. Many nurses believe that it is helpful to become active participants in some formal part of the nursing profession, such as the American Nurses Association (ANA), the National League for Nursing (NLN), or one of the nursing specialty organizations.

Ultimately, health care will be defined and controlled by those wielding the most power. If nurses fail to exert political pressure on health policy makers, they will lose ground to others who are more politically active. It is unrealistic to believe that other stakeholders will take care of nursing while the competition for health care resources increases.

Nurses, like other health care providers, must stand up and compete, negotiate, and collaborate with others who lobby for health care. See Table 7-4.

Power and the Media

People who work in the media recognize the relationship between power and perception. Those who work in advertising, marketing, and public relations understand how media can be used to create or change perceptions. They have long recognized that the public's perception can be created or changed through advertising and marketing campaigns, damage control, timely press releases, and well-orchestrated media events.

The way the media present nursing to the public will empower or disempower nursing. The nursing

TABLE 7-4
Health Care Advocacy and Lobbying Groups

AFL-CIO	Chamber of Commerce
America's Health Insurance Plans	Coalition to Advance Health Care Reform
American Association of Retired Persons	Health Care Equipment Companies
American Hospital Association	National Coalition on Benefits
American Medical Association	National Federation of Independent Business
American Nurses Association	Pharmaceutical Companies
American Public Health Association	National Partnership for Action to End Health Disparities
	Public Health Advocacy—National Association of County and City Health Officials

© Cengage Learning 2014

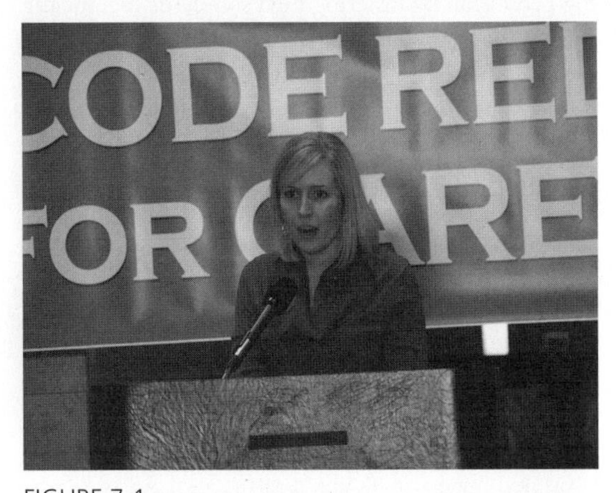

FIGURE 7-1
Utilizing the media to help empower nurses.
(*Source:* Photo used by permission of Minnesota Nurses Association, © 2009. MNA Capitol Rally for Safe Staffing.)

profession has struggled with its public image, visibility, and voice throughout its professional history. There have always been visible and powerful nurses such as Florence Nightingale. While nurses as individuals and as a profession are generally perceived as respected and trusted, they are often not viewed as powerful or able to change or improve the health care system (Fletcher, 2007). The self-image and public image of nurses are interactive, continually influencing each other. The often heard comment, "I am just a nurse," reinforces the public stereotype of nursing as lacking status and power. Both positive and negative images persist in film, television, books, newsprint, and the Internet, although there are more positive images emerging recently (Cohen, 2007; Kalisch, Begeny, & Neumann, 2007; Stanley, 2008). However, news media often ignore nurses when citing experts in health care (Fletcher, 2007). Nurses need to recognize themselves as powerful before they can advocate effectively in the public and political arenas for health care change.

One strategy for empowering nursing is to employ the media to create a stronger, more powerful image of nursing, for example, by writing opinion editorial (op-ed) pieces and letters to the editor for the local newspaper. Examples on a larger scale include a series of television spots promoting a positive nursing image, such as that recently sponsored by the Johnson and Johnson Corporation as part of its Campaign for Nursing's Future (Johnson & Johnson, 2006). Use of digital media is another way to reach individuals and groups to advocate for changes in health care (Galer-Unti, 2010). Examples include:

- Friending and social networking such as Facebook and LinkedIn
- Real-time communications using blast or LISTSERV, e-mail, Twitter, YouTube
- Advocacy channel by developing web portals for reporting the news and educating the public on health issues

- American Nurses Association (ANA), the National League for Nursing (NLN), nursing specialty organizations, e.g., the Emergency Nurses Association.

Dimensions of Nursing

To be politically effective, nurses must be able to clearly articulate at least four dimensions of nursing to any audience or stakeholder: what nursing is; what distinctive services nurses provide to consumers; how nursing benefits consumers, including improvement in nurse-sensitive outcomes; and what nursing services cost in relation to other health care services. Presenting research-based evidence to support the political position of the nursing profession can be a powerful tool. However, stakeholders are often influenced by anecdotal stories or personal testimonies. Table 7-5 addresses the seven essential dimensions of nursing identified by the American Nurses Association (2010).

TABLE 7-5
Essential Dimensions of Nursing

- Providing a caring relationship that enhances healing and health
- Focusing on the full range of experiences and human responses to illness and health within both the physical and social environments
- Appreciating the subjective experience and the integration of such experience with objective data
- Diagnosing and intervening in care by using scientific knowledge, judgment, and critical thinking
- Advancing nursing knowledge through scholarly inquiry
- Influencing social and public policy to promote social justice
- Assuring safe, quality, and evidence-based care

Source: From American Nurses Association. (2010). *Nursing's social policy statement* (3rd ed.). Washington, DC: American Nurses Publishing.

American Nurses Association

The American Nurses Association (ANA) is a full-service professional organization representing the nation's entire RN population whether they are members or not. The ANA is not a collective bargaining agent, though historically it was involved in collective bargaining. It represents 3.1 million RNs in the United States through its 54 constituent state and territorial associations (ANA, 2010). The ANA's mission is "Nurses advancing our profession to improve health for all" (ANA, 2010). The ANA Code of Ethics states, "While seeking to assure just economic and general welfare for nurses, collective bargaining, nonetheless, seeks to keep the interests of both nurses and patients in balance" (ANA, 2010). The ANA represents the interests of nurses in safe, healthy work environments and in many other areas as well. It advances the nursing profession by fostering high standards for nursing practice and lobbies Congress and regulatory agencies on health care issues affecting nurses and the general public. It initiates many policies involving health care reform. It also publishes its positions on issues ranging from whistleblowing to patients' rights. The ANA recently launched a major campaign to mobilize nurses to address the staffing crisis, to educate and gain support from the public, and to develop and implement initiatives designed to resolve the staffing crisis. ANA has created the National Database of Nursing Quality Indicators (NDNQI) that helps show, with the use of data, the link between good nursing care and healthier patients. American Nurses Credentialing Center, a subsidiary of the ANA, created the Magnet Recognition Program to recognize health care organizations that provide the very best in nursing care. Since1994, more than 372 institutions have received this award (ANA, 2010). In 2003, the ANA created a new **workplace advocacy** structure known today as the Center for American Nurses. The ANA feels workplace advocacy is an alternative to unionization and promotes collaboration and communication among nurses. Key ANA programs include: conflict competency training and consultation; workshops and publications on lateral violence and bullying; nurse investor's education project; and the offering of a host of resources through its affiliate, the Institute for Nursing Research and Education (Scott, 2008).

CRITICAL THINKING 7-1

Political conflict occurs because people may hold significantly different or conflicting opinions about any given topic. Consumers may disagree about what health care should be, who should provide it, how much it should cost, and/or who should pay for it. As a new nurse, you have a professional responsibility to promote consumer dialogue and offer creative, thoughtful, and evidence-based solutions to health care problems. Yet nurses disagree with each other in regard to the same issues consumers may have about health care. What do you think your responsibility is as a consumer of health care? What is your responsibility as a health care provider? Do you think your responsibility as a consumer could conflict with your responsibility as a provider?

Workplace Advocacy

The American Nurses Association (ANA), with its partners and through its organizational relationships, is a leader in promoting improved work environments and the value of nurses as professionals, essential providers, and decision makers in all practice settings. The ANA protects, defends, and educates nurses about their rights as employees under the law. It also addresses the growing number of occupational hazards that threaten nurses, such as needlestick injuries, latex sensitivity, back injuries, and violence. Go to http://www.nursing world.org. Click on *health care policy.* Click on *ANA position statements.* Click on *workplace advocacy.*

Collective Bargaining Agents

In **collective bargaining**, the group works with management for what the group desires. If the group cannot achieve its desires through informal collective bargaining with management, the group may decide to use a collective bargaining agent to form a union. In general, nurses who are content in their workplace do not unionize (Forman & Grimes, 2004). It is when nurses feel powerless that they initiate attempts to unionize. Other motivations to unionize include job stress and physical demands (Budd, Warino, & Patton, 2004). Nurses are also motivated to join unions when they feel the need to communicate concerns and complaints to management without fear of losing their jobs. Some nurses believe that they need a collective voice so that management will hear them and changes will be instituted.

Issues that are commonly the subject of collective bargaining include poor wages, unsafe staffing, health and safety issues, mandatory overtime, poor quality of care, job security, and restructuring issues such as cross-training nurses for areas of specialty other than those in which they were hired to practice (United American Nurses, 2006).

Various organizations act as collective bargaining agents for millions of workers including nurses other health care workers, laborers, and specially trained workers such as actors and firefighters. Some of these organizations are the Teamsters Union, the General Service Employees Union, the National Union of Hospital and Health Care Employees, the Service Employees International Union, the United Autoworkers of America, and the United Steelworkers of America. The largest and most recognized national nursing collective bargaining agent is National Nurses United (NNU).

The ANA was part of collective bargaining at the state level through United American Nurses (UAN) until 2003 (Hackman, 2008). Since 2003, the ANA has disaffiliated itself from the UAN and is not a collective bargaining agent (Hackman, 2008). In 1995, the California Nurses Association separated from the existing ANA's California Nurses Association and joined the National Nurses Organizing Committee (NNOC). The NNOC was responsible for mandating, through law, safe patient-nurse staffing ratios in the state of California.

In 2009, the California Nurses Association, the NNOC, the Massachusetts Nurses Association, and UAN (formerly with the ANA) formed National Nurses United (NNU, 2010). Beginning in 2009, the NNU has unionized nurses through collective bargaining at the state and national level (NNU, 2010). It is the only exclusively nurses union that is also a professional association of registered nurses and the only one affiliated with the American Federation of Labor and Congress of Industrial Organizations (AFL-CIO). NNU represents more than 160,000 nurses through collective bargaining in 15 states (NNU, 2010). Its goal is for nurses to improve

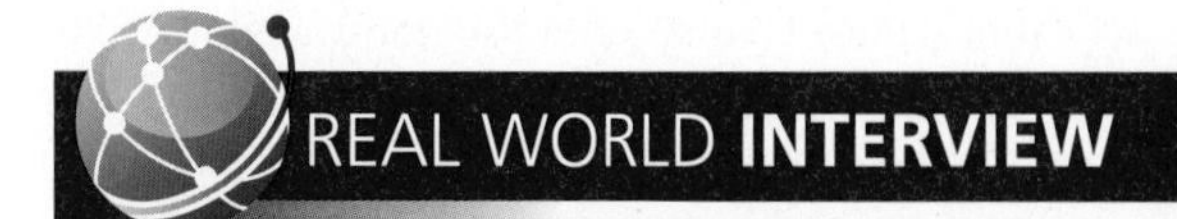

Nurses serve as advocates and allies for consumers by helping consumers obtain what they perceive they need. Nurses have the opportunity to help consumers better understand what is available to them, as well as what they can legitimately expect to get from both the provider and the system. Competent nurses need to work at understanding how the system works, because that is "where they live." Consumers move in and out of the system, so they are not acclimated to the limitations or pathways of the system. The consumer and the nurse become natural allies, whether in a patient care setting or a public policy setting. One of my biggest frustrations is when nurses fail to see themselves as connected to the patient and the whole health care system. Nurses become myopic in their approach to problems in direct patient care, because they do not see that they are a piece of something bigger. No nurse's practice occurs in isolation. We are all part of an interdependent, highly complex system with governing economic and political relationships. I found consumer partnerships to be most useful when working as a lobbyist for the Washington State Nurses Association, because, as nurses, we were able to build politically powerful coalitions with consumer groups and subsequently define the direction of long-term health care policy—specifically, state policies governing the long-term care industry. Because we were successful in partnering with selected consumer interest groups, we were able to assure passage and funding of seven significant legislative bills. These bills included the AIDS Omnibus legislation, a long-term care reform act, and an act enabling nurses to declare a patient dead for the purpose of preventing unnecessary stress, care, and cost to consumers.

ROBERT S. BALL, MSN, RN
Nursing Care Manager
Tacoma, Washington

practice and have a greater voice in decisions that affect patient safety. NNU is considered to be a more aggressive union that has initiated and supported striking for nurses' rights.

Striking

Some nurses are morally opposed to unions because they believe if they are members of a union, they may be forced to strike. In reality, a collective bargaining agent cannot make the decision to strike. The decision to strike is made only if the majority of union members decide to do so. Most nursing collective bargaining agents insert in the contract a no-strike clause, stating that striking is not an option for its members. The union members decide upon the no-strike clause. Provisions set forth in the 1974 Taft-Hartley Amendments to the Wagner Act guarantee the continuation of adequate patient care by requiring the union to provide contract expiration notice and advance strike notice, making mediation mandatory, and giving the hospital or agency the option of establishing a board of inquiry prior to work stoppage.

Recently nurses in Minnesota had a strike for better working conditions. As a result of the strike, nurses gained the ability to refuse new patients to a unit and "close" the unit until staffing situations were addressed.

Advocacy and Moral Courage

As patient advocates, nurses have an ethical and moral duty to protect their patients from actual and potential harm and maintain safety. Some health care professionals may lack **moral courage** when dealing with ethical issues (Murray, 2010). Moral courage involves taking actions when unsafe, illegal, or unethical practice occurs, even if the actions are unpopular or one stands alone, in order to defend patients and maintain ethical standards of care. A nurse's ability to act in a morally courageous manner is contingent on organization support, professional mentoring, and staff development.

Three key areas that require actions of moral courage are unsafe staffing, patient neglect and abuse, and health care fraud. Nurses have a right and responsibility to refuse a patient care assignment that they determine to be unsafe and have the responsibility to report unsafe staffing to their employer and to external bodies if their employer does not comply with safe staffing guidelines (ANA, 2009). See Table 7-6. ANA has many other position statements that relate to patient and health care advocacy. These position statements may be accessed by going to http://www.nursingvoice.org and clicking on *policy statements*.

Many state nurses' associations provide a form that may be used to report unsafe staffing to the nurse's employer. Nurses may also report an incident of unsafe staffing or unsafe patient care to the Joint Commission by submitting a complaint related to an accredited health care facility. The online complaint form is available at http://jcwebnoc.jcaho.org/QMSInternet/IncidentEntry.aspx. Patient neglect and abuse may be reported in the same manner. It may also be reported to the state attorney general under the Vulnerable Adults Act or child abuse laws for individual states. All of these reporting options may be anonymous.

TABLE 7-6
Patient Safety: Rights of Registered Nurses When Considering a Patient Assignment

The American Nurses Association (ANA) upholds that registered nurses—based on their professional and ethical responsibilities—have the professional right to accept, reject, or object in writing to any patient assignment that puts patients or themselves at serious risk for harm. Registered nurses have the professional obligation to raise concerns regarding any patient assignment that puts patients or themselves at risk for harm. The professional obligations of the registered nurse to safeguard patients are grounded in the *Nursing's Social Policy Statement* (ANA, 2003), *Code of Ethics for Nurses with Interpretive Statements* (ANA, 2001b), *Nursing: Scope and Standards of Practice* (ANA, 2004), and state laws, rules, and regulations governing nursing practice.

Source: Excerpt from ANA Position Statement, Patient Safety: Rights of Registered Nurses When Considering a Patient Assignment. (2009) Retrieved November 27, 2011, from http:// nursingworld.org/rnrightsps

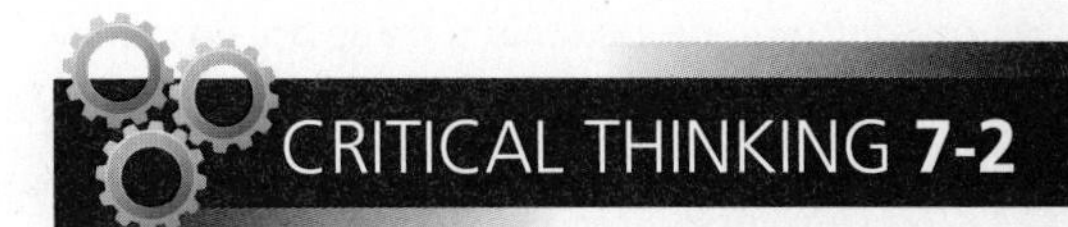

Access, quality, and timing of information available to the public have greatly enhanced the consumer health care movement. Using the Internet, people can do customized searches on practically any health care concern, garner input from a wide audience, and do comparative shopping for services, providers, and products. Several uniform sources of information have been developed for the U.S. health care delivery system. These data sets offer information requested by the decision makers about some predetermined dimension of health care. They also establish standard definitions, classifications, and measurements for making evidence-based decisions. Nursing has been relatively absent from the data sought, collected, and disseminated to the decision makers.

Is there a need for nursing-sensitive consumer outcome measures that can be used by decision makers?

What steps could be taken to make such information available to the public?

Nurses may report health care fraud without fear of retribution under the False Claims Act of 1986 (Weinburg, 2005). This law protects whistle-blowing, the act in which an individual discloses information regarding a violation of a law, rule, or regulation, or a substantial and specific danger to public health or safety. A nurse who suspects health care fraud, which can range from filing false claims to performing unnecessary procedures, may file a *qui tam* lawsuit on behalf of the government or on behalf of the nurse. If the claim is not credible, the nurse remains anonymous, and is thereby protected from any retribution from the employer. If the claim is considered credible, the government will assume all costs for the lawsuit and the nurse will receive 15 to 25 percent of the government's recovery. The government has recouped more than $2 billion since 1995 from whistle-blowers exposing fraud, and over $199 million has been received by whistle-blowers (Weinberg, 2005). You may wish to seek help from an attorney, your state attorney general's office, or your state professional nursing organization. There are five basic steps a nurse should take before deciding to become a whistle-blower (Table 7-7).

As patient advocates, nurses protect patients from known harm. Nurses are often aware of health care fraud in the form of people violating laws or endangering public health or safety. However, some nurses who are aware of health care fraud do nothing because of fear of retribution. Fraud costs the federal government and ultimately costs the taxpayer.

Collective Use of Power

When nurses use collaboration and teamwork to advocate for health care change, they can be more effective than one nurse acting alone. Nurses are dispersed throughout society and health care systems. When nurses band together, they can connect and influence many different segments of society. Nurses can also act in concert with other groups within the community. Individuals and groups are able to act collectively when they share a common goal and are committed to that goal and an action plan. This shared vision and commitment results in group cohesion, the glue that holds individuals and diverse groups together to achieve their common purpose in the face of challenges and adversity. When we act collectively to achieve social, cultural, or political change, this is referred to as "social action." Nurses participate in social action in their role as patient and health care system advocates, a professional and ethical imperative guided by the ANA's *Guide to the Code of Ethics for Nurses* (Fowler & ANA, 2008) and its *Nursing's Social Policy Statement: The Essence of the Profession* (ANA, 2010).

TABLE 7-7
Five Basic Steps to Take Before Deciding to Blow the Whistle

1. Carefully assess the severity and type of problem.
2. Evaluate your priorities and your weaknesses.
3. Identify your reporting options.
4. Plan with an attorney before you act.
5. Identify your supports and be ready to change your life.

Source: Philipsen, N. C., & Soeken, D. (2011). Preparing to blow the whistle: A survival guide for nurses. Journal for Nurse Practitioners, 7(9), 740 -746. Retrieved November 29, 2011, from http://www.medscape.com/viewarticle/751347

Nurses frequently form coalitions or interprofessional partnerships with other health professionals and consumer groups to create a more diverse and more effective power base for social action. While the groups involved in the formation of a partnership do not always agree on every issue, it is important that all of the groups in the partnership agree on specific goals and actions related to their shared health policy interest and agree to disagree respectfully on other issues. Cooperation and compromise are more effective than competition and conflict when trying to achieve shared goals. A partnership takes time and effort to create and sustain. Table 7-8 outlines the steps for creating a partnership with a consumer group. Table 7-9 outlines political strategies that are effective when participating in consumer campaigns.

TABLE 7-8
Steps in Establishing a Partnership with a Consumer Group

Step	Description
1. Listen	Become sensitized to the health care needs and political nature of the potential consumer partner.
2. Study	Seek both representative and opposing perspectives from consumer group meetings, focus groups, relevant literature, and interviews.
3. Assess	Determine the need, value, context, and boundaries for establishing the partnership.

(Continues)

TABLE 7-8 (Continued)

4. Focus	Mutually identify the purpose, and articulate the goals and specific, realistic objectives for the partnership.
5. Compromise	Work through nonessential and noncritical points and issues.
6. Negotiate	Agree on your position and responsibilities in the partnership.
7. Plan	Develop a political strategy for achieving the goals and fulfilling the objectives.
8. Test	Test the political waters. Gather feedback on the plan from key people before taking action.
9. Model	Model the political work. Define the structure for working the political strategy with partners.
10. Direct the political action	Understand the bigger picture, and concentrate on what can be changed.
11. Implement	Line up political support and take action.
12. Network	Be committed to the mutually recognized goal, and consistently work to have an adequate base of support in terms of people, money, and time.
13. Build political credibility	Participate in local, state, and national policy-making efforts that support the partnership and its political agenda.
14. Soothe and bargain	Downplay rivalry, and address conflict in a timely, constructive manner.
15. Report, publicize	Report, publicize, and lobby the group's political cause. Draw public and lobby attention to the needs of the consumer group.
16. Reaffirm, redefine	Regularly evaluate work with the consumer group.

© Cengage Learning 2014

TABLE 7-9
Political Strategies for Mounting Consumer Campaigns

- Lobbying at state and federal levels for health care regulations and guidelines that serve a consumer group's interest
- Consulting with representatives from a consumer group when health care regulations and guidelines are being debated or written
- Monitoring the enforcement of health care regulations and exacting corrective or punitive action when noncompliance occurs
- Encouraging providers and payers to make changes in the delivery of services voluntarily to meet changing consumer demands
- Changing consumer perceptions and behaviors through the distribution of educational materials or other media

© Cengage Learning 2014

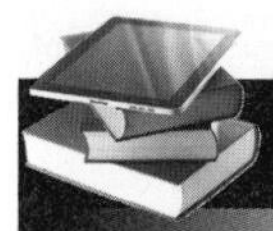

EVIDENCE FROM THE **LITERATURE**

Citation: McDonald, L. (2006). Florence Nightingale as a social reformer. *History Today, 56*(1), 9–15.

Discussion: The purpose of this historical research on the work of Florence Nightingale is to illuminate her work as a social reformer of a public health system. She advocated health promotion and disease prevention based on evidence. Ms. Nightingale extended the use of nurses whom she had trained in hospitals to the care of the poor in pauper houses. She not only placed nurses in these workhouses for the poor, but she lobbied the powerful for passage of laws for the poor. She persuaded key figures to support her ideas for reform. Due to her hard work, the Metropolitan Poor Bill was passed by Parliament in 1867 and followed by other reforms that improved the lot of the poor and infirm in Britain. Ms. Nightingale was able to obtain the support of such powerful and influential people due to her meticulous attention to detail and careful, methodical preparation. Florence Nightingale used what is now dubbed "Nightingale methodology." First, study the best information in print, especially government reports and statistics. Second, interview experts, and if the available information is inadequate, survey others with a questionnaire. When you have a proposed plan, test it at one institution, consult with the practitioners who implemented it, and send out the draft reports for comment before sending the final report out for publication and dissemination to the influential.

Implications for Practice: New nurses often believe that their responsibilities begin and end at the bedside. But historical research demonstrates that from the very beginning of modern nursing, nurses have not only given care but partnered with others to influence public opinion and to change legislation for the benefit of the health care consumer, especially the vulnerable—the poor, the mentally ill, soldiers, and children. So, as a new nurse, you may view yourself as a patient advocate who is willing to join with others through professional associations or consumer groups to improve health care and the system within which it is delivered.

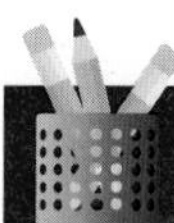

CASE STUDY **7-1**

Maria is a maternity support nurse for First Steps, a specific, state-funded program designed to provide care to underserved and underinsured pregnant women. Maria is in her third year of professional practice and has become highly resourceful as well as able to work in new situations with minimal supervision. Many of her case referrals come through a partnership with the local hospital's Teen Parent Resource Center, which targets girls under 20 who have dropped out of school during their pregnancy.

Many of Maria's patients are from families at high risk for domestic violence and substance abuse. Recently, she was informed that the Teen Parent Resource Center will be discontinuing its partnership with First Steps because of funding issues.

What could Maria do to advocate for continued funding for the Teen Parent Resource Center?

How could she use the Nightingale methodology to research this problem?

What actions might she take?

POLITICS

Politics is predominantly a process by which people use a variety of methods to achieve their goals. These methods inherently involve some level of competition, negotiation, and collaboration for the power to achieve desired outcomes, as well as to protect and enhance the interests of groups or individuals. Nurses who can effectively compete, negotiate, and collaborate with others to get what they want or need tend to develop strong political skills. They have the greatest ability to build strong bases of support for themselves, patients, and the nursing profession. Nurses consistently are rated number one in consumer opinion polls that ask: Who are considered to be trusted professionals? Nurses can garner consumer support for professional nursing positions to help patients and help the profession of nursing by tapping into this strong support. Nursing is important as a profession only as it meets its societal mandate for professional nursing service. Nurses must garner political support to do this most effectively.

Politics exist because resources are limited, and some people control more resources than others. Resources include people, money, facilities, technology, and rights to properties, services, and technologies. Individuals, groups, or organizations that have the ability to provide or control the distribution of desirable resources are politically empowered. The consumer movement in health care is a political movement about health care resources. It reflects consumer perceptions and values and influences patient care delivery.

Stakeholders and Health Care

Control of health care resources is spread among a number of vested interest groups called "stakeholders." Everyone is a stakeholder in health care at some level, but some people are far more politically active about their stake in health care than others. These stakeholder groups include the following: insurance companies; consumer groups; professional organizations, such as the American Nurses Association; and health care groups, such as nurses, doctors, pharmacists, dieticians, physical therapists, administrators, and educational groups. These stakeholders exert political pressure on health policymakers—local, state, and federal legislative bodies—in an effort to make the health care system work to the economic advantage of the stakeholder.

The concept of patient advocacy has been a fundamental aspect of nursing since nursing's beginning. The role of a nurse as a patient advocate has changed as nursing has evolved. Originally, nurses acted as an intermediary and pleader for the patient, and now they act to ensure that the patient's rights to self-determination and free choice are not violated (Rudolph, 2005). Advocacy can be seen as representing the patient to others in the health care organization, which has extended into what has been referred to as cultural brokering or interpreting the health care environment for the patient. There is a strong argument that advocacy actually stems from patient power and consumerism rather than a lack of power or a vulnerability, as some authors have implied (O'Connor & Kelly, 2005).

If a nurse is to act as a patient advocate who interprets the health care environment for the patient and actually guides the patient through the maze, the nurse needs knowledge of the system. Sometimes a nurse's advocating for a patient's rights may be contrary to the wishes of another health care provider or to the organization as a whole. This can be risky for a nurse. Nurses from the beginning of the profession have served as patient advocates. They have acquired the necessary knowledge, and they have taken on the risk. Some early nurses were even jailed for taking unpopular stands. Entry-level nurses need knowledge of the health care organization and the courage of their convictions to act as patient advocates.

Nursing and Political Advocacy

Nurses are the largest health care group, and nurses who are politically active have a definitive voice in their work environments for patient welfare as well as for themselves. Nurses must study the issues, garner political support, and contact policymakers to ensure quality care for patients.

The health of individuals and groups is shaped not only by individual actions but also by society as a whole (Commission on Social Determinants of Health, 2008). The social causes of health are called the "social determinants" of health. For example, people who live in poverty have poorer health and shorter lifespans than those who do not. When societal resources are scarce (i.e., when the country is in an economic downturn), health care resources also become scarce. In the Opening Scenario, Beth was concerned about the mentally ill patients who continued to return to the inpatient unit because of lack of community mental health resources. Every nurse has a story about a patient or family whose health was compromised by lack of funding, health insurance, or lack of health services. Nurses feel a need to advocate for the resources necessary to provide for their patients' well-being. That is a powerful motivation for nurses to expand their role beyond the bedside to the community and to political action.

It is important to understand the political process in order for nurses to be effective political advocates. The political process in the United States exists at all levels of government where laws, regulations, and ordinances are passed and enforced, where taxes are collected, and where resources are allocated by the government to meet the needs of its citizens.

Individuals have diverse views about what the role of government should be in health care; however, the government currently has an active role in funding and providing health care and shaping the health care system. All levels of government are involved to some extent in the health care of its citizens (Table 7-10). The U.S. health care system is a mix of for-profit, nonprofit, and governmental health care systems. Regardless, the government is the single largest provider and payer of health care in the United States including Medicare, Medicaid, the military and Veterans Administration, the U.S. Public Health Services, Indian Health Services, state, city, and county health departments, school health services, and other federal- and state-funded programs.

At the state and national levels of government, the political process includes the electoral process, legislative process, regulatory process, and evaluation process (Table 7-11). Nurses need to be aware of all four processes in order to effectively advocate for health care issues of interest to them. Nurses can participate in the political process as individual citizens, professional nurses, or as elected officials.

Thinking about becoming politically involved can become overwhelming. So, you might want to start by selecting a health issue or service involving your city, county, school district, or state. Once you are comfortable taking actions at the local level, you might expand your horizons to the national or international levels. So, start small and stay local. Become "glocal," which means to think globally about a health care issue but act locally. Choose one health care issue you are passionate about. Make a plan for a year of involvement. You might want to find out the political agenda of your local nursing organization. Gather information from a variety of sources including the positions of groups with views differing from your own. Take a position and set a personal or professional goal for yourself. Develop your action plan. Consider the following actions:

- Discuss your health care issue with families, friends, and peers. Share what you have learned.
- Join one advocacy group (citizen or professional) and go to one meeting.
- Write one letter to the editor of your local paper or to an elected official.
- Contact one elected official.
- Go to one public or community meeting.
- At the end of the year, evaluate:
  - What did you accomplish?
  - How did your actions make a difference?
  - How do you feel about your actions?
  - What might you do the same or differently during the next year?

Develop effective political action strategies. Think about the power of ONE as you prepare to lobby for your health care issue: Use your time and energy wisely.

- ONE issue you feel passionately about
- ONE-minute presentation by phone or in person
- ONE-page letter to send to local newspaper or to elected official
- ONE-page fact sheet to share
- ONE patient or personal story to share

If each nurse used the power of ONE on a health care issue, consider the impact of this type of lobbying on health care today.

TABLE 7-10
Levels of Government and their Authority and Responsibilities

Level of Government	Authority and Responsibilities
Local Level: City, County, Independent School Districts	◆ Taxing authority ◆ Ability to pass ordinances, set policies ◆ Allocate resources ◆ Enforce laws and ordinances ◆ Provide services that protect public's health and safety ◆ Fund and provide health care services: city, county, and school health services
State Government: Three Branches ◆ Bicameral (House and Senate) or Unicameral (House) Legislature ◆ Executive Branch (Governor, Attorney General, Treasurer, Auditor) ◆ Judicial Branch (State Courts)	◆ Taxing authority ◆ Ability to pass and enforce laws, set and enforce policies and regulations ◆ Allocate resources, pass through to local government and private sector ◆ Provide services that protect public's health and safety ◆ Regulate commerce (includes for-profit health care such as hospitals and health care systems, long-term care, managed care organizations, nonprofit health care, pharmacies) ◆ Fund and provide health care services: Medicaid and other funding or services for uninsured, disabled, and elderly; grants to counties, universities, and private health care organizations, state health departments (services at state and county levels)
Federal Government: Three Branches ◆ Legislative—Congress (House and Senate) ◆ Executive—President (Cabinet, Military, Federal Agencies) ◆ Judicial—Supreme Court (Federal Courts)	◆ Taxing authority ◆ Ability to pass and enforce laws, set and enforce policies and regulations (federal laws supersede state laws most of the time) ◆ Allocate resources, pass through to states ◆ Provide services that protect public's health and safety ◆ Establish policies and relationships with international community ◆ Regulate interstate commerce (includes health care systems, pharmaceutical industry, health care technology companies) ◆ Fund and provide health care services: Medicare/Medicaid pass through to states; federal grants to states and universities, military, Veterans Administration, U.S. Public Health Services, Indian Health Services, National Institutes of Health, Health and Human Services, Centers for Disease Control and Prevention, Surgeon General)

© Cengage Learning 2014

TABLE 7-11
The Political Process and Nursing Advocacy

Process	Activities	Nurses' Political Advocacy Actions
Electoral Process	Election of public officials: Candidates present their positions, vie for support, campaign, debate the opposition, run for office.	Candidate selection, endorsement, campaign financing and contributions; Campaign worker: telephoning, mailings, door knocking, signage, rallies, coffee meetings Vote!
Legislative Process	Passage of laws: Issue adoption process includes drafting bills, introducing bills in Senate and House, debating and modifying bills, voting legislation into laws. After bills are passed by legislature, they must be signed by governor or president and funded by legislature.	Lobbying legislators individually, providing expert testimony, providing written and published materials including nursing research, working with legislative staff on bills, serving on legislative staffs, attending hearings, informing and obtaining the support of the public (e.g., letters to the editor, radio call-ins, social media [Facebook, blogs, etc.], town hall meetings)
Regulatory Process	Implementation of laws: Legislature assigns "budget authority" to federal or state agency which promulgates rules, holds hearings, modifies and passes regulations, and implements the law through the regulations. The agency may pass on money to other arms of government or to private organizations, through grants or contracts, to implement projects or programs to carry out the law.	Lobbying agencies with "budget authority," providing expert testimony, providing written and published materials including nursing research, working with agency staff on regulations, serving on boards or committees, attending hearings and community meetings, keeping stakeholders informed, writing grant proposals, carrying out demonstration projects
Evaluation Process	Monitoring and evaluation of laws: State or federal agencies and legislative audit committees monitor implementation of legislation, contracts, grants, and projects. They look at effectiveness of implementation (did it achieve intended purpose?) and efficiency of implementation (were money and resources used appropriately to achieve best outcome?). Outcomes are studied and reported on to legislature in one- or two-year budget cycles of legislature.	Carrying out evaluation and outcome studies, consulting on projects and outcomes, reading reports, attending hearings on whether to endorse or continue funding during next biennium, discussing outcomes with legislators and legislative staff, supporting continuation or denial of continued funding, proposing alternative actions

© Cengage Learning 2014

KEY CONCEPTS

- Effective nurses are powerful. They show objectivity, creativity, and knowledge throughout their practice and regardless of their work setting.
- Sources of power are reward and coercion, legitimacy, expertise, reference, information, and connection.
- The American Nurses Association is a full-service professional organization that represents the nation's entire registered nurse population. Since 2009, National Nurses United (NNU) has a dual role of being a professional organization and a collective bargaining agent for nursing. The ANA is not a collective bargaining agent, but is politically active and lobbies on issues affecting nursing and the general public.
- Nurses demonstrate moral courage when they take actions to improve patient safety, the health care work environment, and to report health care fraud.
- Nurses use collective social action to create change in health care by working together with other nurses and forming partnerships with other stakeholders, professional and consumer groups.
- Nurses use their individual, personal, and professional power by acting as political advocates at the local, state, and national levels. Nurses practice political advocacy when they participate in the political process to improve the health and well-being of their patients, their profession, and the public.

KEY TERMS

coercive power
collective bargaining
connection power
expert power
information power
legitimate power
moral courage
organizational power
personal power
politics
power
professional power
referent power
reward power
sources of power
workplace advocacy

REVIEW QUESTIONS

1. A nurse had an elderly patient fall on her shift last night and is concerned about the frequency of patient falls on the unit. Using professional and organizational sources of power to influence the nursing staff on the unit, what can help to improve practice, decrease falls, and improve safety? Which of the empowerment strategies by the nurse would be most effective in directly achieving these goals? Select all that apply.
   A. Become involved in a consumer group lobbying for safe patient care.
   B. Become a member of a practice committee on the unit dealing with patient falls.
   C. Provide evidence-based care regarding "best practices" in fall prevention.
   D. Become a role model for safe nursing practice when working with patients at risk for falls.
   E. Report nursing staff who do not use "best practices" for fall prevention.
   F. Become a patient advocate at a local church.

2. While speaking to a patient advocate group, the nurse speaker explains that power may be used ethically or unethically. Which example best demonstrates using power in an unethical manner?
   A. Mentoring novice nurses to follow unit policies
   B. Joining a practice committee to enhance her nursing career
   C. Giving staff feedback that they are not using "best practices"
   D. Working on a political campaign of a candidate who shares her views

3. A group of nurses on a unit believe that there is unsafe staffing on the evening shift. This is validated by numerous documented incidents of medications and treatments often being given late and patient complaints of call lights not being answered for 20–30 minutes. The nursing staff has frequently complained to their nurse manager and even the Chief Nursing Officer, but nothing has changed. Which other actions that are supported by professional organizations and government could the nurses take? Select all that apply.

A. Send an incident report to the Joint Commission.
B. Complete an unsafe-staffing report and submit it to the state nursing organization.
C. Send an anonymous letter to the state health department under the Vulnerable Adults Act.
D. Refuse a patient care assignment when assigned more patients than can be cared for safely.
E. File a *qui tam* lawsuit with the government.
F. File a report with the nursing union under the Taft Hartley Act.

4. An area hospital has a string of sentinel events causing unnecessary patient deaths. A consumer group is formed lobbying for safe patient care. The state nurses' association asks to partner with the consumer organization to lobby legislators for mandatory staffing ratios in hospitals. What would the first step be for the nursing organization to take to determine if a partnership would be appropriate?

A. Develop a political strategy for achieving shared goals.
B. Define the structure and boundaries for the two groups to work together.
C. Become sensitized to the issues and views of the consumer group.
D. Poll the nursing organization membership to see if members would support partnership.

5. A patient tells the nurse, "All you nurses are here to look pretty and pick up doctors; you see it on TV all the time." The nurse, a new nursing graduate, is concerned about the way that the media portray nursing. Which action could the nurse take to help improve the image of nursing in the media?

A. Write a letter to the editor of the local paper, identifying herself as a nurse, and complaining about the way nurses are treated in the media.
B. Write the state nursing association asking it to take action and develop a media campaign.
C. Ask patients to write a letter to a local newspaper praising nursing care.
D. Write a letter to the editor of her local paper, identifying herself as a nurse, and advocating for improvements in health care.

6. A nurse executive teaches the roles of the American Nurses Association's 2010 mission to a group of new graduates. While questioning the group on their understanding, which response by a new graduate indicates further teaching is required?

A. "The American Nurses Association is a collective bargaining agent for its members."
B. "The American Nurses Association lobbies Congress and regulatory agencies."
C. "The American Nurses Association credentials nurses in specialty practice."
D. "The American Nurses Association establishes standards for nursing practice."

7. A nurse gains employment at a hospital that is unionized. The nurse asks to speak to the union representative because the nurse has heard that the union benefits nurses by addressing the following: wages, benefits, and mandatory overtime; standards of nursing practice; health and safety issues; restructuring and cross-training; legal representation; unsafe staffing; and poor quality of care. Which areas are indeed included in collective bargaining? Select all that apply.

A. Wages, benefits, and mandatory overtime
B. Standards of nursing practice
C. Health and safety issues
D. Restructuring and cross-training
E. Legal representation
F. Unsafe staffing and poor quality of care

8. Nurses are discussing the option of organizing a union at the hospital where they are employed. Many opinions are discussed. Which response by a nurse best explains the reason professional nurses unionize?
   A. Nurses are usually satisfied with working conditions but want to see what else they could get.
   B. Nurses at the workplace feel powerless and believe a collective voice could help address issues for nurses and improve patient safety.
   C. Nurses like the power of a union so they can strike.
   D. Nurses want a union to get more money and work fewer hours.

9. A home health nurse working in an economically depressed area cares for many patients who cannot afford their medications or basic medical supplies. The nurse speaks with her manager and decides to become more politically active. Which are reasons for nurses to become politically active? Select all that apply.
   A. Patient advocacy is part of the nurse's scope of practice.
   B. The U.S. government is the largest health care provider and health care payer.
   C. Nurses need to be involved in the electoral process.
   D. Because nurses represent only a small percentage of the health care workforce, they need to be as visible as possible.
   E. Federal, state, and local governments pass laws and regulations and allocate resources that affect health care and patients' well-being.
   F. Nurses practice nursing under laws and regulations passed and enforced by Congress, state legislatures, and governmental agencies.

10. A school nurse has a high school student with severe asthma. The student asks the nurse, "Can you help me write a letter to the mayor to ask what we can do to improve the air quality for our town?" Which response by the nurse would be most appropriate?
   A. Write a letter at least five pages long with statistical facts and attach a fact sheet.
   B. Write a one-page letter with key facts and a short story and attach a fact sheet.
   C. Write a letter with a fact sheet.
   D. Write a letter identifying the health issue of concern and demand an appointment.

REVIEW ACTIVITIES

1. Identify nurses you work with who are able to influence others to make changes to improve patient care and safe nursing practice. What types of power do they use? What makes them powerful?
2. Find out who represents nurses at your workplace, clinical site, or local hospital. Are the nurses unionized? Talk with a few nurses about their perspectives on working in unionized versus nonunionized workplaces.
3. Look up your state nurses' association on the Internet. Search for its political platform and agenda for the coming year. Look for the association's position statements and its current lobbying efforts. Compare your state nurses' association's political platform and actions with those of another health care organization such as your state medical association or the state hospital association. How do your own beliefs compare or contrast with those of these organizations? What actions might you take?
4. Find out who your congress people are. Write or e-mail them and find out what health care legislation they are supporting (http://www.house.gov or http://www.senate.gov).

EXPLORING THE WEB

Explore nursing leadership and nursing power. What makes nurses powerful leaders? How are nurses empowered? How are nurses viewed by themselves and others?

- The 25 Most Famous Nurses in History: *http://onlinebsn.org/2009/25-most-famous-nurses-in-history*

- This site has a funny, not scholarly, synopsis of nursing power: *http://www.NursingPower.net*. Go to the site and click on Site Map.
- This is a fun YouTube video about how nurses make a difference in their nursing practice every day. Nurses Making a Difference: *http://www.youtube.com/watch?v=fpSzlFjPoU0&feature=fvw*
- This is a thought-provoking YouTube video about the image of nursing: *http://www.youtube.com/watch?v=qnkmhrneVok&NR=1&feature=endscreen*
- This site critiques and advocates for accuracy in the media's portrayal of the role of nursing and of nurses: *http://www.nursingadvocacy.org*
- What empowers nurses? Watch this video on nursing empowerment and see if you recognize yourself or nurses you know: *http://www.youtube.com/watch?v=lzjbe7ZOCKk&feature=related*
- Find out how young leaders in health care, especially nurses, work together internationally to achieve the UN Millennium Development Goals (MDGs.) Go to AYNLA: *http://www.aynla.org*
- This site supports political power for patients: *http://www.healthcarereform.net*
- This site discusses a variety of nursing resources and issues, including collective power: *http://www.nursingworld.org*

Find out about collective bargaining and workplace advocacy.

- What is the National Labor Relations Board? Go to: *http://www.nlrb.gov*
- Go to this site and search for "workplace advocacy," "collective bargaining," and your state nursing association: *http://www.nursingworld.org*

What nursing health care and consumer organizations might provide current information on health issues and actions? Here are a few.

- American Nurses Association: *http://www.nursingworld.org*
- Sigma Theta Tau International: *http://www.nursingsociety.org*
- American Public Health Association; there is a public health nursing section: *http://www.apha.org*
- American Hospital Association: *http://www.aha.org*
- AARP (American Association of Retired Persons): *http://www.aarp.org*
- Citizen's Council on Health Care: *http://www.cchc-mn.org* and *http://www.cchconline.org*
- Go to the consumer site for combating health-related fraud: *http://www.quackwatch.org*

Read about the U.S. national health goals and action plan for 2020 at Healthy People 2020: *http://www.healthypeople.gov/2020/default.aspx*

- Identify some sites for government bodies and health care agencies.
- U.S. Congress: *http://www.congress.org*
- U.S. Department of Health and Human Services: *http://www.hhs.gov*
- Government consumer health website: *http://www.healthfinder.gov*
- Medicare and Medicaid programs: *http://www.cms.hhs.gov*
- The Library of Congress Thomas site provides a searchable database of federal legislation: *http://thomas.loc.gov*
- The Library of Congress state government information provides state and local government links. Search for state and local government news. *http://www.loc.gov*
- Centers for Disease Control and Prevention: *http://www.cdc.gov*
- Office of the Surgeon General: *http://www.surgeongeneral.gov*
- National Institutes of Health: *http://www.nih.gov*

REFERENCES

American Nurses Association (ANA). (2009). Position statement—Patient safety: Rights of registered nurses when considering a patient assignment. Retrieved November 27, 2011, from http://nursingworld.org/rnrightsps

American Nurses Association (ANA). (2010). *Nursing's social policy statement: The essence of the profession* (3rd ed.). Washington, DC: American Nurses Publishing.

American Nurses Association. (2010a and 2010b). Code of ethics for nurses. Retrieved May 22, 2010, from http://nursingworld.org

Bu, X., & Jezewski, M. A. (2006). Developing a mid-range theory of patient advocacy through competency analysis. *Journal of Advanced Nursing, 57*(1), 101–110.

Budd, K., Warino, L., & Patton, M. (2004). Traditional & nontraditional collective bargaining strategies to improve the patient care environment. *Online Journal of Issues in Nursing, 1*(9). Retrieved September 1, 2012, from http://www.nursingworld.org/ojin/topic23/tpc23_5.htm (2/25/07). Retrieved October 31,2012.

Cohen, S. (2007). The image of nursing: How do others see us? How do we see ourselves? *American Nurse Today, 2*(5), 24–26.

Commission on Social Determinants of Health (CSDH). (2008). *Closing the gap in a generation: Health equity through action on the social determinants of health.* Final Report. Geneva, Switzerland: World Health Organization.

Curtin, L. (1979). The nurse as advocate: A philosophical foundation for nursing. *Advances in Nursing Science, 1*(3), 1–10.

Falk-Rafael, A. (2005). Speaking truth to power: Nursing's legacy and moral imperative. *Advances in Nursing Science, 28*(3), 212–223.

Fisher, J. L., & Koch, J. V. (1996). *Presidential leadership: Making a difference.* Phoenix, AZ: American Council on Education and Oryx Press.

Fletcher, K. (2007). Image: Changing how women nurses think about themselves. Literature review. *Journal of Advanced Nursing, 58*(3), 207–215. doi: 10.1111/j.1365-2648.2007.04285.x

Forman, H., & Grimes, T. C. (2004). The "new age" of union organizing. *Journal of Nursing Administration, 34*(3), 120–124.

Fowler, M. D., (Ed.) & American Nurses Association. (2008). *Guide to the code of ethics for nurses: Interpretation & application.* Atlanta, GA: NursesBooks.org.

French, J. P. R., Jr., & Raven, B. (1959). The bases of social power. In D. Cartwright and A. Zander (Eds.), *Group Dynamics,* (pp. 607–623). New York, NY: Harper and Row.

Galer-Unti, R. (2010). Advocacy 2.0: Advocating in the digital age. *Health Promotion Practice, 11*(6), 784–787.

Gracian, B. (1892). *The art of worldly wisdom.* (J. Jacobs, Trans.) Boston, MA: Dover Publications, 2005. (Original work published 1647).

Hackman, D. (2008). ANA and UAN part ways (American Nurses Association, United American Nurses). Georgia Nursing. Retrieved April 19, 2011, from http://goliath.ecnext.com/coms2/gi_0199- 9596517/ANA-and-UAN-part-ways.html

Hersey, P., Blanchard, K., & Natemeyer, W. (1979). Situational leadership, perception and impact of power. *Group and Organizational Studies, 4,* 418–428.

Johnson and Johnson. (2006). Campaign for nursing's future. Retrieved July 3, 2006, from http://www.jnj.com/our_company/advertising/discover_nursing

Kalisch, B. J., Begeny, S., & Neumann, S. (2007). The image of the nurse on the Internet. *Nursing Outlook, 55*(4), 182–188.

Manojlovich, M. (2007). Power and empowerment in nursing: Looking backward to inform the future. *Online Journal of Issues in Nursing, 12*(1).

McDonald, L. (2006). Florence Nightingale as a social reformer. *History Today 56*(1), 9–15.

Murray, S. (2010). Moral courage in health care: Acting ethically even in presence of risk. *Online Journal of Issues in Nursing, 15*(3), Man 02. Retrieved November 27, 2011, from http://www.nursingworld.org/MainMenuCategories/ANAMarketplace/ANAPeriodicals/OJIN/TableofContents/Vol152010/No3-Sept-2010/Moral-Courage-and-Risk.html

National Nurses United (NNU). (2010). National Nurses United salutes the Minnesota Nurses Association for historic patient care strike of 2010. Retrieved May 7, 2010, from http://www.nationalnursesunited.org

O'Connor, T., & Kelly, B. (2005). Bridging the gap: A study of general nurses' perceptions of patient advocacy in Ireland. *Nursing Ethics, 12*(5), 453–467.

Philipsen, N. C., & Soeken, D. (2011). Preparing to blow the whistle: A survival guide for nurses. *Journal for Nurse Practitioners, 7*(9), 740–746. Retrieved November 29, 2011, from http://www.medscape.com/viewarticle/751347

Ponte, P. R., Glazer, G., Dann, E., McCollum, K., Gross, A., Tyrrell, R., Branowicki, P., et al. (2007). The *power* of professional nursing practice: An essential element of patient and family-centered care. Retrieved November 14, 2011. *The Online Journal of Issues in Nursing, 12*(1), 1–14.

Rudolph, B. J. (2005). *How nurses define the role of patient advocacy.* Unpublished master's thesis, Division of Nursing, Wilmington College, Wilmington, DE.

Rutty, J. (1998). The nature of philosophy of science, theory and knowledge relating to nursing and professionalism. *Journal of Advanced Nursing, 28,* 243–250.

Scott, D. (2008). The Center for American Nurses: Celebrating five years of workforce advocacy. *Nurses First, 1* (1), 5–7.

Seldes, G. (1985). *The great thoughts.* New York, NY: Ballantine Books.

Stanley, D. J. (2008). Celluloid angels: A research study of nurses in feature films 1900–2007. *Journal of Advanced Nursing, 64*(1), 84–95. doi: 10.1111/j.1365-2648.2008.04793.x

United American Nurses (UAN). (2006). Nurses organize. Retrieved February 25, 2007, from http://www.uannurse.org/organizeindex.html

Weinberg, N. (2005, March). The dark side of whistle-blowing. *Forbes,* 90–96.

Wells, S. (1998). *Choosing the future: The power of strategic thinking.* Boston, MA: Butterworth-Heinemann.

Zelek, B., & Phillips, S. P. (2003). Gender and power: Nurses and doctors in Canada. *International Journal for Equity in Health, 2*(1). doi: 10.1186/1475-9276-2-1

SUGGESTED READINGS

American Public Health Association. (2010). Top ten rules of advocacy. Retrieved November 15, 2010, from: http://www.apha.org

Armalegos, J., & Berney, J. (2005). 30 years of collective bargaining autonomy: Voice in practice. *Michigan Nurse, 78*(2), 6–8.

Buresh, B., & Gordon, S. (2005). *From silence to voice: What nurses know and must communicate to the public.* Cornell, NY: ILR Press.

Donelan, K., Buerhaus, P. I., Ulrich, B. T., Norman, L., & Dittus, R. (2005). Awareness and perceptions of the Johnson & Johnson campaign for nursing's future. *Nursing Economics, 23*(4), 150–156,180.

Grindel, C. (2006). The power of nursing: Can it ever be mobilized? *MedSurg Nursing, 15*(1), 5–6.

Hersey, P., Blanchard, P. L., & Johnson, D. E. (2007). Management of organizational behavior. Upper Saddle River, NJ: Prentice Hall.

Hughes, F., Duke, J., Bamford, A., & Moses, C. (2006). Enhancing nursing leadership through policy, politics and strategic alliances. *Nurse Leader, 4*(2), 24–27.

International Council of Nurses. (2008). Promoting health: Advocacy guide for health professionals. Geneva, Switzerland: Author. Retrieved from http://www.whpa.org/PPE_Advocacy_Guide.pdf

Middaugh, D. J., & Robertson, R. D. (2005). Politics in the workplace. *Nursing Management, 14*(6), 393–394.

National Council of State Boards of Nursing. (2010). *Professional boundaries: A nurse's guide to the importance of appropriate professional boundaries.* Retrieved September 28, 2012, from: http://learningext.com/groups/b06e8bc419/summary

Sigma Theta Tau International. (1998). Woodhull study on nursing and the media. Retrieved September 11, 2003, from http://www.nursingsociety.org/media/woodhullextract.html

Vesely, R. (2008). Unleash the energy: Activists, professors try to use their own sphere of influence to affect U.S. health care policy and improve patient care. *Modern Health Care, 38*(17), 6–7.

Vestal, K. (2007). The power and intrigue of workplace politics. *Nurse Leader, 5*(1), 6–7.

LEADERSHIP AND MANAGEMENT OF PATIENT-CENTERED CARE

CHAPTER 8

Delegation of Patient Care

MAUREEN T. MARTHALER, RN, MS, AND
PATRICIA KELLY, RN, MSN

Surround yourself with the best people you can find, delegate authority, and don't interfere as long as the policy you've decided upon is being carried out.

–RONALD REAGAN, 1981

OBJECTIVES

Upon completion of this chapter, the reader should be able to:

1. Discuss concepts of delegation, accountability, responsibility, authority, supervision, competence, and assignment.
2. Utilize the National Council of State Boards of Nursing Delegation Decision-Making Tree.
3. Describe the five rights of delegation.
4. Identify delegation responsibilities of health team members.
5. Identify organizational responsibility and accountability for delegation and the chain of command.
6. Discuss transcultural delegation.

The registered nurse and nursing assistive personnel (NAP) were caring for four patients. One patient's 6 A.M. hemoglobin (Hgb) result was 7.8 gm/dL. The registered nurse notified the health care provider of the abnormally low result. The health care provider prescribed the following: Type and cross-match for two units of packed red blood cells (PRBC), transfuse one unit of packed PRBCs over four hours, check Hgb 30 minutes after the first unit has infused, and call health care provider with results.

Per hospital protocol, two registered nurses checked the unit of blood at the bedside identifying the patient, blood band, blood type, and unit number and expiration date. Prior to initializing the blood transfusion by the nurse, a set of vital signs were obtained by the NAP. Fifteen minutes after the unit of blood was started, a second set of vitals were obtained by the NAP as well. At this time the patient told the NAP that she was feeling warm and her lower back hurt. The NAP opened the window, adjusted the pillow, and returned to her regular duties. An hour later, the nurse entered the room and found the patient covered in a raised red rash and weeping because her back hurt.

Should the registered nurse have checked the patient more often?

What are the responsibilities of the nurse and the NAP in this case?

How could delegation have been appropriately performed in this case?

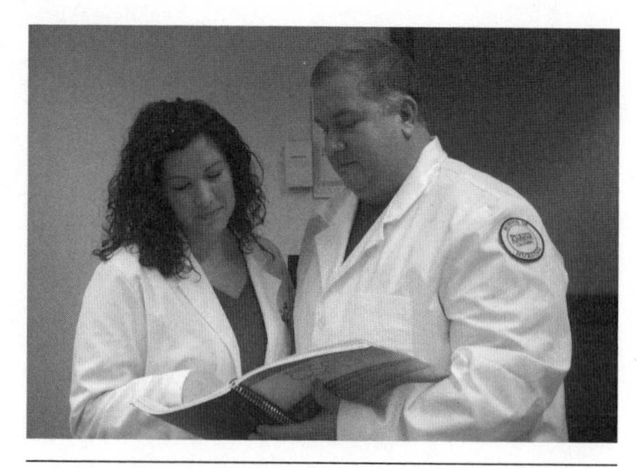

© Cengage Learning 2014

There is more nursing to do than there are nurses to do it. Many nurses are stretched to the limit in the current health care environment, with a greater number of patients, higher acuity of patient illnesses, more technological advances, and increased complexity of therapies. The topic of nursing delegation has never been more timely. Delegation is a process that, when used appropriately, can result in safe and effective patient-centered care. Delegation can free the nurse to deal with more complex patient care needs, promote teamwork and collaboration, develop the skills of nursing assistive personnel (NAP), and promote cost containment for the health care organization. The RN determines appropriate nursing practice by using nursing knowledge, professional judgment, and legal authority to practice nursing. RNs must be familiar with their state's Nurse Practice Act, state laws, professional nursing standards, and agency policies and procedures related to delegation.

The Patient Safety and Quality Improvement Act of 2005 requires health care institutions to make public specified information on staffing levels, patient mix, and patient outcomes, including the number of RNs providing direct care; the numbers of NAP utilized to provide direct patient care; the average number of patients per RN providing direct patient care; the patient mortality rate; the incidence of adverse patient care incidents; and the methods used for determining and adjusting staffing levels and patient care needs.

In addition, health care agencies have to make public their data regarding complaints filed with the state, the Health Care Financing Administration, or an accrediting agency related to Medicare Conditions of Participation. The agency would then have to make public the results of any investigations or findings related to the complaint. Recent studies have demonstrated a direct relationship between RN staffing levels and positive patient outcomes. These outcomes are affected by nursing delegation.

This chapter discusses the concepts of delegation, accountability, responsibility, authority, supervision, competence, and assignment of nurses. It also describes the National Council of State Boards of Nursing Delegation Decision-Making Tree, the five rights of delegation, responsibilities of health team members, the organization's responsibility and accountability related to delegation, and transcultural delegation.

DELEGATION

Florence Nightingale is quoted as saying, "But then again to look to all these things yourself does not mean to do them yourself. . . . But can you not insure that it is done when not done by yourself?" (1859, p. 17). Nursing delegation was discussed by Nightingale in the 1800s and has continued to evolve since then. The American Nurses Association (ANA) and the National Council of the State Boards of Nursing (NCSBN) define **delegation** as the process for a nurse to direct another person to perform nursing tasks and activities (ANA & NCSBN, 2005). In 2006, the ANA and the NCSBN created a joint statement on delegation to support the practicing nurse in using delegation safely and effectively. Two documents that support the joint statement are the ANA Principles of Delegation (2006) and the NCSBN (1997b) Delegation Decision-Making Tree.

Note that state nurse practice acts and laws define the legal parameters for nursing practice. Most states authorize RNs to delegate selected patient care activities. The nursing profession is responsible for determining the scope of nursing practice (ANA and NCSBN, 2006). A scope of practice statement describes the "who," "what," "where," "when," "why," and "how" of nursing practice (ANA, 2010). Competent, appropriately supervised nursing assistive personnel (NAP) are needed in the delivery of affordable, quality health care. The nursing profession defines and supervises the education, training, and utilization of nursing assistants involved in providing direct patient-centered care.

The RN is in charge of patient care and determines the appropriate utilization of any nursing assistive personnel involved in providing direct patient care. All decisions related to delegation are based on the fundamental principles of protection of the health, safety, and welfare of the public. A task delegated to a NAP cannot be redelegated by the NAP. When there is a decision to delegate a nursing task, the decision must be based on and in accordance with standards of practice, policies, and procedures established by the nursing profession, the state nurse practice act, state laws, the agency, and ethical-legal standards of behavior. Standards are written and used to guide both the provision for and evaluation of patient care by RNs and NAP. The nurse who delegates retains accountability for the task delegated (NCSBN, 1995).

The ANA and NCSBN have different constituencies. The constituency of the ANA is state nursing associations and RN members. The constituency of NCSBN is state boards of nursing and all licensed nurses. Although, for the purpose of collaboration, the 2006 Joint Statement refers to registered nurse practice, NCSBN acknowledges that in many states licensed practical nurses/licensed vocational nurses (LPN/LVN) have limited authority to delegate (ANA & NCSBN, 2006).

ACCOUNTABILITY

Accountability is being responsible and answerable for the actions or inactions of self or others in the context of delegation (NCSBN, 1997a).

Licensed-nurse accountability involves compliance with legal requirements as set forth in the jurisdiction's laws and rules governing nursing. The licensed nurse is also accountable for: the safety and quality of the nursing care provided; recognizing limits, knowledge, and experience; and planning for situations beyond the nurse's expertise (NCSBN, 2004). Licensed-nurse accountability includes the preparedness and obligation to explain or justify to relevant others (including the regulatory authority) "the relevant initial and ongoing judgments, intentions, decisions, actions, and omissions . . . and their consequences" (NCSBN, 2004). RNs are accountable for monitoring changes in a patient's status, noting and implementing treatment for human responses to illness, and assisting in the prevention of complications.

The RN assesses the patient, makes a nursing diagnosis, and develops, implements, and evaluates the patient's plan of care. The RN uses nursing judgment and monitors unstable patients with unpredictable outcomes. The monitoring of other more stable patients cared for by the LPN and NAP may involve the RN's direct continuing presence, or the monitoring may be more intermittent. As stated by the American Association of Critical-Care Nurses (AACN) in 2004, the delegation of direct and indirect patient care to other caregivers is reasonable, relevant, and practical.

Nursing tasks that do not involve direct patient care can be reassigned more freely and carry fewer legal implications for RNs than delegation of direct nursing-practice activities. The assessment, analysis, diagnosis, planning, teaching, and evaluation stages of the nursing process may not be delegated to NAP. Delegated activities usually fall within the implementation phase of the nursing process.

RESPONSIBILITY

Responsibility involves reliability, dependability, and the obligation to accomplish work when an assignment is accepted. It is a nursing responsibility to manage the care of a patient whose hands-on care is being performed by nonlicensed nurses' aides (Estate of Travaglini *v.* Ingalls Health, 2009). For example, a NAP is expected to provide the patient with food and water. A NAP does not administer tube feedings but is expected to feed or assist the patient when delegated to do so. After the NAP performs the delegated duties, he or she provides feedback to the nurse about the performance of the duties and the outcome of his or her actions. This feedback is given to the nurse within a specified time frame. Note that feedback is provided in both directions. It is also the RN's responsibility to follow up with ongoing supervision and evaluation of activities performed by non-nursing personnel. The nurse transfers responsibility and authority for the completion of a delegated task, but the nurse retains accountability for the delegation process.

The decision of whether or not to delegate requires the RN's judgment concerning: the condition of the patient; the competence, knowledge, and skill of all members of the nursing team; and the degree of supervision that will be required of the RN if a task is delegated. The RN delegates only those tasks for which she or he believes the NAP has the knowledge and skill to perform, taking into consideration training, culture, experience, and agency policies and procedures. The RN individualizes communication regarding delegation and the patient's situation to the NAP. The communication should be clear, concise, correct, and complete (Hansten & Jackson, 2009). The RN verifies comprehension with the NAP and assures that the NAP accepts the delegation. The NAP is then answerable for his or her actions and the behavior and responsibility that accompany them (NCSBN, 2005). Communication between the RN and the NAP must be a two-way process. The NAP should have the opportunity to ask questions and seek clarification of delegated tasks.

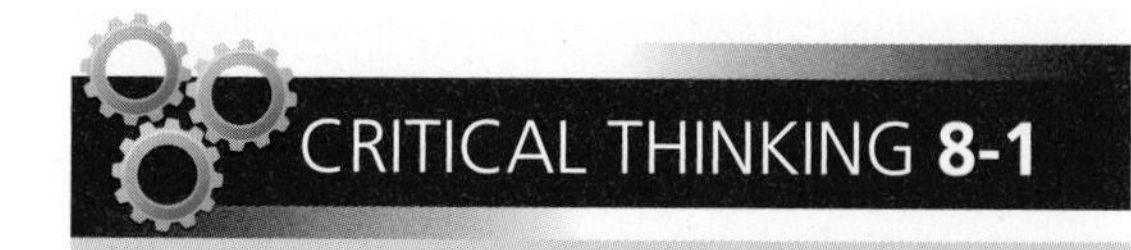

Go to http://www.qsen.org. Click on Quality/Safety Competencies. Then click on Teamwork & Collaboration. Scroll down and click on Staff Work-Around Assignment. Choose a nursing policy or procedure commonly used during clinical, for example, medication administration through a feeding tube. Find the current nursing policy or procedure in place for the agency/unit, observe RNs on the unit performing the identified procedure, discuss why RNs may or may not follow the agency's policy/procedure, reflect on the opportunities and challenges of evidence-based practice and the implementation into actual bedside nursing practice, and discuss what the proper response should be when you as an RN discover unsafe practice that deviates from standards, polices, or procedures.

The RN must ensure that all communication is culturally appropriate and that the person receiving the communication is treated respectfully. Note that delegation involves both individual accountability and organizational accountability. It is inappropriate for employers or others to require nurses to delegate when, in the nurse's professional judgment, delegation is unsafe and not in the patient's best interest. In those instances, the nurse should act as the patient's advocate and take appropriate action to ensure provision of safe nursing care. The RN takes responsibility and accountability for individual nursing practice and determines the appropriate delegation of tasks consistent with the nurse's obligation to provide optimum patient care (ANA, 2006). Two types of patient care activities may be delegated: direct and indirect.

Direct Patient Care Activities

Direct patient care activities include following standards for activities such as assisting the patient with feeding, drinking, ambulating, grooming, toileting, dressing, and socializing. The 2010 Illinois Nurse Practice Act (found at http://nursing.illinois.gov/nursepracticeact.asp) is specific in what the nurse can and cannot delegate. It states: "A registered professional nurse shall not delegate any nursing activity requiring the specialized knowledge, judgment, and skill of a licensed nurse to an unlicensed person, including medication administration." Direct patient-centered care activity may also involve following standards for collecting, reporting, and documenting data related to these activities. This data is reported to the RN, who uses the information to make a clinical judgment about patient care. Activities delegated to a NAP do not include health counseling or teaching, or require independent, specialized nursing knowledge, skill, or judgment.

Indirect Patient Care Activities

Indirect patient-centered care activities are necessary to support patients and their environment and only incidentally involve direct patient contact. These activities assist in providing a clean, efficient, and safe patient care milieu. They typically encompass unit routines such as chore services, companion care, and housekeeping, transporting, clerical, stocking, and maintenance tasks (ANA, 1996).

Underdelegation

Personnel in a new job role such as new nurse managers or new nursing graduates often underdelegate. Believing that older, more experienced staff may resent having someone new delegate to them, new nurses may simply avoid delegation. They may seek approval from other staff members by demonstrating their capability to complete all assigned duties without assistance. New nurses can become frustrated and overwhelmed if they fail to delegate properly. They may, for example, fail to delegate to those with certain responsibilities the appropriate authority to carry them out. Perfectionism and refusal to allow mistakes also can overwhelm new nurses. More-experienced staff members can help new personnel by intervening early on, assisting in the delegation process and clarifying responsibilities (Table 8-1).

Overdelegation

Overdelegation of duties can also be a problem. Delegating duties that are inappropriate for personnel to perform because they have been inadequately educated is dangerous and against the state nurse practice act.

TABLE 8-1
Delegation Checklist

Question	Yes	No
Do you recognize that you retain ultimate responsibility for the outcome of delegated assignments?	_____	_____
Do you spend most of your time completing tasks that require an RN?	_____	_____
Do you trust the ability of your staff to complete job assignments successfully?	_____	_____
Do you allow staff sufficient time to solve their own problems before interceding with advice?	_____	_____
Do you clearly outline expected outcomes and hold your staff accountable for achieving these outcomes?	_____	_____
Do you support your staff with an appropriate level of feedback and follow-up?	_____	_____

(Continues)

TABLE 8-1 (Continued)

Question	Yes	No
Do you use delegation as a way to help staff develop new skills and provide challenging work assignments?	_____	_____
Does your staff know what you expect of them?	_____	_____
Do you take the time to carefully select the right person for the right job?	_____	_____
Do you feel comfortable sharing control with your staff as appropriate?	_____	_____
Do you clearly identify all aspects of an assignment to staff when you delegate?	_____	_____
Do you assign tasks to the lowest level of staff capable of completing them successfully?	_____	_____
Do you support your staff, even when they are learning?	_____	_____
Do you allow your staff reasonable freedom to achieve outcomes?	_____	_____

Source: Compiled with information from Harvard ManageMentor® Skill Pack. (2011). *Improving Productivity: A Harvard ManageMentor Skill Pack.* Boston, MA: Harvard Business School Publishing.

The reasons for overdelegation are numerous. Personnel may feel uncomfortable performing duties that are unfamiliar to them, and they may depend too much on others. They may be unorganized or inclined to either avoid responsibility or immerse themselves in trivia. Overdelegating duties can overwork some personnel and underwork others. See Table 8-2 for other obstacles to delegation.

TABLE 8-2
Obstacles to Delegation

Fear of being disliked	Tendency to isolate oneself and choosing to complete all tasks alone
Inability to give up any control of the situation	Lack of confidence to delegate to staff members who were previously one's peers
Fear of making a mistake	Inability to prioritize using Maslow's hierarchy of needs and the nursing process
Inability to determine what to delegate and to whom	Thinking of oneself as the only one who can complete a task the way "it is supposed" to be done
Inadequate knowledge of the delegation process	Inability to communicate effectively
Past experience with delegation that did not turn out well	Inability to develop working relationships with other team members
Poor interpersonal communication skills	Lack of knowledge of the capabilities of staff, including their competency, skill, experience, level of education, job description, and so on
Lack of confidence to move beyond being a novice nurse	
Lack of administrative support for nurse delegating to LPN and NAP	

© Cengage Learning 2014

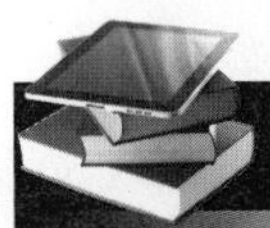

EVIDENCE FROM THE LITERATURE

Citation: Gordon, S. C., & Barry, C. D. (2009). Delegation guided by school nursing values: Comprehensive knowledge, trust, and empowerment. *The Journal of School Nursing, 25*(5), 352–360.

Discussion: As health care institutions in the United States respond to shrinking budgets and nursing shortages by increasing the use of unlicensed assistive personnel (UAP), school nursing practice is changing from providing direct care to supervising activities delegated to UAP. Therefore, delegation is a critical area of concern for school nurses. The purpose of this qualitative research study was to explore values guiding the delegation of health care tasks to UAP in school settings from the perspective of the school nurse.

Implications: Delegation of nursing procedures and medication administration in school is fraught with legal and ethical concerns for the school nurse. Because nurses may be responsible for coordinating care for several school buildings, delegation of nursing care and medication administration has occurred out of necessity. Nurse practice acts in some states, but not all, allow for delegation of medication administration to unlicensed assistive personnel, also known as nursing assistive personnel (NAP).

AUTHORITY

The right to delegate duties and give direction to nursing assistive personnel (NAP) places the RN in a position of authority. Authority identifies the source of the power to act (NCSBN, 1995). **Authority** occurs when a person who has been given the right to delegate, based on the state's nurse practice act, also has the official power from an agency to delegate. Authority given by an agency legitimizes the right of a nurse to give direction to others and expect that they will comply. An understanding of the level of authority at the time the task is delegated and the level of authority that is identified by the state's nurse practice act and the agency's job description prevents each party from making inaccurate assumptions about authority for delegated assignments. Note that there are four possible levels of authority to be used by the RN when delegating a task to another nurse. See Table 8-3.

TABLE 8-3
Levels of Authority

Level	Authority
One	Delegate to collect data to simply find out the facts or assess the situation and report back
Two	Delegate to collect data and make a recommendation back to the RN
Three	Delegate to assess the situation, make a recommendation, report back, and then implement the final RN recommendation
Four	Delegate to carry out the task as he or she believes appropriate

© Cengage Learning 2014

SUPERVISION

NCSBN defines **supervision** as the provision of guidance or direction, oversight, evaluation, and follow-up by the licensed nurse for the accomplishment of a delegated nursing task by assistive personnel. The ANA defines supervision as the active process of directing, guiding, and influencing the outcome of an individual's performance of a task. Both the ANA and NCSBN define supervision as the provision of guidance and oversight of a delegated nursing task (ANA & NCSBN, 2005).

Supervision can be categorized as on-site, in which the nurse is physically present or immediately available while the activity is being performed, or off-site, in which the nurse has the ability to provide direction through various means of written, verbal, and electronic communication (ANA, 1996). On-site supervision generally occurs in the acute care setting where the RN is immediately available. Off-site supervision may occur in community settings.

As a result of the rapidly increasing use of technology in patient care, some operational guidelines for supervision from the ANA are helpful. Ask yourself, Who is in control of the activity? If the RN is responsible, the nurse should incorporate measures to determine whether an activity has been completed in a way that meets expectations. Also ask yourself, How should controls be instituted? Controls must be in place that allow the RN delegating an activity to stop the task when inappropriately done, review the measures taken, and take back control of the task (ANA, 1996).

A nurse who is supervising care will provide clear direction to the staff about what tasks are to be performed for specific patients. The supervising nurse must identify when and how the task is to be done and what information must be collected, as well as any patient-specific information. The nurse must also identify what outcomes are expected and the time frame for reporting results. The nurse will monitor staff performance to ensure compliance with established standards of practice, policy, and procedure. The supervising nurse will obtain feedback from staff and patients and intervene, as necessary, to ensure quality nursing care and appropriate documentation.

Hansten and Jackson (2009) identify three levels of supervision based on the task delegated and the education, experience, competency, and working relationship of the people involved:

- An absence of supervision occurs when one RN works with another RN. Both are accountable for their own practice. When an RN is in a management position (e.g., charge nurse, nurse manager), the RN will supervise other RNs.
- Initial direction and periodic inspection occur when an RN supervises licensed or unlicensed staff, knows the staff's training and competency level, and has a working relationship with the staff. For example, an RN who has worked with a NAP for several weeks is now comfortable giving initial directions to ambulate two new postoperative patients. The RN follows up with an NAP once and as needed during the shift.
- Continuous supervision occurs when the RN determines that the delegate needs frequent-to-continuous support and assistance. This level is required when the working relationship is new, the task is complex, or the delegate is inexperienced or has not demonstrated competency.

ASSIGNMENT

Assignment is defined by both ANA and NCSBN (2005) as the distribution of work that each staff member is to accomplish on a given shift or work period. The NCSBN uses the verb "assign" to describe those situations when a nurse directs an individual to do something the individual is already authorized to do; for example, when an RN directs another RN to assess a patient, the second RN is already authorized to assess patients in the RN scope of practice (ANA & NCSBN, 2005). The 2003 survey by the American Organization of Nurse Executives and McCanis & Monsalve Associates, Inc., states, "Assignments and delegation of activities of care are based on the nurse's assessment of patient needs and are congruent with the caregiver's knowledge and skill."

During a typical shift, patients range from those needing only occasional care to those requiring frequent care. The charge nurse makes out the assignment sheet taking into consideration the skill, knowledge, and judgment of the RNs, LPNs, and NAP. Assignments are given to staff members who have the appropriate knowledge and skill to complete the assignment. They must always be within the legal scope of practice. Assignment sheets are used to identify patient care duties for RNs, LPNs, and NAP. See Figure 8-1.

COMPETENCE

Competence is the ability of the nurse to apply knowledge to interpersonal decision making and psychomotor skills expected for the practice role of a licensed nurse in the context of public health, safety, and welfare (NCSBN, 1995). Competence is

Room/Name	Patient Description	Special Needs
		Report vitals and outcomes to Mary, RN, at 8:30 P.M. Report anything abnormal STAT
2501/Ms. J. D.	68-year-old female, post-op day 1, post-shoulder repair Confused; fall risk; side rails up	Up in chair at 6 P.M. Maintain safety Vitals at 4 P.M. and 8 P.M. check distal pulses Monitor level of consciousness (LOC) Check dressings at 4 P.M. and 8 P.M. Check voiding at 6 P.M. Family at bedside
2502/Mr. D. H.	45-year-old male diabetic, post-op day 1, amputation just below the knee; Insulin sliding scale; Complaining of pain; restlessness; diaphoretic	Vitals and Accucheck STAT and at 4 P.M. and 9 P.M. Up in chair 6 P.M. Pain medication as needed Monitor dressing No pillow under stump
2503/Mr. H. M.	35-year-old male, history of alcohol abuse Complaining of abdominal pain; new hematemesis of coffee-ground fluid; IV of 0.9% normal saline at 125 cc/hour; alert	Vitals Q 15 minutes Monitor LOC, hematemesis, and possible seizures 16 gauge IV, type and crossmatch Possible transfer to ICU
2504/Mr. J. K.	20-year-old male college student, just admitted threatening to commit suicide; alert and oriented	Vitals at 4 P.M. and 8 P.M. Do not leave unattended Maintain safety

FIGURE 8-1

Assignment form.

© Cengage Learning 2014

required to practice safely and ethically in a designated role and setting. Licensed-nurse competence is built upon the knowledge gained in a nursing education program, orientation to specific settings, and the experiences of implementing nursing care. Nurses must: know themselves first, including strengths and challenges; assess the match of their knowledge and experience with the requirements and context of a role; gain additional knowledge as needed; and maintain all skills and abilities needed to provide safe nursing care.

NAP competence is built upon formal training and assessment, orientation to specific settings and groups of patients, interpersonal and communication skills, and the experience of the nurse's aide in assisting the nurse to provide safe nursing care.

Health care organizations require employees to demonstrate that they are competent to perform certain technical procedures and apply specific knowledge to safely care for patients. Written documentation of these competencies is maintained in the employee's personnel file. Most health care organizations require employees to undergo annual competency training for elements of care unique to their practice setting. Annual competency testing for RNs, LPNs, and NAP may include: patient safety, infection control, code blue, medication safety, IV skills, glucose testing, chain of command, HIPAA policies, and restraints.

DELEGATION DECISION-MAKING TREE

The NCSBN has developed a Delegation Decision-Making Tree. Its steps are as follows:

- Assessment of the patient, staff, and context of the situation; planning the delegation based on the patient's needs and available resources
- Communication with the delegate to provide direction and opportunity for interaction during the completion of the delegated task, including any unique patient requirements and characteristics, as well as clear expectations regarding what to do, what to report, and when to ask for assistance
- Surveillance, supervision, and monitoring of the delegation to ensure compliance with standards of practice, policies, and procedures (This includes the level of supervision needed for the particular situation and the implementation of that supervision, including follow-up for problems or a changing situation.)
- Evaluation and feedback to consider the effectiveness of the delegation, including any need to adjust the plan of care to achieve desired patient outcomes (Figure 8-2)

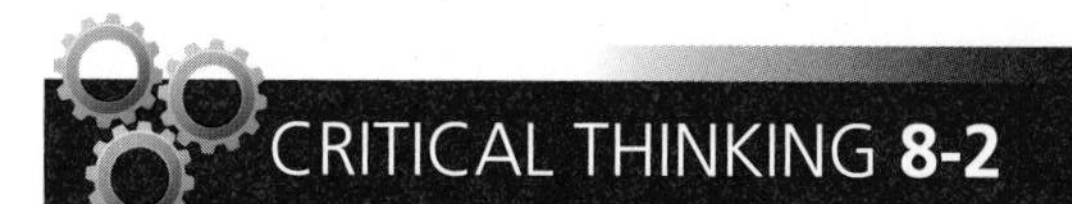

CRITICAL THINKING **8-2**

Identify which members of the health care team may do each of the following nursing activities.

Nursing activity	RN	LPN	NAP
Administer blood to a patient			
Assess a patient going to surgery			
Develop a teaching plan for a newly diagnosed patient with diabetes			
Measure a patient's intake and output			
Provide a bath to an immobilized patient			
Give a dressing change to a patient			
Give patient report when transferring a patient from ICU to a step-down unit			
Give insulin			
Evaluate a patient's DNAR status			
Give an oral medication			
Assist a patient with ambulation			
Give an IM pain medication			

THE FIVE RIGHTS OF DELEGATION

The NCSBN has spelled out Five Rights of Delegation (NCSBN, 1997a) that nurses may apply to their practice. These five rights are the right task, the right circumstance, the right person, the right direction and communication, and the right supervision. See the website for more information at http://www.ncsbn.org. See also Table 8-4.

Knowledge and Skill of Delegation

Note that delegation is not a skill that is simply learned in a classroom. Delegation requires discussion of knowledge and concerns related to delegation, clinical mentorship or practice in responsibilities related to delegation, and discussion of how to handle situations where tasks were not accomplished when delegated. The quality of delegation practices influences patient safety. When delegation is unsuccessful, there is an added work load on the RNs (Potter, Deshield, & Kuhrik, 2010). See Table 8-5.

RESPONSIBILITIES OF HEALTH TEAM MEMBERS

New graduate nurses may feel overwhelmed with their responsibilities and need to delegate patient care. The consequences and likely effects must be considered when delegating patient care. The AACN

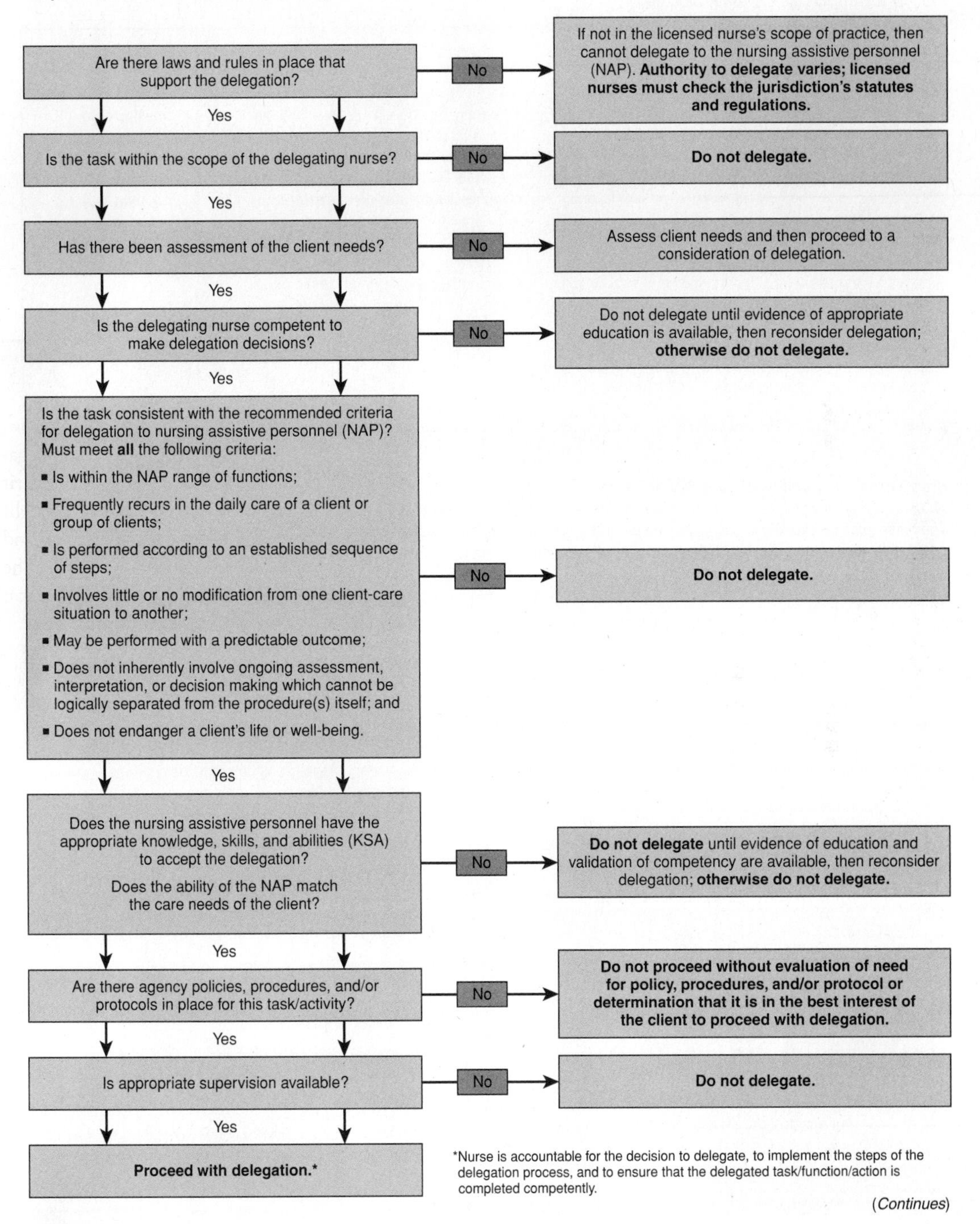

FIGURE 8-2

NCSBN delegation decision-making tree.

Decision Tree – Delegation to Nursing Assistive Personnel (Continued)

Step Two – Communication

Communication must be a two-way process.

The nurse:	*The nursing assistive personnel:*	*Documentation:*

▪ Assesses the assistant's understanding of:
  ▪ How the task is to be accomplished
  ▪ When and what information is to be reported, including:
    ▪ Expected observations to report and record
    ▪ Specific client concerns that would require prompt reporting.
▪ Individualizes for the nursing assistive personnel and client situation
▪ Addresses any unique client requirements, characteristics, and expectations
▪ Assesses the assistant's understanding of expectations, providing clarification if needed
▪ Communicates his or her willingness and availability to guide and support assistant
▪ Ensures appropriate accountability by verifying that the receiving person accepts the delegation and accompanying responsibility.
	▪ Asks questions regarding the delegation and seeks clarification of expectations if needed
	▪ Informs the nurse if the assistant has not done a task/function/activity before, or has only done it infrequently
	▪ Asks for additional training or supervision
	▪ Affirms understanding of expectations
	▪ Determines the communication method between the nurse and the assistive personnel
	▪ Determines the communication and plan of action in emergency situations.
		Timely, complete, and accurate documentation of provided care
		▪ Facilitates communication with other members of the health care team
		▪ Records the nursing care provided.

Step Three – Surveillance and Supervision

The purpose of surveillance and monitoring is related to the nurse's responsibility for client care within the context of a client population. The nurse supervises the delegation by monitoring the performance of the task or function and ensures compliance with standards of practice, policies, and procedures. Frequency, level, and nature of monitoring vary with needs of client and experience of assistant.

The nurse considers the:	*The nurse determines:*	*The nurse is responsible for:*

▪ Client's health care status and stability of condition
▪ Predictability of responses and risks
▪ Setting where care occurs
▪ Availability of resources and support infrastructure
▪ Complexity of the task being performed.
	▪ The frequency of onsite supervision and assessment based on:
	  ▪ Needs of the client
	  ▪ Complexity of the delegated function/task/activity
	  ▪ Proximity of nurse's location.
		▪ Timely intervening and follow-up on problems and concerns. Examples of the need for intervening include:
		  ▪ Alertness to subtle signs and symptoms (which allows nurse and assistant to be proactive, before a client's condition deteriorates significantly)
		  ▪ Awareness of assistant's difficulties in completing delegated activities
		▪ Providing adequate follow-up to problems and/or changing situations, a critical aspect of delegation.

Step Four – Evaluation and Feedback

Evaluation is often the forgotten step in delegation.

In considering the effectiveness of delegation, the nurse addresses the following questions:

- Was the delegation successful?
  - Was the task/function/activity performed correctly?
  - Was the client's desired and/or expected outcome achieved?
  - Was the outcome optimal, satisfactory, or unsatisfactory?
  - Was communication timely and effective?
  - What went well; what was challenging?
  - Were there any problems or concerns; if so, how were they addressed?
- Is there a better way to meet the client need?
- Is there a need to adjust the overall plan of care, or should this approach be continued?
- Were there any "learning moments" for the assistant and/or the nurse?
- Was appropriate feedback provided to the assistant regarding the performance of the delegation?
- Was the assistant acknowledged for accomplishing the task/activity/function?

FIGURE 8-2

NCSBN delegation decision-making tree. (continued)

(*Source:* Reprinted with permission from the National Council of State Boards of Nursing.)

TABLE 8-4
The Five Rights of Delegation

Right Task	Does the delegated task conform to agency-established policies, procedures, and standards consistent with the state's Nurse Practice Act, federal and state regulations and guidelines for practice, nursing professional standards, and the ANA Code of Ethics? Delegated tasks are often repetitive, require little supervision, and are relatively noninvasive.
Right Circumstance	Does the delegated task require independent nursing management? Do the personnel have the education, experience, resources, equipment, and supervision needed to complete the task safely in the current setting and circumstances?
Right Person	Is a qualified, competent person delegating the right task to a qualified, competent person to be performed on the right patient? Is the patient stable with predictable outcomes? Is it legally acceptable to delegate to this LPN or NAP? Do health care personnel have documented knowledge, skill, and competency to do the task?
Right Direction/ Communication	Does the RN communicate the task clearly with standards, directions, specific steps of the tasks, any limitations, and expected outcomes? Are times for reporting back to the RN specified? Is staff understanding of the task clarified? Are staff encouraged to say "I don't know how to do this and I need help," as needed?
Right Supervision	Is there appropriate monitoring, intervention, evaluation, and patient and staff feedback as needed? Are patient and staff outcomes monitored? Does the RN answer staff questions and problem solve as needed? Does the staff report task completion and patient response to the RN? Does the RN provide follow-up teaching and guidance to staff as appropriate? Is there continuous quality improvement of the delegation process and patient care? Are problems, particularly any sentinel events, reported via the chain of command and as needed to the State Board of Nursing and the Joint Commission (JC)?

Source: Adapted from National Council of State Boards of Nursing (NCSBN). (1997a). The Five Rights of Delegation. Retrieved from http://www.ncsbn.org/fiverights.pdf

TABLE 8-5
Nursing Process

Ultimately, some professional activities involving specialized knowledge, judgment, or skill of the nursing process can never be delegated. These include patient assessment, triage, making a nursing diagnosis, establishing nursing plans of care, extensive teaching or counseling, telephone advice, evaluating outcomes, and discharging patients. Delegated tasks are typically those that occur frequently, are considered technical by nature, are considered standard and unchanging, have predictable results, and have minimal potential for risks. As a professional standard for all nurses in all states, the assessment, analysis, diagnosis, planning, teaching, and evaluation stages of the nursing process may not be delegated. Delegated activities usually fall within the implementation phase of the nursing process.

© Cengage Learning 2014

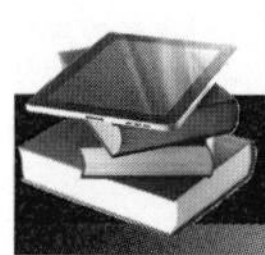

EVIDENCE FROM THE **LITERATURE**

Citation: Bosley, S., & Dale, J. (2008). Health Care Assistants in General Practice: Practical and Conceptual Issues of Skill-Mix Change. *British Journal of General Practice, 58*(547), 118–124.

Discussion: The emergence of health care assistants' (HCAs) (which are synonymous with NAPs in the United States) general practice raises questions about roles and responsibilities, patients' acceptance, cost effectiveness, patient safety and delegation, training and competence, workforce development, and professional identity. There has been minimal research into the role of HCAs and their experiences, as well as those of other staff working with HCAs in general practice.

Implications for Practice: The authors suggest that in the context of changing skill-mix models, viewing roles as fluid and dynamic is more helpful and reflective of individuals' experiences than endeavoring to impose fixed role boundaries. They also conclude that HCAs can make an increasingly useful contribution to the skill mix in general practice, but that more research and evaluation are needed to inform their training and development within the general practice team.

(2004) suggests assessment of five factors that must occur before deciding to delegate:

1. *Potential for Harm:* Determine if there is a risk for the patient in the activity delegated.
2. *Complexity of the Task:* Delegate simple tasks. These tasks often require psychomotor skills with little assessment or judgment proficiency.
3. *Amount of Problem Solving and Innovation Required:* Do not delegate tasks that require a creative approach, adaptation, or special attention to complete.
4. *Unpredictability of Outcome:* Avoid delegating tasks in which the outcome is not clear, causing volatility for the patient.
5. *Level of Patient Interaction:* Value time spent with the patient and the patient's family to develop trust, and so on.

Attention to these five factors will improve patient safety associated with delegation.

Other nursing staff can help new graduates begin to develop their role and learn to delegate by making sure that they introduce all the other department staff and explain their roles to the new nurses. See Figure 8-3 and Table 8-6.

Nurse Manager Responsibility

The nurse manager helps develop staff members' ability to delegate. Guidance in this area is necessary because new graduates, wanting to be regarded favorably, often may try to do everything themselves and not ask for assistance. Orientation will cover staff job descriptions, competency, chain-of-command guidelines, and other delegation resources for the new nurse.

The nurse manager will determine the appropriate mix of personnel on a nursing unit based on the patients' needs, acuity levels, and staff competency. From this personnel mix, the nurse manager will identify who can best perform the direct and indirect nursing duties.

Registered Nurse Responsibility

The registered nurse is responsible and accountable for the provision of nursing care. Although nursing assistive personnel may measure vital signs, intake and output, and other patient status indicators, it is the registered nurse who analyzes these data for comprehensive assessment, planning, nursing diagnosis, implementation, and evaluation of the plan of care.

Elements to Consider

- Federal, state, and local regulations and guidelines for practice, including the state Nurse Practice Act
- Nursing professional standards
- Agency policy, procedure, and standards
- Job description of Registered Nurse, Licensed Practical Nurse/Licensed Vocational Nurse, Nursing Assistive Personnel
- Five rights of delegation
- Ethical-legal standards
- Knowledge and skill of personnel
- Documented personnel competency, strengths, and weaknesses (select the right person for the right job)

RN accountable for application of the nursing process
Assessment and nursing judgment*
Nursing diagnosis
Planning care
Implementation and teaching
RN delegates as appropriate
RN retains accountability
Note that LPNs/LVNs and NAP are also responsible for their actions**

RN

RN assesses, plans, implements, and evaluates care for all patients, especially complex, unstable patients with unpredictable outcomes.

Administer medications, including IV push and IVPBs.

Start and maintain IVs and blood transfusions.

Perform sterile or specialized procedures, for example, Foley catheter and nasogastric tube insertion, tracheostomy care, and suture removal.

Educate patient and family.

Maintain infection control.

Administer cardiopulmonary resuscitation.

Interpret and report laboratory findings.

Implement patient triage.

Prevent nurse-sensitive patient outcomes, for example, cardiac arrest and pneumonia.

Monitor patient outcomes.

LPN/LVN

LPN/LVN cares for stable patients with predictable outcomes. They work under the direction of an RN and are responsible for their actions within their scope of practice.

Gather patient data.

Administer medications.

Implement patient care.

Administer CPR.

Maintain infection control.

Perform sterile procedures and respiratory suctioning.

Provide teaching from standard teaching plan.

Insert Foley catheters; do colostomy care.

Depending on the state and with documented competency, may do the following:**

- Perform specialized procedures, for example, nasogastric tube insertion, tracheostomy care, and suture removal.
- Start and maintain IV therapy.

NAP

NAP assists the RN and the LPN and gives technical care to stable patients with predictable outcomes and minimal potential for risk. NAP work under the direction of an RN and are responsible for their actions within their scope of practice.

Assist with activities of daily living.

Bathe, groom, and dress.

Assist with toileting and bed making.

Perform noninvasive and nonsterile treatments.

Ambulate, position, and transport.

Feed and socialize with patient.

Measure intake and output (I&O).

Document care.

Weigh patient.

Maintain infection control.

Take vital signs.

Depending on the state and with documented competency, may do the following:**

- Perform blood glucose monitoring.
- Administer CPR.
- Perform 12-lead EKGs.
- Perform venipuncture for blood tests.

Evaluation
RN uses judgment and is responsible for evaluation of all patient care.

*Nursing Judgment is the process by which nurses come to understand the problems, issues, and concerns of patients, attend to salient information, and respond to patient problems in concerned and involved ways. Judgment includes both conscious decision making and intuitive response (Benner, Tanner, & Chesla,1996).

**Some variation from state to state and across agencies.

FIGURE 8-3

Considerations in delegation.

© Cengage Learning 2014

TABLE 8-6
Delegation Suggestions for RNs

- Be clear on the qualifications of the delegate, i.e., education, experience, and competency. Require documentation or demonstration of current competence by the delegate for each task. Clarify patient care concerns or delegation problems. Consult ANA position papers at http://www.nursingworld.org and your state board of nursing, as necessary.
- Speak to your delegate as you would like to be spoken to. There is no need to apologize for your delegation. Remember, you are carrying out your professional responsibility. Positively reinforce good attitudes and dependability in your staff.
- Communicate the patient's name, room number, and what you want done and when you want it done. Discuss any changes from the usual procedures that might be needed to meet special patient needs and any potential patient abnormalities that should be reported to you. The expectations for personnel before, during, and after duty performance should be stated in a clear, pleasant, direct, and concise manner.
- Identify realistic, attainable standards that you will use to identify completion of the task. Identify the expected patient outcome.
- Identify the authority necessary to complete the task. Include any limits on the delegate's authority also.
- Verify the delegate's understanding of delegated tasks and have him or her repeat instructions, as needed. Be clear, and welcome lots of questions until you are convinced that the delegate understands what you want done. Verify that the delegate accepts responsibility for carrying out the task correctly. Require frequent mini reports about patients from staff, and include any specific reporting guidelines, times for interventions, and deadlines for accomplishing any tasks.
- As needed, explain to the delegate why the task needs to be done, its importance in the overall scheme of things, and any possible complications that may arise during its performance. Invite questions, and do not get defensive if your delegate pushes you for answers. Seek commitment from your delegate to complete the task according to standards and in a timely fashion.
- Avoid changing standards or removing duties once performance has begun. Removing duties should be done only when the duty is above the level of the delegate, such as when the patient's well-being is in jeopardy because his or her status has changed.
- Provide support, and monitor the task completion according to standards. Make frequent walking rounds to assess patient outcomes. Be sure your delegate has the resources, training, and other help to get the task done.
- Accept minor variations in the style in which the duties are performed. Individual styles are acceptable as long as the duty is performed according to standards. Try to provide for continuity of care by the same staff when possible, and consider the geography of the unit and fair, balanced work distribution among staff when assigning care.
- If the delegate doesn't meet the standards, talk with him or her to identify the problem. If this is not successful, inform the delegate that you will be discussing the problem with your supervisor. Document your concerns, as appropriate. Follow up with your supervisor according to your organization's policy.
- Avoid high-risk delegation. The RN may be at risk if: the delegated task can be performed only by the RN according to law, organizational policies and procedures, or professional standards of nursing practice; the delegated task could involve substantial risk or harm to a patient; the RN knowingly delegates a task to a person who has not had the appropriate training or orientation; or the RN fails to adequately supervise the delegated activity and does not evaluate the delegated action by reassessing the patient (ANA, 1996).

© Cengage Learning 2014

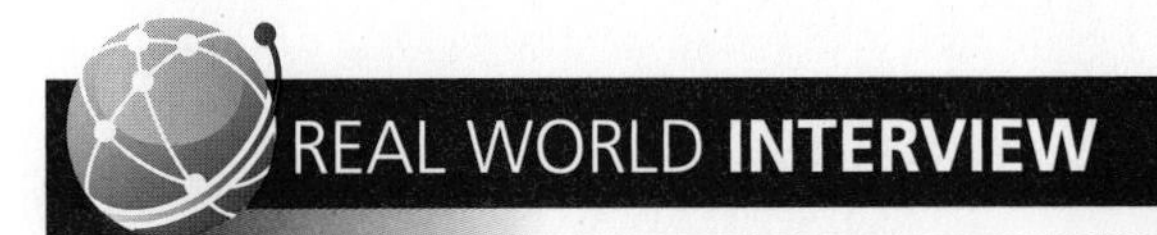

REAL WORLD INTERVIEW

I have been practicing nursing for 31 years, and can honestly say I have seen major changes in nursing delegation through the years. My areas of practice have been in medical-surgical nursing, pediatrics, special care nursery, postpartum, same day surgery, and preoperative health testing/education.

When I began my career as a nurse, I practiced as a team leader. Delegation was a big part of my role as a nurse at that time. Delegation included assigning procedures to LPNs, requesting attention to basic patient needs from nurse assistants, or assistance in contacting physicians, scheduling tests, and obtaining results from the unit secretary. Around 1985, however, we began primary care nursing and my role as an independent caregiver began.

With the onset of primary care nursing, every aspect of my patient's care became my own responsibility. My only assignment of duty when working as a staff nurse after this change went to the unit secretary, or possibly to a new RN in my unit whom I was precepting. I always worked beside the nurse I was orienting, so any procedure she carried out was under my direct supervision. I also assigned duties to my fellow RNs when working in a role as charge nurse. In this capacity, I coordinated and supervised the delivery of nursing care in the unit and delegated nursing tasks to nursing assistants.

Today, I still work independently, but collaborate with fellow RNs preparing patient records, gathering pre-op test results, interviewing patients, obtaining medical histories, and providing preoperative teaching to surgical patients and patients coming in for interventional radiology procedures. I also work with the anesthesiologists reviewing the patients' medical records to ensure all necessary testing has been done in accordance with their status prior to OR. Therefore, the only real delegation in my job at this time is to the unit secretary to request assistance in collecting test results done outside our facility, preadmission orders, and medical/cardiac clearances as needed.

MARGIE PALERMO, RN
Homer Township, Illinois

Many nurses are reluctant to delegate. This is reflected in NCSBN research findings, a review of the literature, and anecdotal accounts from nursing students and practicing nurses. Many factors contribute to this reluctance, for example, not having had educational opportunities to learn how to work with others effectively, not knowing the skill levels and abilities of nursing assistive personnel, the fast work pace, and the rapid turnover of patients. At the same time, NCSBN research shows an increase in the complexity of the nursing tasks performed by assistive personnel. With demographic changes and the resultant increase in the need for nursing services, combined with the nursing shortage, nurses need to lean upon the support of nursing assistive personnel (ANA, NCSBN, 2005).

Licensed Practical/Vocational Nurse Responsibility

Licensed practical/vocational nursing (LPN/LVN) caregivers who have undergone a standardized training and competency evaluation are able to perform duties and functions that NAPs are not allowed to do. LPNs/LVNs usually care for stable patients with predictable outcomes, though they may help the RN with seriously ill patients in ICU. The LPN does not do initial patient assessment, but after the RN has completed the patient's initial assessment and the plan of care, the LPN does the ongoing assessment, monitoring vital signs, medication, administration, breath sounds, and so on. In nursing homes in some states, the LPN may assume the charge-nurse role

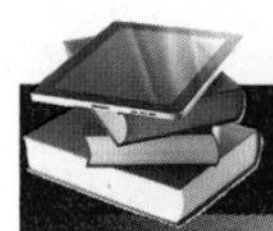

EVIDENCE FROM THE LITERATURE

Citation: Nursing and Midwifery Council (2008, May). Advice on Delegation for Registered Nurses and Midwives. Retrieved October 31, 2011, from http://www.nmc-uk.org

Discussion: This article provides advice on delegation to nurses and midwives in the United Kingdom (U.K.). Nurses in the United States can also use this advice. The Nursing and Midwifery Council is the United Kingdom's regulatory body organization for nursing and midwifery. The primary purpose of the Council is to protect the public. This role is similar to that of the state boards of nursing in the United States. "Nonregulated personnel"is the term in the U.K. for "NAP." The term "registrant" is the U.K. term for "nurse." When a nurse or midwife has authority to delegate tasks to another, he or she will retain responsibility and accountability for that delegation. A nurse or midwife may delegate an aspect of care only to a person deemed competent to perform the task. The nurse or midwife should be sure that the person to whom care has been delegated fully understands the nature of the delegated task and what is required. Where another person such as an employer has the authority to delegate an aspect of care, the employer becomes accountable for that delegation. The nurse or midwife will, however, continue to carry the responsibility to intervene if he or she feels that the proposed delegation is inappropriate or unsafe. The decision whether or not to delegate an aspect of care or to transfer and/or rescind delegation is the primary responsibility of the nurse or midwife and is based on his or her professional judgment. Nurses and midwives have the right to refuse to delegate if they believe it would be unsafe to do so or if they are unable to provide or ensure adequate supervision. Those delegating care and those assuming delegated duties should do so in accordance with robust local employment practice in order to protect the public and support safe practice.

Implications for Practice: The decision to delegate is made either by the nurse, midwife, or by the employer. It is this decision maker who is accountable for the decision. Health care can sometimes be unpredictable. It is important that the person to whom an aspect of care is being delegated understands his or her limitations. He or she must know when not to proceed should circumstances affecting the task change. No one should feel pressured into either delegating or accepting a delegated task. When pressure is felt, advice should be sought, as appropriate, from either the nurse or the midwife's professional manager.

with an on-site supervising RN. LPNs report their findings to the RN. The RN is still primarily responsible for overall patient assessment, nursing diagnosis, planning, implementation, and evaluation of the quality of care delegated.

NAP Responsibility

According to the ANA (2006), if the RN knows or reasonably believes that the nursing assistant has the appropriate training, orientation, and documented competencies, then the RN can reasonably expect that the NAP will function in a safe and effective manner.

NAP cannot be assigned to assess or evaluate responses to treatment because that is the role of the RN. It may be more cost effective to have NAP perform non-nursing duties than to have nurses perform them. NAP can deliver supportive care. They cannot practice nursing or provide total patient care.

If LPNs or NAPs perform poorly, the RN should tell them about the mistakes privately, as much as possible, in a supportive manner with a focus on learning from them. If the LPN or NAP performs in an inappropriate, unsafe, or incompetent manner, the RN must intervene immediately and stop

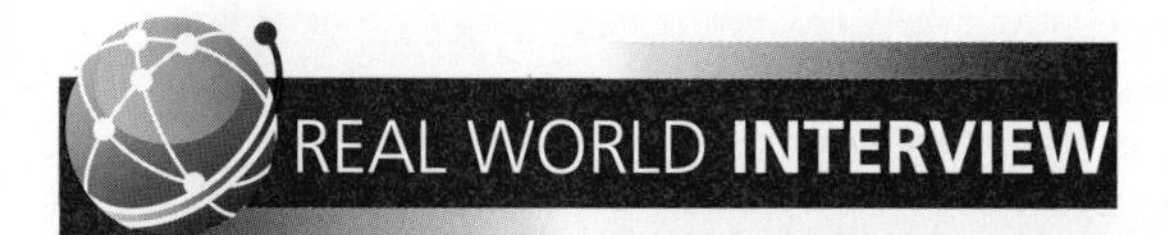

On my labor and delivery unit we are very busy. We deliver 30 to 40 babies a day. We are a hard-working team and help each other all the time. I assign IV starts, blood draws, medication administration, patient ambulation/positioning and tasks associated with delivery to other nurses. I delegate to the patient care technician infant vitals and measurements, maternal blood draws, and transportation to postpartum.

ALISSA COWAN, RNC

the unsafe activity, counsel the LPN or NAP, document the facts, and report to the nurse manager, as appropriate.

ORGANIZATIONAL ACCOUNTABILITY FOR DELEGATION

Organizational accountability for delegation requires providing sufficient resources, including the following: sufficient staffing with an appropriate staff mix; documenting competencies for all staff providing direct patient care; ensuring that the RN has access to information regarding all staff competencies; providing opportunities for continuing staff development; creating an environment conducive to teamwork, collaboration, and patient-centered care; and developing organizational policies on delegation with the active participation of all nurses. These policies on delegation must acknowledge that delegation is a professional nursing right and responsibility. Note that chief nursing officers are responsible for establishing systems to assess, monitor, verify, and communicate ongoing competence requirements in areas related to delegation, both for RNs and for other nursing staff. The organization is accountable for delegation through the allocation of resources to ensure sufficient staffing so that the RN can delegate appropriately. The organization must also ensure that the educational needs of NAP are met through the implementation of a system that allows for nurse input. See Table 8-7.

Chain of Command

The RN, including the new graduate nurse, is accountable to the charge nurse and nurse manager of the unit. The nurse manager is accountable to the chief nursing officer, for example, the vice president of nursing. The chief nursing officer is accountable to the chief executive officer of the hospital, who is accountable to the board of directors. The board of directors is accountable to the community it serves and often to another, larger hospital corporation, as well as to the state nursing and licensing boards and the accreditation agency. See Figure 8-4.

TABLE 8-7
Organizational Elements Needed for Efficient Delegation

- Describe a formal, nurse handoff process that includes the NAP, including change of shift and taking breaks.
- Have clear job descriptions and ongoing licensing and credentialing policies for RNs, health care providers, LPN/LVNs, NAP, and other health care staff. The organization must ensure that all staff members are safe, competent practitioners before assigning them to patient care. Orient staff to their duties, chain of command, and the job descriptions of RN, LPN, and NAP.
- Facilitate clinical and educational specialty certification and credentialing of all health care practitioners and staff.

(Continues)

TABLE 8-7 (Continued)

- Provide standards for ongoing supervision and periodic licensure/competency verification and evaluation of all staff.
- Provide access to professional health care standards, policies, procedures, library, Internet, and medication information with unit availability and efficient library and Internet access.
- Facilitate regular evidence-based reviews of critical standards, policies, and procedures.
- Have clear policies and procedures for delegation and chain-of-command reporting lines for all staff from RN to charge nurse to nurse manager to nurse executive and, as appropriate, to risk management, the hospital ethics committee, the hospital administrator, nursing and medical practitioners, the chief of the medical staff, the board of directors, the State Licensing Board for Nursing and Medicine, and the Joint Commission. See Figure 8-3 for an illustration of one such organizational chain of command.
- Provide administrative support for supervisors and staff who delegate, assign, monitor, and evaluate patient care.
- Clarify health care provider accountability; e.g., if a medical or nursing practitioner or physician assistant delegates a nursing task to NAP, the health care provider is responsible for monitoring that care delivery. This must be spelled out in hospital policy. If the RN notes that the NAP is doing something incorrectly, the RN has a duty to intervene and to notify the ordering practitioner of the incident. The RN always has an independent responsibility to protect patient safety. Blindly relying on another nursing or health care provider is not permissible for the RN.
- Provide education and standards for regular RN evaluation of NAP and LPN/LVN, and reinforce the need for NAP and LPN/LVN accountability to the RN. RNs must delegate and supervise. They cannot abdicate this professional responsibility.
- Develop a physical, mental, and verbal "No Abuse" policy to be followed by all professional and nonprofessional health care staff. Follow up on any problems.
- Consider applying for magnet status for your facility. This status is awarded by the American Nurses Credentialing Center to nursing departments that have worked to improve nursing care, including the empowering of nursing decision making and delegation in clinical practice.
- Monitor patient outcomes, including nurse-sensitive outcomes, staffing ratios, and other quality indicators, as well as develop ongoing clinical quality improvement practices. Benchmark with national groups.
- Maintain ongoing monitoring of incident reports, sentinel events, and other elements of risk management and performance improvement of the process and outcome of patient care.
- Develop systematic, error-proof systems for medication administration that ensure the six rights of medication administration, i.e., the right patient, right medication, right dose, right time, right route, and right documentation. Develop safe, computerized, order-entry systems.
- Provide documentation of routine maintenance for all patient care equipment.
- Attain the JC Patient Safety Goals (http://www. jointcommission.org).
- Develop intrahospital and intra-agency safe-transfer policies.

© Cengage Learning 2014

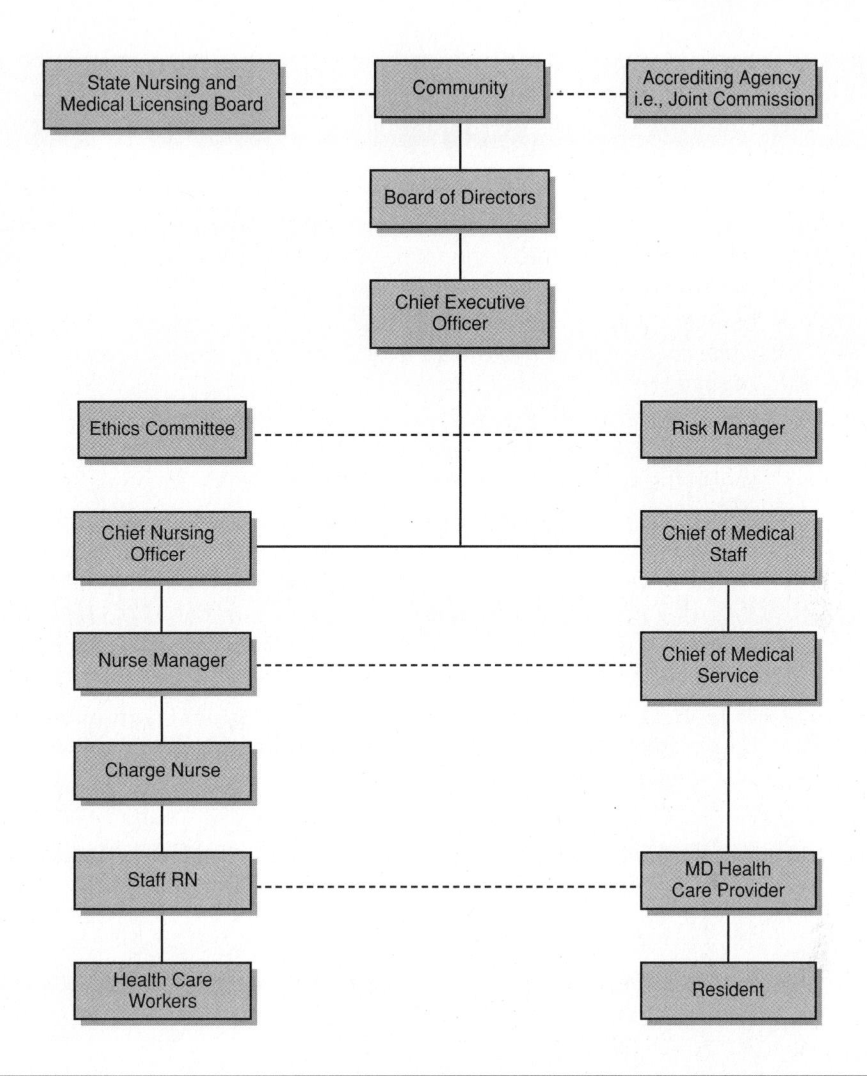

FIGURE 8-4

Chain of command.

© Cengage Learning 2014

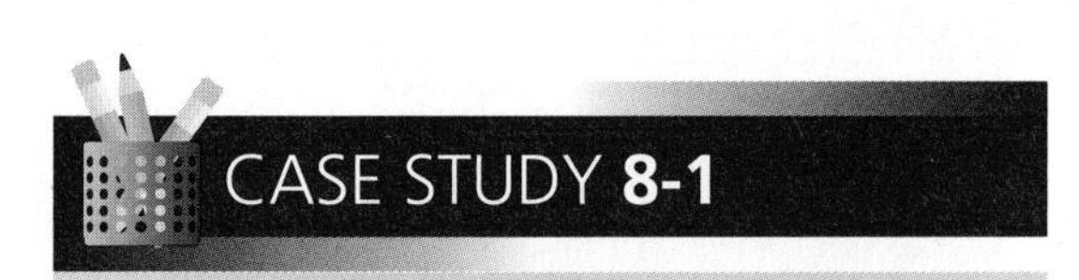

A newly oriented charge nurse is working with an RN, NAP, an LPN/LVN, and a sitter. Which person will you have do the P.M. care for all patients, pass water, answer call lights, and pick up supplies? Which person will be assigned to give the medications and change dressings?

TRANSCULTURAL DELEGATION

Nurses and patients come from diverse cultural backgrounds. Transcultural delegation requires that personnel perform duties with this cultural diversity taken into consideration. Poole, Davidhizar, and Giger (1995) suggest there are six cultural phenomena to be considered when delegating to a culturally diverse staff: communication, space, social organization, time, environmental control, and biological variations. See Table 8-8.

TABLE 8-8
Cultural Phenomena

Phenomena	Example
Communication	Consider cultural communication elements such as volume, dialect, use of touch, context of speech, and kinesics such as gestures, stance, and eye behavior as you delegate patient care to staff.
Space	Consider physical closeness. Some cultures prefer to stand close physically while communicating. Others prefer to maintain more physical distance between themselves and others.
Social Organization	When communicating with patients, consider that cultures vary in the amount of close social supports they maintain with family and others. Note that staff also vary in the amount of social support that they need from other health care staff.
Time	Cultures vary in their past, present, or future orientation. Note that some cultures focus on maintaining past traditions, while other cultures focus on the current activities of today. Still other cultures focus on preparing for the future.
Environmental Control	Note that cultures with an internal locus of control plan and take action. They do not rely on luck or fate. Cultures with an external locus of control wait for fate and luck to determine and guide their actions.
Biological Variations	Note that there are cultural and biological variations in attributes such as physiological strength, stamina, and susceptibility to disease. Consider these as you delegate patient care to staff.

© Cengage Learning 2014

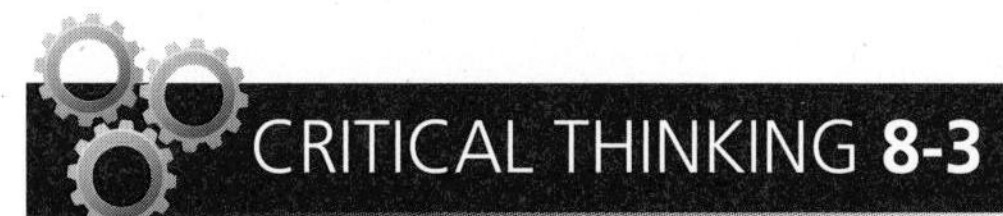

CRITICAL THINKING 8-3

The RN continuously monitors unstable, complex patients who have threats to their airway, breathing, circulation, or safety. Examples of these patients might include a patient on a ventilator and an unconscious patient. The RN can assign care of stable patients to the LPN and delegate to the NAP. What are some examples of unstable patients who would not be assigned to LPNs?

KEY CONCEPTS

- Delegation is the transfer of responsibility for the performance of a task from one individual to another while retaining accountability for the outcome.
- Accountability is being responsible and answerable for the actions or inactions of self or others.
- Responsibility involves reliability, dependability, and the obligation to accomplish work when one accepts an assignment. Responsibility also includes each person's obligation to perform at an acceptable level to which they have been educated.

- Authority occurs when a person who has been given the right to delegate based on the state's Nurse Practice Act also has the official power from an agency to delegate.
- The RN is accountable for the delegation and performance of all nursing duties.
- Transcultural delegation is encouraged to provide a patient with optimal care.
- Assignment is the distribution of work that each staff member is to accomplish on a given shift or work period. It is often identified on an assignment sheet.
- Organizations interested in quality patient care provide staff with guidelines on how to use the chain of command, clear standards, and other resources to achieve quality outcomes.
- The NCSBN Delegation Decision-Making Tree is a useful tool when developing skill in delegating patient care.
- All members of the health care team must fulfill their delegated responsibilities.
- Note that the assessment, analysis, diagnosis, planning, teaching, and evaluation stages of the nursing process may not be delegated. Delegated activities usually fall within the implementation phase of the nursing process.
- In a hospital, NAP and LPNs/LVNs are accountable to the RN.
- According to the NCSBN, supervision is the provision of guidance or direction, oversight, evaluation, and follow-up by the licensed nurse for accomplishment of a nursing task delegated to NAP.
- The five rights of delegation are the right task, the right circumstance, the right person, the right direction and communication, and the right supervision.
- Competence is the ability of the nurse to act with and integrate the knowledge, skills, values, attitudes, abilities, and professional judgment that underpin effective and quality nursing and is required to practice safely and ethically in a designated role and setting.

KEY TERMS

accountability
assignment
authority
competence
delegation
responsibility
supervision

REVIEW QUESTIONS

1. The nurse has become incredibly busy with discharging two patients and expecting a new admission any minute. The following list is tasks that need to be completed right away for the group of patients. What task can be delegated to the NAP to best assist the nurse in managing patient care?
   A. Remove sutures and drain from an incision on the left wrist of the patient to be discharged.
   B. Provide tracheostomy care on one of the patients.
   C. Sit with a patient recently diagnosed with Crohn's disease who is crying.
   D. Transport a patient to X-ray on a cardiac monitor.

2. A nurse from the intensive care unit has been asked to work on a medical-surgical unit. What information will the nurse need in regard to working with NAP on a medical-surgical unit? Select all that apply.
   A. Documentation of license
   B. Training received
   C. Orientation received
   D. Competencies documented
   E. Usual patient load for NAPs
   F. Number of previous rotations on the medical-surgical unit

3. When a nurse considers delegating a task to assist in the care of a patient, what five rights should be utilized?
   A. Right task, right circumstance, right person, right direction/communication, and right supervision
   B. Right room, right time, right person, right documentation, and right directions
   C. Right patient, right chart, right physician, right results, and right information
   D. Right person, right patient, right task, right documentation, and right time frame

4. The staff working on the unit includes three RNs, one LPN, and one NAP for 25 patients. What assignment is the most appropriate for the LPN?
   A. Pass water to all of the patients on the unit.
   B. Pass oral medications to a group of patients.
   C. Admit a new patient by completing the history and physical.
   D. Obtain a urine sample from a Foley catheter from a patient who is not assigned to them.

5. What is the most appropriate task for the NAP to perform once delegated by the nurse to assist in patient care?
   A. Administer a soapsuds enema to a patient who is constipated.
   B. Notify the family of a patient who has died.
   C. Reinforce teaching a patient who is a recent above-the-knee amputee (AKA).
   D. Press the silence button on the beeping feeding pump until the RN arrives.

6. What parts of the nursing process cannot be delegated? Select all that apply.
   A. Assessment
   B. Nursing diagnosis
   C. Plan/Outcome
   D. Interventions
   E. Evaluation

7. The charge nurse delegated to the NAP six patients to provide A.M. care. Several hours later, one of the patients called the nurses' station stating they had not had their bed changed or a bath. The charge nurse went to the patient's room and verified the patient's complaint. What should the nurse do next in this situation?
   A. Ask all of the patients if they have received their medications.
   B. Follow the NAP the next day to observe completion of the tasks delegated.
   C. Discuss with the NAP the recent complaint by the patient.
   D. Disregard the patient's complaint and provide A.M. care.

8. A NAP who works on the unit is also a nursing student. She asks the nurse if she can flush an IV site after the antibiotic infuses. The NAP wants to know as much or even more than her fellow students and would hope for more opportunities like this. Which statement by the nurse is correct to the nursing student who is working as a NAP to complete this delegated task?
   A. "Sure you can, as long as you have been taught how to flush an IV site."
   B. "No, not as a NAP."
   C. "Yes, as long as the tubing is identified as the antibiotic tubing to be flushed."
   D. "Yes, as long as I am with you."

9. A new nurse asks the charge nurse, "How do I know what I can and cannot delegate?" What is the best reply for the charge nurse to give to the new nurse?
   A. "If you follow the five rights of medication administration, you should be fine."
   B. "If you review our state's list of standards, laws, and guidelines for delegation, they will guide you. It is nice to know every state has a list of standards, laws, and guidelines for delegation."
   C. "You will not be delegating; only the charge nurse delegates, so there is nothing to worry about."
   D. "Delegation takes time and practice to learn what you can and cannot delegate."

10. Which barriers can an RN experience when delegating? Select all that apply.
   A. There is insufficient evidence of education, certification, and validation of the NAP.
   B. There are policies, procedures, and/or protocols in place for delegation to NAP that vary state to state.
   C. The delegated tasks are not universal in all agencies and states.
   D. The new nurse views delegation as the inability of the RN to complete the care.
   E. The person being delegated to is not receptive to the person delegating.
   F. The agency's organizational leadership does not support maintaining the education and preparation to delegate.

REVIEW ACTIVITIES

1. You are caring for a new patient in Room 2510. You are trying to decide whether to delegate his care to NAP Jill or to NAP Penny. Use the NCSBN Delegation Decision-Making Tree to decide.
2. During your clinical rotation, answer the following questions: What tasks did your patients require that could have been delegated? How effective was a nurse in delegating tasks who was responsible for your patient?
3. Review the job descriptions of NAP and RNs in the institution in which you are doing your clinical rotation. Compare the job descriptions. Do the job descriptions identify what the NAP can do? What the RN can do?

EXPLORING THE WEB

✦ Go to your favorite search engine such as *http://www.google.com* and type in "How to use RSS feeds." Create a Rich Site Summary (RSS) feed. By setting up an RSS you can store all of your favorite bookmarks. Create a category such as "delegation," and all links placed in the RSS feed will be updated automatically. No more "Page Not Found" when going back to a website or pdf previously book marked.

✦ Go to *http://www.nursingworld.org* and read the American Nurses Association and the National Council of State Boards of Nursing joint statement on Social Network Guidelines. The impact of sharing patient-sensitive information and ways to avoid it can be found in this white paper.

✦ Go to *http://www.ncsbn.org* to follow results of a study of new nurses as they "Transition to Practice." Three states are participating in this longitudinal study that will end in 2014.

✦ Go to *http://managementhelp.org* This site gives the nurse an alternative way to look at delegating from a management perspective.

REFERENCES

American Association of Critical, Care Nurses (AACN). (2004). *AACN delegation handbook.* Aliso Viejo, CA: Author.

American Nurses Association (ANA). (1996). *Registered professional nurses and unlicensed assistive personnel* (2nd ed.). Washington, DC: Author.

American Nurses Association (ANA). (2006). *Principles for delegation.* Silver Spring, MD: Author.

American Nurses Association (ANA). (2009). *Code of ethics for nurses with interpretive statements.* Silver Spring, MD: Author.

American Nurses Association (ANA). (2010). Recognition of a nursing specialty, approval of a specialty nursing scope of practice statement, and acknowledgment of specialty nursing standards of practice. Retrieved from http://www.nursingworld.org/3Sbooklet

American Nurses Association (ANA) and the National Council of State Boards of Nursing (NCSBN). (2005). Joint statement on delegation. Retrieved September 1, 2012, from http://www.ncsbn.org/Joint_statement.pdf

American Organization of Nurse Executives and McCanis & Monsalve Associates, Inc. (2003). *Healthy work environments: Striving for excellence* (Vol. 2). Retrieved September 1, 2012, from http://www.mcmanis-monsalve.com/assets/publications/healthy_work_environments_full.pdf

Benner, P., Tanner, C. A., & Chesla, C. A. (1996). *Expertise in nursing practice: Caring clinical judgment and ethics.* New York City, NY: Springer Publishing Company.

Bosley, S., & Dale, J. (2008). Health care assistants in general practice: Practical and conceptual issues of skill-mix change. *British Journal of General Practice, 58*(547), 118–124.

Gordon, S. C., & Barry, C. D. (2009). Delegation guided by school nursing values: Comprehensive knowledge, trust, and empowerment. *The Journal of School Nursing, 25*(5), 352–360.

Hansten, R., & Jackson, M. (2009). *Clinical delegation skills,* (4th ed.). Sudbury, MA: Jones and Bartlett Publishers.

Harvard ManageMentor® Skill Pack. (2011). *Improving productivity: A Harvard ManageMentor skill pack.* Boston, MA: Harvard Business School Publishing.

Joint Statement on Delegation. ANA and NCSBN. (2005). Reprinted and used by permission of the National Council of State Boards (1997).

Kalisch, J. B., & Lee, K. H. (2010). Nurse staffing levels and teamwork: A cross-sectional study of patient care units in acute care hospitals. *Journal of Nursing Scholarship, 43*(1), 82-88.

National Council of State Boards of Nursing (NCSBN). (1995). Delegation concepts and decision-making process, NCSBN position paper. Retrieved September 1, 2012, from http://www.ncsbn.org/323.htm#Delegation_Decision-Making_Process

National Council of State Boards of Nursing (NCSBN). (1997a). The five rights of delegation. Retrieved September 1, 2012, from http://www.ncsbn.org/fiverights.pdf

National Council of State Boards of Nursing (NCSBN). (1997b). *Delegation decision-making tree.* Chicago, IL: Author.

National Council of State Boards of Nursing (NCSBN). (2004). *Working with others: NCLEX-RN test plan.* A position paper. Chicago, IL: Author.

National Council of State Boards of Nursing (NCSBN). (2005). *Working with others: Delegation and other health care interfaces.* Chicago, IL: Author.

Nightingale, F. (1859). *Notes on nursing: What it is and what it is not.* London, England: Harrison & Sons.

Nursing and Midwifery Council. (2008, May). Advice on delegation for registered nurses and midwives. Retrieved October 31, 2011, from http://www.nmc-uk.org

Poole, V., Davidhizar, R., & Giger, J. (1995). Delegating to a transcultural team. *Nursing-Management 26*(8), 33–34.

Potter, P., Deshield, T., & Kuhrik, M. (2010). Delegation practices between nurses and nursing assistive personnel. *Journal of Nursing Management, 18*(2), 157–165.

Reagan, R. (1981). Retrieved September 30, 2010, from http://thinkexist.com/quotation/surround_yourself_with_the_best_people_you_can/223798.html

SUGGESTED READINGS

American Association of Critical-Care Nurses. (2009). Synergy™ model for patient care. Retrieved October 29, 2010, from http://www.aacn.org/wd/certifications/content/synmodel.pcms?menu=certification

American Nurses Association. (2009). *Guide to the code of ethics for nurses: Interpretation and application.* Silver Spring, MD: Author.

Barra, M. (2011). Nurse delegation of medication pass in assisted living facilities: Not all medication assistant technicians are equal. *Journal of Nursing Law, 14* (1), 3–10.

Beattle, L. (2009). New health care delivery modes are redefining the role of nurses. Retrieved October 15, 2010, from: http://www.nursezone.com/Nursing-News-Events/more-features/New-Health-Care-Delivery-Models-are-Redefining-the-Role-of-Nurses_29442.aspx

Berman, A., & Snyder, S. (2012). *Kozier & Erb's fundamentals of nursing: Concepts, process, and practice* (8th ed.). Philadelphia, PA: Prentice Hall.

Bittner, N. P. & Gravlin, G. (2009). Critical thinking, delegation, and missed care in nursing practice. *Journal of Nursing Administration, 39*(3), 142–146.

Brinkert, R. (2010). A literature review of conflict communication causes, benefits, and interventions in nursing. *Journal of Nursing Management, 18*, 145–156.

Dufault, M., Duquette, C. E., & Ehmann, J. (2010). Translating an evidence-based protocol for nurse-to-nurse shift handoffs. *World Views on Evidence-Based Nursing, 2*(7), 59–75.

Institute of Medicine (IOM). (2011). *The future of nursing: Leading change, advancing health.* Washington, DC: The National Academies Press.

Manojlovich, M., Barnsteiner, J., Bolton, L. B., Disch, J., & Saint, S. (2008, Jan.). Nursing practice and work environment issues in the 21st century: A leadership challenge. *Nursing Research, 57*(1), S11–S14. doi:10.1097/01.NNR.0000280648.91438.fe

Marquis, B. L. & Huston, C. J. (2009). *Leadership roles and management functions in nursing: Theory and application,* (6th ed.). Philadelphia, PA: Wolters, Kluwer, Lippincott, Williams, & Wilkens.

McKenna, H., Thompson, D., Watson, R. (2007). Health care assistants: An oxymoron? *International Journal of Nursing Studies, 44*(8), 1283–1284.

Nelson, G. A., King, M. L., & Brodine, S. (2008, February). Nurse-physician collaboration on medical-surgical units. In *MedSurg Nursing.* Retrieved July 4, 2011, from http://findarticles.com/p/articles/mi_m0FSS/is_1_17/ai_n24964202/?tag=mantle_skin;cont 35(10), 16-17

Thungjaroenkul, P., Cummings, G., & Embleton, A. (2007). The impact of nurse staffing on hospital costs and patient length of stay: A systematic review. *Nursing Economic$, 25*(5), 255–266. Retrieved September 1, 2012, from EBSCO*host.*

CHAPTER 9

Effective Staffing

DEBORAH ERICKSON, RN, PHD; ANNE BERNAT, RN, MSN, CNAA; MARY L. FISHER, RN, PHD, CNAA, BC; AND BETH VOTTERO, RN, PHD, CNE

Best-practice staffing provides timely and effective patient care while providing a safe environment for both patients and staff as well as promoting an atmosphere of professional nursing satisfaction.

–RAY, C. E., JAGIM, M., AGNEW, J., INGLASS-MCKAY, J., & SHEEHY, S. (EMERGENCY NURSES ASSOCIATION, 2003)

OBJECTIVES

Upon completion of this chapter, the reader should be able to:

1. Discuss how staffing needs are determined.
2. Calculate full-time equivalents (FTEs) needed to staff a typical inpatient nursing unit.
3. Discuss appropriate units of service used to measure nursing need by unit type.
4. Identify patient classification systems.
5. Review considerations in developing a staffing pattern.
6. Discuss staff scheduling on a patient care unit.
7. Discuss the role of nurse staffing in achieving quality nurse-sensitive outcomes.
8. Compare and contrast models of care delivery and their impact on patient outcomes.
9. Discuss care delivery management tools, such as clinical pathways, case management, and disease management.

You are a new nurse on a 30-bed medical unit that uses primary nursing as the care delivery model. There are 40 employees who work full and part time on this unit with vacancies for eight additional full-time staff. The current schedule does not accommodate any 12-hour shifts. There are five long-term staff members who are threatening to leave if they are forced to work 12-hour shifts. You have heard there are several new graduates who will come to work on the unit only if there are 12-hour shifts.

How can the needs of both groups of staff be accommodated?

What effect would hiring new graduates have on scheduling?

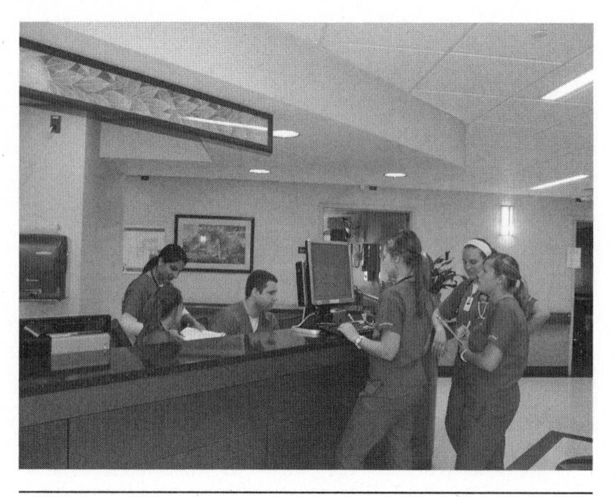

© Cengage Learning 2014

The ability of a nurse to provide safe and effective care to a patient is dependent on many variables. These variables include the knowledge and experience of the staff, the severity of illness of the patients, patient dependency for daily activities, complexity of care, the amount of nursing time available, the care delivery model, care management tools, patient classification systems, and organizational supports in place to facilitate care. This chapter explores these factors, how they affect planning for staffing, scheduling staff, and patient outcomes associated with staffing factors. It also reviews the models of care delivery that can be used with various patient populations and their impact on patient outcomes.

DETERMINATION OF STAFFING NEEDS

Nurse staffing has varied widely since the inception of nursing as a profession. Nursing staffing ratios have ranged from a ratio of one nurse to many soldiers, as in Florence Nightingale's time, to today when you may see a ratio of one nurse to one patient in a critical care area. Gaining an understanding of the key terms—full-time equivalents (FTEs), productive time, nonproductive time, direct and indirect care, nursing workload, and units of service—is necessary for understanding staffing patterns.

FTEs

A **full-time equivalent** (FTE) is a measure of the work commitment of a full-time employee. A full-time employee has traditionally worked five days a week for 40 hours per week for 52 weeks a year. This amounts to 2,080 hours of work time (Figure 9-1). A full-time employee who works 40 hours a week is referred to as a 1.0 FTE. An employee who works 36 hours (three 12-hour shifts) is considered full time for benefit purposes in many agencies, but is assigned 0.9 FTE for budgeting purposes (36/40 = 0.9 FTE). A part-time employee who works five days in a two-week period is considered a 0.5 FTE. FTE calculation is used to mathematically describe how much an employee works (Figure 9-2). Understanding FTEs is essential when moving from a staffing plan to the actual number of staff required.

FTE hours are a total of all paid time. This includes worked time as well as non-worked time.

5 days per week	×	8 hours per day	=	40 hours per week
40 hours per week	×	52 weeks per year	=	2,080 hours per year

FIGURE 9-1
Calculation of full-time equivalent hours.
© Cengage Learning 2014

1.0 FTE = 40 hours per week or five 8-hour shifts per week

0.8 FTE = 32 hours per week or four 8-hour shifts per week

0.6 FTE = 24 hours per week or three 8-hour shifts per week

0.4 FTE = 16 hours per week or two 8-hour shifts per week

0.2 FTE = 8 hours per week or one 8-hour shift per week

FIGURE 9-2

FTE calculation for varying levels of work commitment.

© Cengage Learning 2014

Vacation time	15 days	or	120 hours
Sick time	5 days	or	40 hours
Holiday time	6 days	or	48 hours
Education time	3 days	or	24 hours
Total nonproductive time		=	232 hours

2,080 − 232 = 1,848 hours of productive work time available for each staff member with these benefits.

FIGURE 9-3

Calculation of productive and nonproductive time.

© Cengage Learning 2014

Hours worked and available for patient care are designated as **productive hours**. Benefit time such as vacation, sick time, and education time is considered **nonproductive hours**. When considering the number of FTEs you need to staff a unit, you must count only the productive hours available for each staff member. Available productive time can be easily calculated by subtracting benefit time from the time a full-time employee would work (Figure 9-3). These figures vary greatly depending on institutional policy and availability of human resource benefits.

In this case, a full-time registered nurse (RN) would have 1,848 hours per year of productive time available to care for patients.

Employees who work with patients can be classified into two categories: those who provide direct care and those who provide indirect care. **Direct care** is time spent providing hands-on care to patients. **Indirect care** is time spent on activities that are patient related but are not done directly to the patient. Documentation, time consulting with people in other health care disciplines, and time spent following up on problems are good examples of indirect care. Even though RNs, licensed practical nurses (LPNs), and nursing assistive personnel (NAP) engage in indirect care activities, the majority of their time is spent providing direct care; therefore, they are classified as direct care providers. Nurse managers, clinical specialists, unit secretaries, and other support staff are considered indirect care providers because the majority of their work is indirect in nature and supports the work of the direct care providers.

Units of service include a variety of volume measures that are used to reflect different types of patient encounters as indicators of nursing workload (Figure 9-4). Volume measures are used in budget negotiations to project nursing needs of patients and to ensure adequate resources for safe patient care.

The majority of nurses practice on inpatient units; therefore, further calculations for this chapter's examples will be in nursing hours per patient day. **nursing hours per patient day (NHPPD)** is the amount of nursing care required per patient in a 24-hour period and is usually based on midnight census and past unit needs, expected unit practice trends, national benchmarks, professional staffing standards, and budget negotiations. NHPPD reflects only productive nursing time needed. Calculation of NHPPD is displayed in Figure 9-5.

Unit Type	Unit of Service
Inpatient Unit	Nursing Hours Per Patient Day (NHPPD)
Labor and Delivery	Births
Operating Room	Surgeries/Procedures
Home Care	Patient Visits
Emergency Services	Patient Visits

FIGURE 9-4

Units of service—volume measures by unit type.

© Cengage Learning 2014

20 patients on the unit

5 staff × 3 shifts = 15 staff

15 staff each working 8 hours = 120 hours available in a 24-hour period

120 nursing hours ÷ 20 patients = 6.0 NHPPD

FIGURE 9-5

Calculation of nursing hours per patient day (NHPPD).

© Cengage Learning 2014

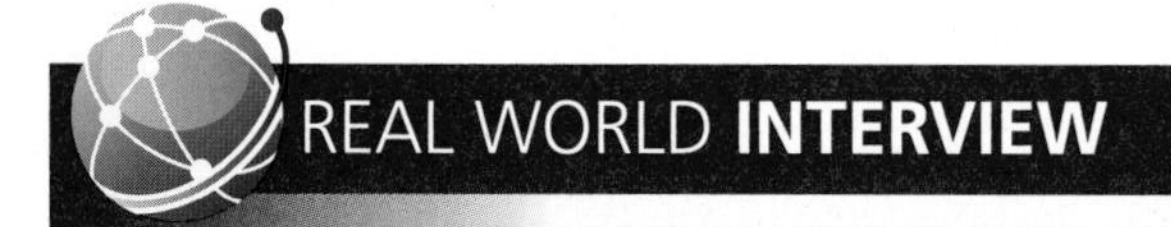

Given the need for staffing and financial accountability, I used spreadsheet software to improve the development of staffing patterns in our facility. We had been using a pencil and paper template for managers to use to develop staffing patterns. This manual template concentrated on the weekday staffing needs and applied an overall factor to calculate weekend and benefit time. The FTE number provided did not address orientation and educational needs for any of the staff or benefit needs for the weekend staff. Although these staffing patterns were used to project the number of FTEs needed and the distribution of employees to staff the nursing unit, they were not used to drive the budgeted quota for the unit.

Using a computer software program, I developed a spreadsheet template the managers could use to accurately project FTEs needed to meet the staffing pattern. This computerized approach allows for weekday and weekend staffing to be considered independently, allowing for any differences in census or direct NHPPD. A benefit-time factor, tailored to our organization's specific benefit package for each skill level, is used to calculate the number of FTEs needed to staff for benefit time. Benefit time is now calculated for weekday and weekend staffing coverage for a 24/7 operation. Additionally, an orientation and educational factor is used to calculate the FTEs needed to provide coverage. For the first time, benefited time off and orientation time are built into each unit's staffing pattern. Additionally, direct and indirect NHPPD are automatically calculated as the staffing pattern is changed, and the calculated FTE needs can be compared to the current budgeted quota for variances.

Overall, this template has been accepted as a valid management tool, has standardized inclusion of nonproductive time into FTE budgets, and has given managers a simple tool to develop new staffing patterns. It has also helped in raising the accountability of managers, in that it helps them develop workable staffing patterns for which they can be held accountable.

BARBARA LEAFER, RN, BS

Fiscal Administrator for Patient Care

Albany, New York

Nurse Intensity

Nurse intensity is "a measure of the amount and complexity of nursing care needed by a patient" (Adomat & Hewison, 2004, p. 304). Nurse intensity is dependent on many factors that are difficult to measure: severity of illness, patient dependency for activities of daily living, complexity of care, and amount of time needed for care (Beglinger, 2006). It is vital that nurses measure nurse intensity because staffing needs vary not only with the number of patients being cared for, but also with the type of care provided for each of those patients (Unruh & Fottler, 2006).

Patient turnover affects nurse intensity. Patient turnover is a measure reflecting patient admission, transfer, and discharge, all of which entail RN-intensive procedures. As the health care industry pushes to reduce costs through shorter lengths of stay, these RN-intensive procedures related to patient turnover consume an increasing proportion of the hospital stay. An example of this is in a 2009 study; Downing and others note a decrease in length of stay after surgery for breast cancer from 9.8 days in 1990 to 5.2 days in 2005 (2009). As length of stay shortens, the intensity and need for NHPPD increases.

Patient Classification Systems

A **patient classification system (PCS)** is a measurement tool used to articulate the nursing workload for a specific patient or group of patients over a specific period of time. The measure of nursing workload that is generated for each patient is called the **patient acuity**. PCS data can be used to predict the amount of nursing time needed based on the patient's acuity. As a patient becomes sicker, the acuity level rises, meaning the patient requires more nursing care (see Table 9-1). As a patient's acuity level decreases, the patient requires less nursing care. In most patient classification systems, each patient is classified using weighted criteria that then approximate the nursing care hours needed for the next 24 hours.

Because patient care is dynamic, it is impossible to capture future patient care needs using a one-time measure. Criteria reflect care needed in assessment, bathing, mobilizing, supervision, monitoring, evaluation, and so on. In most cases, patients are classified once a day; using the midnight census to budget for the next 24 hours underestimates the cost of nursing services (Beswick, Hill, & Anderson, 2010). The ideal PCS produces a valid and reliable rating of individual patient care requirements, which are matched to the latest clinical technology and caregiver skill variables. These systems are generally applied to all inpatients in an organization. Other PCS systems exist to measure the workload associated with patient visits in the emergency department (ED) or in clinic environments based on relative weights for visit lengths as well as complexity of care. There are two different types of classification systems: factor and prototype. A patient *factor* system assigns a time or weight to reflect the amount of time needed to perform a nursing task. The time or weight factor assigned for different nursing activities can be changed over time to reflect the changing needs of the patients or hospital systems. A *prototype* classification system allocates nursing time to large patient groups based on an average of similar patients. For example, specific **diagnostic-related groups (DRGs)** have been used as groupings of patients to which a nursing acuity is assigned based on past organizational experience. DRGs are patient groupings established by the federal government for reimbursement purposes. DRGs are sorted by patient disease or condition. This model assumes that, on average, this measure will reflect the nursing care required and provided. The data are then used by hospitals in determining the cost of nursing care and negotiating contracts with payers for specific patient populations. Both classification systems have advantages and disadvantages. No perfect system exists, as patients are unique and changes can happen in moments in the hospital environment.

TABLE 9-1
Comparative Values of Acuity and Care Hours

PCS Acuity	Care Hours
1	3.00
2	3.60
3	6.00
4	9.99
5	15.00

© Cengage Learning 2014.

Utilization of Classification System Data

Patient classification data are valuable sources of information, a form of informatics, for all levels of an organization. On a day-to-day basis, acuity data can be utilized by staff and managers in planning nurse staffing over the next 24 hours. Acuity data and NHPPD are concrete data parameters that are used to educate staff on how to adjust staffing levels. For example, for an acuity range of 1.0 to 1.10, the RN staffing may be five RNs on day shifts. For an acuity of 1.10 to 1.15, the RN staffing on day shifts might be six RNs. Experienced staff have the knowledge to manage staffing to acuity levels given the information, boundaries, and authority to do so. In many organizations, a central staffing office monitors the census and acuity on all units and deploys nursing resources to the areas in most need using the classification system data and recommended staffing levels. The manager reviews the results of staffing over the past 24 to 48 hours to adjust staffing to patient requirements. In critical care environments, managers may review the staffing each shift, and even within the shift, because of quick acuity changes in the critical care population. At the unit level, acuity data are also essential in preparing month-end justification for variances in staff utilization. If your average acuity has risen, then there is often a rise in NHPPD to accommodate the increased patient needs.

At an organizational level, acuity data have been used to cost out nursing services for specific patient populations and global patient types. This information is also very helpful in negotiating payment rates with third-party payers such as insurance companies to ensure that reimbursement reflects nursing costs. In most organizations, the classification or acuity data are also used in preparation of the nursing staffing budget for the upcoming fiscal year. The data can be benchmarked with other organizations to lend credence to any efforts to change nursing hours. Finally, patient acuity data and NHPPD can be used to develop a staffing pattern. Patient classification and NHPPD data provide an enormous amount of information that serves a multitude of needs.

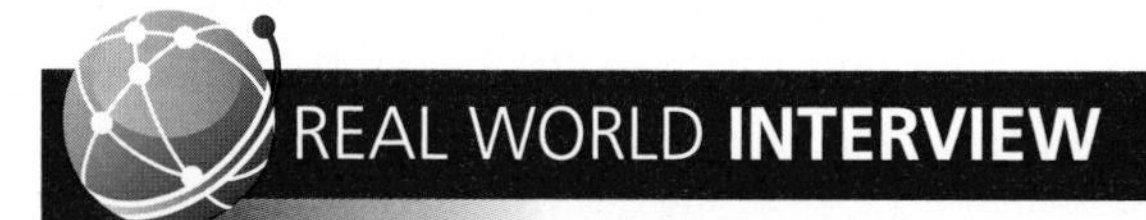

As a manager of an intensive care unit, I can say that self-scheduling has greatly increased my staff's satisfaction with their schedules. I think the biggest factor in the success of our process was the initial buy-in from the staff. Before implementing, staff were surveyed to assess their commitment to making the process work. I was looking for 60 to 75 percent buy-in before implementation and found greater than 70 percent. A second critical factor was having clear guidelines for the process. These included timelines for how and when staff can sign up for time and how time off is prioritized.

During implementation, we learned many things. One key factor was that staff needed to have confrontation and negotiation skills in order for this process to work. Inevitably there were situations when someone had to change their schedule. When confrontation and negotiation did not take place, there were periods of short staffing and patient care needs not being met. We also learned that this is a time-consuming process. It takes about 16 hours per month for the self-scheduling committee to put the schedule together.

Another key element I found was the manager had to maintain accountability for staffing. I meet with the scheduling committee regularly and oversee the orientation of new staff to the self-scheduling process. I sign off on every schedule to ensure that the schedule maintains appropriate staffing levels at all times. I found that I needed to identify trends that may be affecting staffing and assist the staff in addressing the trends. I also work with the staff on the implementation of any new program that affects the schedule. The weekend program is a good example of this. I worked with the staff to ensure there were appropriate guidelines for staff receiving a reduced weekend commitment. And finally, the most important role I play is to be very clear about the expectations for all—the committee, the staff, and myself. This scheduling process has been one of the most positive qualities of work-life efforts for my staff.

ROB ROSE, BSN, MSN
Nurse Manager, Cardiopulmonary Surgery Intensive Care Unit
Albany, New York

CONSIDERATIONS IN DEVELOPING A STAFFING PATTERN

Benchmarking is a tool used to compare productivity across facilities to establish performance goals and improve outcomes. Often, benchmarking data provide only comparable unit-of-service performance and do not reflect quality-of-care indicators that can link quality patient care outcomes to productivity measures. In developing a staffing pattern that leads to a budget, it is important to benchmark your planned NHPPD against other organizations with similar patient populations as part of evidence-based decision making (EBD-M). Purchased patient classification systems often offer acuity and NHPPD benchmarking data from around the country as part of their system. This kind of data can be helpful in establishing a starting point for a staffing pattern or as part of justification for increasing or reducing nursing hours. Caution must be used, however, because each organization has varying levels of support in place at the unit level for the nurse. For example, a nursing unit that has dietary aides from the dietary department who distribute and pick up meal trays would need less nursing time than a unit that had no external support for this activity. Practice differences such as these contribute significantly to differences in hours of care from one organization to another.

Regulatory Requirements

Generally speaking, there are few regulatory requirements related to nurse staffing. The 42 Code of Federal Regulations (Centers for Medicare & Medicaid Services, 2007) requires Medicare-certified hospitals to have adequate numbers of direct care providers, leaving it up to the states to determine appropriate staffing. Three methods are used to comply with the Code, namely, placing accountability on the hospital, mandating ratios through legislation, and requiring public reporting of staffing levels.

Fifteen states and the District of Columbia have enacted legislation and/or enacted regulations that address nurse staffing (ANA, 2011). The American Nurses Association (ANA, 2012) promotes a legislative model that empowers nurses to create staffing plans specific for their unit, patient population, and nursing skill mix. In June 2010, the ANA introduced federal regulation, the Registered Nurse Safe Staffing Bill, whereby hospital staffing committees must comprise at least 55 percent direct care nurses (ANA, 2012). In 1999, California became the first state to mandate development of nurse-to-patient ratios. There is considerable controversy within the nursing profession over regulating nurse staffing. There are nurses who are adamant that they need to be protected by law with stipulated staffing levels. There are other nurse leaders who are concerned that the mandated staffing levels would soon become the maximum staffing levels rather than the minimum.

The Joint Commission (JC) surveys hospitals on the quality of care provided. The JC does not mandate staffing levels, but does assess staffing effectiveness. JC standards on staffing require organizations to monitor a correlation between two clinical and two human resource indicators; for example, HNPPD against hospital-acquired pressure ulcer occurrence or NHPPD against falls. Findings must then be used to adjust staffing levels.

Skill Mix

Skill mix is another critical element in nurse staffing. **Skill mix** is the percentage of RN staff compared to other direct care staff, licensed professional nurses (LPNs) and nursing assistive personnel (NAP). For example, in a unit that has 40 FTEs budgeted, with 20 of them being RNs and 20 FTEs of other skill types, the RN skill mix would be 50 percent. If the unit had 40 FTEs, with 30 of them being RNs, the RN skill mix would be 75 percent. The skill mix of a unit should vary according to the care that is required and the care delivery model utilized. For example, in a critical care unit, the RN skill mix will be much higher than in a nursing home where the skills of an RN are required to a much lesser degree.

Staff Support

Another important factor to consider in developing a staffing pattern is the support in place for the operations of the unit or department. For instance, does your organization have a systematic process to deliver medications to the department or do unit personnel have to pick up patient medications and narcotics? Does your organization have staff to transport patients to and from ancillary departments? The less support available to your staff, the more nursing hours have to be built into the staffing pattern to provide care to patients.

Historical Information

As you consider the many variables that affect staffing, it helps to ask the following questions: What has worked in the past? Was the staff able to provide the care that was needed? How many patients were cared for? What kind of patients were they? How many staff were utilized and what kind of staff were they? This kind of information can help to identify operational issues that would not be apparent otherwise. For example, it is important to review any data on quality or staff perceptions regarding the effectiveness of any previous staffing plans. This information will allow you to calculate previous NHPPD and outcomes for comparison to your current staffing plans. History is a valuable tool that we often overlook as we plan for the future.

ESTABLISHING A STAFFING PATTERN

A **staffing pattern** is a plan that articulates how many and what kind of staff are needed by shift and day to staff a unit or department. There are basically two ways of developing a staffing pattern. It can be generated by determining the required ratio of staff to patients; nursing hours and total FTEs are then calculated. It can also be generated by determining the nursing care hours needed for a specific patient or patients and then generating the FTEs and staff-to-patient ratio needed to provide that care. In most cases, you would use a combination of methods to validate your staffing plan.

Staffing an Inpatient Unit

An **inpatient unit** is a hospital unit that is able to provide care to patients 24 hours a day, 7 days a week. Establishing a staffing pattern for this kind of unit utilizes all the data discussed in the previous sections. Using data from all your sources, you can build a staffing plan that you believe will meet the needs of the patients, the inter-professional staff, and the organization. To illustrate the concept of calculating a staffing plan, we will use a typical medical unit with 24 beds and an average daily census (ADC) of 20 (Figure 9-6). ADC is calculated by taking the total number of patients at census time, usually midnight, over a period of time (e.g., weekly, monthly, or yearly) and dividing by the number of days in the time period. Many institutions budget their staffing based on ADC and then adjust for patient census and acuity changes. To fully understand the complexity of decisions involved in staffing, you must review the Models of Care Delivery section later in this chapter. Allocating FTEs cannot be separated from an intelligent understanding of how patient care is delivered and how to use the right mix of staff, collaboration, and teamwork to accomplish that patient care.

SCHEDULING

Scheduling of staff is the responsibility of the nurse manager. The nurse manager must ensure that the schedule places the appropriate staff on each shift for safe, effective patient care. There are many issues to consider as staff are scheduled: patient needs and acuity, the number of patients, the experience of the staff, and the supports available.. The combination of these factors determines the number of staff to be scheduled on each shift.

Patient Need

Patient classification systems do not tell you when the nursing activity will take place over the next 24 hours. In addition to planning for the acuity of the patients, the staffing plan must support having staff working when the work needs to be done. A good example of this would be an oncology unit in which chemotherapy and blood transfusions typically occur on the evening shift. In this scenario, staffing in the evening may need to be higher than for other shifts to support these nurse-intensive activities.

Experience and Scheduling of Staff

Each nurse is different regarding his or her knowledge base, experience level, and critical-thinking skills. A novice nurse takes longer to accomplish the same

Scenario: A 24-bed medical unit where the ADC is 20 and NHPPD is budgeted at 8.

Step 1:

Formula: Number of patients × NHPPD = care hours per day = shifts needed per 24 hours

Example: $20 \times 8 = \frac{160 \text{ care hours per 24-hour day}}{8} = 20$ eight-hour shifts needed per 24 hours

Step 2:

Allocate 20 staff to the unit by shift and skill mix, based on when and how care is provided.

	% of Staff Per Shift	# of Staff	RN	Tech/Unit Clerk
Days	40	8	4	4
Evenings	35	7	4	3
Nights	25	5	4 12	1 8 (Total 20)

Step 3:

Calculate FTE to cover staff days off. (Calculations are in parentheses in the matrix below.)

Formula: $\frac{\text{Number of staff needed per shift} \times \text{Days of needed coverage}}{\text{Number of shifts each FTE works}}$

Example: $\frac{4 \times 7}{5} = 5.6$

	% of Staff Per Shift	# of Staff	RN	Tech/Unit Clerk
Days	40	8	4 (5.6)	4 (5.6)
Evenings	35	7	4 (5.6)	3 (4.2)
Nights	25	5	4 (5.6) 12 (16.8)	1 (1.4) 8 (11.2) = 20 (28)

Step 4:

Provide coverage for benefit time off, e.g., vacation, educational time, etc. Managers and other support staff are often not replaced on their days off.

Formula: Productive hours/budgeted nonproductive hours = percent of nonproductive hours × total FTE = additional FTE needed to cover benefits

Productive + nonproductive FTE to cover each week = Grand Total FTE

Example: 2080/232 = 0.11 × 28 = 3.08

3.08 + 28 = 31.08 Grand Total FTE

FIGURE 9-6

Staffing plan template for an inpatient unit.

© Cengage Learning 2014

task than an experienced nurse. An experienced RN can handle more in terms of workload and acuity of patients. If a nursing unit requires special skills or competencies, you would also want to plan for additional nursing hours, so that staff with those particular skills are scheduled when the patient care needs may arise. The underlying principle of good staffing is that the patients you serve come first. This may dictate some undesirable shifts, but there must be appropriate numbers and kinds of staff on hand to care for the patients you serve. Staff are plotted out across a staffing sheet (Figure 9-7).

The scheduled days should be assigned so that there are an even number of staff available across the week. Typically, the spread of FTEs across the 24-hour period falls within the following guidelines: days 33 percent to 50 percent, evenings 30 percent to 40 percent, and nights 20 percent to 33 percent. The spread is based on patient need.

Options in Staffing Patterns

To attract and retain employees, organizations offer traditional and flexible schedules to meet organizational and employee needs. Traditional staffing patterns are generally eight-hour shifts, 7 A.M. to 3:30 P.M., 3 P.M. to 11:30 P.M., and 11 P.M. to 7:30 A.M. A full-time employee works 10 eight-hour shifts in a two-week period. The start time of eight-hour shifts may vary by organization or by unit and patient need. For example, emergency departments are typically busiest during the evening into the night hours. An eight-hour shift for the ED may be 7 P.M. to 3 A.M. to cover the peak activity times.

In recent years, new options in scheduling have emerged. Twelve-hour shifts have become very popular across the country. In many organizations, employees can work less than 40 hours per week and get full-time benefits. In one example, a nurse could work three 12-hour shifts per week and have four days off and be full time. Another popular option is weekend programs. Weekend program staff work two 12-hour shifts every weekend and are paid a rate that would make the 24 hours of work equal to 40 hours of work. Some of these programs include full-time benefits as well. These programs are expensive, but they can be helpful. See Figure 9-8. Note that any time you implement a scheduling plan, it is critical to assess what the effect will be on the care of patients.

The number of staff shift-handoff reports per day also affects patient care. A shift-handoff report occurs any time the nurse caring for a group of patients reports off to the nurse on an oncoming shift. Such shift-handoff reports are opportunities for missed communication and errors in patient care. In eight-hour shifts, there are three shift-handoff reports per 24 hours, whereas, in twelve-hour shifts, there are only two shift-handoff reports. The use of SBAR (situation, background, assessment, and recommendation) as a frame-work for communication helps communication between nurses regardless of the number of shift-handoff reports.

Self-Scheduling

Self-scheduling is a process in which unit staff take leadership in creating and monitoring the work schedule while working within defined guidelines. Often, there is a staffing committee that is part of unit-shared governance, which is a unit model where staff manage professional practice through unit committees. Increasing staff control over their schedule is a major factor in nurse job satisfaction and retention and has been associated with reductions in sick time usage. The nurse manager retains an important role in self-scheduling through mentoring, providing open communication, and holding everyone to equal expectations. To ensure that patient care needs are met, there must be structure to a self-scheduling program. This is often achieved by a unit committee, made up of staff that report to the nurse manager. It is important to spell out the roles and responsibilities of all of the unit-based committee—the chairperson if there is one, the staff, and the manager. Generic boundaries need to be established regarding fairness, fiscal responsibility, evaluation of the self-scheduling process, and the approval process. Table 9-2 spells out specific issues that must be addressed.

Informatics Support for Evidence-Based Staffing

Information technology can provide innovative solutions to support evidence-based nurse staffing. Hospitals currently capture data electronically from

<table>
<tr><th></th><th>Monday
04</th><th>Tuesday
05</th><th>Wednesday
06</th><th>Thursday
07</th><th>Friday
08</th><th>Saturday
09</th><th>Sunday
10</th><th>Monday
11</th><th>Tuesday
12</th><th>Wednesday
13</th><th>Thursday
14</th><th>Friday
15</th><th>Saturday
16</th><th>Sunday
17</th></tr>
<tr><td>Melinda</td><td>A</td><td></td><td>D</td><td>A</td><td></td><td>D</td><td>D</td><td></td><td></td><td>D</td><td>D</td><td>D</td><td>A</td><td></td></tr>
<tr><td>Carlos</td><td></td><td>8.00
1900</td><td></td><td></td><td>N</td><td>N</td><td>N</td><td></td><td>8.00
1900</td><td></td><td>A</td><td></td><td></td><td></td></tr>
<tr><td>Tabitha</td><td>12.00
0900</td><td></td><td>A</td><td></td><td>D</td><td>12.00
0900</td><td>12.00
0900</td><td>12.00
0900</td><td></td><td>A</td><td></td><td>N</td><td></td><td></td></tr>
<tr><td>Susan</td><td>D</td><td>8.00
1100</td><td></td><td>E</td><td>E</td><td>E</td><td>P</td><td>vac</td><td></td><td>8.00
1100</td><td>E</td><td>E</td><td>P</td><td></td></tr>
<tr><td>Barbara</td><td></td><td>14.00
2400</td><td>13.00
2400</td><td>13.00
2400</td><td>A</td><td></td><td></td><td></td><td>14.00
2400</td><td>13.00
2400</td><td>13.00
2400</td><td></td><td>D</td><td>A</td></tr>
<tr><td>Rosemary</td><td>D</td><td>D</td><td>D</td><td>D</td><td></td><td>E</td><td></td><td></td><td>A</td><td>N</td><td>N</td><td></td><td>E</td><td></td></tr>
<tr><td>Robert</td><td>N</td><td>N</td><td>N</td><td>N</td><td></td><td></td><td>N</td><td>N</td><td>N</td><td>N</td><td>N</td><td></td><td></td><td>N</td></tr>
<tr><td>Jacqueline</td><td>E</td><td>E</td><td>P</td><td></td><td>E</td><td></td><td>E</td><td></td><td>E</td><td>E</td><td>E</td><td>P</td><td></td><td>P</td></tr>
<tr><td>Marcella</td><td></td><td>D</td><td></td><td>D</td><td>D</td><td>D</td><td>A</td><td></td><td>D</td><td></td><td></td><td>D</td><td></td><td></td></tr>
<tr><td>Nirmala</td><td>P</td><td></td><td></td><td>E</td><td>8.00
0800</td><td></td><td>E</td><td>P</td><td></td><td></td><td>E</td><td>8.00
0800</td><td></td><td>E</td></tr>
<tr><td>Gary</td><td></td><td>E</td><td>E</td><td></td><td>E</td><td>N</td><td></td><td>E</td><td>E</td><td>E</td><td></td><td>12.00
1500</td><td></td><td></td></tr>
<tr><td>Irma</td><td>N</td><td>N</td><td>N</td><td></td><td>N</td><td>P</td><td>P</td><td>N</td><td>N</td><td>P</td><td></td><td>P</td><td></td><td></td></tr>
<tr><td>Toni</td><td>8.00
0730</td><td>8.00
0730</td><td>8.00
0730</td><td>8.00
0730</td><td>8.00
0730</td><td></td><td></td><td>8.00
0730</td><td>8.00
0730</td><td></td><td>8.00
0730</td><td>A</td><td>N</td><td></td></tr>
</table>

The 1st number in a square is the number of hours scheduled; the second number is the shift start time in military time.

Standard Work Assignments

D 0700–1500
E 1500–2300
N 2300–0700
A 0700–1900
P 1900–0700

FIGURE 9-7

Excerpt from schedule for an emergency department showing great variation in shift design.

© Cengage Learning 2014

Weekend staff working at $42 an hour × 24 hours = $1,008 per weekend

Regular staff working at $25 an hour × 24 hours = $600 per weekend

Difference in cost = $408 per weekend option FTE

Six weekend option staff members at $1,008 would cost $2,448 more than regular staff per weekend;

$2,448 × 52 weekends a year would cost $127,296 more than regular staff annually.

FIGURE 9-8

Annual cost of a weekend option program for one nursing unit.

© Cengage Learning 2014

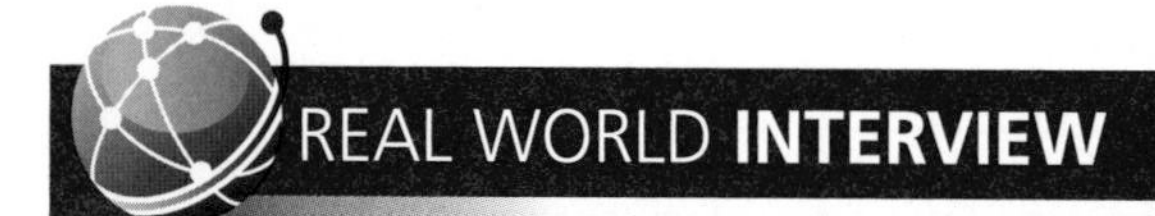

REAL WORLD INTERVIEW

We have developed a nursing practice quality scorecard. The scorecard is a tool to display data on our three organizational priorities: mission, customer orientation, and cost-effectiveness. By looking at measures in all three arenas, we can see how we are doing in these areas. We also can see if changes made in one arena positively or negatively affect the other measures. To look at nursing's mission for nursing practice, we track and trend several of the American Nurses Association national indicators. We track medication errors, patient falls, restraints, nosocomial pressure ulcers, and urinary tract infections. For customer satisfaction, we measure overall satisfaction with nursing care provided and how well patients' pain was controlled. For cost-effectiveness, we track nursing hours per patient day. All of these measures are tracked and trended on control charts every three months. The specific data is trended, and measures that are greater than two standard deviations from the target are identified as potential points to be reviewed for identification of opportunities for improvement.

One of the areas we chose to target for improvement was medication errors. It became evident that the most prominent reason for medication errors was delayed and omitted medications. Further investigation proved that the procedures for obtaining medications were unclear and outdated. We have written new procedures to specify responsibilities of the nursing staff and the pharmacy staff. We are now monitoring our rate of medication errors to see if our changes have made any improvement in the error rate.

Another example of use of the scorecard was in review of our pressure ulcer rate. We found there was an increase in the incidence of pressure ulcers. In review of causes, we found that the reporting system had been revised to include all stages of skin breakdown. Since the reporting change, we have seen an increase in the number of pressure ulcers reported. This is a positive change, as we now have accurate data on which to target our improvement efforts.

Lessons that we have learned in the development of the scorecard are that we needed to set improvement targets earlier in the process to push the search for opportunities for improvement. We also learned that many of these measures are not well defined, and, therefore, benchmarking to other organizations is difficult. We continue to strive for further improvement and utilize the scorecard to measure our success and look for opportunities for improvement. Reviewing nursing outcome data for the entire nursing division has been a powerful tool to ensure that care provided is meeting expected outcomes, and it allows us to benchmark our outcomes to other organizations.

LOUANN VILLANI, RN, BSN

Nursing Quality Specialist

Albany, New York

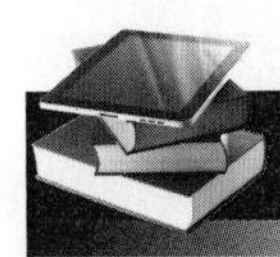

EVIDENCE FROM THE **LITERATURE**

Citation: Kane, R. L., Shamliyan, T. A., Mueller, C., Duval, S., & Wilt, T. J. (2007). The association of registered nurse staffing levels and patient outcomes: Systematic review and meta-analysis. *Medical Care, 45*(12), 1195–1204.

Discussion: A total of 2,858 studies were considered for this review, with 96 studies meeting the inclusion criteria. Findings suggested that an increase of one RN FTE per patient day was associated with a 9 percent reduction in ICU deaths and a 6 percent reduction in medical unit deaths. In addition, consistent and significant reductions in patient adverse events such as a 30 percent reduction in hospital-acquired pneumonia in ICU patients, a 16 percent reduction in failure to rescue in surgical patients, and a 49 percent reduction in nosocomial infections were also identified. On the other hand, one additional patient per shift resulted in an 8 percent increase in hospital-related mortality across the health care setting. Of interest, ". . . nurse-sensitive adverse events including falls, pressure ulcers, and urinary tract infections did not demonstrate a consistent association with staffing levels" (p. 1201). Causal relationships between outcomes and RN experience, competence, knowledge and education level, work environment, quality of medical care, collaboration practices, nurse retention, and job satisfaction were identified but not measured in this study.

The review found that fixed minimum RN-to-patient ratios did not always realize patient safety benefits, primarily because individual patient needs and acuity were not taken into consideration. Patient acuity-based staffing was found to be used inconsistently in the studies, largely due to the varying types and use of classification systems. The effect of public reporting of staffing on quality of care is not known at this time; there is a need for more research in this area. Pay for performance is promoted to encourage quality, but until more research is conducted, its effects are not well understood.

Implications for Practice: There is a strong association between RN staffing and hospital-related mortality and other outcomes. Study findings encourage health care organizations to critically review current RN staffing, mindful of all causal relationships between patient outcomes and nurse staffing.

a variety of sources, for example, admissions, discharges, transfers, call-light timing, computerized charting of risk assessments, and nurse profiles. Some organizations even use infrared signals to identify the nurse's location on the unit. When all of this data is combined, informatics provides meaningful information on nursing care needs, supply of qualified nurses, and quality of care outcomes (Hyun, Bakken, Douglas, & Stone, 2008).

Standardizing how computer programs collect and represent data allows different computer programs to work together. For example, data is collected and reported from a variety of sources such as pagers, laboratory, nurse charting, glucometers, call-light timing, and medication barcode and administration. The ability of each system to interact with the other and provide data on real-time care provision by nurses provides information on the actual workload of nurses. Computer systems can pull the pieces of data together in real time and combine them with historical trends to help inform staffing decisions.

For example, a medical-surgical unit experiences multiple patient admissions, discharges, and transfers during a Monday shift. In the morning, the 30-bed unit has 26 beds occupied. Computerized staffing identifies six potential discharges and seven surgical admissions. In addition, the average number of call-light signals is 67.3 per shift, with the length of time spent with the patient at 8.9 minutes per call. The computerized staffing program warns that there are four experienced nurses and one new nurse scheduled for the day shift. Another computerized warning shows that a surgeon is back from vacation, the emergency department (ED) is full, and historically Mondays have an ED admission rate of 4.2 patients. The ability to utilize informatics to access real-time information on variables that impact

TABLE 9-2
Issues To Be Spelled Out in Self-Scheduling Guidelines

1. Scheduling period: Is the scheduling period two-, four-, or six-week intervals?
2. Schedule timeline: What are the time frames for both staff and per diem workers to sign up for regular work, special requests, and overtime?
3. Staffing pattern: Will 8- or 12-hour shifts, or both, be used?
4. Weekends: Are staff expected to work every other weekend? If there are extra weekends available, how are they distributed?
5. Holidays: How are they allocated?
6. Vacation time: Are there restrictions on the amount of vacation during certain periods?
7. Unit vacation practices: How many staff from one shift can be on vacation at any time?
8. Requests for time off: What is the process for requesting time off?
9. Short-staffed shifts: How are shifts that are short-staffed handled?
10. On call, if applicable: How do staff get assigned or sign up for on-call time?
11. Cancellation guidelines: How and when do staff get canceled for scheduled time if they are not needed?
12. Sick calls: What are the expectations for calling in sick, and how are these shifts covered?
13. Military/National Guard leave: What kind of advance notice is required?
14. Schedule changes: What is the process for changing one's schedule after the schedule has been approved?
15. Shifts defined: What are the beginnings and endings of available shifts?
16. Committee time: When does the self-scheduling committee meet and for how long?
17. Seniority: How does it play into staffing and request decisions?
18. Staffing plan for crisis/emergency situations: What is the plan when staffing is inadequate?
19. Job sharing: Who can participate? When?

© Cengage Learning 2014.

staffing during a shift from a variety of sources assists in determining appropriate staffing needs.

Computerized programs that support staffing allow for automated staff scheduling, online staff bidding for shifts, and prompt notification of open shifts. Over the past decade, computerized programs have advanced to include sophisticated patient tracking throughout the hospital and identification of appropriate extended care placement for patient case management. The future of informatics promises to bring innovative solutions to support staffing and improve quality care outcomes.

NURSE-SENSITIVE PATIENT OUTCOMES

Nurse-sensitive patient outcomes such as patient length of stay and incidence of hospital-acquired pneumonia, postoperative infections, nosocomial bloodstream infections, cardiac arrest, respiratory failure, and odds of failure to rescue are negatively affected when nurse staffing is inadequate (Kane et al., 2007).

Nurse Staffing and Nurse Outcomes

In addition to patient outcomes, nurse outcomes should also be measured. Staff's perception of the adequacy of staffing should be tracked. Nurse perception of staffing effectiveness must be monitored by hospitals seeking magnet status. Initiating such measures might lead to comparisons for benchmarking best practice in the future and linking RN staffing perception to patient outcomes (Shirey & Fisher, 2008). There should be the ability for staff to communicate both in written and verbal form regarding staffing concerns. In addition, actual staffing compared to recommended staffing should be tracked. This will give clues to other staffing issues. Medication errors is another measure that has been linked with inadequate NHPPD. When resources are scarce, data are imperative to drive needed changes. The outcomes of ineffective staffing patterns and nursing care can be devastating to patients, staff, and the organization.

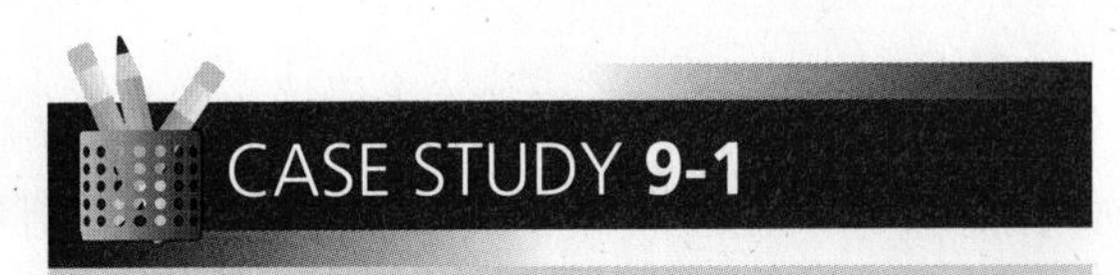

CASE STUDY 9-1

You are working on a patient care unit that is planning to begin doing its own scheduling. Using Figure 9-7, make a schedule for your unit. Identify the number of nurses budgeted for each day. Develop a plan to allocate these nurses to cover 24 hours a day, 7 days a week of patient care for two weeks.

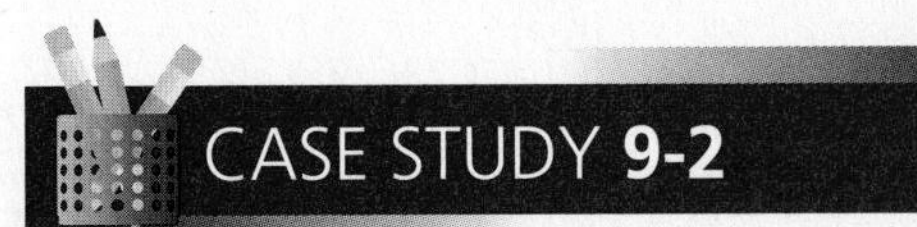

CASE STUDY 9-2

The nurse manager discusses the topic of starting self-scheduling at your staff meeting. What information will the staff need to consider before making the decision to adopt self-scheduling for your unit? What are advantages of this method of scheduling? What are the disadvantages?

MODELS OF CARE DELIVERY

To ensure that nursing care is provided to patients, the work must be organized. A **nursing care delivery model** organizes the work of caring for patients. The decision about which nursing care delivery model is used is based on the needs of the patients and the availability of competent staff in the different skill levels.

Case Method and Total Patient Care

In the case method, the nurse has one patient whom the nurse cares for exclusively. Total patient care is the modern-day version of the case method. In **total patient care**, the nurse is responsible for the total care for the nurse's patient assignment for the shift the nurse is working. The RN is responsible for several patients. The RN can assign patient care to the LPN or delegate to the NAP, but the RN retains accountability for the patient's care. LPNs and NAP work under the direction of the RN, but they must complete their assignments.

Advantages and Disadvantages

The advantage of total patient care and the case method for patients is the consistency of one individual caring for patients for an entire shift. This enables the patient, nurse, and family to develop a relationship based on trust. This model provides a greater number of RN hours of care than other models. The nurse has more opportunity to observe and monitor progress of the patient. A disadvantage is that these models utilize a high level of RN nursing hours and are more costly to deliver care. This level of RN intensity is not always warranted in patients with low acuity.

Functional Nursing Care

Functional nursing divides the nursing work into functional duties. These duties are then assigned to one of the team members. In this model, each care provider has specific duties or tasks he or she is responsible for. For instance, a typical assignment of labor for RNs is medication nurse or admission nurse. Decision making is usually at the level of the head nurse or charge nurse (Figure 9-9).

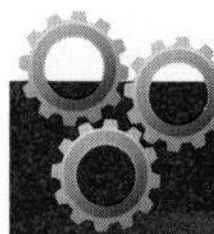

CRITICAL THINKING 9-1

Recently, you have been part of a unit committee that is reviewing data on your unit's pressure ulcer rates. In researching further, you discover that your unit's rates are significantly higher than those of other units. Staffing on your unit has been stable and in accordance with the staffing plan. The staff are experienced, and, in fact, they include some of the longest-tenured staff in the hospital.

Why is the pressure ulcer rate higher than that of other units?

What could your committee do to investigate this nurse-sensitive outcome further?

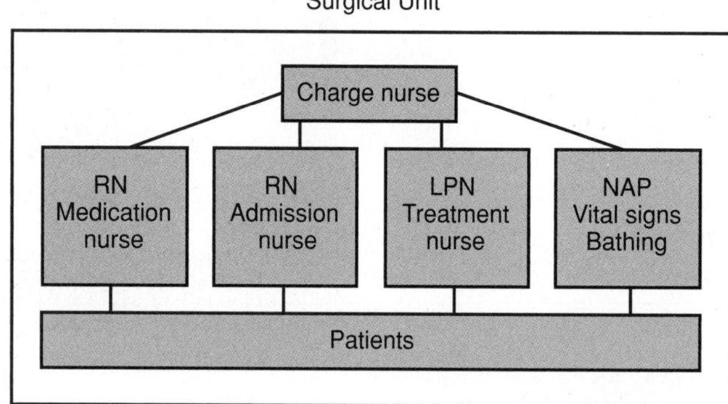

FIGURE 9-9

Functional nursing model.

© Cengage Learning 2014

Advantages and Disadvantages

In this model, care can be delivered to a large number of patients. This system utilizes other types of less-skilled health care workers when there is a shortage of RNs. Patients are likely to have care delivered to them in one shift by several staff members. To a patient, care may feel disjointed. Staff must be aware of this disadvantage and collaborate on ways to eliminate this outcome.

Team Nursing

Team nursing is a care delivery model that assigns staff to teams that then are responsible for a group of patients. A unit may be divided into two teams, and each team is led by a registered nurse. The team leader supervises and coordinates all the care provided by those on his or her team. The inter-professional team is most commonly made up of LPNs and NAP, but occasionally there is another RN. Care is divided into the simplest components and then assigned to the appropriate care provider. In addition to supervision duties, the team leader also is responsible for providing professional direction to those on the team regarding the care provided (Figure 9-10).

A **modular nursing** delivery system is a kind of team nursing that divides a geographic space into modules of patients, with each patient module cared for by a team of staff led by an RN. The modules may vary in size, but typically there is one RN with an LPN and nursing assistant to make up the module. In this case, the RN is responsible for the overall care of the patients in his or her module.

Advantages and Disadvantages

In team nursing and modular nursing, the RN is able to get work done through others, but patients

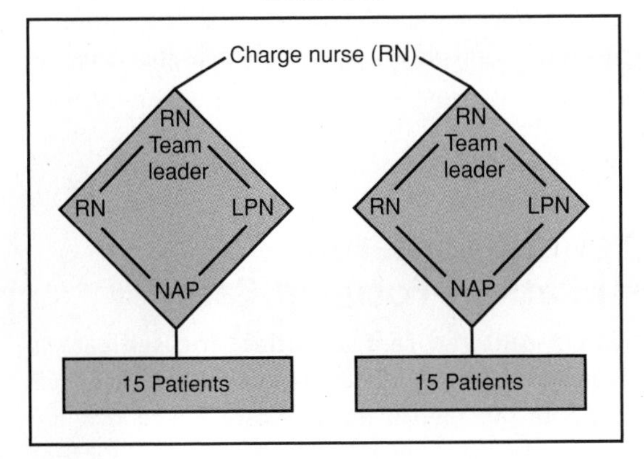

FIGURE 9-10

Team nursing model.

© Cengage Learning 2014

sometimes receive fragmented, depersonalized care. Communication, collaboration and teamwork in these models is complex. There is shared responsibility and accountability, which can cause confusion and lack of accountability. These factors may contribute to RN dissatisfaction with these models. These models require the RN to have very good delegation and supervision skills.

Primary Nursing

Primary nursing is a care delivery model that clearly delineates the responsibility and accountability of the RN and designates the RN as the primary provider of care to patients. Primary nursing is a form of the case model that consists of four elements. These are allocation and acceptance of individual responsibility for the decision making to one individual; assignments of daily care by the case method; direct person-to-person communication; and operational responsibility of one person for the quality of care administered to patients on a unit 24 hours a day, 7 days a week. Patients are assigned a primary nurse who is responsible for developing with the patient a plan of care that is followed by other nurses caring for the patient. Nurses and patients are matched according to needs and abilities. Patients are assigned to their primary nurse regardless of unit geographic considerations. In the primary nursing model, the role of the head nurse changes to one of leader by empowering the staff RNs to be knowledgeable about their patients and to direct the care of their primary patients. The primary nurse has the authority, accountability, and responsibility to provide care for a group of patients. Associate nurses care for the patient when the primary nurse is not working. Several associate nurses are assigned to each patient (Figure 9-11).

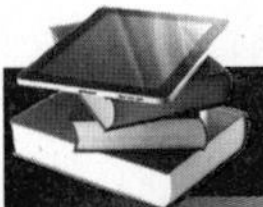

EVIDENCE FROM THE **LITERATURE**

Citation: Garrett, C. (2008). The Effect of Nurse Staffing Patterns on Medical Errors and Nurse Burnout. *AORN Journal, 87*(6), 1191–1204.

Discussion: This literature review explored the effect nurse-staffing patterns have on medical errors, fatigue, and nurse burnout. An unrealistic workload, including overtime, rotating shifts, and working 12.5 hours or longer, may lead to fatigue, burnout, absenteeism, job dissatisfaction, and increase the risk of making medication errors. While some hospitals use mandatory overtime to cover nurse vacancies, this practice produces fatigue and nurse burnout. Low nurse-to-patient ratios can lead to nurses not finishing nursing tasks and account for an increase in patient mortality and failure to rescue. Where there were high rates of RN staffing, patients experienced reduced rates of hospital stay, UTIs, pneumonia, shock, and upper gastrointestinal bleeding.

Implications for Practice: Nurse-staffing patterns can have both positive (with more staff) and negative (with less staff) effects on patient outcomes. Hospital administrators need to work with nurse leaders: to examine how health care is delivered; to assure that nurse staffing levels and working conditions are adequate; to avoid low nurse retention rates; and to promote safe and effective patient care.

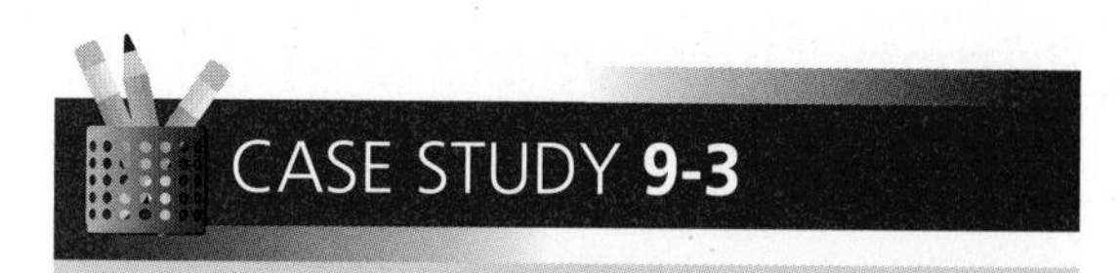

CASE STUDY 9-3

As a new RN graduate, you have just finished orientation, having worked closely with your mentor. You have been scheduled to work the 3–11 shift and carry a full load of patients. As the only new graduate working this shift, you begin to feel anxious and have doubts about your abilities. To whom should you go to discuss your feelings? What concerns would the nurse manager have about this situation? What can you do to prepare for this experience?

Advantages and Disadvantages

An advantage of this model is that patients and families are able to develop a trusting relationship with one primary nurse. There is defined accountability and responsibility for the nurse to develop a plan of care with the patient and family. The approach to care is holistic, which facilitates continuity of care rather than a shift-to-shift focus. Nurses, when they have adequate time to provide necessary care, find this model professionally rewarding because it gives the authority for decision making to the nurse at the bedside.

Disadvantages include a high cost because there is a higher RN skill mix. With no geographical boundaries within the unit, nursing staff may be required to travel long distances at the unit level to care for their primary patients. Nurses often perform functions that could be completed by other staff. And finally, nurse-to-patient ratios must be realistic to ensure there is enough nursing time available to meet the patient care needs.

Patient-Centered or Patient-Focused Care

Patient-centered care or **patient-focused care** is designed to focus on patient needs rather than staff needs. In this model, required care and services are brought to the patient. In the highest evolution of this model, all patient services are decentralized to the patient area, including radiology and pharmacy services. Staffing is based on patient needs. In this model, there is an effort to have the right person doing the right thing. Care teams are established for a group of patients. The care teams may include other disciplines such as respiratory or physical therapists. In these teams, disciplines collaborate to ensure that patients receive the care they need. Staff are kept close to the patients in decentralized work stations. For example, on a rehabilitation unit, physical therapists may be members of the care team and work at the unit level rather than in a centralized physical therapy department (Figure 9-12). Reiling, Hughes, & Murphy

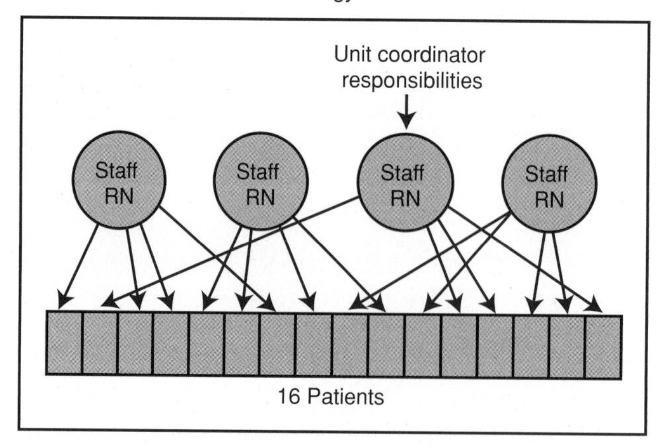

FIGURE 9-11

Primary nursing model.

© Cengage Learning 2014

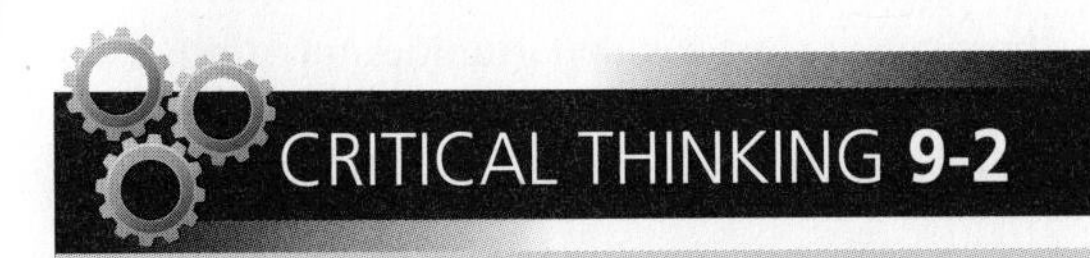

What is safe nurse staffing?

What are the benefits to patients when staffing levels are appropriate?

(2008) have put attention to the actual physical design of patient care areas to improve safety. They state that a badly designed environment that is not nurse and patient friendly can cause safety problems and impede quality care. Conversely, well-designed patient care units help improve quality and safety.

Advantages and Disadvantages

The pros of this system are that it is most convenient for patients and expedites services to patients. But it can be extremely costly to decentralize major services in an organization. A second disadvantage is that some staff have perceived the model as a way of reducing RNs and cutting costs in hospitals. In fact, this has been true in some organizations, but many other organizations have successfully used the patient-centered model to have the right staff available for the needs of the patient population.

Patient Care Redesign

In the 1990s, pressure to reduce health care costs was significant. Hospitals bore the brunt of this pressure. During that decade, patient care redesign was an initiative to redesign how patient care was delivered. The industry learned a lot about how care is delivered as it struggled with the redesign process. In addition to cost reduction, the redesign movement goals included making care more patient-centered and not caregiver-centered. This was accomplished by reducing the number of caregivers with which each patient had to interface and by organizing care around the patients, thus encouraging greater patient satisfaction. The concept is one of having caregivers cross-trained so they can intervene in more patient situations without having additional resources from outside the care team to assist. Examples include having the team members (e.g., RNs and cross-trained care technicians) draw lab specimens instead of having a phlebotomy team come to the unit, or team members doing their patients' breathing treatments instead of calling respiratory therapy to come to the unit. Team control of these functions allowed the functions to occur when patients needed them and not at the convenience of outside departments.

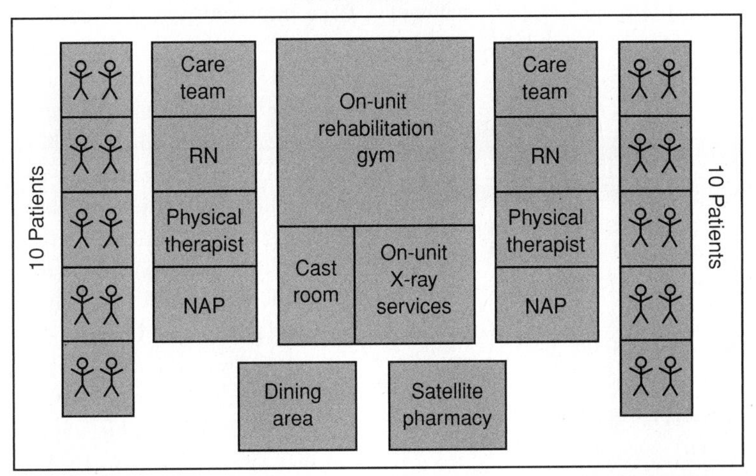

FIGURE 9-12

Patient-centered care model.

© Cengage Learning 2014

Many of these value-added changes in care attributed to the patient care redesign movement of the 1990s continue to this day as good practices within patient-centered care. Other aspects of redesign have not survived. Those redesign projects that failed to assist caregivers to change their roles or failed to consider unit culture in the patient care redesign were frequently not successful.

CARE DELIVERY MANAGEMENT TOOLS

In 1983, the federal government established diagnostic-related groups (DRGs) as a payment system for hospitals. In DRGs, the national average **length of stay (LOS)** for a specific patient type is used to determine payment for that grouping of Medicare patients. LOS refers to the average number of days a patient is hospitalized from day of admission to day of discharge. In DRGs, hospitals are paid the same amount for caring for a DRG patient group regardless of the actual LOS of the specific patient. This prompted initiatives in hospitals to reduce LOS and reduce hospital costs. There are further adjustments to costs based on patient comorbidities, that is, additional conditions (e.g., diabetes or hypertension) that add to the complexity of care needed by, for example, a patient with heart disease. Hospitals were able to benchmark their LOS for specific patient populations against a national database published through the Medicare DRG system.

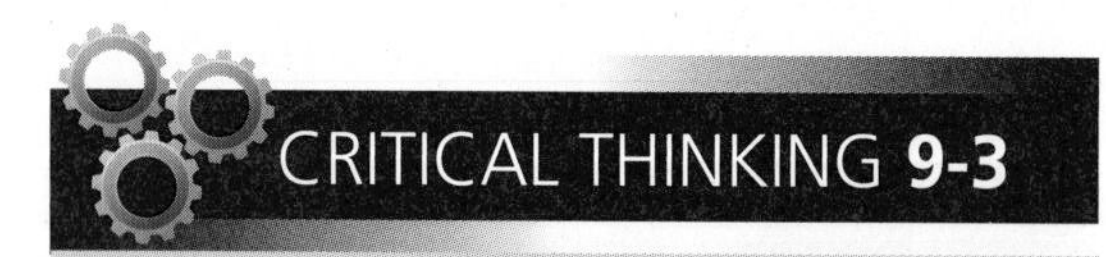

CRITICAL THINKING 9-3

The nurse manager brings the following issue to the nursing unit's governance committee of which you are a member. Over the past three months, two staff nurses have called in sick at least one day out of four weekends that they were scheduled to work.

What are the issues to be considered?

What are possible solutions?

How would you handle this situation if you were the nurse manager?

As hospitals looked for opportunities to reduce costs through reduction in the LOS, clinical pathways and case management surfaced as significant strategies.

Clinical Pathways

Clinical pathways are a strategy used to reduce LOS, enhance outcomes, and contain costs. **Clinical pathways** are care management tools that outline the expected clinical course and outcomes for a specific patient type. Clinical pathways take a different form in each organization that develops them. Typically they are pathways that outline the normal course of care for a patient. Pathways are often done by day, and expected outcomes are articulated for each day. It is the expected outcomes that patient progress is measured against. In some organizations, the pathways include multidisciplinary orders for care, including orders from nursing, medicine, and other allied health professionals such as physical therapy and dietary services. This serves to further expedite care for patients. Figure 9-13 provides an excerpt from a clinical pathway.

These pathways can be used by nursing and medical practitioners and case managers to care for the patient and measure the patient's progress against expected outcomes. Any variance in outcome can then be noted and acted upon to get the patient back on track.

Case Management

Case management is a second strategy to improve patient care and reduce hospital costs through coordination of care. Typically a case manager is responsible for coordinating care and establishing goals from preadmission through discharge. In the typical model of case management, a nurse is assigned to a specific high-risk patient population or service, such as cardiac surgery patients. The case manager has the responsibility to work with all disciplines to facilitate care. For example, if a postsurgical hospitalized patient has not met ambulation goals according to the clinical pathway, the case manager would work with the physician and nurse to determine what is preventing the patient from achieving these goals. If it turns out that the patient is elderly and is slow to recover, they may agree that physical therapy would be beneficial to assist this patient in ambulating. In other models, the case management function is provided

Clinical Pathway: Lower Extremity Revascularization
EXCERPT

ADDRESSOGRAPH

DAILY ANTICIPATED OUTCOMES							
POD2	**Date/Time /Init When met**	**POD3**	**Date/Time /Init When met**	**POD4**	**Date/Time /Init When met**	**POD5**	**Date/Time /Init When met**
Patient rates pain 0-2 on pain scale 0-10 using po analgesia.		Graft signal present with doppler.		Graft signal present with doppler.		Graft signal present with doppler.	
Graft signal present with doppler.		Incisional edges will be approximated without drainage.		Able to participate in self-care and adjunct therapies.		Ambulates independently.	
Patient will verbalize knowledge of plan of care, testing and treatment.		Site of invasive devices without signs of infection.		Patient viewed diet video.		Patient/significant other will verbalize understanding of activity/diet restrictions, medication use, wound management.	
Ambulate in hall Q I D.		Ambulates in hall Q I D.					
Tolerates po solids.		Patient/significant other will describe appropriate problem-solving skills to decrease anxiety.				Completed nutrition posttest.	
Voiding without difficulty.		Rehab referral started: _yes _no					
		Family support available at discharge, specify ______ ______					

TO BE KEPT IN PROGRESS NOTE SECTION OF CHART AT ALL TIMES.

FIGURE 9-13

Example of a clinical pathway.
(*Source:* Courtesy of Albany Medical Center, Albany, NY.)

by the staff nurse at the bedside. This works well if the population requires little case management, but if the patient population requires significant case management services, there needs to be enough RN time allocated for this activity. In addition to facilitating care, the case manager usually has a data function to improve care. In this role, the case manager collects aggregate data on patient variances from the clinical pathway. The data are shared with health care clinicians who participate in the clinical pathway and are then used to explore opportunities for improvement in the pathway or in hospital systems.

Disease Management

Increasingly, health care centers are developing disease management (DM) programs. Disease management is a "systematic, population-based approach to identify persons at risk, intervene with specific programs of care, and measure clinical and other outcomes" (Epstein & Sherwood, 1996). An objective of disease management is cost containment, and research indicates that this is occurring. Patients, whose chronic diseases are managed by nurses, often have lower numbers of patient readmissions and costs.

DM can be as simple as a pharmaceutical pamphlet describing how best to use a medication, or as complex as nurse managers developing individualized care plans and regularly contacting patients to ensure compliance with the plans.

Disease management strategies use a variety of methods, including telephone, the Internet, and in-person visits, to keep high-risk, high-cost patients out of the hospital. These DM strategies collect data from and send reminders to patients who need constant monitoring. They also provide information systems that help caregivers develop care plans and gather data for clinical improvement initiatives.

KEY CONCEPTS

- To plan nurse staffing, you must understand and apply the concepts of full-time equivalents (FTEs) and nursing hours per patient day (NHPPD).
- Determination of the number of FTEs needed to staff a unit requires review of patient classification data, NHPPD, regulatory requirements, skill mix, staff support, historical information, and the physical environment of the unit.
- In developing a staffing pattern, additional FTEs must be added to a nursing unit budget to provide coverage for days off and benefited time off.
- Scheduling of staff is the responsibility of the nurse manager, who must take into consideration patient need and acuity, volume of patients, budget, and the experience of the staff.
- Self-scheduling can increase staff morale and professional growth, but requires clear boundaries and guidelines to be successful.
- Evaluating the outcomes of your staffing plan for patients, staff, and the organization is a critical activity that should be done regularly.
- Case management and clinical pathways are care management tools that have been developed to improve patient care and reduce hospital costs.

KEY TERMS

benchmarking
case management
clinical pathways
diagnostic-related groups (DRGs)
direct care
full-time equivalent
functional nursing
indirect care
inpatient unit
length of stay (LOS)
modular nursing
nonproductive hours
nursing care delivery model
nursing hours per patient day (NHPPD)
patient acuity
patient-centered care
patient classification system (PCS)
patient-focused care
primary nursing
productive hours
self-scheduling
skill mix
staffing pattern
team nursing
total patient care
units of service

REVIEW QUESTIONS

1. Patient classification systems measure nursing workload required by the patient. The higher the patient's acuity, the more care the patient requires. Which of the following statements is a weakness of classification systems?
   A. Patient classification data are useful in predicting the required staffing for the next shift and for justifying nursing hours provided.
   B. Patient classification data can be utilized by the nurse making assignments to determine what level of care a patient requires.
   C. Classification systems typically focus on nursing tasks rather than a holistic view of a patient's needs.
   D. Aggregate patient classification data are useful in costing out nursing services and for developing the nursing budget.

2. If your RN staff members receive 4 weeks of vacation and 10 days of sick time per year, how many productive hours would each RN work in that year if she utilized all of her benefited time?
   A. 2,080 productive hours
   B. 1,840 productive hours
   C. 1,920 productive hours
   D. 1,780 productive hours

3. Patient outcomes are the result of many variables, one being the model of care delivery that is utilized. From the following scenarios, select which is the *worst* fit between patient need and care delivery model.
   A. Cancer patients being cared for in a primary-nursing model
   B. Rehabilitation patients being cared for in a patient-centered model
   C. Medical intensive care patients being cared for in a team-nursing model
   D. Ambulatory surgery patients with a wide range of illnesses being cared for in a functional-practice model

4. The medical-surgical unit provides 200 hours of care daily to 20 patients. Their NHPPD is which of the following?
   A. 1
   B. 10
   C. 20
   D. 200

5. When calculating paid nonproductive time, which should the nurse manager consider?
   A. Overtime pay and evening and night shift differential
   B. Total hours available to work
   C. Insurance benefits and educational hours
   D. All hours that are paid but not worked in the assigned unit

6. As a new manager learning about staffing patterns and schedules, which is the most important variable that affects staffing patterns and schedules?
   A. Organizational philosophy
   B. Budget allocation and restrictions
   C. Delivering safe, quality patient care
   D. Personnel policies regarding shift rotation

7. A new graduate asks the manager what she meant when she mentioned "benchmarking." Which response is most correct?
   A. A comparison of productivity data for similar nursing units
   B. A method to measure cost of care
   C. A comprehensive measure of good quality
   D. A set of written standards of care

8. Which statement best explains how informatics supports staffing?

A. Determining the flow of information throughout the organization
B. Organizing data from multiple sources into information for taking action
C. Facilitating the development of an individualized care model
D. Reinforcing staffing without considering variables

9. In developing a staffing plan for your unit, which of the following considerations would you include? Select all that apply.

A. Data from census and staffing from the past quarter
B. Benchmark against the organization's NHPPD from the previous year's data
C. Presence of a mini pharmacy on your unit that stocks medications
D. The hiring of three new nurses for your unit
E. Your hospital is located in Modesto, California
F. The scope of practice for nursing assistive personnel on your unit

10. Which of the following would you take into account when developing a staffing schedule starting next week and running for six weeks? Select all that apply.

A. An RN took four vacation days last month and has three days scheduled this month.
B. An RN comes out of nursing orientation next week.
C. There is scheduled maintenance on the water system for six rooms next week.
D. The unit secretary is scheduled for vacation and a float-pool secretary will take that place next week.
E. There are 22 nurses with over 10 years' experience on the unit.
F. A hospital-wide lift team will start in two weeks.

REVIEW ACTIVITIES

1. How do you know whether the outcomes of your staffing plan are positive? What measures do you have available in your organization that indicate your staffing is adequate or inadequate?
2. You are a nurse on a new unit for psychiatric patients. What should be considered in planning for FTEs and staffing for this unit?
3. You are a new nurse and you have increasing concerns regarding the staffing levels on your unit. You are becoming increasingly anxious each time you go to work. What should you do?

EXPLORING THE WEB

- Mandated staffing levels: *http://www.nursingworld.org*
  Go to "staffing issues"on the menu and review the legislative agenda for the ANA regarding staffing. Also review data on the ANA's latest staff survey.
- Nursing quality measures: *http://www.mriresearch.org*. Search for "quality measures."
- Staffing effectiveness: *http://www.jointcommission.org*
  Type "staffing effectiveness"into the search box, and read about staffing effectiveness standards issued by the JC.
- Staffing and quality: *http://www.ahrq.gov*
  This government site of the Agency for Healthcare Research and Quality provides evidence-based analysis of clinical issues. Look in the section on Quality and Patient Safety. You can also search using the term "safe staffing."

REFERENCES

Adomat, R., & Hewison, A. (2004). Assessing patient category/dependence systems for determining the nurse/patient ratio in ICU and HDU: A review of approaches. *Journal of Nursing Management, 2*(5), 299–308.

American Nurses Association (ANA). (2011). Safe staffing saves lives. *Nursing World*. Retrieved October 23, 2011, from http://safestaffingsaveslives.org/whatisanadoing/statelegislation.aspx?css=print

American Nurses Association (ANA). (2012). Safe staffing: The Registered Nurse Safe Staffing Act, H.R. 876/S.58. *Nursing World*. Retrieved October 4, 2012, from http://nursingworld.org/safestaffingfactsheet.aspx

Beglinger, J. E. (2006). Quantifying patient care intensity: An evidence-based approach to determining staffing requirements. *Nursing Administration Quarterly, 30*(3), 193–202.

Beswick, S., Hill, P. D., & Anderson, M. A. (2010). Comparison of nurse workload approaches. *Journal of Nursing Management, 18*, 592–598.

Centers for Medicare & Medicaid Services. (2007). The 42 code of federal regulations. Retrieved October 1, 2012, from http://ecfr.gpoaccess.gov/cgi/t/text/text-idx?c=ecfr&tpl=/ecfrbrowse/Title42/42cfr483_main_02.tpl

Downing, A., Lansdown, M., West, R., Thomas, J., Lawrence, G., & Forman, D. (2009). Changes in predictors and length of stay in hospital after surgery for breast cancer between 1997/98 and 2004/05 in two regions of England: A population-based study. BMC Health Service Research. doi: 10.1186/1472-6863-9-202.

Epstein, R. S., & Sherwood, L. M. (1996). From outcomes research to disease management: A guide for the perplexed. *Annals of Internal Medicine, 124*, 835–837.

Garrett, C. (2008). The effect of nurse staffing patterns on medical errors and nurse burnout. *AORN Journal, 87*(6), 1191–1204.

Hyun, S., Bakken, S., Douglas, K., & Stone, P. W. (2008). Evidence-based staffing: Potential roles for informatics. *Nursing Economics, 26*(3), 151–173.

Kane, R. L., Shamliyan, T. A., Mueller, C., Duval, S., & Wilt, T. J. (2007). The association of registered nurse staffing levels and patient outcomes: Systematic review and meta-analysis. *Medical Care, 45*(12), 1195–1204.

Ray, C. E., Jagim, M., Agnew, J., Inglass-McKay, J., & Sheehy, S. (2003). ENA's new guidelines for determining emergency department nurse staffing. *Journal of Emergency Nursing, 29*(3), 245–253.

Reiling, J., Hughes, R. G., & Murphy, M. R. (2008). The impact of facility design on patient safety. In R. G. Hughes (Ed.), *Patient safety and quality: An evidence-based handbook for nurses*. Agency for Healthcare Research and Quality. Retrieved October 4, 2012, from http://www.ahrg.gov/qual/nurseshdbk

Shirey, M. R., & Fisher, M. L. (2008). Leadership agenda for change: Toward healthy work environments in acute and critical care. *Critical Care Nurse, 28*(5), 66–79.

Unruh, L. Y., & Fottler, M. D. (2006). Patient turnover and nursing staff adequacy. *Health Services Research, 47*(20), 599–612.

SUGGESTED READINGS

Brennan, C. W., & Daly, B. J. (2009). Patient acuity: A concept analysis. *Journal of Advanced Nursing, 65*(5), 1114–1126.

Kalisch, B. J., & Lee, K. H. (2011). Nurse staffing levels and teamwork: A cross-sectional study of patient care units in acute care hospitals. *Journal of Nursing Scholarship, 43*(1), 82–88.

Kirschling, J. M., Colgan, C., & Andrews, B. (2011). Predictors of registered nurses' willingness to remain in nursing. *Nursing Economics, 29*(3), 111–117.

Needleman, J., Buerhaus, P., Pankratz, S., Leibson, C. L., Stevens, S. R., & Harris, M. (2011). Nurse staffing and inpatient hospital mortality. *New England Journal of Medicine, 364*(11), 1035–1045.

Welton, J. M., Zone-Smith, L., & Bandyopadhyay, D. (2009). Estimating nursing intensity and direct cost using the nurse-patient assignment. *The Journal of Nursing Administration, 39*(6), 276–284.

Whitehead, D. K., Weiss, S. A., & Tappen, R. M. (2010). Essentials of nursing leadership and management. Philadelphia, PA: F. A. Davis Company. Retrieved October 1, 2012, from http://www.ebscohost.com

Windle, P. E. (2008). Addressing the nurse staffing shortage. *Journal of PeriAnesthesia Nursing, 23*(3), 209–214.

CHAPTER 10

Budget Concepts for Patient Care

CORINNE HAVILEY, RN, MS, PHD; LAURA J. NOSEK, RN, PHD; IDA M. ANDROWICH, RN, BC, PHD, FAAN; AND KIM AMER, RN, PHD

The purpose of creating and analyzing records of what transpires in hospitals is to know how the money is being spent; whether it is, in fact, doing good, or whether it is doing mischief.

—FLORENCE NIGHTINGALE, 1859

OBJECTIVES

Upon completion of this chapter, the reader should be able to:

1. Discuss national and international perspectives on the cost of health care.
2. Discuss budgets commonly used for planning and management.
3. Describe key elements that influence budget preparation.
4. Identify revenue and expenses associated with the delivery of nursing service

You are assigned to a patient care unit for your clinical experience. You are wondering what types of services are provided to patients on this unit. You talk with your instructor and the nursing manager of the unit. Together, you review the unit's scope of service and budget.

What kinds of nursing services are provided to patients on this unit?

How does the unit's budget help ensure the provision of high-quality, safe nursing care for patients on this unit?

Does the unit share how it measures the budget to make sure that they are using their resources efficiently?

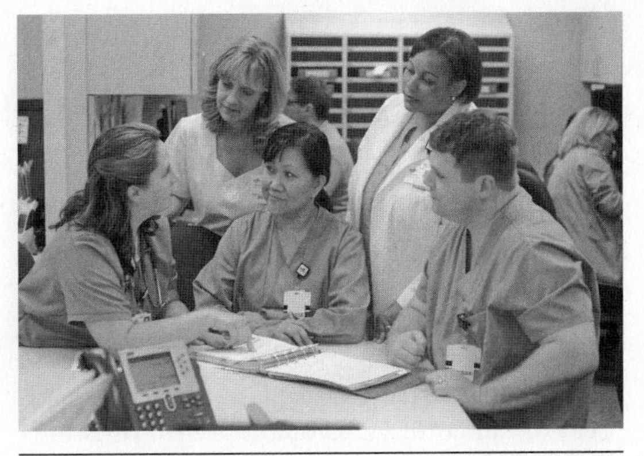

Source: Photo by Bart Harris photography. Used with permission of Central DuPage Hospital.

Regardless of how expert, creative, collaborative, and altruistic a health care system may be, it cannot function without money. Securing the bottom line is basic to achieving the mission of providing health care. Nurses need to understand concepts of budgeting and economics to help secure this bottom line. **Economics** is the study of how scarce resources are allocated among possible uses in order to make appropriate choices among the increasingly scarce resources.

The study of economics is based on three general premises: (1) scarcity—resources exist in finite quantities and consumption demand is typically greater than resource supply; (2) choice—decisions are made about which resources to produce and consume among many options; and (3) preference—individual and societal values and preferences influence the decisions that are made. In a traditional market economy, the sellers sell to the buyers who buy, with each trying to maximize their gains from the transactions. Health care does not fit well in this model. For example, consider the concept of price elasticity, which is related to the price that an individual is willing to pay for a given item. Normally, as the price goes up, the demand goes down. When the purchase is health care, however, the price may be viewed as irrelevant to the decision to purchase. Think of a wristwatch that you might always purchase for $10, would likely not buy at $100, and would never consider at $1,000. Now, imagine that instead of a wristwatch, the item in question is a medication or therapy needed to save your sick child. Now the consideration of price in the decision-making process is likely quite different. Thus, health care is much less "elastic" with reference to price from many other consumer goods.

Another aspect of health care's difference from the traditional economic model relates to the knowledge of options and payment mechanisms available to the consumer. In a typical market, the buyer is also the payer. In health care, the health care provider (buyer) ordering a hospitalization or treatment is a doctor or nurse. The provider is not the payer, nor is the patient (buyer) who is using the hospital or treatment the payer. The actual payer is the third-party reimburser (insurance company or government). Consequently, the financial impact of the decision on the provider (buyer) and the patient user (buyer) is skewed. Neither of these buyers is the payer.

This chapter presents basic health care budgeting and economics concepts that are important to the novice nurse entering clinical practice. Included are perspectives on national and international costs of health care. Additionally, hospital departmental budgets will be explored along with the key elements that influence budget preparation, including revenue and expenses associated with the delivery of patient care. Finally, monitoring of a budget will be reviewed as it relates to the scope of service unique to different units and departments.

NATIONAL AND INTERNATIONAL PERSPECTIVES ON THE COST OF HEALTH CARE

The United States health care industry has experienced intense consumer-, insurer-, and government-generated examination of quality and cost in recent years. Consumers, insurers, and the government expect expeditious diagnosis and treatment of disease, measurable positive patient outcomes, error reduction, and a consistent and competent workforce in spite of waning financial reimbursement, professional provider shortages, and staff dissatisfaction with the work environment (Kimball, 2005). Health care spending has continued to increase, outpacing incomes in most westernized countries.

There is mounting pressure in the United States as one result of the economic downturn to manage the rising costs of health care while ensuring that value and choice are maintained. U.S. health care costs are reported as two times higher than other wealthy nations (Davis et al., 2007). Health care needs are a topic of tremendous scrutiny because of concerns related to how to pay for these services.

According to the Commonwealth Fund (2011), health care spending comprises 16 percent of the U.S. gross domestic product (GDP). The U.S. percentage of GDP health care spending has increased at a fast rate from 9 percent in 1980 to 16 percent of GDP in 2009. Health care spending per capita in the United States is close to double that of many other countries (Figure 10-1).

What is very important to note is that U.S. performance measures are not surpassing other countries as they relate to mortality rates amenable to health care. Since the 2006 Commonwealth Fund National Scorecard, the United States has fallen into last place among 16 industrialized countries on national rates of "mortality amenable to health care"—deaths before age 75 that are caused by at least partially preventable or treatable conditions such

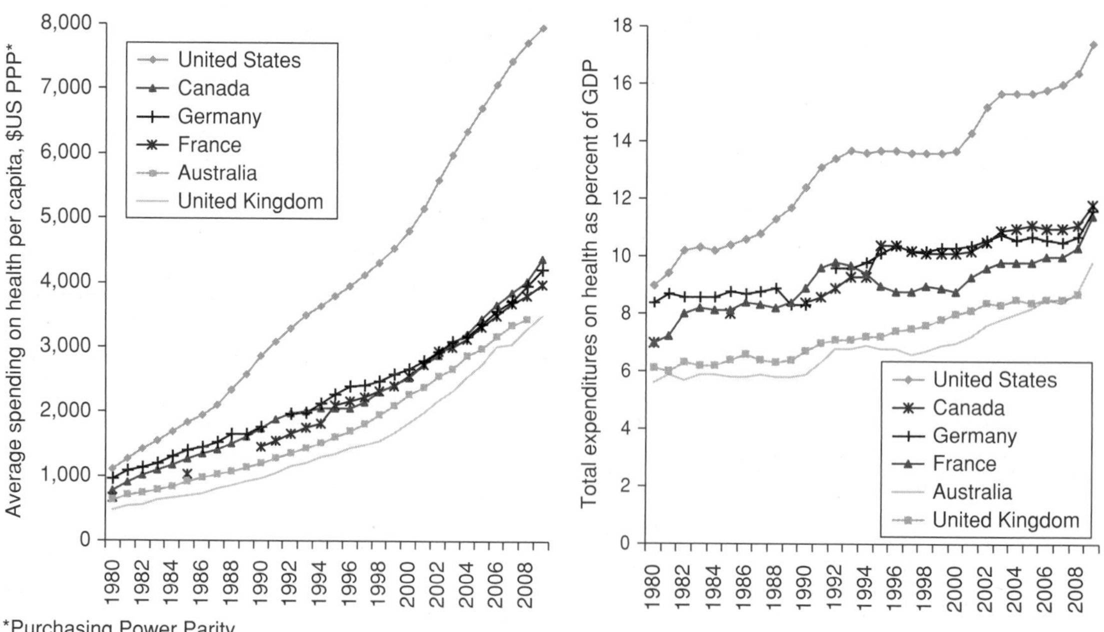

FIGURE 10-1

International comparison of spending on health, 1980–2009.

(*Source:* Commonwealth Fund National Scorecard on U.S. Health System Performance. (2011). Retrieved January 3, 2012, from http://www.commonwealthfund.org/~/media/Files/Publications/Fund%20Report/2011/Oct/1500_WNTB_Natl_Scorecard_2011_web.pdf)

as bacterial infections, screenable cancers, diabetes, heart disease, stroke, or complications of common surgical procedures. While the U.S. rate improved 21 percent between 1997–98 and 2006–07 (from 120 to 96 deaths per 100,000), rates improved by 32 percent, on average, in the other countries. The United States lagged markedly in preventing or delaying deaths among people under age 65 (Figure 10-2).

Higher spending does not match up with better outcomes. In a recent study examining a comparison of six indicators (access, quality care, efficiency, equity, healthy lives, and health expenditures per capita), the United States ranked last in contrast with five westernized countries (Davis et al., 2007). Health care costs continue to rise and there is significant consumer dissatisfaction.

In an effort to contain costs, one U.S. government payer source, the Centers for Medicaid & Medicare Services (CMS), has developed quality criteria to measure and pay hospitals related to patient care in the past several years. Hospitals are now required by the CMS to report their performance on specific health care quality measures.

The CMS Hospital Inpatient Quality Reporting (Hospital IQR) program was mandated by the Medicare Prescription Drug Improvement and Modernization Act (MMA) of 2003, and the Deficit Reduction Act of 2005. The CMS Hospital IQR program requires hospitals to submit quality measurement data for common health problems and diseases for patients who use Medicare, for example, patients with pneumonia, myocardial infarction, or heart failure. Hospitals that do not participate can receive an annual reduction of 2 percent in hospital reimbursement.

Some of these quality measures include inpatient satisfaction rates and compliance with core measures. **Core measures** are a set of quality health care indicators established using evidence-based practice that have been shown to reduce the risk of patient complications, prevent illness reoccurrences, and otherwise treat the majority of patients who come to a hospital for treatment of a condition or illness, for example, quality health care indicators for patients with acute myocardial infarction, heart failure, surgical infection prevention, hospital-based inpatient psychiatric services, hospital outpatient department measures, immunization, perinatal care, pneumonia,

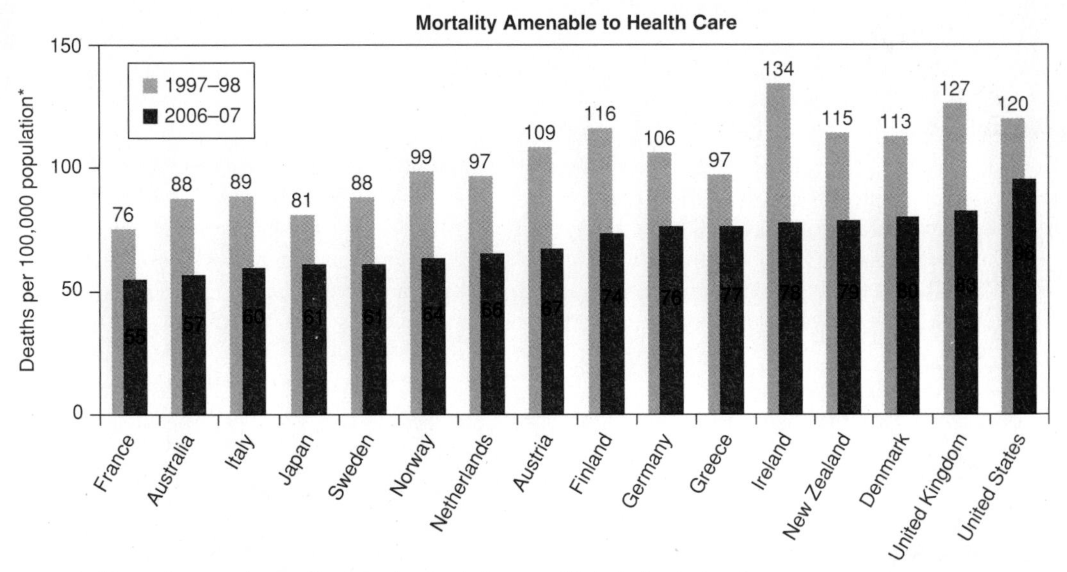

FIGURE 10-2

Mortality amenable to health care.

(*Source:* Commonwealth Fund National Scorecard on U.S. Health System Performance. (2011). Retrieved January 3, 2012, from http://www.commonwealthfund.org/~/media/Files/Publications/Fund%20Report/2011/Oct/1500_WNTB_Natl_Scorecard_2011_web.pdf.)

stroke, surgical care improvement project, and venous thromboembolism. Core measures can be viewed at: http://www.jointcommission.org/core_measure_set/. Hospital performance measures are available on a website for public viewing: http://www.hospitalcompare.hhs.gov. Note that hospital performance is variable related to conforming to the expectations of managing core measures (Curry et al., 2011).

Additionally, hospital reimbursement has been eliminated for certain "never events." **Never events** are preventable, serious events that should never occur in a hospital and include items such as patient incidence of pressure ulcers, surgery on the wrong leg, and so on. The National Quality Forum initially defined 27 such never events in 2002 and revised and expanded the list in 2006. The list is grouped into six categorical events: surgical, product or device, patient protection, care management, environmental, and criminal events Agency for Healthcare Research and Quality(AHRQ). (2006) Never Events. retrieved November 8, 2012 from http://www.psnet.ahrq.gov/primer.aspx?primerID=3. primer.aspx?primerID=3. There are also CMS plans to reduce hospital reimbursement rates based upon patient readmission rates, for example, readmission of a patient for the treatment of congestive heart failure.

As these reimbursement challenges continue, hospitals need to manage their financial health in order to prosper in the future. That is why creating and managing a budget is so important (Curry et al., 2011).

THE COST EQUATION: MONEY = MISSION = MONEY

The mission statement of any health care business or unit describes the purpose for existence of the business or unit and the rationale that justifies that

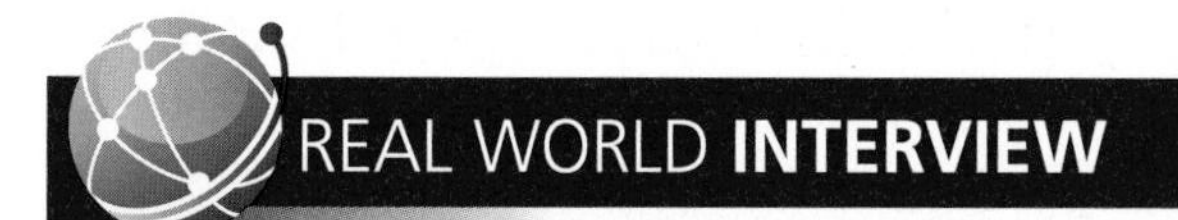

REAL WORLD INTERVIEW

Perhaps the most challenging part of the budget process in health care is finding an efficient and effective method to enlist the involvement and intellectual capital of our staff. Labor costs, on average, constitute 60 percent of a department's budget. Balancing the budget and obtaining staff nurse input for key budget decisions about their practice is imperative. Our organization uses a value analysis program (VAP) to ensure efficient staff involvement in decisions about the products and services that staff members use in their daily practice.

Our value analysis program ensures that, whenever quality is equivalent, cost is the greater factor in making a decision about products and services. The VAP is brought to life through our value analysis teams (VAT) for key areas, for example, medical-surgical units and the operating room. Nurses lead and participate in these teams. The VATs align with our organization's commitment to thoughtful stewardship in providing the highest-quality health care to our patients. The nurses on the VATs are supported by the purchasing and finance departments with financial and utilization data. These nurses explore literature on best practices and national standards such as those of the Oncology Nursing Society.

Recently, one medical-surgical VAT identified an opportunity to reduce the inventory of selected medical-surgical supplies on their unit. They looked at the amount of supplies used per day, decided on the appropriate inventory, and achieved an immediate cost savings of $4,500. They set a targeted cost savings and continue to monitor their progress through a budget dashboard that reports average daily costs of supplies. They make adjustments as needed.

Our staff feels a commitment to the VAT process and realizes the importance of their input into decision making. The organization identifies the value of staff involvement in this process and incorporates this into our budget cycle.

BARBARA BUTURUSIS, RN, MSN
Executive Director, Cancer Services
Loyola University Medical Center
Maywood, Illinois

existence. The mission directs decision making about what is or is not within the purview of the business or unit. The vision statement is a logical extension of the mission into the future and establishes long-range goals for the business or unit. Once the vision is established and the business can articulate where it wants to go, a strategic plan that identifies how to achieve the vision or how to accomplish the goals is developed. There must be cohesion and consistency across the mission, vision, and strategic plan for the business or unit to successfully achieve its mission. There must also be money, for without it no mission can be accomplished.

Business Profit

Revenue (income) minus cost (expense) equals profit. Profit is not restricted to for-profit businesses. "Profit" is not a dirty word. All businesses must realize a profit to remain in business. In for-profit businesses, a portion of the profit is distributed to stockholders in appreciation for their investing in the business and the remainder is used to maintain and grow the organization. In non-profit businesses, there are no stockholders to share the profit, so all of it is fed back into the business for maintenance and growth.

Not-for-profit organizations desiring a purer image than the term "profit"engenders refer to their profit as a contribution to **margin**, with the rule of thumb being to secure 4 to 5 percent of the total budget as profit or margin. A truism of business is: no margin, no mission. Mission and margin are strategically and operationally linked by the reality that resources are required to carry out the organization's strategic plan and achieve its mission. Without margin, or with limited margin, there would be a lack of money to replace worn-out equipment, to establish new services or enlarge existing services in response to changing community needs for health care, to purchase state-of-the-art technology, to improve salaries, to maintain existing buildings or undertake new construction, and to replace heating and lighting systems. Failure to maintain such infrastructure can impair the organization's ability to be competitive, resulting in failure to meet its mission and, eventually, organizational failure.

Right to Health Care at Any Cost

The American belief system has held that every individual has a right to all the knowledge, skill, and technology related to health care at any cost, although certain factors such as race, location, and income have had an effect on the availability of health care. In an attempt to ease the burden of health care costs, the U.S. government stepped up in 1965 and enacted Titles XVIII and XIX, amendments to the Social Security Act, commonly referred to as Medicare and Medicaid, which provide health care coverage for the elderly and the indigent, respectively. CMS. (2011). Medicare and Medicaid, Brief summaries. Retrieved November 8, 2012, from http://www.cms.gov/Research-Statistics-Data-and-Systems/Statistics-Trends-and-Reports/MedicareProgramRatesStats/Downloads/Medicare-MedicaidSummaries2011.pdf.

In 1993, the Oregon Health Plan, the state's Medicaid program, introduced health care rationing. It was intended to make health care more available to the working poor while rationing benefits. The system involves a treatment schedule that lists 649 potentially covered procedures. The state pegs the number of procedures the state will cover to the available funds. Patients requiring procedures above the cut-off line are out of luck. As of October 2010, only the first 502 treatments were covered. The Oregon Health Plan also rations covered procedures under certain circumstances. Chemotherapy, for instance, is not provided if it is deemed to have a 5 percent or less chance of extending the patient's life for 5 years, meaning that a patient whose life might be extended a year or two with chemotherapy

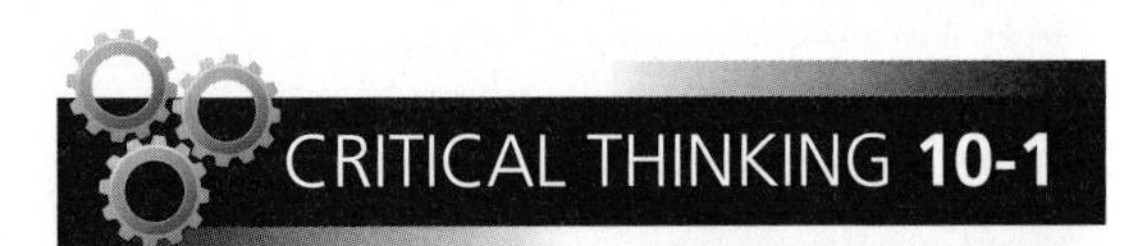

You notice that a colleague frequently does not record patient charge items for elderly patients. When you inquire about it, you are told that your colleague feels sorry for those on fixed incomes and wants to save them money. Who pays when your colleague does this?

may not receive it (Oregonian PolitiFact Oregon, 2011). Neonates who are born with a weight of less than 500 grams are not provided intensive care, because the outcomes are very poor with such extreme prematurity. While controversial, many believe that citizens, patients, and health care providers must develop clear criteria for how health care dollars should be spent, as money for health care is not limitless. End-of-life care is the most expensive, and potentially the least effective if patients languish on long-term life support.

Information Technology, Salary, and Medication Costs

Close examination of a health care budget often reveals that although the nursing payroll is the most expensive payroll item and the most expensive operating budget item, the most expensive item on the total budget is often diagnostic, implantable pacemakers ($4,218), CT scanners ($1,081,200), and MRI equipment ($1,674,322) Modern Healthcare. (2012).

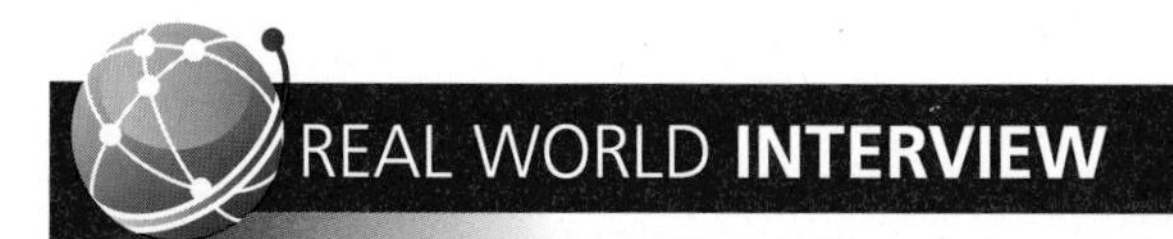

REAL WORLD INTERVIEW

In order to be successful, all health care organizations need to strategize regarding financial performance. Nursing managers receive training to develop unit budgets based on long-range financial planning and organizational goals. Staff nurses, as well, need to have input into the budget process. The budget is developed based upon a projected average daily census or number of procedures. Patient acuity is also taken into consideration, along with the patient population. Patient acuity is based on the severity of the patient's illness and the nursing time that is needed to meet the patient's needs, that is, the time it takes to frequently monitor vital signs, intake and output, and to give additional nursing support to the patient with feeding tubes, frequent suctioning, and so on. Many organizations compare their operations against national benchmarks using the daily nursing care hours required for different types of nursing units and patient populations. Organizations may rely on the finance department to forecast increased patient volume, and the need for growth in patient care programs and patient service lines. The nurse at the bedside is very valuable in providing input into the budgetary process. This is accomplished by evaluating appropriate nurse/patient ratios for their patient populations, examining patient acuity, and assisting in projecting appropriate staffing levels for various work shifts and days of the week. Nurses at the bedside can also identify additional support needs as well as equipment needs. This all helps with budget planning. The use of staffing guidelines, that is, the number of nurses needed to care for a specific number of patients or patients with various acuity levels, as well as the use of reports that measure nursing productivity, helps the staff nurse to participate in managing the staffing budget on a daily basis. Giving nurses at the bedside the autonomy to flex the number of staff either up or down as appropriate, and using patient census and patient acuity as key measures, promotes accountability and ownership of appropriate staffing decisions. Based on the census and patient acuity on the unit as well as on the patient-expected admissions, transfers, and discharges, nurses can plan staffing patterns for the oncoming work shift. This is called "flexing up and down." It includes floating staff to units that need more help, and utilizing a float pool of both available staff and agency or registry staff when needed for patient care. Nursing productivity measures the direct patient care hours and the indirect hours, which include education time, orientation time, and sick and vacation time. This also needs to be calculated at budget time.

CAROL PAYSON, MSN, RN
Director of Surgical Services
Northwestern Memorial Hospital
Chicago, Illinois

The high cost of technology has been recognized by regulatory agencies for many years. In pursuit of cost control in hospitals, the states independently established laws more than 30 years ago creating Certificate of Need (CON) agencies to oversee, regulate, and approve major technology and construction expenditures. A secondary goal was to ensure equitable distribution of and access to high-end technology across the state. The CON approach was not successful because it focused only on hospitals and provided no incentives to change either physician or patient behavior. Hospitals were given spending limits, but there was no incentive for physicians to change their practice, so they did not. Without incentives, patients' expectations and demands for care also remained unchanged. More recently, managed care programs have exerted oversight of the use of complex, expensive technology by requiring justification and approval prior to its use for payment to occur. Also, there has been a movement toward rationing the most expensive technology to those with the ability and willingness to pay for it over and above their health insurance coverage. The best-selling book *Who Lives? Who Dies? Ethical Criteria in Patient Selection* by John Kilner (1990) underscores public and professional concern about health care rationing. We have begun to see managed care programs become more lenient in response to a public and professional outcry about who possesses the appropriate expertise to make clinical decisions.

Cost of Medications and Health Care Executive Salaries

Medications are a significant item in the overall budget. A recent health care website visit identified the drug charges found in Table 10-1. Also note the health care compensations shown in Table 10-2.

Nursing Cost

Fiscally, most organizations view nursing as a cost center that does not independently generate revenue. Although some deviation from that fiscal philosophy may occur when selected nursing practitioners are permitted by law to bill directly for their unique professional services, the cost of providing nursing care (wages, benefits, selected supplies and equipment, overhead) is commonly bundled into a catchall (room or per diem) cost that assumes that every patient consumes identical nursing resources each day. Such a view is not only antiquated, it is incorrect. Nursing care is not an identical product delivered in assembly-line fashion. It varies remarkably in intensity, in depth, and in breadth across patients, consistent with their unique, individual dependency needs.

Access to a high degree of nursing care is an important reason for hospitalization. When access to both nursing care and medical technology is needed, hospitalization is unquestionably appropriate. Consequently, the revenue generated from hospitalization is, in fact, payment primarily for consumption of medical technology and nursing services and should be recognized as such.

TABLE 10-1
Cost of Selected Medications

Drug	Strength	Price
Acyclovir	200 mg capsules	$14.99 for 30 capsules
Advair Diskus	28 250-50 mcg/dose Aerosol Disp Pack	$105.99 each pack
Lipitor	10 mg tablets	$114.99 for 30 tablets
Lisinopril	2.5 mg tablets	$12.99 for 30 tablets
Lorazepam	0.5 mg tablets	$14.99 for 30 tablets
Nexium	20 mg delayed release capsules	$201.00 for 30 capsules

Source: http://www.drugstore.com, accessed 11.11.2011

TABLE 10-2
Health Care Compensation

Position	Salary	Source
CEO—MD	$393,152 median	http://www.beckershospitalreview.com/compensation-issues/physician-executive-compensation-how-are-top-physician-leaders-paid.html Cejka Physician Executive Compensation Survey 2011
CEO—Children's hospitals	$1,965,682 average	http://www.kaiserhealthnews.org/Stories/2011/September/28/Chart-CEO-Pay-Packages.aspx
CEO—Trevor Fetter, Tenet Healthcare	$5.85 million (2010)	http://www.forbes.com/lists/2011/12/ceo-compensation-11_Trevor-Fetter_3519.html Forbes CEO Compensation Survey
CEO—Miles White, Abbott Labs	$15.51 million	http://www.forbes.com/sites/christopherhelman/2011/10/12/americas-25-highest-paid-ceos/ Forbes America's Highest Paid Chief Executives 2011
CEO—Richard Bracken, HCA	$38.2 million	http://www.modernhealthcare.com/article/20110815/MAGAZINE/308159978/?template=printpicart *Modern Healthcare*, August 15, 2011
Medical Director	$269,050 median	http://www.beckershospitalreview.com/compensation-issues/physician-executive-compensation-how-are-top-physician-leaders-paid.html Cejka Physician Executive Compensation Survey 2011
Cardiology	$422,291 median	http://cejka.force.com/PhysicianCompensation#compdata AMGA Physician Compensation Survey excerpt
Family Medicine	$208,658 median	http://cejka.force.com/PhysicianCompensation#compdata AMGA Physician Compensation Survey excerpt
Emergency Care	$285,910 median	http://cejka.force.com/PhysicianCompensation#compdata AMGA Physician Compensation Survey excerpt

(Continues)

TABLE 10-2 (Continued)

Position	Salary	Source
Dentist	$167,389 median	http://www.cejkasearch.com/view-compensation-data/mid-level-compensation-data/ AMGA Mid-Level Compensation Data 2009
Pharmacist	$104,260	http://www.bls.gov/K12/science/02.htm
Nurse Practitioner	$86,410 median	http://www.cejkasearch.com/view-compensation-data/mid-level-compensation-data/ AMGA Mid-Level Compensation Data 2009
Physical Therapist	$69,397 median	http://www.cejkasearch.com/view-compensation-data/mid-level-compensation-data/ AMGA Mid-Level Compensation Data 2009
Registered Nurse	$67,720 mean	http://www.bls.gov/oes/current/oes291111.htm Occupational Employment and Wages, May 2010 29-1111 Registered Nurses?
Nursing Aide	$24,010 median	http://www.bls.gov/ooh/healthcare/nursing-assistants/htm

© Cengage Learning 2014

USE OF THE COMPUTER TO CAPTURE NURSING COSTS

Many hospitals are beginning to examine the use of computerization to capture nursing costs. Computers will be much better able to assist in measuring the nursing resources expended on each patient when algorithms are developed that account for the cognitive and assessment work of nurses, as well as the physical care. At that point, the computer should be able to track sophisticated data on nursing resource usage by a patient. With computers, nurses record not only when they are with each patient but also what they are doing for each patient. The specific cost of the nurse's care can be calculated by having the computer multiply the time spent with the patient by the salary of the nurse providing the care. When nurses are doing some indirect activities, such as documentation, the computer can also assign that cost to the appropriate patient, because the documentation is being done on the computer. The system will need a fast way to record data so that it does not greatly increase the documentation work of the nurse. Radio frequency identification (RFID) chips may eventually assist with that task. An RFID chip embedded in the nurse's name tag can be detected by a sensor in the door frame. The sensor is a data receiver that transmits information to the computer. It records the times of the nurse's entry into and exit from the patient's room and links that information with the patient's hospital ID number. RFID technology is still under development (Finkler and McHugh, 2008).

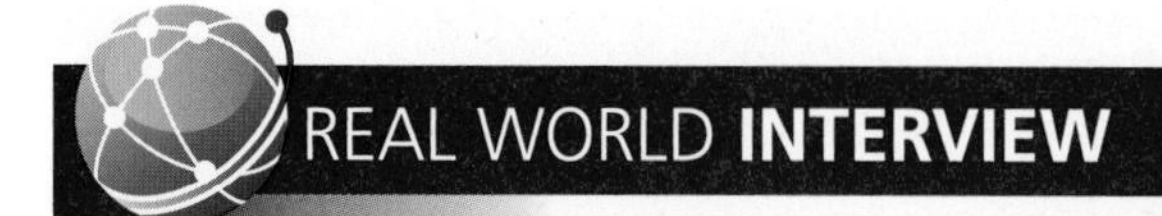

The staff nurse plays a critical role in assisting the unit manager in planning department budgets. Without appropriate planning, department budgets are at risk of not meeting the organization's budget targets. It is important that staff both provide input regarding the current environment and also discuss with the unit manager the goals and objectives for the upcoming fiscal year. Historic data related to patient volume, revenue, and expense is a starting point. However, new programs and services need to be anticipated. In addition, practice changes, safety and quality initiatives, changes in patient populations, and patient acuity must all be considered in the planning process. Unit equipment requirements are another important piece that must be included in capital budget planning.

Ideally, staff nurse input is given on an ongoing basis to the unit manager so that by the time budget planning is started, the unit manager has received comprehensive feedback from many staff who are working different shifts. In addition to assisting with planning, the staff nurse is responsible for managing resources on a daily basis. Resource management is done through supply management and labor management. Nurses work to utilize supplies efficiently and minimize waste. This assists the organization to meet budget targets and reduces unnecessary costs for the patient. Labor costs account for a significant percentage of most nursing budgets. Overtime management is one way in which the staff nurse can assist in meeting the unit budget targets on a daily basis. The staff nurse role is multidimensional. The nurse is not only a clinical care provider but is also a financial manager of the organization's use of resources on a daily basis.

ANNE K. ANDERSON, RN, BSN, MHSA
Director, Patient Care Services Operations
Central DuPage Hospital
Winfield, Illinois

TYPES OF BUDGETS

Health care organizations use several types of budgets to help with future planning and management. A **budget** is a plan that provides formal quantitative expression for acquiring and distributing funds over the ensuing time period (generally one year). A budget is based on what is known about how much was spent in the past and how that will inevitably change in the coming year. The types of budgets are operational, capital, and construction.

Operational Budget

An **operational budget** accounts for the income and expenses associated with day-to-day activity within a department or organization. Revenue generation is based on billable services and expenses associated with equipment, supplies, staffing, and other indirect costs. Revenue may be based on the number of days that a patient stays on an inpatient unit or the number of hours spent in a procedure room. Revenue may also be based on the types of procedures delivered to a patient. Depending on reimbursement rates and requirements, expenses are sometimes bundled or included into a procedure or room charge, for example, an admission packet that includes a washbasin, cup, soap holder, and so on. In other situations, supply items may be billed separately, such as IV start kits, or leukocyte removal filters.

Capital Budget

A **capital budget** accounts for the purchase of major new or replacement equipment. Equipment is purchased when new technology becomes available or when older equipment becomes too expensive to maintain because of age-related problems such as inefficiencies resulting from the decreased speed of equipment or increased downtime (amount of time it is out of service for repairs). Sometimes equipment maintenance is cost-prohibitive due to the expense and limited availability of replacement parts. Other times equipment may become antiquated because of its inability to deliver service consistently, meet industry or regulatory standards, or provide high-quality outcomes.

Construction Budget

A **construction budget** is developed when renovation or new structures are planned and generally includes labor, materials, building permits, inspections, equipment, and so on. If it is anticipated that a department will need to close during construction, then projected lost revenue is accounted for in the budget. Revenue and expenses may also be shifted to another department that absorbs the services on a temporary basis.

BUDGET OVERVIEW

An operational budget is a financial tool that outlines anticipated revenue and expenses over a specified period. A process called **accounting**, which is an activity that managers engage in to record and report financial transactions and data, assists with budget documentation. Budgets serve as standards to plan, monitor, and evaluate the performance of a health care system. Budgets account for the income generated as compared to the expenses needed to deliver the service. **Profit** is determined by the relationship of income to expenses and results when the income is higher than the expenses.

Budgets make the connection between operational planning and allocation of resources. This is especially important because health care organizations measure multiple key indicators of overall performance. These key indicators can be illustrated in a dashboard. A **dashboard** or balanced scorecard is a documentation tool providing a snapshot image of pertinent information and activity reflecting quality performance at a particular point in time. Figure 10-3 shows the dashboard of two separate units: the emergency department and a medical unit. **Variance**, or the difference between what was budgeted and the actual result, can be tracked.

Budget Preparation and Scope of Service

Formulating a budget involves a systematic approach that begins with preparation. Budgets are generally developed for a 12-month period and are monitored monthly. The yearly cycle can be based on a fiscal year as determined by the organization (e.g., September 1 through August 31) or a calendar year (e.g., January 1 through December 31). Shorter- or longer-term budgets may also be developed depending on the organizational planning process.

Prior to the beginning of the budget year, most organizations devote approximately six months to preparing and developing the operational budget. To prepare a budget, organizations gather fundamental information about a variety of elements that influence the organization, including patient demographic and marketing information such as age, race, sex, and income; competitive analysis; regulatory influences; strategic plans; goals; and history. Additionally, it is helpful to review the department's scope of service (Table 10-3).

Marketing

Marketing is the process of creating a product or health care service for patients, and it uses the four "P"s of marketing, that is, Patient, Product, Price, and Placement, to place desirable health care services or products in desirable locations at a price that benefits both patients and the health care facility. In this way, the health care facility, the patient, and the community benefit. Marketing of services does have a price tag, such as the cost of advertising campaigns on television and radio. Using printed materials, mailing information to patient residences, and advertising in journals, magazines, and newspapers are all examples of ways to educate and stimulate the public for future referrals for health care services. Once marketing strategies are implemented, most organizations attempt to measure their effectiveness, or return on investment.

Pulling together demographic information relative to the population that the organization serves is most helpful because it identifies unique market characteristics, such as age, race, sex, and income that

Metric	Target Performance	1-Jan	1-Feb	1-Mar	1-Apr	1-May	1-Jun
Efficiency							
Emergency Department							
Last year volume	64,904	5353	4917	5922	5798	6297	5540
Current volume	63,750	5540	5183	5434	5281	5670	5563
Medicine Unit							
Bed Request to Bed Assigned (in Minutes)	30 min	40	38	38	37	31	20
Bed Assigned to Patient Placement (in Minutes)	30 min	60	55	50	63	58	46
Patient Satisfaction - Scores in Percentile Rank							
Emergency Department							
Overall Quality of Care	85	99.5	88.5	92.2	63.9	92.9	92.2
Discharge Calls - % Attempted	90%	81%	77.0%	79.1%	74.8%	75%	67%
Medicine Unit							
Overall Quality of Care	85	85.0	82.5	84.5	85.5	90	80.6
Discharge Calls - % Attempted	90%	90.0%	60.0%	56.0%	78.8%	80%	70%
Regulatory Compliance & Quality							
Emergency Department							
Misidentified Specimens	0	4	0	5	0	1	1
Moderate Sedation Flow Sheet Documentation	95%	91%	96%	89%	94%	94%	96%
Total Narcotic Discrepancies	0	7	7	6	6	15	8
Number of Discrepancies Resolved	100%	7	7	6	6	15	8
Narcotic Counts	100%	100%	90%	86%	80%	82%	100%
Medicine Unit							
PNI (Pneumonia Core Measures) - Misses	0	2	0	0	0	0	0
AMI (acute myocardial infarction core measures) - Misses	0	1	0	2	1	0	1
Stroke Tool Compliance	100%	75%	83%	44%	86%	88%	100%
Hand Hygiene Compliance	90%	96%	76%	80%	75%	79%	89%

FIGURE 10-3 (*Continues*)

Dashboard, emergency department and medical unit.

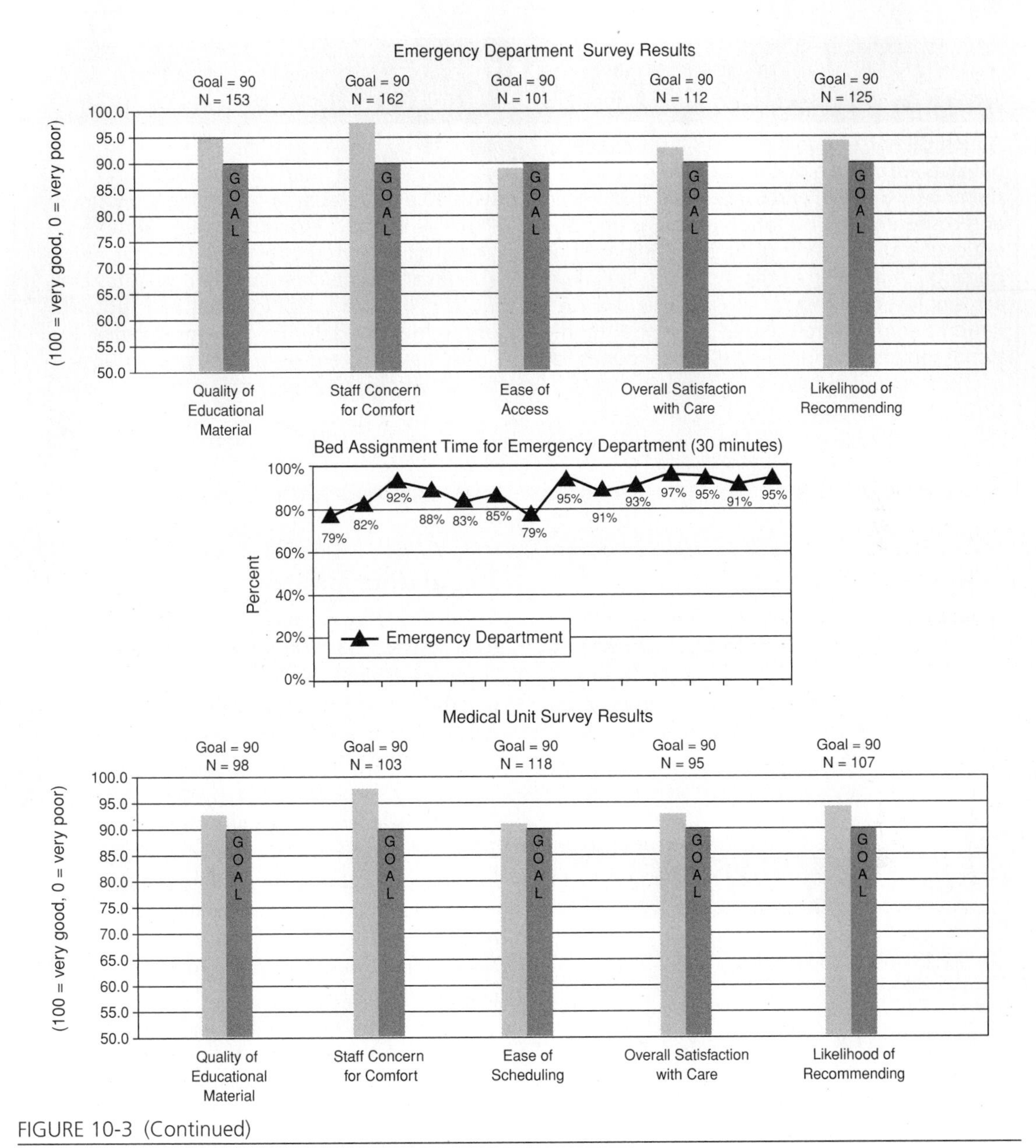

FIGURE 10-3 (Continued)

Dashboard, emergency department and medical unit.

(*Source:* Adapted with permission of Central DuPage Hospital, Winfield, Illinois.)

influence patient behavior. Marketing strategies are built around the population types that an organization is attempting to attract. For example, if a hospital is opening an open heart or transplant department, then outreach activities might be developed to attract those patients who can benefit from the open heart or transplant department screening, prevention, or treatment services.

TABLE 10-3
Medical Nursing Unit, Scope of Service

A medical nursing unit provides high-quality, patient-centered, safe care to hospitalized patients with acute or chronic medical problems, such as congestive heart failure, diabetes, pulmonary disease, and cancer. The unit, equipped with 30 private beds, a full kitchen, a lounge, and conference/consultation rooms, is operational 24 hours per day, 7 days per week. Patient education and support groups are held routinely in the library located directly on the unit. Team nursing is employed as the model of care. Nurses, patient care technicians, and unit secretaries are employed, with a social worker and diabetes educator providing additional patient support. Patients admitted to the unit for longer than 48 hours are discussed during daily interprofessional rounds. The interprofessional rounds include: case management personnel; psychosocial counselors; and nutrition, nursing, and medical staff. Staff discuss patient problems to facilitate future care, including discharge planning.

© Cengage Learning 2014

Competitive Analysis

A competitive analysis is important because it probes how the competition is performing as compared to other health care organizations. A competitive analysis examines other hospitals' or practices' strengths and weaknesses, in addition to details such as location and new or existing services and technology. Table 10-4 presents a competitive analysis of three different hospitals.

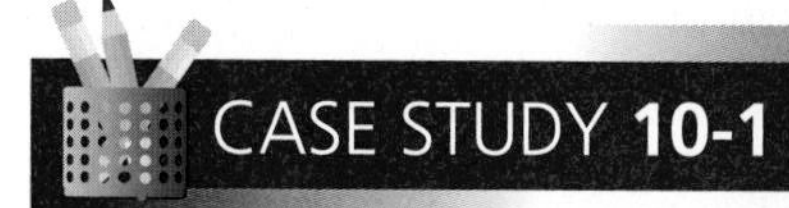

The manager from an inpatient unit asks for staff input into identifying ways to decrease use of health care supply and paper items. These items have been identified as being in excess of the budget by 10 to 20 percent during the past three months. This is the first time that the staff have been involved in helping with cost containment. Clinical nurses and assistants have been invited to participate.

When approaching an analysis of health care supply use, what might be the first step in the process? If you were to break the staff into workgroups, which members should be chosen to analyze the use of clerical supplies? How would you proceed if you were trying to determine the supply costs associated with starting an IV with continuous intravenous infusions and medications? Would nursing and pharmacy be helpful in this process?

Regulatory Influences

Regulatory requirements and reimbursement rates have an effect on financial performance. Regulatory changes are influenced by several governing bodies. A government agency that has high visibility in the area of reimbursement is the Centers for Medicare & Medicaid Services (CMS), whose mission is to ensure health care security for beneficiaries. CMS (http://www.cms.hhs.gov) administers federal control, quality assurance, and fraud and abuse prevention for Medicare, Medicaid, and the State Children's Health Insurance Program (SCHIP). Under the aegis of the Department of Health and Human Services, it is also responsible for coordinating health care policy, planning, and legislation.

Other regulatory bodies play a role in reimbursement by ensuring that federal and state laws are adhered to through approval and accreditation. For example, the Food and Drug Administration (http://www.fda.gov) regulates the use of drugs, food products, and medical devices in the United States. If equipment or drugs under its jurisdiction are not approved, then organizations cannot bill for their use, by law. The Joint Commission (JC) (http://www.jointcommission.org) accredits hospitals and health care agencies to ensure that they meet specific standards. Medicare & Medicaid will not reimburse for services unless a hospital is accredited by the JC.

TABLE 10-4
Competitive Analysis of Three Hospitals

Competitive Analysis: Hospital A

Location: Rural—100 miles from metropolitan area

Affiliation: Currently negotiating with three academic hospitals

General clinical description:

- Scattered bed approach to inpatient oncology
- Ambulatory chemotherapy clinic
- Many of the same physicians on staff at Hospital J

Radiation capability: None—refers to Hospital J

Support services: Cancer screenings offered sporadically

Miscellaneous:

- Tumor board
- Cancer committee

Competitive Analysis: Hospital B

Location: Suburb of large metropolitan city

Affiliation: University hospital

General clinical description:

- Dedicated oncology inpatient unit
- Ambulatory chemotherapy department
- Comprehensive breast center
- Head and neck oncology team

Radiation therapy:

- Linear accelerator—two units
- High dose rate
- Intraoperative radiation therapy
- Stereotactic radiosurgery

Support services:

- Home infusion and home care program
- Hospice care program
- Annual cancer awareness fair
- Support group—general cancer patients

Miscellaneous:

- Tumor registry
- Tumor board
- Committee on cancer

(Continues)

TABLE 10-4 (Continued)

- Head and neck patient conferences
- Stereotactic radiosurgery conferences

Competitive Analysis: Hospital C

Location: Urban city with a population of 150,000

Affiliation: For-profit corporation

- Medical oncology affiliation with University K
- Radiation Therapy Department affiliation with University K Radiation Therapy Department

General clinical description:

- Dedicated inpatient medical oncology unit
- Dedicated inpatient surgical oncology unit
- Four-bed autologous and stem cell bone marrow transplant unit (Eastern Cooperative Oncology Group Referral Center for autologous bone marrow transplants)
- Coagulation laboratory
- Therapeutic Pheresis
- Pain clinic
- Oncology clinic
- Oncology rehabilitation
- Breast cancer rehabilitation program
- Ambulatory care chemotherapy unit
- Medical oncologist on staff at two hospitals

Radiation therapy:

- Linear accelerator
- Stereotactic radiosurgery
- Hyperthermia
- Brachytherapy

Support services:

- Home health and hospice program
- Cancer registry
- Cancer committee
- Physician update—quarterly cancer newsletter
- Cancer information line
- Cancer advisory council
- Cancer Survivor's Day offered annually
- Cancer screenings offered routinely
- Cancer support group—general cancer patients

© Cengage Learning 2014

Regulatory requirements may change regarding who may deliver a specific service and in what type of setting; for example, a procedure may have to be done in the hospital rather than in a practitioner's office if it is to be reimbursed by the insurance company. Medicare & Medicaid change their reimbursement rates periodically. Total and partial coverage of specific procedures can change and may not be predictable from year to year.

Managed care organizations and insurance companies typically negotiate rates on a yearly basis, which can affect hospital revenue. Consumers' willingness to pay out of pocket when not covered by insurance affects revenue as well.

Strategic Plans, Goals, and History

During the budget preparation phase, it is important to examine the history of an individual nursing unit or hospital thoroughly. These nursing or hospital units, departments, or sections, commonly called **cost centers**, are used for organizational purposes to track financial data. Each department or cost center defines its own scope of service, goals, and strategic plans. This is an ongoing, ever-changing process.

Revenue Projections

Revenue is income generated through a variety of means, including billable patient services, investments, and donations to the organization. Specific unit-based revenue is generated through billing for services such as X-rays, invasive diagnostic or therapeutic procedures, drug therapy, surgical procedures, and physical therapy. Revenue can also be generated through the delivery of multiple services over time, such as hourly rates for chemotherapy administration or blood transfusions. The specific number and types of services and procedures have to be projected for the budget. The payments received by hospitals often do not equal the actual hospital or unit charges for the services rendered. For example, there may be a fixed or flat reimbursement rate per case regardless of how long the patient stays in the hospital or how much the hospital pays for the service. If the costs exceed the reimbursement rate, then the provider absorbs the remaining costs.

It is important to note that the reimbursement rates of third-party payers affect revenue and can change from year to year. Uniform rates are often used, which transfers significant financial risk to the provider. Medicare & Medicaid, managed care companies, and insurance companies dictate or negotiate rates with health care organizations that may include discounts or allowances. Payers determine what costs are allowable for procedures, visits, or services. Payment schedules vary from state to state and among plans. Additionally, the rates can change monthly such as with the ambulatory payment classification (APC) system from Medicare, which applies to the outpatient setting.

Another payment classification system called diagnosis-related groups (DRGs) is used to group inpatients into categories based upon the number of inpatient days, age, complications, and so on. Reimbursement covers room and board, tests, and therapy during a predetermined length of stay.

Some patients will not have health care insurance nor the ability to pay their bills. Therefore, the hospital may receive only a portion of the payment for services, if any.

Typically, organizations will review their payer mix to determine the percentage of patients carrying different types of health care coverage (Figure 10-4). The proportions help measure the anticipated dollars to be received for services delivered and projections for the coming year.

If charges for patient care are negotiated with a third-party payer, such as insurance companies and

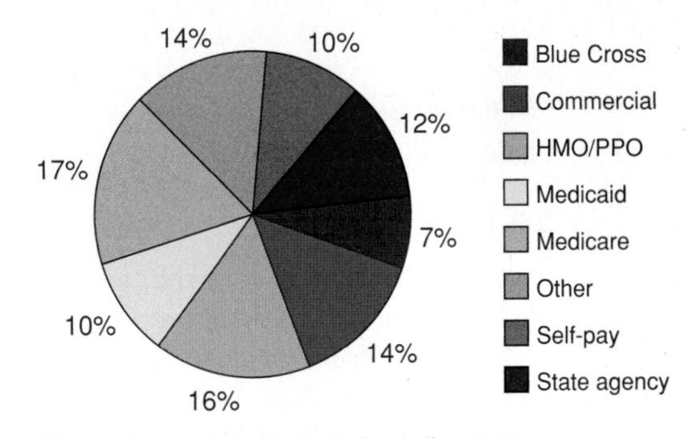

The reimbursement rates vary depending upon the payer. For example, Medicare may reimburse 40% of charges, Medicaid's rate may be 30%, and managed care may be at 60%. Factoring in reimbursement rates leads to profit and loss calculations for an organization.

FIGURE 10-4

Inpatient payer mix.

© Cengage Learning 2014

TABLE 10-5
Total Charges—Central Line Placement $500,000

Third-Party Payer Reimbursement	Rate (Measured in % of Charges)	Expected Reimbursement
Managed Care	60%	$300,000
Medicare	40%	$200,000
Medicaid	30%	$150,000

© Cengage Learning 2014

managed care corporations, they are pre-established and are not negotiable once established. Third-party payers often impose a penalty fee, as a disincentive, if a health care organization changes a charge under contract. The penalty often exceeds the charge amount and will usually create a loss for the organization.

The following illustrates the differences in reimbursement related to a procedure. The charge for a central line placement is $2,500, which includes the use of the fluoroscopy equipment, supplies, nursing, and technical time. If a hospital places 200 central lines per year, then the anticipated total revenue is $500,000. The breakdown of third-party payers becomes important because the total revenue does not mean that the hospital will be reimbursed for the full amount of $500,000. Third-party payers typically contract with health care organizations for the amount that the third-party payer is willing to pay or reimburse. Table 10-5 demonstrates the potential reimbursement rates based upon varying third-party payers.

Expense Projections

Expenses are determined by identifying the costs associated with the delivery of service. Budget expenditures are resources used by an organization to deliver services and may include supplies, staffing, labor, equipment, utilities, and miscellaneous items. See Figure 10-5.

Staffing

The amount and types of staff are often accounted for in a staffing model. The model outlines the number of staff required based upon a primary statistic such as procedures or patients. Figure 10-6 illustrates a sample staffing model.

Staffing ratios and salary data are particularly important because of the cost factor. Specialty salaries fluctuate, depending upon supply and demand (Ponti, Germain, & Mouton, 2010). When there are shortages of certain staff, the salary tends to increase. Additionally, a health care organization may change its benefits, offering a more attractive package that includes: continuing education; paid time off for education, vacation, sick time, or personal needs; or professional membership expenses (Cohen, 2010). Institutions may also look for alternative ways to supplement or deliver services during staff shortages. This means that supplemental staff—professional agency nurses, nurses from in-house registries, or patient care technicians—may be hired at a different salary rate. It is important to note whether a unit has had historical difficulty retaining or recruiting staff. Recruitment and retention, especially attracting, interviewing, hiring, and orienting staff, require dollars. For example, it has been estimated that the turnover cost per nurse, including advertising, recruitment, orientation, and time to fill the vacancy, can equate to a reported range from $22,000 to $66,000 (Jones, 2008) and as high as $88,000 (Krsek 2011). The average cost to educate a nurse during a six-week orientation period is more than $6,000. Not only the salary but also benefits and unproductive time are frequently factored into a salary package, and they need to be included in the budget (Table 10-6).

Direct and Indirect Expenses

Expenses can be further broken down into direct and indirect. **Direct expenses** are those expenses directly associated with the patient, such as medical

Monthly Variance Report*								
	MTD Actual	MTD Budget	Variance	Variance from budget	YTD Actual	YTD Budget	Variance	Variance from budget
Volume - visits	450	500	(50)	-0.10	2905	2885	20	0.01
Gross Revenue	$576,317	$407,312	$169,005	0.41	$1,656,194	$1,235,149	$421,045	0.34
Gross Revenue per Unit of Service	$411.00	$429.40	$(18.40)	-0.04	$570.37	$428.06	$142.31	0.33
Total Expense per Unit of Service	$130.26	$120.31	$(9.95)	(0.08)	$114.06	$120.87	$6.81	0.06
Supply Expense per Unit of Service	$13.74	$23.94	$10.20	0.74	$12.93	$23.93	$11.00	0.85
Total FTEs	10.90	11.00	0.10	0.01	10.61	11	0.39	0.04

	MTD Actual	Staffing Matrix (Fixed) Budget	Productivity	YTD Actual	Staffing Matrix (Fixed) Budget	Productivity
Paid Hours per Unit of Service	1.99	1.98	99.50%	1.92	2	104.17%
Worked Hours per Unit of Service	1.75	1.79	102.29%	1.7	1.81	106.47%

Finance / Action Steps

Volume is slightly down MTD (month to date), but still over budget YTD (year to date). Total expenses are slightly above budget for this month due to changing process for ordering but these expenses are still in line YTD. Plan: Although productivity is strong the department will continue to focus on reducing staffing when volumes are down. Anticipate additional efficiencies with implementation of the charging system which is anticipated to improve revenue capture.

FIGURE 10-5 *(Continues)*

Monthly variance report, emergency department.

Patient Satisfaction / Action Steps

Patient satisfaction overall quality of care rating for this month is at target; however, the quarter results are trending downward. The staff is focusing on total time spent in the department and have developed multiple tools to help patients understand how long it takes to complete a procedure.

Quality Initiatives / Action Steps

The staff is currently working on documentation of services and trauma flow sheet requirements. Audits have been completed to ensure that the staff is in compliance. Action plans are being initiated to educate staff so that lab compliance can be improved. Core measures are strong; time to EKG and CT are at target.

* Values are for instructional purposes only.

FIGURE 10-5 (Continued)

Monthly variance report, emergency department.
(*Source:* Adapted with permission of Central DuPage Hospital, Winfield, Illionois.)

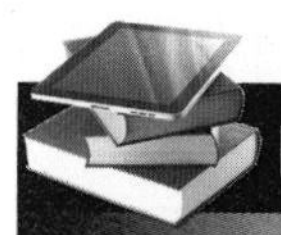

EVIDENCE FROM THE **LITERATURE**

Citation: Goetz, K., Janney, M., & Ramsey, K. (2011). When nursing takes ownership of financial outcomes: Achieving exceptional financial performance through leadership, strategy, and execution. *Nursing Economics, 29* (4), 173–182.

Discussion: Accountability is the key to ensuring that there is a culture that focuses on financial performance as well as quality improvement. This article presents outcomes achieved over a four-year period related to improving nurse-sensitive quality indicators while at the same time reducing overall nursing expenses by $10 million within a large academic hospital. Through the use of standardizing processes, central line associated blood stream infections were reduced by 79 percent, hospital-acquired pressure ulcers were reduced by 66 percent, and patient falls were reduced by 23 percent. Cost savings were achieved by revamping the new nurse orientation to reduce the number of hours required during orientation by 25 percent. This led to a cost savings of $300,000. Additionally, the organization created a sense of urgency when the nursing units were not meeting budget expectations. They used immediate feedback and analysis to get their units back on track so that the financial goals could be met. Another important strategy shared was the elimination of a high-cost weekender program (nurses were paid significantly higher if they worked only weekends, e.g., Friday through Sunday). At one point in the organization's history, there was difficulty finding staff to fill weekend shifts. Now, however, staff were willing to rotate in order to cover all needed shifts.

Implications for Practice: Nursing leadership is responsible for not only the practice of nursing but also for the fiscal and business management of an organization. Utilizing multiple improvement projects targeting varying areas with rigorous follow-through can reduce costs associated with health care and improve the quality of care delivered.

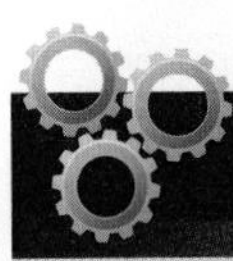

CRITICAL THINKING 10-2

You work in an emergency department (ED) that sees 6,000 patients a month. Patients are charged $200.00 per visit plus charges for tests and medications. Thus, these 6,000 patients can generate $1,200,000 in gross revenue for the hospital. Consider that there are 15 RNs making $30.00 per hour and six MDs making $150.00 per hour working each shift. Salaries for the RNs total $324,000. Salaries for the MDs total $648,000. The total monthly salary for these two groups is $972,000. Of the 6,000 patients, 50 percent have Medicare & Medicaid, 45 percent are covered by managed care or insurance, and 5 percent have no insurance. Thus, just 95 percent of patients can pay their bills. The other 5 percent of patients' bills are written off by the hospital as bad debt.

Medicare & Medicaid or managed care or insurance companies often pay only 55 percent of the bills for these patients. They may deny payment for 45 percent of the bills. Thus, for the $1,140,000 billed (95% of $1,200,000), the hospital will receive approximately $627,000 (55% of the $1,140,000 billed). Approximately $513,000 of the bill will not be paid by Medicare & Medicaid or managed care or insurance companies. Consider the following:

What other expenses besides salary must the hospital pay out of the $627,000 that it receives? Consider hospital space, liability insurance, technology costs, and so on. Consider that the hospital will also be partially reimbursed for all services delivered during the patient's visit.

Notice the effect that increasing the volume of patients has on your budget figures. What happens to your budget if the patient volume goes to 8,000 patient ED visits per month and staffing stays the same?

Are patients receiving useful information about future illness prevention and healthy living practices in the ED?

Is this a cost-effective way to deliver health care?

How could we better serve the health care needs of Americans?

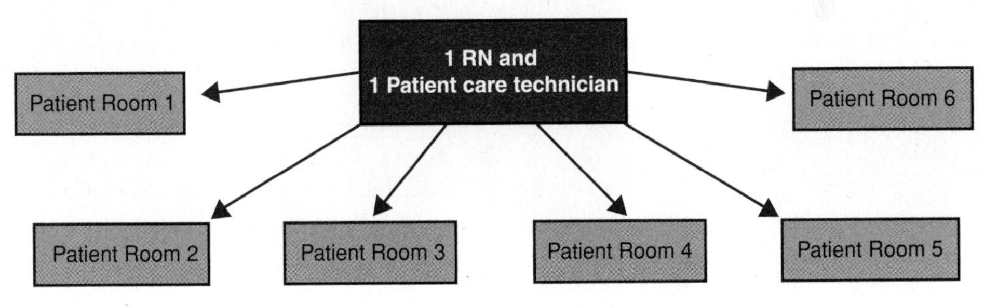

FIGURE 10-6

Inpatient staffing model.

© Cengage Learning 2014

and surgical supplies, wages, and drugs. **Indirect expenses** are expenses for items such as utilities—gas, electric, and phones—that are not directly related to patient care but are necessary to support care. Other support functions frequently charged to a department that are not specifically related to patient care delivery are housekeeping, maintenance, materials management, and finance.

TABLE 10-6
Unproductive Time

Unproductive Time	Number of Hours	Salary*
Vacation	168	$5,376
Holiday	56	$1,792
Sick	40	$1,280
Personal	24	$ 768
Education	8	$ 256
Total	296	$9,472

© Cengage Learning 2014
*Salary dollars are based upon an average rate of $32.00 per hour. Remember to calculate the number of hours times $32.00. The salary dollars change depending upon pay rate and shifts; for example, day shift versus evening shift differential or 10- and 12-hour shift rates.

Fixed and Variable Costs

Fixed costs are those expenses that are constant and are not related to productivity or volume. Examples of these costs are building and equipment depreciation, utilities, fringe benefits, and administrative salaries. **Variable costs** fluctuate depending upon the volume or census and types of care required. Medical and surgical supplies, drugs, laundry, and food costs often increase the volume.

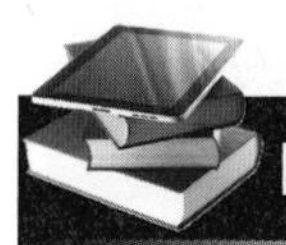

EVIDENCE FROM THE **LITERATURE**

Citation: Aiken, L. H., Sloan, D. M., Cimiotti, J. P., Clarke, S .P., Flynn, L., Seajo, J. A., Spetz, J., & Smith, H. L. (2010). Implications of the California Nurse Staffing Mandate for other states. *Health Research and Educational Trust.* doi:10.1111/j.1475-6773.2010.01114.x

Discussion: The article discusses survey data from hospital staff nurses in California, Pennsylvania, and New Jersey. Nursing workloads and patient outcomes including mortality, failure to rescue, and satisfaction were compared between the California nurses with mandated ratios and the Pennsylvania and New Jersey nurses. On average, the patient workload was one less patient for California nurses in intensive care units and two less patients on medical-surgical units. This workload appeared to influence patient mortality, and the nurses in California had lower burnout levels and lower job dissatisfaction. The California nurses also reported better quality of care for their patients.

Implications for Practice: This survey of RNs in California, New Jersey, and Pennsylvania explored self-reported patient workload, staffing ratios, and quality of care of patients. California nurses had lower patient workloads and less mortality for patients. Using a predictive model, the authors adjusted the lower risk of death that could have been experienced if lower patient workloads were implemented in Pennsylvania and New Jersey. The predictive model revealed 13.9 percent fewer deaths in New Jersey and 10.6 percent fewer deaths in Pennsylvania. The authors recommend multiple strategies for improving nurse staffing, such as mandatory reporting of nurse staffing or a mandated process for determination of staffing. Whether the exact number of patients per nurse is mandated or the hospital provides a reliable and safe staffing plan to provide the best quality and safest care, nurses must be aware of the research on this topic and be ready to discuss it with hospital administrators and decision makers.

BUDGET APPROVAL AND MONITORING

Once developed, budgets are submitted to administration for review and approval, and the entire health care team is then responsible for ensuring that expenses are kept within the budgeted amount. The manner in which this is accomplished depends on the organization. Some institutions request that budget dashboards (Figure 10-7) be developed reflecting monthly departmental activity at a glance. Note that one can review patient volume/access, patient satisfaction, human resources staffing, expenses, and budget using this dashboard monthly. Variance reports or dashboards may be posted so that all staff members have an opportunity to review the budget and participate in any needed improvement.

Year to Date						
Volume/Access						
Department	Cost Center	Volume Year to Date	Percentage Budget Variance	Percentage Variance from Last Year	Days to Next Appointment/ Available Bed	
GI Laboratory	1265	6,706	16	23	3	
Medical Unit	7095	9,705	18	28	1	
Patient Satisfaction						
	Overall Score		Percentile	Percentile	Results Reporting	
Department	Actual	Target	Actual	Target	Average Report Turnaround Time	Reports > 24
GI laboratory	90.5	91.70	90	95	28	20%
Medical unit	89	90.00	88	92	NA	NA
Human Resources						
					Employee Performance	
		Actual	Vacancies	Turnover	Staff Performance Reviews on Time	
Department	Manager	FTEs Year to Date	Year to Date	Rate	> 30 Days	
GI laboratory	1	33.00	0.4	8%	0	
Medical unit	1	45.00	6	12%	1	
Expenses						
				Supply	Productivity	
		Percentage of Budget Compared to Actual	Percentage Variance from Budget Year to Date	Variance from Budget Year to Date	Variance from Last Year	
Department						
GI laboratory	250	(5.00)	11.00	unfavorable	unfavorable	
Medical unit	118	8.00	12.00	favorable	unfavorable	
Capital Budget						
Line Items	Number	Year	Budgeted	Expensed	Balance	
GI lab						
7 Video endoscopes	10002895	2001	112,550.00	109,389.19	14,226.00	
Endoscopy travel cart	30256409	2001	2,750.00	0.00	32,750.00	
Scopes	89756452	2001	38,255.00	35,225.00	1,199.00	
Comments						
Financial improvement plan ongoing in GI lab: Interventional charges have been adjusted and cost reduction/inventory control is being explored with materials management.						
Medical nursing unit has achieved highest overall patient satisfaction goal. Multidisciplinary conferences are being held every other day to focus on patient care issues.						

FIGURE 10-7

G1 laboratory and medical unit dashboard.

(*Source:* Adapted with permission of Northwestern Memorial Hospital, Chicago, Illinois.)

Staff can meet to discuss implementation or reinforcement of strategies that can positively affect the dashboard. Following are examples of such strategies:

- Analyze time efficiency of staff involved in patient care.
- Plan for supplies needed for every patient encounter and consciously eliminate unnecessary items.
- Learn how a department is reimbursed for services delivered, identifying covered and excluded expenses.
- Explore new products with vendor representatives, and network with colleagues who have tried both new and modified products.
- Reduce the length of stay by troubleshooting early.
- Enhance productivity through rigorous process improvement.
- Ensure that staff have the right tools and that the tools are ready when needed.
- Track various steps in patient care that are time consuming or problematic for a unit (e.g., communication from front desk to recovery room, staff response to patient call lights, number of staff responding to an emergency code).
- Acquire a working knowledge of how a department/unit monitors financial and quality indicators, and participate in the development of action plans to increase patient satisfaction or to create the "best patient experience."

KEY CONCEPTS

- ✦ Nurses play an integral role in the development, implementation, and evaluation of a unit or departmental budget.
- ✦ Hospitals use several types of budgets to help with future planning and management. These include operational, capital, and construction budgets.
- ✦ The budget preparation phase is one of gathering data related to a variety of elements that influence an organization, including demographic information, marketing, competitive analysis, regulatory influences, and strategic plans. Additionally, it is helpful to understand the department's scope of service, goals, and history.
- ✦ Once background data have been gathered, the development of the budget can follow. This includes projecting revenue and expenses.
- ✦ Expenses are determined by identifying the cost associated with the delivery of service. Expenditures are resources used by an organization to deliver services and may include labor, supplies, equipment, utilities, and miscellaneous items.
- ✦ Once developed, budgets are submitted to administration for review and final approval. The approval process may take several months as the unit budgets are combined to determine the overall budget for the health care organization.
- ✦ Health care economics is grounded in past values and culture. Nearly 150 years ago, Florence Nightingale recognized that the resources being used to care for sick people ought to be tracked and analyzed to improve clinical and business outcomes.
- ✦ In the United States, multiple payer sources exist to pay for health care.
- ✦ Health care costs vary significantly both nationally and internationally.
- ✦ The ability to track and manage both cost and quality is critical to achieve an organization's economic and quality goals.

KEY TERMS

accounting
budget
capital budget
construction budget
core measures
cost centers
dashboard
direct expenses
economics
fixed costs
indirect expenses
margin
never events
operational budget
profit
revenue
variable costs
variance

REVIEW QUESTIONS

1. The purpose of nurse budget monitoring is which of the following?
   A. Keep expenses above budget
   B. Maintain revenue above the previous year's budget
   C. Ensure revenue stays below budget
   D. Manage revenue and control expenses during a predefined time frame

2. Revenue and expense are typically tracked by a nurse on a patient care unit using which of the following tools?
   A. Strategic planning
   B. Competitive analysis
   C. Operational budget
   D. Construction budget

3. Cost centers are used to do which of the following?
   A. Develop guidelines for budgeting
   B. Track surgery schedules
   C. Log patient complaints
   D. Monitor financial data in a department or unit

4. Nurses review operational budgets for which of the following reasons?
   A. Monitor demographic information related to patients on their units
   B. Monitor regulatory requirements for nurses
   C. Monitor a competitor's behavior
   D. Monitor revenue and expenses

5. Economics is the study of which of the following?
   A. The cost-quality interface
   B. Cost accounting
   C. The cost of doing business
   D. How to manage scarcity of resources

6. Which of the following are indirect expenses?
   A. Salary of staff providing care
   B. Gas, electric, phones
   C. Medical supplies
   D. Monitoring equipment

7. Examples of capital budget items include which of the following? Select all that apply.
   A. Gauze and tape
   B. Forceps
   C. MRI scanner
   D. Paper supplies
   E. Mammogram equipment
   F. Brain scanner

8. What types of indicators are typically displayed on dashboards in hospital settings? Select all that apply.
   A. Patient satisfaction
   B. Financial performance
   C. Quality performance
   D. Staff satisfaction
   E. Patient outcomes
   F. Patient medications

REVIEW ACTIVITIES

1. Review Figure 10-4. Construct a competitive analysis for two nursing units where you are doing your clinical experience. What did you observe?
2. Look around your clinical agency. Do you see any dashboards? What do they reveal about your agency?
3. Interview the nurse manager of a health care organization to gain an understanding of how various costs are managed. Use the following questions to guide the interview:

   What method is used to measure nursing cost?

   How are contracts with various insurers such as Medicare, Medicaid, Blue Cross, and managed care discounted?

   What percentage of profit did the organization make last year, and how was it allocated?

   Which professional services are billed directly?

EXPLORING THE WEB

- Go to the site for the Joint Commission and look for budgeting-related information: *http://www.jointcommission.org*
- Review the site for the American Organization of Nurse Executives: *http://www.aone.org*
- Visit the site for nurse-sensitive outcomes: *http://www.nursingworld.org*
- Review these sites for helpful information. What did you find there?

  Healthcare Financial Management Association: *http://www.hfma.org*

  American College of Healthcare Executives: *http://www.ache.org*

  Centers for Medicare and Medicaid Services: *http://www.cms.hhs.gov*

  Agency for Healthcare Research and Quality: *http://www.ahrq.gov*

- Search an alternate government bureau site to see what professionally relevant information you can find: *http://www.bls.gov*

- Search the following sites for information of interest to nurses:
  http://www.florence-nightingale.co.uk
  http://www.aahn.org
  http://www.webmd.com
  http://www.medexplorer.com
  http://www.healthology.com
  http://www.medicarerights.org

REFERENCES

Agency for Healthcare Research and Quality (AHRQ). (2006) Never Events. retrieved November 8, 2012 from, http://www.psnet.ahrq.gov/primer.aspx?primerID=3

Aiken, L. H., Sloan, D. M., Cimiotti, J. P., Clarke, S. P., Flynn, L., Seajo, J. A., Spetz, J., & Smith, H. L. (2010). Implications of the California Nurse Staffing Mandate for other states. *Health Research and Educational Trust.* doi:10.1111/j.1475-6773.2010.01114.x

America's Highest Paid Chief Executives. (2011). *Forbes.* Retrieved October 1, 2012, from http://www.forbes.com/sites/ christopherhelman/2011/10/12/americas-25-highest-paid-ceos/

AMGA Physician Compensation Survey excerpt. (2011). Retrieved October 1, 2012, from http://cejka.force.com/PhysicianCompensation#compdata

Cejka Physician Executive Compensation Survey. (2011). Retrieved October 1, 2012, from http://www.beckershospitalreview.com/compensation-issues/physician-executive-compensation-how-are-top-physician-leaders-paid.html

Centers for Medicare & Medicaid Services (CMS). Retrieved October 1, 2012, from http://www.cms.hhs.gov

CMS. (2011). Medicare and Medicaid, Brief summaries. Retrieved November 8, 2012, from http://www.cms.gov/Research-Statistics-Data-and-Systems/Statistics-Trends-and-Reports/MedicareProgramRatesStats/Downloads/MedicareMedicaidSummaries2011.pdf

Cohen, J. (2010). How many nurses does your hospital need? *Nursing Management, 41*(6), 20–25.

Commonwealth Fund on a High Performance Health System. (2011). make it November 30, 2011, from http://www.commonwealthfund.org

Compare Drug Prices. Retrieved November 11, 2011, from http://www.drugstore.com. Click on "Compare drug prices."

Curry, L., Spatz, E., Cherlin, E., Thompson, J., Berg, D., Ting, H., Decker, C., Krumholz, H., & Bradley, E. (2011). What distinguishes top-performing hospitals in acute myocardial infarction mortality rates? *Annals of Internal Medicine, 154,* 384–390.

Davis, K., Schoen., C., Schoenbaum, S., Doty, M., Holmgren, A., Kriss, J., & Shea, K. (2007). Mirror, mirror on the wall: An international update on the comparative performance of American health care. The Commonwealth Fund. Retrieved November 3, 2011, from http://www.commonwealthfund.org

Deficit Reduction Act of 2005. Public Law 109-171, 109th Congress. Retrieved November 8, 2012, from http://www.gpo.gov/fdsys/pkg/PLAW-109publ171/html/PLAW-109publ171.htm

Drugstore.com. (2011). Retrieved November 11, 2011 from, http://www.drugstore.com

Finkler, S. A., & McHugh, M. L. (2008). *Budgeting concepts for nurse managers.* St. Louis, MO: Saunders.

Goetz, K., Janney, M., & Ramsey, K. (2011). When nursing takes ownership of financial outcomes: Achieving exceptional financial performance through leadership, strategy, and execution. *Nursing Economics 29*(4), 173–182.

Health Care Spending in the United States and Selected OECD Countries. (2011). Snap Shots Health Care Costs, Kaiser Family Foundation. Retrieved October 1, 2012, from http://www.kff.org/insurance/snapshot/OECD042111.cfm

Jones, C. (2008). Revisiting nurse turnover costs: Adjusting for inflation. *The Journal of Nursing Administration 38*(1), 11–18.

Kaiser Health News. (2011). Chart: CEO Pay Packages, Ranked By Hospital Revenue. Retrieved November 8, 2012 from, http://www.kaiserhealthnews.org/Stories/2011/September/28/Chart-CEO-Pay-Packages.aspx

Kilner, J. F. (1990). *Who lives? Who dies? Ethical criteria in patient selection.* New Haven, CT: Yale University Press.

Kimball, B. (2005). Cultural transformation in health care. The Robert Wood Johnson Foundation. Retrieved from http://www.rwjf.org/quality/product

Krsek, C. (2011, April). Investing in nursing retention is a smart move in today's economy. *American Nurse Today, 6*(4). Retrieved October 1, 2012, from http://www.americannursetoday.com/article.aspx?id=7704&fid=7658

Medicare Prescription Drug, Improvement, and Modernization Act of 2003. Public Law 108-173, 108th Congress. Retrieved November 8, 2012, from http://www.gpo.gov/fdsys/pkg/PLAW-108publ173/html/PLAW-108publ173.htm

Modern Healthcare. (2012).The Modern Healthcare/ECRI Institute Technology Price Index. Retrieved from, http://www.modernhealthcare.com/section/technology-price-index#, accessed October 23, 2012.

Nightingale, F. (1859). *Notes on hospitals; Being two papers read before the National Association for the Promotion of Social Science, at Liverpool in October, 1858. With evidence given to the Royal Commissioners on the State of the Army in 1857* (2nd ed.). London, England: Parker.

Oregonian PolitiFact Oregon. (2011). Truth-o-Meter. update, Feb. 21, 2011. Retrieved Februrary 21, 2011, from http://politifact.com/oregon/statements/2011/feb/19/wesley-smith/one-pundit-says-oregon-health-plan-rations-covered

Ponti, M., Germain, M., & Mouton, L. (2010). Budgets: Planning, executing and managing into the future. *Nursing Management, 41*(9), 35–38.

US Dept. of Labor Statistics. (2012). Retrieved November 8, 2011 from, http://www.bls.gov/oes/current/oes291111.htm

SUGGESTED READINGS

Hughes, R. G. (2008.) Nurses at the “sharp end” of patient care. In R. G. Hughes (Ed.), *Patient safety and quality: An evidence-based handbook for nurses.* Prepared with support from the Robert Wood Johnson Foundation. AHRQ Publication No. 08-0043. Rockville, MD: Agency for Healthcare Research and Quality. Retrieved September 20, 2012, from http://www.ncbi.nlm.nih.gov/books/NBK2672

Hughes, R. G. (Ed.). (2008) *Patient safety and quality: An evidence-based handbook for nurses.* Prepared with support from the Robert Wood Johnson Foundation. AHRQ Publication No. 08-0043. Rockville, MD: Agency for Healthcare Research and Quality.

McHugh, M., Kang, R., & Hasnain-Wynia, R. (2009). Understanding the safety net: Inpatient quality of care varies based on how one defines safety-net hospitals. *Medical Care Research and Review, 66*(5), 590–605.

Michael , F. & Minch, F.M. (2012). Thoughts on transparency–and a few final words. *Tennessee Medicine. 105*(5):5.

Porter, M. (2010). What is value in healthcare? *The New England Journal of Medicine, 363*, 2477–2481.

CHAPTER 11

Strategic Planning and Organizing of Patient Care for Quality and Safety

JOSEPHINE REIDY, RN, MSN; AMY ANDROWICH O'MALLEY, RN, MSN; IDA M. ANDROWICH, RN, BC, PHD, FAAN; AND KATHLEEN F. SELLERS, RN, PHD

There is no more powerful engine driving an organization towards excellence and long-range success than an attractive, worthwhile, achievable vision for the future widely shared.

–BURT NENUS, VISIONARY LEADERSHIP, 1995

OBJECTIVES

Upon completion of this chapter, the reader should be able to:

1. Understand the importance of an organization's mission and philosophy and the impact of these on the structure and behavior of the organization.
2. Review the strategic-planning process.
3. Articulate the importance of aligning the organization's strategic vision both with its philosophy, mission, and values and with the goals and values of the communities and stakeholders served by the organization.
4. Discuss common organizational work structures and work processes used to meet desired organizational outcomes.
5. Discuss high-reliability organizations and a culture of safety.
6. Identify the 14 Forces of Magnetism.
7. Describe elements of the magnet model.

When questions and answers were entertained at an open Nursing Forum at Peace Memorial Hospital, a medical-surgical nurse stated a concern. She stated that an increased number of medical patients with secondary psychiatric diagnoses were being admitted to the medical-surgical unit requiring 1:1 nursing assistive personnel (NAP) as sitters with patients until a psychiatric consult was completed. A long discussion followed at the Nursing Forum addressing patient safety and quality of care. A few weeks later, a subcommittee was formed to research and investigate alternative solutions to this situation. After several months, the subcommittee recommended that the mental health unit (MHU) be redesigned to accommodate medical-surgical and telemetry-psychiatric patients on the MHU. The nursing director of the MHU had participated in the subcommittee. She was recommended to oversee the development of the modifications and additions to be completed on her unit. It was thought that these revisions would enhance patient and staff safety, increase quality of care and performance, improve staff productivity and unit revenue, and lead to positive patient outcomes. Resources for unit design, staff education and competencies, and provisions of a culture of safety with quality-focused care were made available. The goal was to maintain the institution's mission in conjunction with the understanding that the investment would enhance organizational value.

What unit structures and patient care work processes need to be put in place?

What outcomes should you expect to see and monitor?

How will nursing competency and continued professional growth be attained on the new mental health unit?

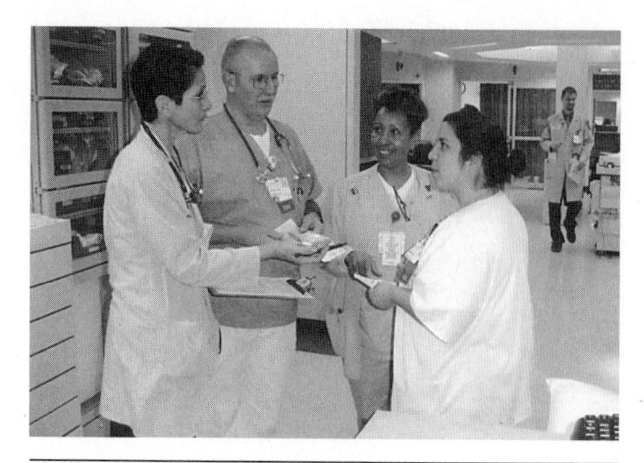

© Cengage Learning 2014

Nursing leaders in health care face a multitude of challenges when doing strategic planning and organizing patient care for quality and safety to achieve important organizational goals. Implementing strategic plans that ensure quality, safety, regulatory compliance, and cost effectiveness can be a difficult task for even the most experienced leader. Nurses serve as informants to provide first-hand information about organizational features and relationships, from which aspects such as organizational support, staffing, and quality of care can be measured. These measures have proven to be a reliable and valid instrument to measure the nursing practice environment and have been used in many studies, across many countries, and with different systems. (Cheung, R. D., Aiken, L. H., Clarke, S. P., & Sloane, D. M. (2010).). Although many health care organizations collect large sets of data and are beginning to use scientific methods to improve the services they render, these activities are typically fragmented, isolated from day-to-day nursing management, and lack alignment with organizational strategy. It is critical that nurses be a part of the institutional decision-making process about strategic planning for quality, patient safety, and planning for the future.

The 2004 Institute of Medicine (IOM) report *Keeping Patients Safe: Transforming the Work Environment of Nurses* found that nurses, who comprise the largest segment of the health care workforce and spend the most time providing direct care to patients, are indispensable to patient safety and quality (Khoury, Blizzard, Moore, & Hassmiller, 2011). An earlier IOM report, *To Err Is Human: Building a Safer Health System* (1999), stated that preventable adverse events cause between 44,000 and 98,000 deaths each year, at an annual cost of between $37.6 billion and $50 billion. These IOM reports have changed the way we view quality and patient safety. It is now generally understood that patient safety is dependent on the implementation of inter-professional collaborative teams and patient care delivery systems that address the realities of practice and patient care. These patient care delivery systems often have errors occur in them.

Errors often occur as a result of system failure rather than human failure. Recent research studies stress that the way a nurse's work is organized is a major determinant of patient welfare. Consequently, nurses must be prepared to be able to implement sound models for the effective delivery of patient care.

Current nursing leadership must embrace future leaders of the nursing profession to mentor and educate these novices. This will help these future leaders acquire the understanding, knowledge, and skill to improve health care. Providing safe, quality health care requires technical expertise, the ability to think critically, experience, and clinical judgment. A high-performance expectation of nurses is dependent upon nurses' continual learning, professional accountability, independent and interdependent decision-making, and creative problem-solving abilities (Benner, Hughes, & Sutphen, 2008).

This chapter discusses the importance of an organization's philosophy and mission and the steps in the strategic-planning process. It notes the importance of aligning the organization's strategic plan both with its philosophy, values, and mission, and with the goals and values of the communities and stakeholders served by the organization. The chapter reviews common organizational work structures and work processes used to meet desired organizational outcomes. It discusses high-reliability organizations, a culture of safety, the 14 Forces of Magnetism, the Magnet Model, and the historical evolution and significance of magnet hospitals.

STRATEGIC PLANNING

The purpose of strategic planning is twofold. First, it is important that everyone have the same plan for where the organization is headed, and second, a good plan can help to ensure that the needed resources and budget are available to carry out the initiatives that have been identified as important to the organization. A clear plan allows the nurse manager to select from among seemingly equal alternatives based on the alternatives' potential to move the organization toward the desired end goal. As Lewis Carroll observed in *Alice's Adventures in Wonderland*, "If you don't know where you are going, any road will do." A health care organization needs to have a good idea of where it fits into its environment and what types of programs and services are needed and demanded by its customers or stakeholders. This is true at the organization's board level as well as at the patient care unit level. It is important that a nurse manager have an understanding of which programs and services are valued by a patient population. The nurse manager can then help plan for how the patient care unit's ongoing activities can serve that population and fit in with the overall strategy of the larger organization.

As outlined in Figure 11-1, strategic planning starts with: clarifying the organization's philosophy and values or what is important to the organization; identifying the mission of why the organization exists; articulating a vision and goals for what the organization wants to be; conducting an environmental assessment, or SWOT assessment, which examines the Strengths, Weaknesses, Opportunities, and Threats of the organization. The SWOT assessment is useful both for initial brainstorming and for more formal planning (Figure 11-2). This information provides data that then drive the development of three- to five-year strategic plans for the organization. Tactics are then created and prioritized. Finally, goals and objectives are concretized into annual, operating work plans for the organization, which can be measured. This same process is used for unit or departmental strategic planning. In developing a strategic plan, unit staff must also examine their organization's mission, vision, goals, and annual operating plans. Unit strategic plans should be congruent with and support the mission and vision of the organizational system of which they are a part. Therefore, communication with the nursing leadership responsible for the unit and the nursing staff is essential to achieve success.

Community and Stakeholder Assessment

A frequently overlooked but highly important area for analysis is the stakeholder assessment. A stakeholder is any person, group, or organization that has a vested interest in the program or project under review. Stakeholders in health care include people such as patients, nursing and medical practitioners, community representatives, insurance companies, hospital/agency

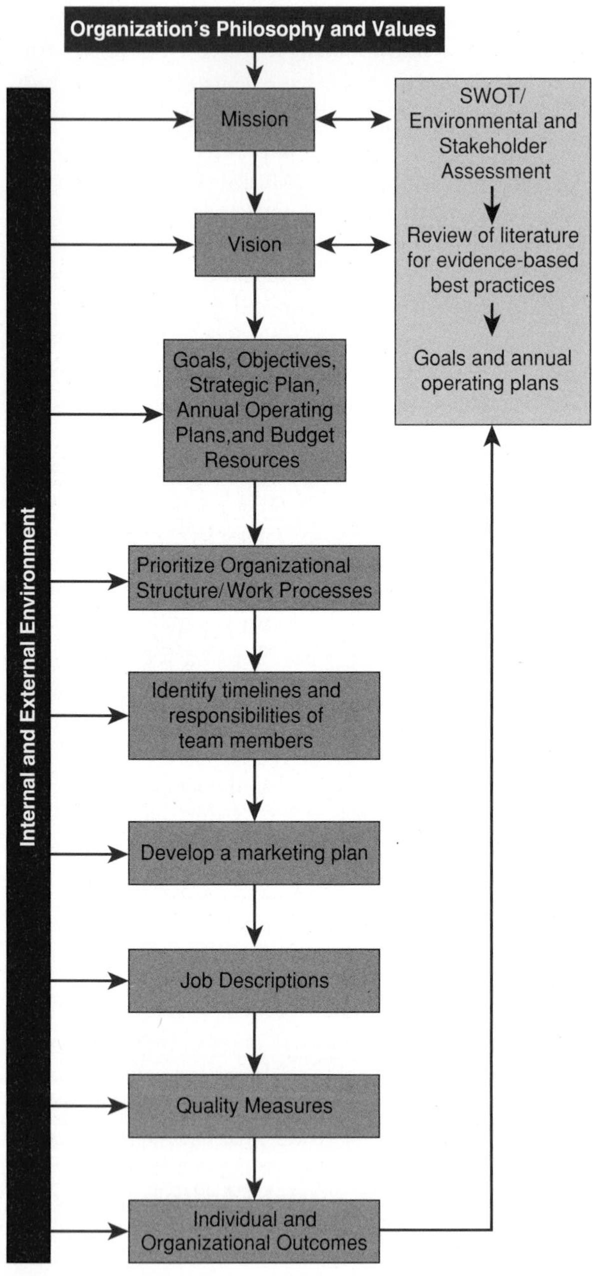

FIGURE 11-1
Strategic planning.
© Cengage Learning 2014

administrators, federal and state accreditation agencies, pharmaceutical companies, and technology and equipment companies. A **stakeholder assessment** is a systematic consideration of all potential stakeholders to ensure that the needs of each of these stakeholders are incorporated in the planning phase of a program, project, or quality initiative. For a program to be successful, engaging and involving all stakeholders is essential. This is true whether the stakeholders are in the community or they are the unit staff who will be affected by a proposed strategic plan. This fact has been reported by Hughes, who identifies the need to "engage all the right stakeholders (ranging from senior management to staff)." Hughes further states that there is a need for staff "to be involved and supported to actively make the change and to be the champion and problem solver within departments for the interventions to succeed" (Hughes, p 101 2008).

An environmental assessment (SWOT analysis) of the type of undergraduate nursing education that would be needed for the 21st-century professional nurse led one school of nursing to begin planning a curriculum revision that would incorporate the increasing emphasis on community-focused care. This assessment of the environment led faculty to understand that new models for clinical education will be needed to promote improved and expanded linkages between education and practice. It is important that the internal environment as well as the external environment be carefully assessed. Whereas the external environmental assessment is broad based and attempts to view opportunities and threats that could impact the organization, the internal assessment seeks to inventory the organization's strengths and weaknesses.

Additional Methods of Strategic Planning Assessment

A number of other strategic-planning assessment methods can be used in the strategic-planning process. These methods include surveys and questionnaires, focus groups and interviews, use of advisory boards, review of literature on similar programs, and review of best practices. Frequently, surveys or questionnaires are used when there is a large

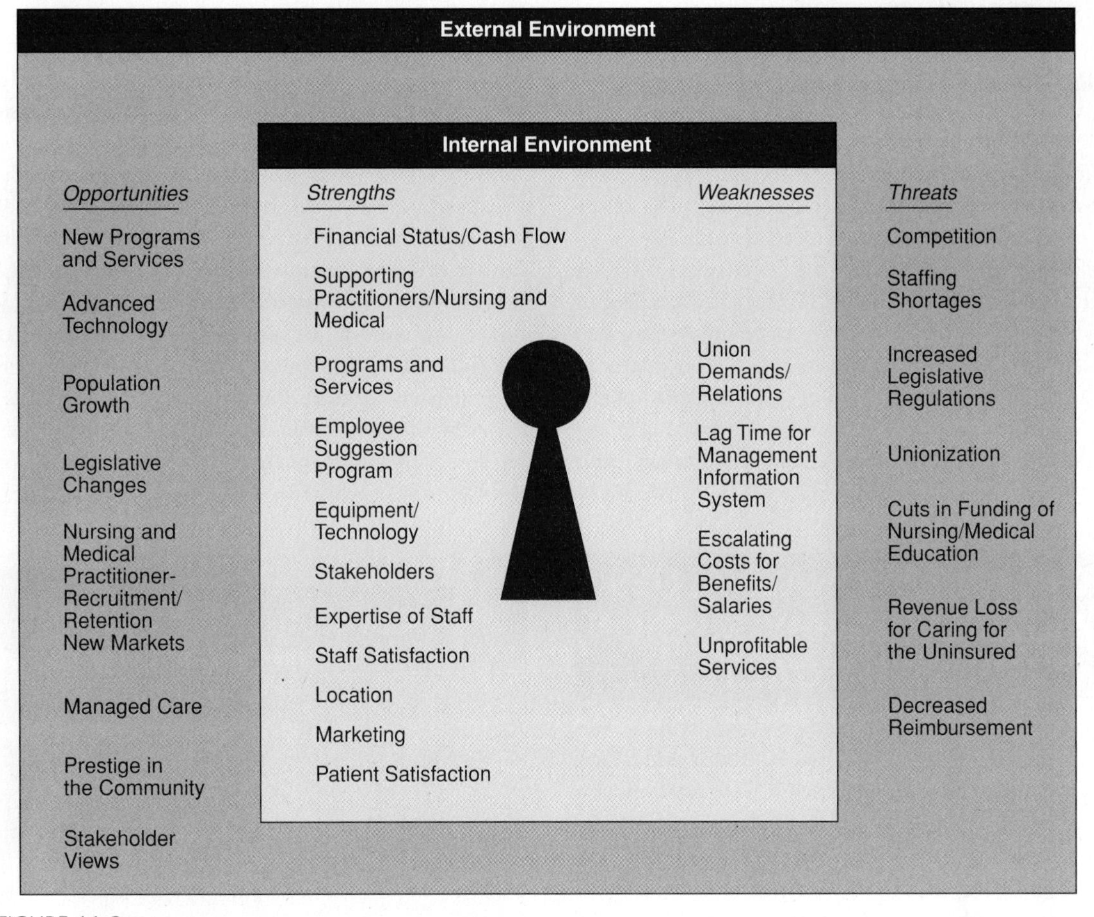

FIGURE 11-2

Key to success in strategic planning: SWOT assessment.

(*Source:* Compiled with information from Jones, R., & Beck, S. (1996). *Decision Making in Nursing.* Clifton Park, NY: Delmar Cengage Learning.)

number of stakeholders in order to get a general idea of the options available. For example, staff might be polled to see whether they would attend a continuing education program and which days and times would be most desirable. **Focus groups** are small groups of individuals selected because of a common characteristic who meet in a group and respond to questions about a topic in which they have interest or expertise, for example, patients with a recent diagnosis of diabetes. These patients might be asked to come together to discuss their diabetes experiences at an institution in the hope that the discussion will lead to insights or information that could be used by the institution for improving diabetic care or marketing diabetic services in the future. Focus groups are usually more time consuming and expensive to conduct than surveys or questionnaires. Focus groups work best when the topic is broad and the options are not clear.

Large projects often benefit from the formation of an advisory board selected from various stakeholders affected by a proposed program. The advisory board does not have formal authority over the proposed program but does make recommendations and suggestions. Because the advisory board is deliberately selected to reflect representation from various stakeholders and areas of expertise, it is expected that the advisory board will be able to identify potential concerns and provide sound guidance for the proposed program. A review of literature on similar programs should be completed as part of strategic planning for any new program. This review of literature allows the project team to identify similar programs, their structures and organization, potential problems, pitfalls, and successes. The review of literature is an ongoing process that includes identifying programs, searching the literature for successes and issues, and then refining the program ideas. Identifying best practices or evidence-based innovations that have been adopted with success by other organizations can facilitate strategic planning. Consequently, nurses planning to develop a new program need to carefully examine the existing evidence and best practices prior to beginning strategic planning.

ORGANIZATIONAL VALUES AND PHILOSOPHY, MISSION, VISION, AND GOALS

Every organization has a guiding philosophy and values, mission, and vision. The philosophy and values of the organization are reflected in its formal mission statement. Typically, this mission statement provides the reader with an indication of the behavior and strategic actions that can be expected from that organization. Most health care organizations have mission statements that speak to providing high quality or excellence in patient care. Some mission statements focus exclusively on providing care, whereas others assume a broader view and include the education of health care professionals and the promotion of research as contributing to their broader mission. The mission of still other organizations may focus on providing community outreach and population-based services to a specific community or a population within a community.

Mission Statement

The **mission statement** is a formal expression of the purpose or reason for the existence of the organization. It is the organization's declaration of its primary driving force and the manner in which it believes care should be delivered. An institution's mission statement defines how it is unique and different from other organizations that provide a similar service. Mission statements with phrases such as "without consideration for ability to pay," or "with respect for the dignity of each elderly resident," or "provide a brighter future for all children," or "provide vigorous rehabilitation to maximize each individual's utmost potential" provide clues as to the type of service that you could expect from an organization. In the best of worlds, there is congruence between the mission and goals of the organization (Table 11-1). Sometimes, organizations get into trouble when they move too far afield of their core mission. Consequently, each new project needs to be evaluated in light of its congruence with the main mission that has been identified. It is fine for an organization to move to another project, but

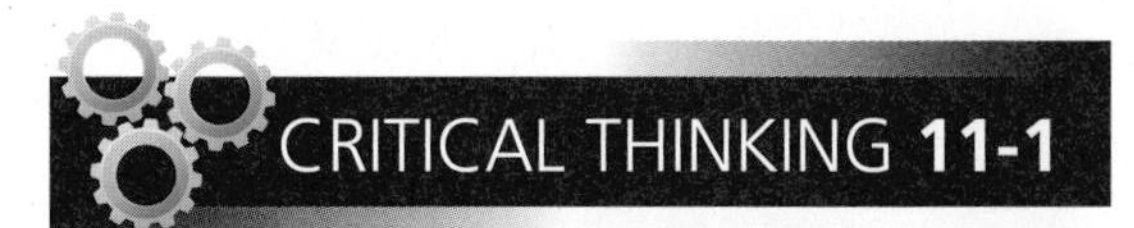

Examine these two mission statements and then respond to the questions that follow.

Hospital A: "Our mission is to ensure the highest quality of care for the patients in our community. We believe that each patient has the right to the most innovative care that current science and technology can provide. To that end, we have assembled a world-renowned medical staff who will strive to ensure that the latest developments in medical science are used to combat disease."

Hospital B: "Our mission is to provide excellence in care to all. Our health care staff, nursing and medical practitioners, and other professionals believe that care can best be provided in an atmosphere of collaboration and partnership with our patients and community. We believe in education—for our patients, for our staff, and for future health care providers. At all times we strive for optimal health promotion and the prevention of disease and disability."

Which of these institutions do you think would be more likely to have a patient lecture series on living with diabetes? Value the contributions of nursing? Provide experimental therapy for cancer? Be open to scheduling routine patient care visits for uninsured patients?

TABLE 11-1
Mission, Goals, and Quality Measures

Mission

The People's Choice Health Care Center provides excellent health care to all patients through partnerships with patients and the community and collaboration with nursing and medical practitioners and other health care staff. We believe in continuous education for patients, health care staff, and future health care providers. We are committed to optimal health care promotion and prevention of disease and disability.

Goals

1. Collaborate with all interprofessional health care staff to improve patient care
2. Deliver patient-centered care
3. Monitor patient satisfaction scores
4. Increase number of emergency room visits
5. Increase use of computers by all staff
6. Increase funding for staff's continuing education
7. Increase number of specialty certifications of staff
8. Monitor nurse-sensitive patient outcomes, such as incidence of cardiac arrest, urinary tract infections, upper GI bleeding, thrombophlebitis, and failure to rescue
9. Increase use of evidence-based guidelines and practices for safe, high-quality patient care delivery
10. Achieve national patient safety goals
11. Improve performance on Joint Commission core measures

Nursing-Sensitive Care Performance Measures. (The National Quality Forum [NQF], 2004.)

1. Falls prevalence
2. Falls with injury
3. Restraint prevalence (vest and limb only)
4. Skill mix (RN, LPN, NAP, and contract)
5. Nursing care hours per patient day (RN, LPN, and NAP)
6. Practice Environment Scale—Nursing Work Index (composite and 5 subscale measurements)
7. Voluntary turnover

Quality Measures for Emergency Department

Customer/Patient

1. Deliver patient-centered care
2. Improve patient-satisfaction scores
3. Increase in customer returns, when required
4. Decrease in patient complaints
5. Increase in market share

(Continues)

TABLE 11-1 (Continued)

6. Decrease in repeat visits of patients with asthma, heart failure, pneumonia, etc.
7. Develop patient-education materials for well and ill children and adults
8. Develop evidence-based standards for care of patients with heart failure, acute myocardial infarction, pneumonia, cardiac arrest, UTI, upper GI bleeding, and thrombophlebitis, etc.
9. Review all emergency department deaths
10. Improve working relationships of all interprofessional health care staff
11. Increase use of computers by all staff
12. Increase funding for staff's continuing education
13. Increase number of specialty certifications of staff
14. Increase use of evidence-based guidelines and practices for safe, high-quality patient care delivery
15. Achieve national patient-safety goals
16. Improve all nursing- sensitive patient care outcomes
17. Improve performance on Joint Commission core measures

Financial

1. Increase use of computers and electronic health records
2. Monitor budget compliance
3. Improve nurse staffing ratios
4. Develop computerized order-entry system for medications

Internal Processes

1. Achieve 90% on key performance improvement measures
2. Decrease sick time and overtime by 10%
3. Increase number of nursing research and evidence-based practice projects
4. Achieve Magnet status
5. Increase use of best-practice educational materials by all patients and staff
6. Increase participation of all interprofessional team in quality improvement activities
7. Arrange for all staff to attend one outside conference yearly
8. Set up nursing journal club meetings monthly
9. Set up interprofessional team committee on medication administration safety
10. Review policies for adherence to evidence-based practice standards

Employee Growth and Learning

1. 50% of the nursing department joins a professional nursing association
2. All nurses working in the emergency room are certified in ACLS, PALS, etc.
3. One-third of nurses are continuing their nursing education
4. 50% of all staff are cross-trained and can work in the ICU and ER
5. 90% of employees state they are very satisfied with their work

(Continues)

TABLE 11-1 (Continued)

6. 90% of staff are retained
7. All nurses are able to use the computer to access and record patient information, to search literature, etc.
8. 20% of nursing staff present a community program yearly on topics such as care of the patient with an acute myocardial infarction, stroke, etc.
9. Each staff member compiles a professional portfolio, including evidence of quality patient outcomes, patient-centered care, interprofessional teamwork, evidence-based practice, quality improvement, patient safety, etc.

© Cengage Learning 2014

only if the new project is in line with the mission. Otherwise, there is a risk that the new program will drain energy from the main mission of the organization.

Vision Statement

A vision statement identifies how the people of the organization plan to actualize the mission. It portrays what people think of the organization and how the organization envisions itself to be in three to five years. Even though it is focused on the future, a vision statement is written in the present tense, using action words, as if the vision had already been achieved. In health care, a vision statement describes a balance of addressing the needs of the providers, the patients, and the environment.

Goals and Quality Measures

The next step in the planning process is for the organization and the work unit to develop goals and quality measures that reflect the mission. A **goal** is a specific aim or target that the unit wishes to attain within a specified time span (e.g., one year). Measures of the goal may reflect finances, customer satisfaction and services, internal operating efficiency, and learning and growth (Norton & Kaplan, 2001). See Table 11-1.

Planning Goals

After all strategic goals and objectives have been identified, they need to be prioritized according to strategic importance, resources required, and time and effort involved. A timeline should be set. This will allow a thoughtful evaluation of each goal and objective and the degree to which each can be implemented in the specified time frame with the available resources. Realistic timelines and individual responsibilities must be developed, specified, clarified, and communicated to all stakeholders. This will help to avoid misunderstandings and unmet expectations.

Developing a Marketing Plan

If part of strategic planning involves new programs, the strategic plan, goals, and objectives will need to be communicated to all involved constituencies. Such communication will be needed, for example, when an institution is planning to implement a new health care information system to ensure that it remains competitive in the market. Designing, implementing, training, and evaluating this new system will require substantive changes in work flow and in the way that employees carry out their day-to-day work processes. If there has not been adequate thought given to communication across the organization about the project, there is less chance of success and a greater risk of poor cooperation.

A marketing plan ensures that all stakeholders have the needed information. Marketing is the process of creating a product of health care services for patients, and it uses the four "P"s of marketing, namely, Patient, Product, Price, and Placement, to place desirable health care service or products in desirable locations at a price that benefits both patients and the health care facility. In this way, the health care facility, the patient, and the community benefit. Marketing of services does have a price tag, such as the cost of advertising campaigns on television and radio. Using printed materials, mailing information to patient residences, and advertising in journals, magazines, and newspapers are all examples of ways to educate and stimulate the public for

TABLE 11-2
Structure and Work Process Examples to Decrease Negative Postoperative Outcomes

Structure	Process
1. Increase RN staffing on the unit	1. Review patient care routines/standards for pre-op care (e.g., teaching about coughing and deep-breathing exercises, early ambulation) to decrease negative outcomes.
2. Increase number of incentive spirometers	2. Review patient care routines/standards for teaching patients about incentive spirometer use to decrease negative outcomes.
3. Etc.	3. Etc.

© Cengage Learning 2014

TABLE 11-3
Surgical Unit, Individual RN's Daily Routines/Standards Excerpt

0700	Shift handoff report
0715	Patient rounds
0730	Review postoperative care routines/standards and patient care with nursing assistive personnel (NAP). See Table 11–4.
0800	Give patient medications
0900	Document/monitor care and assist NAP. Use additional patient care standards as needed.
Etc.	

© Cengage Learning 2014

TABLE 11-4
Surgical Unit, Nursing Assistive Personnel (NAP) Routines/Standards Excerpt

0700	Monitor patient call lights during shift handoff report
0715	Take vital signs/pass fresh water
0730	Review postoperative routines/standards and patient care with RN to include: ◆ Ambulating assigned patients at 0800, 1200 ◆ Turning, coughing, and deep-breathing patients at 0800, 1000, 1200, 1400 ◆ Giving all baths and linen changes to assigned patients by 1100
Etc.	

© Cengage Learning 2014

future referrals for health care services. Once marketing strategies are implemented, most organizations attempt to measure their effectiveness, or return on investment.

Structures, Processes, and Outcomes

As discussed in Chapter 13, Quality Improvement and Evidence-Based Patient Care, an organization or patient care unit must structure the unit's environment and develop work processes to achieve quality outcomes. For example, if an organization seeks to improve all patient care outcomes, the postoperative surgical unit in that organization may develop environmental structures and work processes to improve outcomes similar to Table 11-2.

Each nurse and nursing assistive personnel on the surgical unit must review patient care routines/standards to achieve the organization and unit goals. See Tables 11-3 and 11-4.

REAL WORLD INTERVIEW

Strategic planning and organizing patient care are critical issues in the field of clinical information systems. The strategic-planning process consists of several phases, each of which requires specific activities for designing and implementing an electronic health record. One important area to consider is the selection of a standardized, coded nursing terminology for documenting patient care. I recommend that the Clinical Care Classification (CCC) system (http://www.sabacare.com) or another similar system be selected as the terminology of choice. It is important to select a research-based and ANA-recognized documentation terminology such as the CCC, The Nursing Interventions Classification (NIC) (http://www.nursing.uiowa.edu/cncce/nursing-interventions-classification-overview), Nursing Outcomes Classification (NOC) (http://www.nursing.uiowa.edu/cncce/nursing-outcomes-classification-overview), the Omaha System (http://www.omahasystem.org), or the International Classification for Nursing Practice (http://www.icn.ch/pillarsprograms/international-classification-for-nursing-practice-icnpr/). These allow nurses to document nursing diagnoses, nursing interventions and actions, and patient outcomes. This documentation is critical in the development of a computerized information system that supports and informs nursing practice.

VIRGINIA K. SABA, EdD, RN, FAAN, FACMI
Developer and Consultant CCC System
Distinguished Scholar, Adjunct
Georgetown University
Washington, D.C.

PLANNING FOR PATIENT SAFETY

Five essential elements are required in planning for patient safety and quality improvement. These elements include: fostering and sustaining a culture of change and safety; developing and clarifying an understanding of problems; involving key stakeholders; testing change strategies; and continuously monitoring performance and reporting findings to sustain needed change. Organizations that plan for patient safety and quality improvement accomplish their objectives by focusing on the needs of the total care delivery system, not just focusing on a single, isolated, patient safety and quality improvement need. Selected tools are often used in combination to plan for patient safety and quality improvement and may include Plan-Do-Study-Act (PDSA) (discussed in Chapter 13); Six Sigma; and the Define, Measure, Analyze, Improve, and Control (DMAIC) process. Six Sigma involves improving, designing, and monitoring a work process to minimize or eliminate waste while optimizing satisfaction and increasing financial stability. The baseline performance of a work process before quality improvement is compared with the work process after piloting potential solutions for quality improvement. One component of Six Sigma uses the DMAIC approach, where a quality need is identified, historical data about the need is reviewed, and the scope of expectations to meet the need is defined. Next, quality performance standards are measured, sources of performance variability are analyzed, and needed improvements are identified. As the needed improvement is implemented, data are collected to assess how well the change is working. To support this assessment, validated quality control measures are developed to assure the quality of the new improvement.

Lean Production System

The Lean Production System overlaps with the Six Sigma methodology, but differs from it in that the Lean Production System is driven by the identification of customer needs. It aims to improve health care processes by removing activities that are nonvalue-added or wasteful. It depends on root-cause analysis to investigate errors, improve quality, and prevent similar errors.

Factors involved in the successful application of the Lean Production System in health care are: eliminating unnecessary daily activities associated with overcomplicated health care work processes, workarounds, and rework; involving front-line staff throughout the Lean Production System; and rigorously tracking problems as they are experimented with throughout the problem-solving process (Hughes, 2008).

Root-Cause Analysis

Root-cause analysis (RCA) is a problem-solving approach used in a health care system to focus on identifying and understanding all the underlying causes of an event as well as potential events that were prevented. The Joint Commission (JC, 2010) requires RCA to be performed in response to all sentinel events. Based on the results of the RCA, JC expects the organization to develop and implement an action plan consisting of improvements designed to reduce future risk of sentinel events and to monitor the effectiveness of those improvements.

RCA is a reactive assessment that begins after an error, retrospectively outlining the sequence of events that led to the problem and identifying all root causes of the error to completely examine it. RCA can be used to identify trends and assess risk. It can be used whenever an error is suspected. RCA focuses on the understanding that system factors, rather than individual factors, are likely the root cause of most errors. The aim of RCA is to uncover the underlying causes(s) of an error by looking at all contributing factors, for example: lack of education, drug errors, not checking a patient's identification band, or two patients in the same hospital with the same last name. Those involved in an RCA investigation ask a series of key questions, including what happened, why it happened, what were the most dominant factors that caused it to happen, why those factors occurred, and what systems and processes underlie those factors. Answers to these questions help identify safety barriers and causes of problems so that similar problems can be prevented in the future. Often, it is important to also consider events that occurred immediately prior to the error in question, because other factors may also have contributed to the error. The final step of a traditional RCA is developing recommendations for system and process improvement(s), based on the findings of the investigation (Hughes, 2008).

A similar problem-identifying procedure is the critical incident technique in which, after an event occurs, information is collected on the causes and actions that led to the critical incident event. Ideally, an inter-professional team trained in RCA and the critical incident technique identifies major findings from the RCA or critical incident technique and increases the validity of the findings.

Failure Modes and Effects Analysis

Failure modes and effects analysis (FMEA) is an evaluation technique used to identify and eliminate known and/or potential failures, problems, and errors from a system, design, work process, and/or service before they actually occur. FMEA was developed for use by the U.S. military and has been used by the National Aeronautics and Space Administration (NASA) to predict and evaluate potential failures and unrecognized hazards and to proactively identify steps in a work process that could reduce or eliminate future failures. The goal of FMEA is to prevent errors by attempting to identify all the ways a work process could fail, estimate the probability and consequences of each failure, and then take action to prevent the potential failures from occurring. In health care, FMEA focuses on the system of care and uses an interdisciplinary team to evaluate a work process from a quality improvement perspective (Hughes, 2008).

HIGH-RELIABILITY ORGANIZATIONS—A CULTURE OF SAFETY

High-reliability organizations have generated much interest from nurses in recent years. Nurses want to know how to halt the alarming rate of health care errors and preventable complications and develop health care systems that are safe for patients. High-reliability organization theory (HROT) is a framework describing characteristics of high-risk, yet safe, systems. HROT was developed in non-health care systems such as nuclear submarines, aircraft carriers, and aviation. In these systems, a small slip or error could lead to a catastrophic event. HROT describes five characteristics of high-reliability systems, including preoccupation with failure, reluctance to simplify, sensitivity to operations, commitment to resilience, and deference to expertise (Kemper & Boyle, 2009). Within highly reliable systems, a unique teamwork culture called a "culture of safety" operates. An organization's **culture of safety** is the result of their shared values and behaviors that demonstrate communication based on mutual trust, agreement on the importance of safety, and confidence in the ability to prevent errors through the use of known safety practices (Kemper & Boyle 2009). Organizations that want to develop high reliability and a culture of safety take these actions:

- Determine areas of high risk; for example, monitor patient outcomes and use survey tools such as the Denison Organizational Culture Model (DOCS) and the National Database of Nursing Quality Indicators (NDNQI) RN Survey (NDNQI, 2006).
- Develop action plans to improve performance in weak areas of practice.
- Ask staff to speak up if they witness an unsafe practice.
- Learn from errors and near misses. Focus on analysis of system problems, not on blaming individuals.
- Evaluate the culture of safety and consider use of the following:
  - Hospital Survey on Patient Safety Culture
  - Nursing Home Survey on Patient Safety Culture
  - Safety Climate Survey
  - Safety Attitude Questionnaire
- Enhance teamwork skills. Consider use of TeamSTEPPS.
- Safeguard patients (Kemper & Boyle, 2009). Use standardized approaches to common procedures; develop decision aids, e.g., an operating room checklist, standing orders; develop system redundancy, e.g., use of two nurses to confirm that the correct type of blood is being hung for a patient; develop patient care bundles that are a collection of best practices for a particular patient condition, e.g., a ventilator bundle (Sanford, 2010).

High-reliability organizations will encourage all staff to use their professional judgment and assess each patient individually. Not all patients fit the standard.

A Just Culture and the Role of the System

In the past, nurses and other health care providers often attempted to work more safely by working more carefully and by retraining, counseling, or disciplining workers involved in errors. The prevailing thought at the time was that individual workers were solely accountable for the outcomes of patients under their care, even if the underlying work processes for achieving those outcomes were not under their direct control. Perfect performance was expected and felt to be achievable through education, professionalism, vigilance, and care (ISMP, 2006). Little thought was given to the health care system's contribution. The effect was to cause fear of retribution, ranging from undue embarrassment to employment and/or licensure termination. Workers were afraid to report their own errors or those of a colleague. Enormous opportunities to learn about risks and implement health care system changes to reduce the chance of error were missed.

By the mid-1990s, a culture shift to a "no-blame" culture occurred, in which there was general agreement that even the most experienced, knowledgeable, vigilant, and caring workers could make mistakes that could lead to patient harm. There was recognition that workers who made honest errors were not always completely blameworthy, nor was there much benefit to punishing them for these unintentional acts (ISMP, 2006). The problem with the "no-blame" concept is that it failed to confront individuals who willfully (and often repeatedly) made unsafe choices, knowingly disregarding a risk that most peers would recognize as being likely to lead to a bad outcome (ISMP, 2006).

A new, just culture is emerging in health care that is about creating an environment where staff can raise their hands when they have seen a risk or made a mistake. It is a culture that rewards reporting and puts a high value on open communication and is hungry for knowledge to improve quality and safe care. It is also about having a well-established system of accountability. A just culture must recognize that, while we as humans are fallible, we do generally have control of our behavioral choices, whether we are a nurse, doctor, executive, or a nurse manager. Just culture flourishes in an organization that understands the concept of shared accountability—that good system design and good behavioral choices of staff together produce good results. It has to be both (ISMP, 2006).

Organizational Culture

Organizational culture consists of the deep underlying assumptions, beliefs, and values that are shared by members of the organization and that typically operate unconsciously. Effective organizations that demonstrate high levels of four important cultural traits can be measured. The four cultural traits are: (1) adaptability, with the measures of creating change, customer focus, and organizational learning; (2) involvement, with the measures of empowerment, team orientation, and capability development; (3) consistency, with the measures of core values, agreement, and coordination and integration; and (4) mission, with the measures of strategic direction and intent, goals and objectives, and vision (Denison Consulting, 2012). The DOCS items were developed to address those aspects of organizational culture that had demonstrated links to organizational effectiveness, such as having a shared sense of responsibility, possessing consistent systems and procedures, being responsive to the market, and having a clear purpose and direction for the organization.

ORGANIZATIONAL STRUCTURE

Organizations are structured or organized to facilitate the execution of their mission, goals, reporting lines, and communication within the organization. This is true of entire organizations as well as individual nursing units. There are a number of ways to describe organizational structures that involve classifying them by identifying selected characteristics. Each of these characteristics tends to exist on a continuum. For example, under the category of type or level of authority in an organizational structure, a highly bureaucratic, highly authoritarian structure is at one end of the continuum and a highly democratic, participative structure is at the other end. The highly authoritarian model is seen in the military and is well suited for the purposes of the military. When decisions need to be made quickly, with clarity and not with challenges or discussion, as in a battle situation, a highly authoritarian organizational structure works well.

Types of Organizational Structures

Most often the existing organizational structures are communicated by means of an organizational chart. Figure 11-3 is an example of an organizational chart for a nursing home. This organization has a tall, bureaucratic structure with many layers in the hierarchy or chain of command, and a centralized, formal authority in the board of trustees. It represents a functional, formal, top-down reporting structure (Shortell & Kaluzny, 2006). Note it is the board of directors that delegates to the chief executive officer. The chief executive officer delegates to the two vice presidents. The vice president of Patient Care Services oversees five directors, namely, the directors of Social Work, Rehabilitation and Recreation, Pharmacy, Nursing, and Health Records. The nurse managers (NMs) of Unit A and Unit B report to their nursing director. The charge nurse reports to the NM of Unit B. The treatment nurse and the medication nurse report to the charge nurse. In this functional design, the division of labor is such that each individual may be so focused on a specific area that he or she has little perspective about the overall picture. For example, a treatment nurse may focus only on treatments and have little information about the total patient.

Matrix Structure

Today, given the greater complexity of the health care system, more organizations are using matrix structures. Figure 11-4 shows a matrix design (Shortell & Kaluzny, 2006).

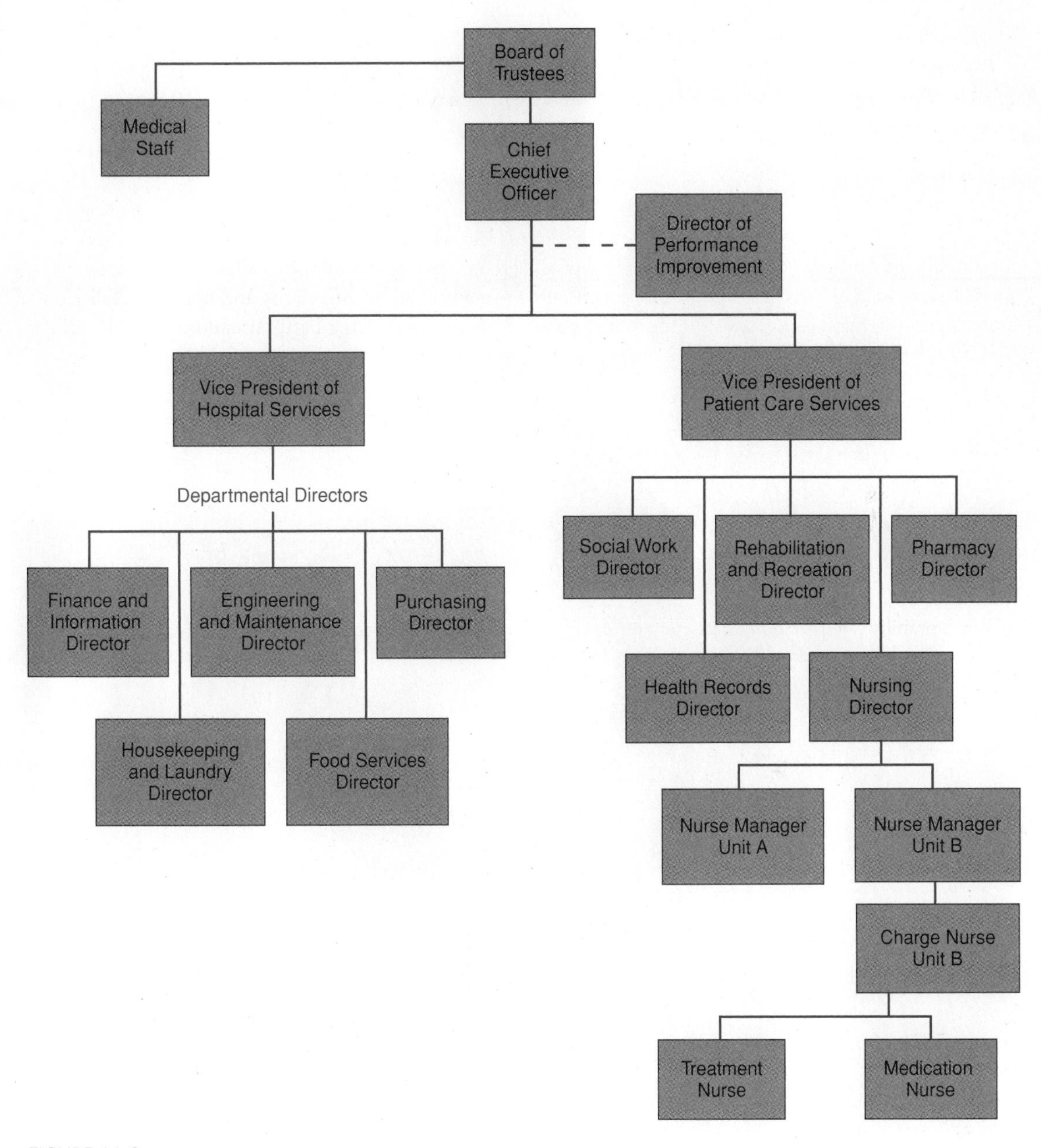

FIGURE 11-3

A functional design: nursing home.

(*Source:* Shortell, S., & Kaluzny, A. (2006). *Health care management: Organization design and behavior* (5th ed.). Clifton Park, NY: Delmar Cengage Learning.)

Flat Versus Tall Structure

Organizations are considered flat when there are few layers in the reporting structure. A tall organization would have many layers in the chain of command. An example of a flat organizational structure in a hospital would be one director of nursing with two

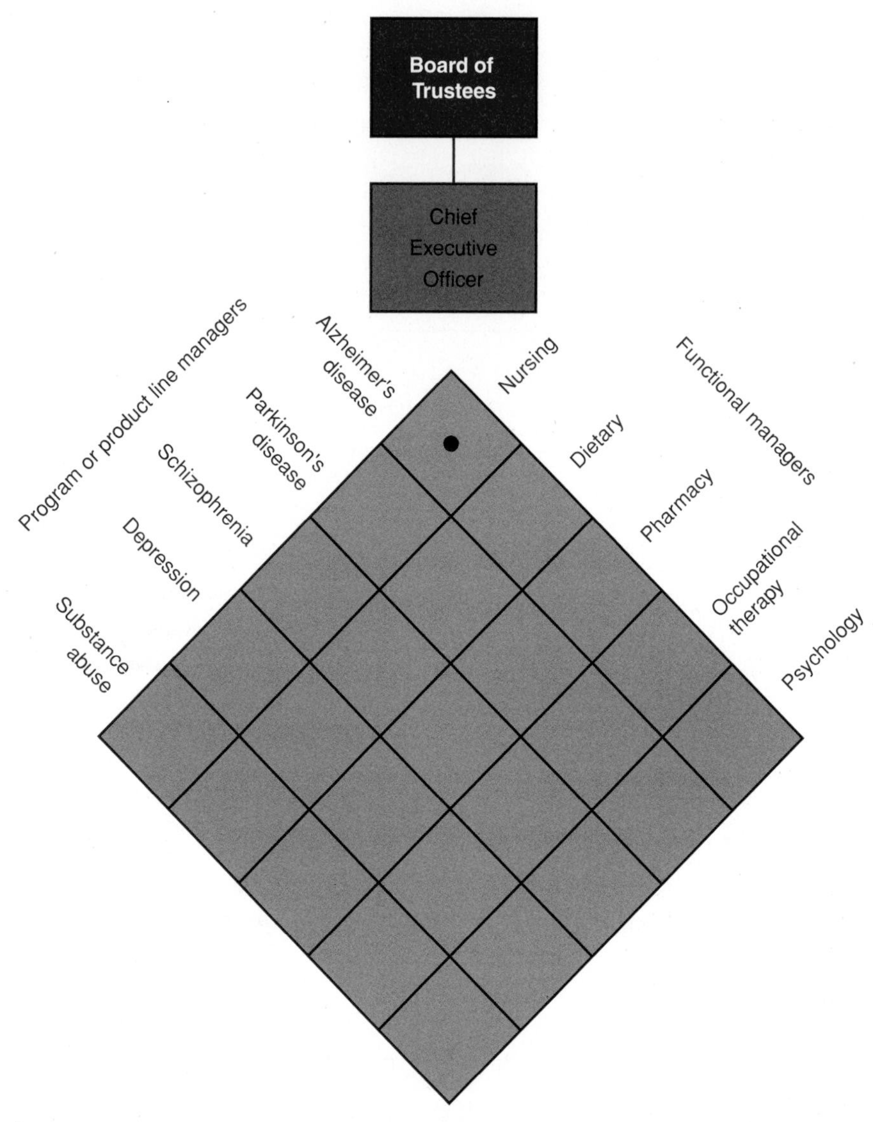

FIGURE 11-4

Matrix design: a psychiatric center. An individual worker in this example is part of the Alzheimer's program, as well as a member of the nursing department.

(*Source:* Shortell, S., & Kaluzny, A. (2000). *Health care management: Organization design and behavior* (4th ed.). Clifton Park, NY: Delmar Cengage Learning.)

head nurses reporting to her, one for maternal and child patient care units and one for medical-surgical patient care units (Figure 11-5). Contrast this flat type of structure in Figure 11-5 with the functional, tall, bureaucratic structure in Figure 11-3, which has many layers.

Decentralized versus Centralized Structure

The terms "centralized" and "decentralized" refer to the degree to which an organization has spread its lines of authority, power, and communication. A tall, bureaucratic design such as that in Figure 11-3

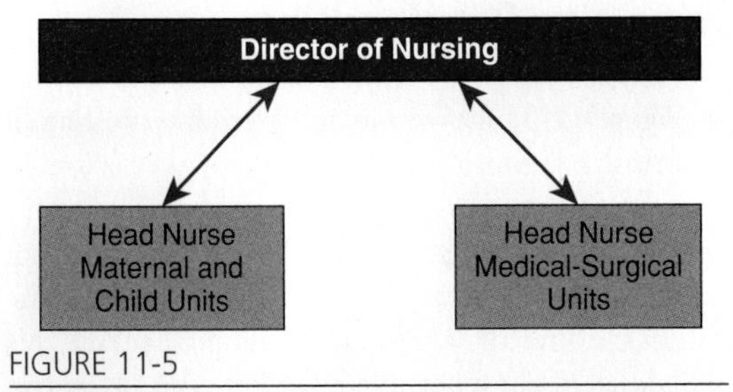

FIGURE 11-5

Example of a flat organizational structure.

© Cengage Learning 2014

would be considered highly centralized. A matrix design such as that in Figure 11-4 would be on the decentralized end of the continuum. As can be seen in Figure 11-4, the nursing manager can interface with the Alzheimer's disease program manager without going through a central, hierarchical core, as would happen in a bureaucratic structure like that in Figure 11-3.

Other characteristics or attributes can be used to assess organizations. Many typologies exist that may be used for this purpose. For example, Shortell and Kaluzny (2006) suggest using external environment, mission/goals, workgroups/work design, organizational design, interorganizational relationships, change/innovation, and/or strategic issues to review different health service organizations.

Division of Labor

The way the labor force is divided or organized has an impact on how the mission is accomplished. There are a number of ways to divide the workload in an organization. The important consideration is that the manner in which the work is divided should match the goals of the organizational unit and should contribute maximally to the efficient, effective attainment of the desired outcomes.

For example, in the matrix structure shown in Figure 11-4, the structure is less important, and the workforce roles and reporting relationships are based on the project or task to be accomplished, rather than on a rigid hierarchy. An example of this is the planning involved in the preparation for a Joint Commission (JC) planning review. The JC team could be composed of various individuals at varying levels of responsibility and from programs across the organization, but they could interact with staff at all levels and report as a task force at a high level in the organization.

Span of Control

The term "span of control" is used to designate the number of individuals who report to one person. If the span of control is too narrow, an organization may become top heavy, and much time may be wasted in unnecessary communications up and down the chain of command, resulting in lost efficiency. On the other hand, if the span of control is too broad, it is difficult for one manager to give adequate attention to the support and development of all the individuals who report to him or her.

Division of Labor by Geographic Area

Care delivery divided according to geography or location can be efficient. It might consist of the hospital and ambulatory care or, at smaller unit levels, the North Team and the West Team. Frequently, care provided by home health agencies is divided by geographic district for efficiency in travel. At the health care system level, geographical division could mean that each major area, such as the hospital or the clinics, would have separate supporting services, such as two pharmacies, one in the outpatient clinic and one in the hospital. Both clinic and inpatient areas could, and often do, have separate medical records departments. An obvious concern in such arrangements is lack of coordination and duplication of services.

Division of Labor by Product or Service

Sometimes, care delivery is organized around product lines or service lines. This is a type of functional division of work, but it is based on a patient's diagnosis or the specialty care required by a patient. For example, there might be a cardiology service line, a woman's health service line, and an oncology service line, all of them with both inpatient and outpatient services. This can lead to improved quality of care and decreased confusion for the patient, because the information and protocols used in the outpatient side would be consistent with the information and protocols used in the hospital and across the entire health care system. Figure 11-6 demonstrates a product line design (Shortell & Kaluzny, 2006).

Roles and Responsibilities

Note that exact roles and responsibilities within each level and division are not defined on the organizational charts beyond specifying the given division, for example, nursing. Scope of responsibilities, specific duties, and specific job requirements are found in documents such as individual job or position descriptions.

Reporting Relationships

An organizational chart, such as the one that appears in Figure 11-3, allows you to determine the formal reporting relationships, which are shown with a solid line. Sometimes dotted lines are used in an organizational chart to depict dual or secondary reporting relationships. An example of this in Figure 11-3 is the role of the director of performance improvement. This individual might report directly to the chief executive officer but also have position accountabilities to the board of trustees. The formal reporting relationships may or may not reflect the actual communications

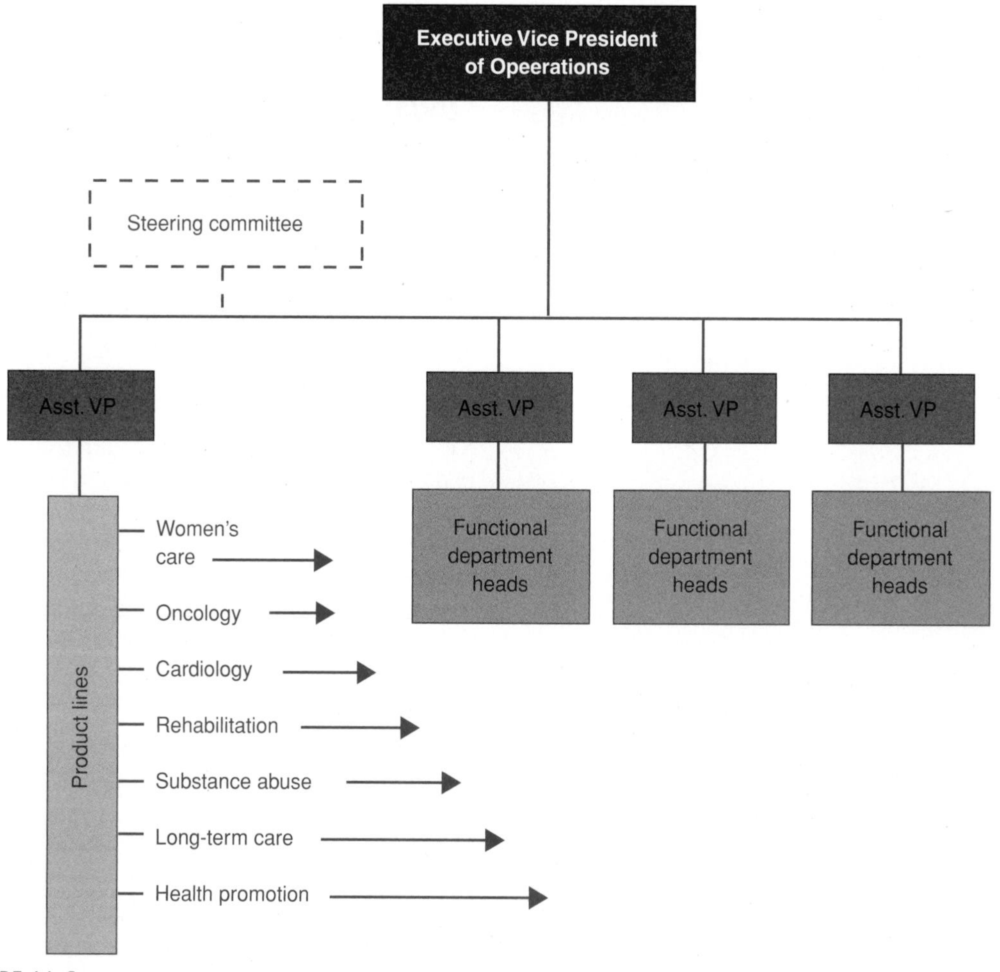

FIGURE 11-6

Product line design.

© Cengage Learning 2014

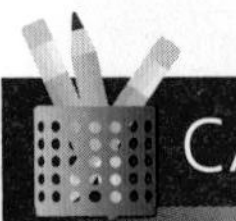

CASE STUDY 11-1

You are a staff nurse working as part of the interprofessional orthopedic team. You notice that there are an increasing number of diabetic patients being admitted for elective total hip surgery. Because the length of stay is so short and your team has a surgical focus in caring for patients, the patients' underlying diabetes and other chronic diseases have not been a focus on the unit. However, you are aware that the larger organization is beginning to evaluate how different populations of patients, such as diabetics, are cared for across the continuum of care.

What should you do to improve care for your patients?

What steps would you take to do this?

that occur within the institution. For example, information may be communicated outside the formal reporting relationships. This method of information sharing is often referred to as the "grapevine." An example of grapevine communication is when a nurse has a personal friend who is in a high administrative position who shares confidential information about pending budget cuts with her.

SHARED GOVERNANCE

Shared governance is an organizational framework grounded in a philosophy of decentralized leadership that fosters autonomous decision making and professional nursing practice (Porter-O'Grady, Hawkins, & Parker, 1997). Shared governance, by its name, implies the allocation of control, power, or authority (governance) among mutually (shared) interested, vested parties (Stichler, 1992).

In most health care settings, the vested parties in nursing fall into two distinct categories: (1) nurses practicing direct patient care, such as staff nurses; and (2) nurses managing or administering the provision of that care, such as managers. In shared governance, a nursing organization's management assumes the responsibility for organizational structure and resources. Management relinquishes control over issues related to clinical practice. In return, staff nurses

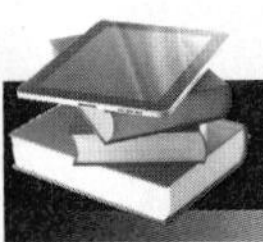

EVIDENCE FROM THE LITERATURE

Citation: Dansky, K. H., Vasey, J., & Bowles, K. (2008). Impact of telehealth on clinical outcomes in patients with heart failure. Clinical Nursing Research, 17(3), 182-199.

Discussion: The purpose of this study was to determine the effects of telehomecare on hospitalization, emergency department (ED) use, mortality, and symptoms related to sodium and fluid intake, medication use, and physical activity.

The authors studied two hundred eighty four patients with heart failure and noted the effects of telehomecare on health services utilization and mortality and changes in self-reported symptoms. They found that after sixty days of telehealth services, the telehomecare patients had statistically-significant, lower rates of rehospitalization and emergency department use. Differences were statistically significant at 60 days but not 120 days. The technology enables frequent monitoring of clinical indices and permits the home health care nurse to detect changes in cardiac status and intervene when necessary.

Implications for Practice: The trend toward the increased use of technology has created a need for nurses to learn additional methods of delivering nursing care. Nurses need to become educated on the benefits and responsibilities of providing care using telehealth. This method of health care provision will require different skills in patient assessment, patient education, and equipment utilization.

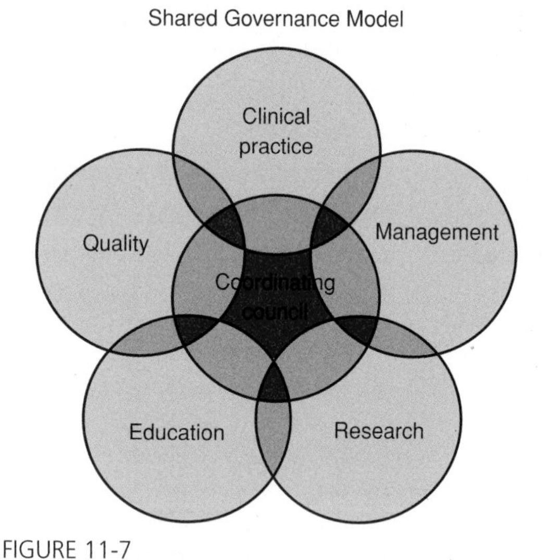

FIGURE 11-7

A shared governance model.

© Cengage Learning 2014

accept the responsibility and accountability for their professional practice.

Unit-based shared governance structures are most successful if there is an organization-wide structure of shared governance in place that unit-based functions can coincide with. Organizational-shared governance structures are usually council models that have evolved from preexisting nursing or institutional committees. In a council structure, clearly defined accountabilities for specific elements of professional practice have been delegated to five main arenas: clinical practice, quality, education, research, and management of resources (Porter-O'Grady et al., 1997). Figure 11-7 illustrates a shared governance model.

Purposes of the Shared Governance Councils

The purpose of the clinical practice council is to establish nursing practice standards for a unit. The purpose of the quality council is to make recommendations about hiring, promoting, and credentialing nursing staff, and to oversee the unit quality management initiatives. The purpose of the nursing education council is to assess the learning needs of the unit staff and develop and implement evidence-based programs to meet these needs.

The research council advances research utilization with the intent of incorporating evidence-based findings into the clinical nursing standards of practice. The research council may also coordinate research projects if advanced practice nurses practice at the institution. The purpose of the management council is to ensure that the standards of nursing practice and governance agreed upon by unit staff are upheld and that adequate resources are available to deliver patient care. The purpose of the nursing coordinating council is to facilitate and integrate the activities of the other councils.

MAGNET HOSPITALS

A **magnet hospital** is a health care organization that has met the rigorous nursing excellence requirements of the American Nurses Credentialing Center (ANCC), a division of the American Nurses Association (ANA). Magnet designation is a voluntary credentialing process. Achieving magnet designation represents the highest level of recognition that the ANCC accords to health care organizations that provide the services of registered professional nurses (ANCC, 2008). As a testament to the increasing recognition given to magnet hospitals, *U.S. News and World Report* now includes magnet designation in its criteria for its annual Best Hospitals of America list (© *U.S.News & World Report. (2012).*). Two decades of research by Kramer and Schmalenberg (2002) suggests that nurses in magnet facilities indicate high levels of job satisfaction because they perceive that magnet practice environments allow nurses the ability to give quality patient care.

History of Magnet Designation

In 1983, the American Academy of Nursing (AAN), an organization affiliated with the ANA, appointed a Task Force on Nursing Practice in Hospitals. The purpose of the task force was to identify workplace characteristics that were successful in recruiting and retaining hospital nurses. The task force studied 163 hospitals in the United States, based on their reputation for successfully attracting and retaining nurses and for the delivery of high-quality nursing care. Of the 163 hospitals studied, 41 (25%) were described as magnet hospitals (McClure, Poulin, Sovie, & Wandelt, 1983). A magnet designation was earned through demonstrated high nurse satisfaction, low nurse turnover, and low nurse vacancy rates. Interestingly, the 41 original magnet hospitals were able to recruit and retain nurses despite: concurrent health care industry changes in the payment system; an unprecedented number of hospital mergers, acquisitions, and consolidations; and a major nursing shortage. The AAN's 1983 study concluded that the 41 original magnet hospitals shared a set of core organizational attributes that were desirable. The study stimulated additional independent research that provided further evidence to highlight the achievement of superior outcomes in magnet hospitals.

By June 1990, the ANA established the ANCC as a separate, incorporated, nonprofit organization that was to serve as the credentialing arm for magnet hospitals. The initial proposal for the Magnet Recognition Program was approved by the ANA board of directors in December 1990. The magnet program proposal indicated that it would be built upon the 1983 AAN magnet hospital study. Further, the magnet program would use the 1999 *ANA Scope and Standards for Nurse Administrators*, now in its third revision (ANA, 2009), as a baseline for program development.

The ANCC Magnet Facilities

The University of Washington Medical Center in Seattle became ANCC's first magnet facility in 1994. By 1998, 13 more hospitals achieved magnet designation. By 2010, there were more than 300 magnet-designated facilities. Hundreds of facilities are continuously in the pipeline, seeking to become magnet hospitals. To date, the Magnet Recognition Program has been expanded to include both acute care hospitals and long-term facilities. The Magnet Recognition Program reviews applications from both U.S. and international health care organizations.

Of the 5,815 hospitals in the United States (American Hospital Association, 2009), 372 (or 6.4%) are magnet-designated facilities (ANCC, 2010). This figure is rising daily. Community hospitals, teaching hospitals, and hospital systems, large (more than 1,000 beds) and small (less than 100 beds), in rural and urban settings, have achieved magnet recognition. Although pursuing magnet designation is an individual organizational decision, implementing the magnet standards in hospital settings can potentially benefit institutions, independent of whether or not they achieve magnet designation (Miller & Anderson, 2007).

There are 14 Forces of Magnetism. They are the outcomes of innovative and dynamic implementation of the Scope and Standards for Nurse Administrators by visionary nurse leaders creating supportive and collegial environments for nursing practice (ANCC, 2008). Magnet designation requires the full expression of the 14 Forces of Magnetism. This means that facilities seeking magnet designation must show evidence to support the existence of all the Forces of Magnetism in the organization. An emerging body of literature exists, including: help in navigating the magnet journey (Goode et al., 2005; Ellis & Gates, 2005; Havens & Johnston, 2004; Shirey, 2004); articles that describe the magnet application process (Bumgarner & Beard, 2003; Bliss-Holtz, Winter, & Scherer, 2004); articles that provide guidance in meeting difficult standards (Messmer, Jones, & Rosillo, 2002; Turkel, Reidinger, Ferket, & Reno, 2005; Turkel, Ferket, Reidinger, & Beatty, 2008); help in documenting the Forces of Magnetism (Shirey, 2005; Drenkard, 2005; Poduska, 2005); sources assisting with the magnet journey (Broom & Tilbury, 2007), the magnet site visit (Conerly & Thornhill, 2009), and the redesignation preparation (Upenieks & Sitterding, 2008).

A New Magnet Model

In 2004, the magnet program underwent a comprehensive evaluation using an independent consultant external to ANCC (Triolo, Scherer, & Floyd, 2006). The evaluation process ended in 2005, culminating with 22 evidence-based recommendations. In 2008, a new magnet model was developed that incorporated scholarly review and statistical analysis (Wolf, Triolo, & Ponte, 2008) and affirmed what the magnet program represents. The new magnet model emphasizes five new components within global issues in nursing and health. Although the program continues to incorporate the Forces of Magnetism, the new model eliminates redundancy within the 14 Forces

(ANCC, 2008). The five components are: transformational leadership; structural empowerment; exemplary professional practice; new knowledge, innovation, and improvements; and empirical quality results. Overarching the new magnet model components is an acknowledgment of Global Issues in Nursing and Health Care. While not technically a model component, this category includes the various factors and challenges facing nursing and health care today.

Magnet Appraisal Process

Magnet-aspiring organizations generally begin the magnet process by purchasing the most current issue of the Magnet Recognition Program® Manual - Recognizing Nursing Excellence(ANA, 2008). This manual guides the aspiring magnet organization's chief nursing officer (CNO), magnet program coordinator, and magnet steering-team members in pursuing the magnet journey.

The magnet appraisal process consists of four sequential phases: application, evaluation, site visit, and award decision. Additionally, the magnet process considers feedback acquired from public comment opportunities.

The application phase involves review of the application manual and the decision to apply for magnet designation. Early in the magnet journey, organizations will need to establish a database to collect data on nursing-sensitive indicators, that is, measures that reflect the outcome of nursing actions. Joining the National Database of Nursing Quality Indicators (NDNQI, 2006) is a means to achieve this data-collection requirement. Membership in the NDNQI is beneficial, because it provides organizations with the capability to benchmark data on nursing-sensitive indicators gathered at the unit level. Benchmarking is the process of comparing outcomes with those of similar organizations to identify and establish best practices. Organizations will also conduct a gap analysis in the application process. A gap analysis is an assessment of the differences between the expected magnet requirements and the organization's current performance of those requirements. A gap analysis serves as a tool that provides direction in developing the necessary activities to bridge any gaps.

The evaluation phase occurs following the written application and submission of the aspiring hospital's magnet evidence. This evidence and documents are reviewed by a team of ANCC magnet appraisers who independently score the evidence for magnetism.

Arrangements for a site visit by the magnet appraisal team will follow if the written documentation earns the necessary points to score at a level of excellence. While on site, the magnet appraisers visit the units of the organization where nurses work, to verify the content of the written magnet evidence previously submitted and scored. Following the site visit, the appraisal team prepares a consensus report summarizing the written documentation review and the site visit findings.

The award decision involves review of the consensus report by ANCC's Commission on Magnet Recognition. Magnet awards are made when the Commission members agree that the evidence reflects magnet-defined excellence in an organization's nursing services (ANCC, 2008). After magnet designation is conferred, facilities must maintain compliance with the magnet standards to sustain the magnet workplace culture and to position the organization for magnet redesignation. Magnet hospitals submit annual reports for interim reporting and repeat the original application, evaluation, and site visit activities every four years for the redesignation process.

PROFESSIONAL NURSING PRACTICE

The quality of a professional nursing practice environment is crucial in attracting and retaining professional nurses. Nurse leaders play a key role in creating practice environments that are supportive of and conducive to professional nursing practice. Magnet hospitals represent one example of supportive and collegial work environments that are both high-performance and high quality-of-work-life organizations for nurses and other health care professionals. These desired work environments do not happen overnight. They require significant investment of time, energy, and resources by individuals, groups, and organizations. Although the investment required to create magnet workplaces is significant, the rewards to individuals, groups, and organizations are even greater. Ultimately, the investment in building supportive and collegial work environments results in organizational effectiveness, a key desired outcome of organizational behavior.

KEY CONCEPTS

- Strategic planning is a process that is designed to achieve goals in dynamic, competitive environments through the allocation of resources.
- A stakeholder assessment is a systematic consideration of all potential stakeholders to ensure that the needs of each of these stakeholders are incorporated in the planning phase. For a program to be successful, the involvement of those who will be affected is essential.
- Magnet hospitals are known to have supportive and collegial work environments for nurses and may be classified as both high-performance and high-quality-of-work-life environments.
- In the face of a highly competitive health care industry, health care leaders have a compelling obligation to create highly reliable, supportive, and collegial work environments that are conducive to maintaining a culture of safety for patients and retaining nurses within the profession.
- The 14 Forces of Magnetism are configured into five magnet model components within global issues in nursing and health care.
- Shared governance is an organizational framework grounded in a philosophy of decentralized leadership that fosters autonomous decision making and professional nursing practice.
- The mission statement reflects an organization's philosophy and values and provides the reader with an indication of the behavior and actions that can be expected from that organization.
- A health care organization needs to have a good idea of where it fits into its environment and what types of programs and services are needed and demanded by its customers or stakeholders.
- The purpose of planning is twofold. First, it is important that everyone has the same idea or vision of where the organization is headed; second, a good plan can help to ensure that the needed resources are available to carry out the initiatives that have been identified as important to the unit or agency.
- Organizations are structured or organized in a manner that is designed to facilitate the execution of their mission and their strategic plans.

KEY TERMS

culture of safety
focus groups
goal
magnet hospital
mission statement
shared governance
stakeholder assessment

REVIEW QUESTIONS

1. A subcommittee of nurses has convened to describe the institution's purpose and philosophy. Which of the following documents would they begin with to start the process?
   A. The organizational chain of command
   B. The organizational chart
   C. The mission statement
   D. The strategic plan

2. A nurse on the pediatric unit has been asked to join a team of professionals to identify both strengths and weaknesses in the internal environment, and opportunities and threats in the external environment. Which analysis format would the nurse choose?
   A. Strategic plan analysis
   B. SWOT analysis
   C. Performance improvement analysis
   D. LEAN Production System methodology analysis

3. A visitor stops the nurse in a hall and inquires as to the meaning of the posting labeled "vision statement." The nurse replies with which of the following? A vision statement:
   A. Is an advertisement for the hospital.
   B. Reflects the organization's vision for the future.
   C. Is a six-month goal statement that staff work on.
   D. Is a quality improvement initiative.

4. A nurse evaluating an organization's potential for long-term success knows that high-performance environments offer a competitive advantage. Which of the following examples illustrate a high-performance organization? Select all that apply. The organization:
   A. Partners with a technology center that readily integrates new and emerging technologies into clinical practice.
   B. Demonstrates a commitment to continuous quality improvement.
   C. Controls information available to employees and follows the company policy that "what employees don't know won't hurt them."
   D. Develops a succession strategy that supports promotions from within.
   E. Plans for the education of future leaders within the organization.
   F. Seeks outside candidates for all managerial positions.

5. The LEAN Production System methodology is driven by which of the following?
   A. Financial profit escalation
   B. Identification of customer needs and the improvement of work processes by removing activities that are nonvalue-added
   C. Solutions for quality improvement
   D. System and work process review

6. Which of the following most accurately characterizes why magnet hospitals may be classified as high-performance organizations?
   A. High-performance organizations and magnet hospitals possess no similarities, and therefore this association in terminology is not well founded.
   B. High-performance organizations such as magnet hospitals recognize the importance of attracting and retaining talented employees.
   C. High-performance organizations such as magnet hospitals are known for high employee turnover.
   D. High-performance organizations such as magnet hospitals focus on maintaining the status quo and benefit from the fact that they do not experience change or turmoil.

7. Demonstrating that all the 14 Forces of Magnetism exist in an organization is crucial to meeting magnet requirements. As a staff nurse working on a magnet committee, you have been asked to help evaluate the magnet evidence to be submitted with the hospital's magnet application. Which of the following information pieces is not evidence to support professional development, a Force of Magnetism?
   A. Documentation of annual nurse-certification preparation courses offered in all the nursing specialty areas within the hospital
   B. Access to Web-based educational programs for nurses working in both the unit and in their own homes
   C. A 12-month financial report that details on a unit-by unit basis the economic support provided to all staff nurses on that unit for attending educational programs outside the health care organization
   D. A statement describing how decision making is done by the medical staff

8. A primary goal for creation of the Magnet Recognition Program is which of the following?
   A. To start the reengineering effort in the health care industry
   B. To promote excellence in the delivery of nursing services to patients
   C. To increase the incidence of medication-error reporting
   D. To promote staff and physician satisfaction

9. SWOT stands for which of the following?
   A. Strengths, weaknesses, opportunities, threats
   B. Strengths, worries, outcomes, threats
   C. Strengths, weaknesses, opportunities, treatment
   D. Structures, worries, outcomes, threats

10. The strategic planning process typically considers which of the following? Select all that apply.
   A. Values clarification
   B. Mission definition
   C. Vision statement
   D. Annual budget
   E. Performance improvement plan
   F. SWOT analysis

REVIEW ACTIVITIES

1. Write a beginning mission statement and strategic plan for your professional nursing career. What might they include?
2. You are asked to plan for the advisory board for your institution's proposed hospice program. How would you go about determining whom to include on the advisory board? What groups of professionals and consumers would you want to see represented on a hospice advisory board?
3. To learn more about the magnet eligibility criteria, access and review the document entitled Organization Eligibility Requirements (ANCC, 2012). To access the document, go to http://www.nursecredentialing.org/Magnet/Application-Process/JourneytoMagnetExcellence/JourneyCategory/Eligibility-Requirements/Journey-OrgEligibilityRequirements. Search for Organization Eligibility Requirements. After you have found the document, use the document to familiarize yourself with the magnet requirements that must be in place to achieve magnet designation. How do you see your current health care work environment meeting the specified requirements?

EXPLORING THE WEB

- Upon completion of your nursing degree, you plan to interview for a position at an area hospital. In preparation for your interview, you want to understand the mission as well as other information about that institution. Today that information is readily available on the Web. For example, if you are planning to apply at Loyola University, Chicago, go to *http://luc.edu.* Click on Mission and Identity. Review the University Mission Statement.
- Agency for Healthcare Research and Quality (AHRQ): *http://www.ahrq.gov.* Explore the various elements of the website.
- Institute of Medicine: *http://www.iom.edu.* Explore the various elements of the website.
- National Student Nurses Association (NSNA) Career Center: *http://www.nsna.org*
- Visit the website for the nursing profession's honor society: *http://www.nursingsociety.org.* This site provides weekly information from Sigma Theta Tau International. What did you see there that may be helpful to you in your practice?

REFERENCES

American Hospital Association (AHA). (2009). Statistics and studies: Fast facts on U.S. hospitals. Retrieved July 24, 2010, from http://www.aha.org/aha/resource-center

American Nurses Association (ANA). (2008). Magnet Recognition Program® Manual - Recognizing Nursing Excellence. Retrieved November 14, 2012 from, http://www.nursesbooks.org/Main-Menu/Magnet/Magnet-Recognition-Program-Manual-Recognizing-Nursing-Excellence-.aspx

American Nurses Association (ANA). (2009). *Scope and standards for nurse administrators* (3rd ed.). Washington, DC: American Nurses Publishing.

American Nurses Credentialing Center (ANCC). (2004). *Magnet recognition program: Application manual 2005.* Washington, DC: American Nurses Credentialing Center.

American Nurses Credentialing Center (ANCC). (2008). Modifying the magnet model: The shape of things to come. *American Nurse Today, 3*(7), 22.

American Nurses Credentialing Center (ANCC). (2010). Nurse opinion questionnaire. Retrieved July 24, 2010, from http://www.nursecredentialing.org/magnet/nurseopinionsurvey.aspx

American Nurses Credentialing Center (ANCC). (2012). Organization eligibility requirements. Retrieved October 6, 2012, from http://www.nursecredentialing.org/Magnet/Application-Process/JourneytoMagnet Excellence/JourneyCategory/Eligibility-Requirements/Journey-OrgEligibilityRequirements

Benner, P. E. Hughes,R.G., & Sutphen, M. (2008). Clinical Reasoning, Decision making, and Action: Thinking Critically and Clinically. in Hughes, R. G. Ed. (2008). Patient safety and quality: An evidence-based handbook for nurses. AHRQ Publication No. 08-0043. Rockville, MD: Agency for Healthcare Research and Quality. Retrieved November 14, 2012 from http://www.ahrq.gov/qual/nurseshdbk/

Best hospitals 2010–2011: The honor roll. *U.S. News & World Report.* Retrieved October 1, 2012, from http://health.usnews.com/healthnews/best-hospitals/articles/2010/07/14/best-hospitals-2010-11-the-honor-roll.html

Bliss-Holtz, J., Winter, N., & Scherer, E. M. (2004). An invitation to magnet accreditation. *Nursing Management, 35*(9), 36–43.

Broom , C., & Tilbury, M.S. (2007). Magnet Status: A Journey, Not a Destination. Journal of Nursing Care Quality. June 2007, 22(2), 113–118.

Bumgarner, S. D., & Beard, E. L. (2003). The magnet application. *Journal of Nursing Administration, 33*(11), 603–606.

Carroll, L. (2009). Alice's Adventures in Wonderland and Through the Looking-Glass. Oxford University Press.

Cheung, R. D., Aiken, L. H., Clarke, S. P., & Sloane, D. M. (2010). Nursing care and patient outcomes: International evidence. National Institutes of Health.

Conerly, C., & Thornhill, L. (2009). Magnet site visit preparation. *Nursing Management, 40*(7), 41, 42, 44, 46–48.

Dansky, K. H., Vasey, J., & Bowles, K. (2008). Impact of telehealth on clinical outcomes in patients with heart failure. Clinical Nursing Research, *17*(3), 182 –199.

Denison Consulting. (2012). Denison organizational culture survey (DOCS). Retrieved October 1, 2012, from http://www.denisonconsulting.com/model-surveys/denison-model/organizational-culture

The Denison Organizational Culture Model. Retrieved November 14, 2012 from, http://www.denison consulting.com/model-surveys/denison-model/organizational-culture.

Drenkard, K. N. (2005). Sustaining Magnet: Keeping the forces alive. *Nursing Administration Quarterly, 29*(3), 214–222.

Drenkard, K. (2011). A force to be reckoned with! The international attraction of Magnet status. PACEsetterS. March 2011, *8*(1), 10 -13. Retrieved November 14, 2012 from, http://www.nursingcenter.com/lnc/journalarticle?Article_ID=1147946

Ellis, B., & Gates, J. (2005). Achieving Magnet status. *Nursing Administration Quarterly, 29*(3), 241–244.

Goode, C. J., Krugman, M. E., Smith, K., Diaz, J., Edmonds, S., & Mulder, J. (2005). The pull of magnetism: A look at the standards and the experience of a Western academic medical center hospital in achieving and sustaining magnet status. *Nursing Administration Quarterly, 29*(3), 202–213.

Havens, D. S., & Johnston, M. A. (2004). Achieving magnet hospital recognition: Chief nurse executives and magnet coordinators tell their stories. *Journal of Nursing Administration, 34*(12).

Hughes, R. G. (2008). *Patient safety and quality: An evidence-based handbook for nurses.* AHRQ Publication No. 08-0043, April 2008. Rockville, MD: Agency for Healthcare Research and Quality. Retrieved November 14, 2012, from http://www.ahrq.gov/qual/nurseshdbk

Institute for Safe Medication Practice (ISMP). (2006, September 7). Our long journey towards a safety-minded just culture: Part I: Where we've been. Retrieved October 1, 2012, from http://www.ismp.org/newsletters/acutecare/articles/20060907.asp

Institute of Medicine. (IOM). (1999). *To err is human: Building a safer health system.* Washington, DC: National Academies Press.

Institute of Medicine. (IOM). (2004). *Keeping patients safe: Transforming the work environment of nurses.* Washington, DC: National Academies Press.

Joint Commission (JC). (2010). *Comprehensive accreditation manual for hospitals: The official handbook.* Chicago, IL: Author. Retrieved August 15, 2010, from http://www.jointcommission.org

Jones, R., & Beck, S. (1996). *Decision Making in Nursing.* Clifton Park, NY: Delmar Cengage Learning.

Kane, R. L., Shamliyan, T. A., Mueller, C., Duval, S., & Wilt, T. J. (2007). The association of registered nurse staffing levels and patient outcomes: Systematic review and meta-analysis. *Medical Care, 45*(12), 1195–1204.

Kemper, C., & Boyle, D. K. (2009, April). Leading your organization to high reliability. *Nursing Management,* 14–18.

Khoury, C., Blizzard, R., Wright Moore, L., & Hassmiller, S. (2011, July/August). Nursing leadership from bedside to boardroom: A Gallup national survey of opinion leaders, vol. 41 (7/8), 299–305. Retrieved October 6, 2012, from http://www.nursingcenter.com/lnc/static?pageid=1236963

Kramer, M., & Schmalenberg, C. (2002). Magnet hospitals: What makes nurses stay? *Nursing 2004, 34*(6), 50–54.

Kramer, M., & Schmalenberg, C. (2004). Magnet hospitals: What makes nurses stay? *Nursing 2004, 34*(6), 50–54.

McClure, M., Poulin, M., Sovie, M., & Wandelt, M. (1983). *Magnet hospitals: Attraction and retention of professional nurses.* American Academy of Nursing Task Force on Nursing Practice in Hospitals. Kansas City, MO: American Academy of Nursing.

Messmer, P. R., Jones, S. G., & Rosillo, C. (2002). Using nursing research projects to meet magnet recognition program standards. *Journal of Nursing Administration, 32*(10), 538–543.

Miller, L., & Anderson, F. (2007). Lessons learned when Magnet designation is not received. *Journal of Nursing Administration, 37*(3), 131–134.

National database for nursing quality indicators (NDNQI). (2006). Retrieved May 6, 2006, from http://www.nursingquality.org

Norton, D. P., & Kaplan, R. W. (2001). *The strategy-focused organization.* Boston, MA: Harvard Business School.

Plan-Do-Study-Act (PDSA) (Tague, 2004). (discussed in Chapter 13); Six Sigma (Webber & Wallace, 2006); and the Define, Measure, Analyze, Improve, and Control (DMAIC) process (Webber & Wallace, 2006).

Poduska, D. D. (2005). Magnet designation in a community hospital. *Nursing Administration Quarterly, 29*(3), 223–227.

Porter-O'Grady, T., Hawkins, M. A., & Parker, M. L. (1997). *Whole-systems shared governance.* Gaithersburg, MD: Aspen Publishers.

Sanford, K. D. (2010). Designing more reliable nursing systems. Healthcare Financial Management Association. Retrieved December 28, 2010, from http://www.hfma.org/Publications/E-Bulletins/Business-of-Caring/Archives/2010/Spring/Designing-More-Reliable-Nursing-Systems

Shirey, M. R. (2004). Preparing an organization for achieving magnet designation. (Fellow project, 2004). American College of Health Care Executives, Chicago, IL.
Shirey, M. R. (2005). Celebrating certification in nursing: Forces of magnetism in action. *Nursing Administration Quarterly*, 29(3), 245–253.
Shortell, S., & Kaluzny, A. (2000). *Health care management: Organization design and behavior* (4th ed.). Clifton Park, NY: Delmar Cengage Learning.
Shortell, S., & Kaluzny, A. (2006). *Health care management: Organization design and behavior* (5th ed.). Clifton Park, NY: Delmar Cengage Learning.
Stichler, J. F. (1992). A conceptual basis for shared governance. In N. D. Como & B. Pocta (Eds.), *Implementing shared governance: Creating a professional organization* (pp. 1–24). St. Louis, MO: Mosby.
Tague, N.R. (2004). Plan-Do-Study-Act (PDSA). The Quality Toolbox, Second Edition, ASQ Quality Press. 390-392. Retrieved November 14, 2012 from http://asq.org/learn-about-quality/project-planning-tools/overview/pdca-cycle.html.
Triolo, P. K., Scherer, E. M., & Floyd, J. M. (2006). Evaluation of the Magnet recognition program. *Journal of Nursing Administration, 36*(1), 42–48.
Turkel, M. C., Ferket, K., Reidinger, G., & Beatty, D. E. (2008). Building a nursing research fellowship in a community hospital. *Nursing Economics, 26*(1), 26–34.
Turkel, M. C., Reidinger, G., Ferket, K., & Reno, K. (2005). An essential component of the Magnet journey: Fostering an environment for evidence-based practice and nursing research. *Nursing Administration Quarterly, 29*(3), 254–262.
Upenieks, V. V., & Sitterding, M. (2008). Achieving magnet redesignation: A framework for cultural change. *Journal of Nursing Administration, 38*(10), 419–428.
Urden, L. D., & Monarch, K. (2002). The ANCC Magnet recognition program: Converting research into action. In M. L. McClure & A. S. Hinshaw (Eds.), *Magnet hospitals revisited: Attraction and retention of professional nurses* (pp. 103–115). Washington, DC: American Nurses Publishing.
U.S. News Best Hospitals 2012-13. Retrieved November 14, 2012 from http://health.usnews.com/best-hospitals/rankings
Von Thaden, T. L., & Gibbons, A. M. (2008) *The Safety Culture Indicator Scale Measurement System (SCISMS).* Technical Report HFD-08-03/FAA-08-02. Savoy, IL: University of Illinois, Human Factors Division.
Webber, L. & Wallace, M. (2006). Quality Control for Dummies. (15 December 2006). 42 –43.
Wolf, G., Triolo, P., & Ponte, P. R. (2008). Magnet recognition program: The next generation. *Journal of Nursing Administration. 38*(4), 200–204.

SUGGESTED READINGS

Agency for Healthcare Research and Quality (AHRQ). (2010a). TeamSTEPPS. Retrieved December 28, 2010, from http://teamstepps.ahrq.gov
Agency for Healthcare Research and Quality (AHRQ). (2010b). Nursing home survey on patient safety culture. Retrieved December 28, 2010, from http://www.ahrq.gov/qual/patientsafetyculture/nhsurv index.htm
Agency for Healthcare Research and Quality (AHRQ). (2010c). Hospital survey on patient safety culture. Retrieved December 28, 2010, from http://www.ncbi.nlm.nih.gov/pmc/articles/PMC2912897
Agency for Healthcare Research and Quality (AHRQ). (2010d). Safety climate survey. Retrieved December 28, 2010, from http://ahrq.gov/downloads/pub/advances/vol4/Connelly.pdf
Agency for Healthcare Research and Quality (AHRQ). (2010e). Safety attitude questionnaire. Retrieved December 28, 2010, from http://psnet.ahrq.gov/resource.aspx?resourceID=3601
Furman, C., & Caplan, R. (2007). Applying the Toyota production system: Using a patient safety alert system to reduce error. *Joint Commission on Quality and Patient Safety, 33*(7), 376–386.
Germaine, J. (2007). Six Sigma plan delivers stellar results. *Materials Management in Health Care*, 20–26.
Harrington, L. (2007). Quality improvement research and the institutional review board. *Journal of Healthcare Quality, 29*(3), 4–9.
Lynn, J., Baily, M. A., Bottrell, M., et al. (2007). The ethics of using quality improvement methods in health care. *Annals of Internal Medicine, 246,* 666–673.

Middleton, S., Chapman, B., Griffiths, R., et al. (2007). Reviewing recommendations of root-cause analyses. *Australian Health Review, 31*(2), 288–295.

National Healthcare Disparities Report. (2006). Rockville, MD: Agency for Healthcare Research and Quality. Retrieved March 16, 2008, from http://www.ahrq.gov/qual/nhdr06/nhdr06.htm

National Healthcare Quality Report. (2006). Rockville, MD: Agency for Healthcare Research and Quality. Retrieved March 16, 2008, from http://www.ahrq.gov/qual/nhqr06/hrqr06.htm

CHAPTER 12

Time Management and Setting Patient Care Priorities

TANYA L. TOTH, RN, MSN, MBA, HCM, CNOR, CRNFA;
AND PATSY MALONEY, RN-BC, MSN, MA, EDD, NEA-BC

We realize our dilemma goes deeper than shortage of time; it is basically a problem of priorities. We confess, we have left undone those things that we ought to have done; and we have done those things which we ought not to have done.

—CHARLES E. HUMMEL, 1967

OBJECTIVES

Upon completion of this chapter, the reader should be able to:

1. Discuss concepts of time management.
2. Describe strategies for setting priorities.
3. Discuss shift handoff report and making assignments.
4. Use time management strategies to find personal time for lifelong learning.

Inez has just completed her medical-surgical orientation as a new graduate registered nurse. This evening is her first solo shift, but she is frightened and feels like she is holding up the world on her new graduate shoulders. Although she feels that everything rests on her, she is not really alone. Inez and Carole, the other RN, along with one certified nursing assistant, are responsible for 12 possible patients on this section of the unit. Currently, 10 patients are in this section, but a new admission is on the way, another patient is returning from surgery, the dinner trays are arriving, and Inez has medications to pass. Just as the dinner trays arrive, a patient's family member runs out to Inez and states that her mom is confused and incontinent and has pulled out her IV.

What would you do if you were Inez?

What would .you do first?

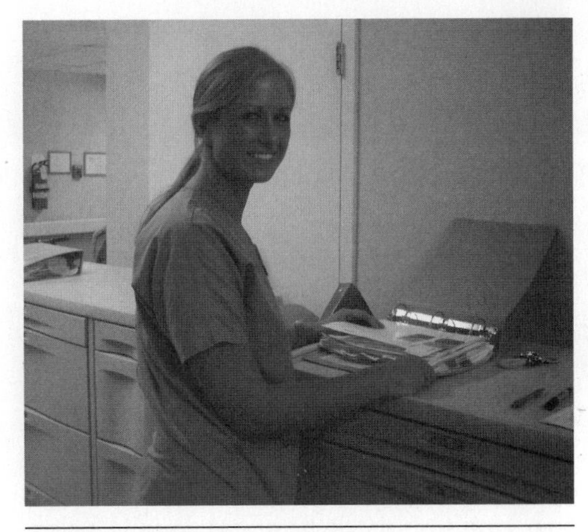

© Cengage Learning 2014

Many nurses become nurses out of idealism. They want to help people by meeting all their needs. Unfortunately, most new graduates find it impossible to meet all or even most of their patients' needs. Needs tend to be unlimited, whereas time is limited. In addition to the direct patient care responsibilities, there are shift responsibilities, charting, doctors' orders to be transcribed or checked, medications to be given, and patient reports to be given.

New graduates often go home feeling totally inadequate. They wake up remembering what they did not accomplish. One young nurse shared with tears in her eyes that once, when she answered a call bell late in her shift, the patient requested a pain medication. She went to the narcotics cabinet to get the medication, but was interrupted by an emergent situation. When she arrived home, she was so exhausted that she fell asleep rapidly, only to awaken with the realization that she had not returned with her patient's medication. Her guilt was tremendous. She had gone into nursing to relieve pain, not to ignore it.

Time management allows the novice nurse to prioritize care, decide on outcomes, and perform the most important interventions first. Time management skills are important not just for nurses on the job, but for nurses in their personal lives as well. They allow nurses to make time for fun, friends, exercise, and professional development. This chapter discusses concepts of time management and strategies for setting priorities when delivering nursing care. Shift handoff report and strategies to enhance personal productivity are also discussed.

TIME MANAGEMENT CONCEPTS

Time management has been defined as "a set of related common-sense skills that helps you use your time in the most effective and productive way possible" (Mind Tools, 2006). In other words, time management allows us to achieve more with our time. Time management requires self-examination of what pursuits are really important, analysis of how time is currently being used, and assessment of the distractions that have been siphoning time from more important pursuits (Maloney, 2012).

A simple principle, the **Pareto Principle**, states that 20 percent of focused effort produces 80 percent of results, or, conversely, that 80 percent of unfocused effort produces 20 percent of results (Pareto Principle, 2008) (Figure 12-1).

With the Pareto Principle in mind, it is important to recognize that more is achieved through an emphasis on achieving outcomes and goals than through an emphasis on the process of task completion.

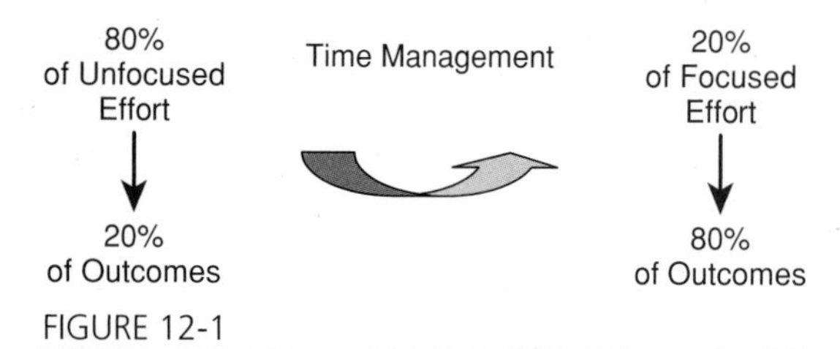

FIGURE 12-1
The Pareto principle.
© Cengage Learning 2014

Long-term goals must be determined. It is often best to break long-term goals down into smaller achievable goals that are the steps toward larger long-term goals. Long-term goals cannot be achieved overnight. Long-term goals should be written down in a planner or in a personal electronic device. Even though these long-term goals are written, they should remain flexible. Flexibility should be built into any goal orientation. There may come a time when the goals are no longer realistic or should be shifted to a more realistic goal as circumstance changes (Reed & Pettigrew, 2006).

Analysis of Nursing Time

Analysis of nursing time use is an important step in developing a plan to effectively use time. As organizational employees, nurses are expected to complete their work assignment efficiently to support the organization's goal of a positive profit margin. The emphasis is on standardization and efficiency, and time is a resource that costs money (Jones, 2010). Nurses often undervalue their time. Consider salary and benefits. Benefits are frequently forgotten, but they add 15 to 30 percent to salary. If a nurse is making $26 an hour, benefits add $3.90 to $7.25 to the hourly cost of a nurse's time. The value of nursing time in this example, excluding what the organization is paying in workers' compensation and payroll taxes, is $29.90 to $33.25 an hour. The organization has also invested in nurse recruitment, orientation, and development, which easily can exceed $20,000 per nurse. Nursing time is a valuable commodity. Keeping this in mind will be invaluable when considering work that can be delegated to personnel who receive less compensation, or when considering spending time on completing a task that does not support achieving an outcome.

Use of Time

Numerous studies have shown how nurses use their time. A time study completed by Heindrich, Chow, Skierczynski, and Lu (2008) had similar findings to previous time studies except for a significant decrease in nonproductive personal time, from 13–20 percent to only 6 percent. Unit-related activities and non-nursing practices filled 13 percent of nursing time in this study. Documentation accounted for the largest proportion of time, at approximately 25 percent, followed by care coordination and patient care activities, each accounting for 14 percent (Figure 12-2).

How do you use your time? Memory and self-reporting of time have been found to be unreliable. Staff are often unaware of time spent socializing with colleagues, making and drinking coffee, snacking, and other nonproductive time. Self-reporting of time is not recommended for estimating the total number of activities or the average time an activity takes to complete (Barrero et al., 2009).

Begin the task of prioritizing your activities for goal attainment by using a priority matrix. The priority matrix involves assigning one's activities into four categories. The priority time management matrix (Table 12-1) lists many of the daily activities of a nurse and assigns each activity to one of the four quadrants. Tasks that need to be prioritized are placed in one of four quadrants:

1. Important and urgent
2. Important but not urgent
3. Not important but urgent
4. Not important and not urgent

The goal is to shift high-priority activities to the second quadrant, to which your important but not urgent activities are assigned. This shift is accomplished through anticipatory planning with a focus on minimizing emergencies, controlling time wasters, and establishing realistic deadlines.

Compare your current time management principles to Table 12-1. What steps must you take to move your most important activities to quadrants 1 and 2? What can you do to control the number of activities that are classified as urgent? Time wasters fall into the fourth quadrant labeled "not important" and "not urgent."

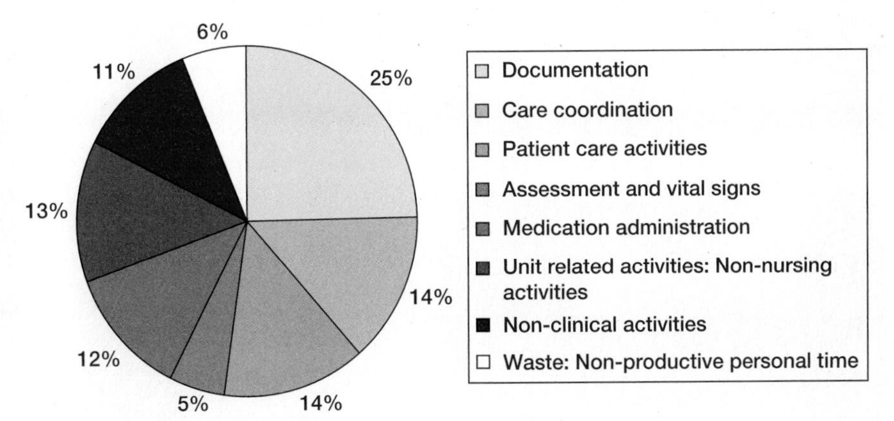

FIGURE 12-2

Use of nursing time.

(*Source:* Compiled with information from Hendrich, A., Chow,M.P., Skierczynski,B.A., & Lu, Z. (2008). A 36-hospital time and motion study: How do medical-surgical nurses spend their time? The Permanente Journal, 12(3). Retrieved April 5, 2011, from http://xnet.kp.org/permanentejournal/sum08/time-study.html/clinicalTOC.html)

TABLE 12-1
Priority Time Management Matrix

	Urgent	Not Urgent
Important	◆ Patient/personal emergencies, e.g., crises, unanticipated problems, emergency patient admissions to the unit) ◆ Impending deadlines, e.g., physician orders, patient reassessments	◆ Scheduled visits ◆ Relationship building ◆ Team meetings ◆ Restocking supplies ◆ Completing reports
Not Important	◆ Most interruptions ◆ Some telephone calls, mail, or meetings	◆ Unplanned telephone calls or e-mails ◆ Tasks without deadlines or time limits ◆ Doing the work of others ◆ Failing to properly delegate ◆ Excessive socializing and other time wasters

© Cengage Learning 2014

An **activity log** is a time management tool that can assist the nurse in determining how both personal and professional time is used. The activity log (Table 12-2) should be used for several days. Behavior should not be modified while keeping the log. The nurse should record every activity, from the beginning of the day until the end.

After filling out the activity log for several days, a nurse needs to review it and ask herself how the Pareto Principle would apply. Has 20 percent of the

TABLE 12-2
Work Activity Log

Time	Name of Activity (Medication administration, vital signs, bed-making, patient transport, etc.)	Time Required and Feelings (Energetic, bored, etc.)	Could be better done by someone else? Who? (LPN, nursing assistant, housekeeper, etc.)	Toward what outcome achievement? (Increase in patient's functional status, prevention of complications, etc.)
0500	Treadmill	30 min – energetic	Keep for self	Fitness
0530	Shower and breakfast	45 min – energetic	Keep for self	Health
0600	Drive to work	10 min – alert	Keep for self	Get to work
0700	Hand off shift report	15 min – alert	Keep for self	Patient identification
0730	Patient rounds/ planning	15 min – alert	Keep for self	Prioritize patients
0800	Etc.			
0830				
0900				
0930				
1000				
1030				
1100				
Etc.				

© Cengage Learning 2014

effort resulted in 80 percent of the outcome achievement? If the activities have not achieved the desired outcomes, the nurse needs to change activities and focus on priorities. Analysis of the activity log will allow the separation of essential professional activities from activities that can be performed by someone else (Grohar-Murray, DiCroce, & Langan, 2010; Sullivan & Decker, 2009). She should start by noticing her most energetic time of day. Activities that take focus and creativity should be scheduled at high-energy times and dull, repetitive tasks at low-energy times. Scheduling time for proper rest, exercise, and nutrition allows for quality time.

Create More Time

There are three major ways to create time. One is to delegate work to others or hire someone else to do work. Another is to eliminate chores or tasks that add no value. The last way is to get up earlier in the day. When a person delegates a task, he or she cannot control when and how the task is completed. Initially, it may take more time to get others to do the chore than to just do it, but this investment of time should save the investor time and energy in the future. If a chore is boring and mundane, it makes more sense to work an hour more at a job one enjoys in order to pay for someone else to do unrewarding, boring work.

SETTING PRIORITIES

To plan effective use of time, nurses must understand the big picture and decide on priority outcomes. Start by reviewing the big picture. No nurse works in isolation. Nurses should know what is expected of their coworkers, what is happening on the other shifts, and what is happening in the agency and the community. If the previous shift was stressed by a crisis, a shift may not get started as smoothly (Hansten & Jackson, 2009). If areas outside of the unit are overwhelmed, someone might be moved to assist on the overwhelmed unit. When nurses take the big picture into consideration, they are less likely to be frustrated when asked to assist others. They can also build into their time management plan the possibility of giving and receiving assistance.

First Priority: Life-Threatening Conditions with ABCs

Life-threatening conditions include patients at risk to themselves or others and patients whose vital signs and level of consciousness indicate potential for respiratory or circulatory collapse (Hansten & Jackson, 2009). A patient whose condition is life threatening is the highest priority and requires monitoring until transfer or stabilization. Life-threatening conditions can occur at any time during the shift and may or may not be anticipated.

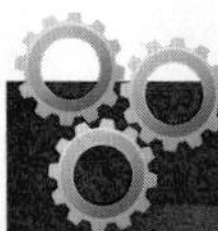

CRITICAL THINKING 12-1

The relationship between personal lifestyle and the incidence of several diseases has been demonstrated. Many health promotion programs include the expectation that people invest in themselves. Do you invest in yourself with your daily activities to promote: higher education; planned savings; healthy eating; regular exercise; deferred gratification; avoidance of smoking, tanning booths, drugs, and excessive alcohol consumption; regular physical checkups? Do you know people who seem to live only from one day to the next because their perspective of time is in the immediate and they do not seem to recognize the benefits of setting priorities and doing long-term planning?

Getting up one hour earlier in the day for a year can free up 365 hours, or approximately nine weeks a year, extra time that can be used to enrich life. After several days of rising an hour earlier, an individual may feel tired and respond to the fatigue by going to bed a little earlier (Mind Tools, 2006). This may be a good strategy for many people, especially those who are not productive in the evening and spend time doing activities that are minimally rewarding such as watching television. If a person does not get to bed earlier, though, and the end result of getting up early is fatigue, the strategy is not beneficial (Maloney, 2012).

A quick guide to assessing life-threatening emergencies is as simple as ABC. A stands for Airway. Is the airway open and patent or in danger of closing? This is the highest priority for care. B stands for Breathing. Is there respiratory distress? C stands for Circulation. Is there any circulatory compromise? This method is a way of prioritizing actions. Although there is clearly an order of importance, ABC is often assessed simultaneously while observing the patient's general appearance and level of consciousness (Figure 12-3 and Tables 12-3 and 12-4). Patients with life-threatening conditions or potentially life-threatening conditions usually have an IV access line and receive continuous monitoring of their cardiac rhythm, blood pressure, pulse, respiration, and oxygen saturation level. Their temperature and urinary output is monitored closely as well.

Second Priority: Measures Essential to Safety

Measures that are essential to safety are very important and include those responsibilities that ensure the availability of life-saving monitoring, medications, and equipment, and that protect patients from infections and falls. They include asking for assistance or providing assistance during two-people transfers or turning and movement of heavy patients (Hansten & Jackson, 2009). They also include monitoring the patient for the prevention of adverse nurse-sensitive outcomes. Nurse-sensitive patient outcomes are those outcomes that improve if there is a greater quantity or quality of nursing care—e.g., incidence of pressure ulcers, falls, and intravenous infiltrations (Vanhook, 2007).

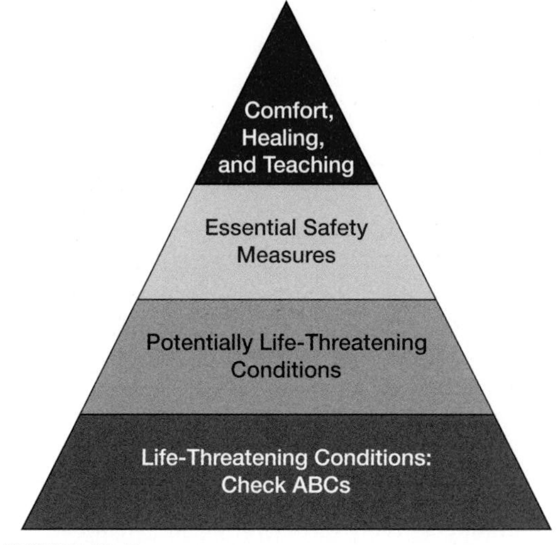

FIGURE 12-3
Prioritization triangle.
© Cengage Learning 2014

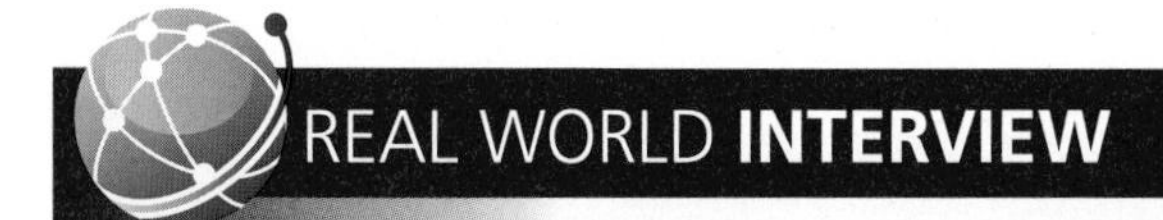

REAL WORLD INTERVIEW

I am sometimes assigned to work in the triage section where patients are seen when they first enter the emergency department (ED). It can be really nerve-wracking at times, with everyone needing or wanting to be cared for immediately. The principles of setting priorities really come in handy in this situation. I decide which patient will be cared for in the ED first based on priorities. If a patient has a life-threatening attack on their ABCs, such as an asthma attack, chest pain, significant alteration in vital signs, or significant bleeding, I arrange for this patient to be cared for immediately. My next priority is to ensure safety for my patients. I constantly monitor all the patients in the triage area of the ED until they can be seen. I want to be sure that their condition remains stable and that they are safe while waiting to be seen. I also think it is important to keep the patients who are waiting informed as to how patients are seen and cared for in the ED. When patients see that we care for them based on how ill they are, they don't seem to mind waiting as much when someone who is sicker is cared for first. Of course, they all want to be cared for reasonably quickly. That is my goal also!

PATRICIA KELLY, RN
Chicago, Illinois

TABLE 12-3
Top-Priority Patient Care Groups

Top-priority patient care groups	
Respiratory	◆ Airway compromise ◆ Severe respiratory distress, inadequate breathing ◆ Critical asthma ◆ Chest trauma with respiratory distress
Cardiovascular	◆ Cardiac arrest ◆ Shock or hypotension ◆ Exsanguinating hemorrhage
Neurological	◆ Major head injury ◆ Unconscious or unresponsive ◆ Active seizure state
Musculoskeletal	◆ Major trauma ◆ Traumatic amputation—extremity ◆ Major cold injury—hypothermia
Skin	◆ Burn, >25% body surface area (BSA) or airway involvement
Gastrointestinal	◆ Difficulty swallowing, with airway or respiratory compromise ◆ Abdominal trauma, penetrating or blunt
Gynecological	◆ Vaginal bleeding, patient with abnormal vital signs
Hematologic/Immunologic	◆ Anaphylaxis
Endocrine	◆ Hypoglycemia—altered consciousness
Infection	◆ Septic shock
Child or elder abuse	◆ Unstable situation or conflict

Source: Compiled with information from Hendrich, A., Chow, M. P., Skierczynski, B. A., & Zhenqiang, Z. (2008). A 36-hospital time and motion study: How do medical-surgical nurses spend their time? *The Permanente Journal, 12*(3). Retrieved from April 5, 2011, http://xnet.kp.org/permanentejournal/sum08/time-study.html/clinicalTOC.html

Third Priority: Comfort, Healing, and Teaching

Activities that provide comfort, healing, and teaching lead to outcomes that relieve symptoms and/or lead to healing. They are the activities that, if omitted, will hinder the patient's recovery. These essential activities include those that provide comfort, promote healing, and relieve symptoms, such as pain, nausea, and so on—and those activities, including teaching, that promote healing, such as providing nutrition, activity, positioning, and medication administration.

Vaccaro (2007) states that prioritizing has several traps that nurses should avoid. Frequently, nurses act on the "doing whatever hits first" trap. This means that a nurse may respond to things that happen first. For example, a nurse at the beginning of the day shift chooses to fill out the preoperative checklist for a

TABLE 12-4
Setting Priorities for Safe Patient Outcomes

- First Priority—ABCs. Remember Maslow's (1970) Hierarchy of Human Needs. Assess physiological needs first. See high-priority unstable patients who have any threats to their ABCs first (i.e., airway, breathing, and circulation). These patients require nursing assessment, judgment, and evaluation until transfer or stabilization. Life-threatening conditions can occur at any time during the shift and may or may not be anticipated. Notice your patient's level of consciousness and general appearance. Remember that all equipment and observations used to support and monitor the status of patients' ABCs are also a high monitoring priority (e.g., monitoring suicide threats, vital signs, level of consciousness, neurological status, skin color and temperature, pain, IV access, cardiac monitor, oxygen, suction, and urine output).
- Second Priority—Safety. Next, assess Maslow's second level of human needs (i.e., safety and security). Are there any threats to patient safety and security such as threats of violence, need for fall prevention, infection control, and so on? See these patients next.
- Third Priority—Comfort, healing, teaching, and other needs. Assess the patients' other needs and prioritize using Maslow's hierarchy. These patient needs may also include love and belonging, self-esteem, and self-actualization. What do the nursing and medical standards of care include, e.g., comfort, ambulation, positioning, and teaching? Stable patients who need standard, unchanging procedures and have predictable outcomes are seen last. Monitoring ABCs and patient safety is always top priority!

© Cengage Learning 2014

patient going to surgery the next day, rather than assess the rest of his or her patients first.

The second trap is "taking the path of least resistance." In this trap, nurses may make the flawed assumption that it is easier to do a task rather than delegate it when they could be completing another task that only nurses can complete. For example, a nurse who is admitting a patient needs the patient's vital signs and weight, baseline assessment, and patient orders. The first two tasks can be delegated to nursing assistive personnel (NAP) so that the nurse may complete the baseline assessment of the patient and then call the nursing or medical practitioner for orders.

The third trap is "responding to the squeaky wheel," wherein nurses feel compelled to respond to whatever need has been vocalized the loudest. In this case, the nurse may choose to respond to a family member who has come to the nursing station every half hour with some concern. To appease the family member, the nurse may take time to focus on one of his or her many verbal concerns and overlook a more pressing patient need elsewhere.

The fourth trap is called "completing tasks by default." This trap occurs when nurses feel obligated to complete tasks that no one else will complete. A common example of this trap is emptying the garbage when it is full instead of asking housekeeping to do it.

The last trap is "relying on misguided inspiration." The classic example of this trap is when nurses feel "inspired" to document findings in the chart and avoid taking care of a higher priority responsibility. Unfortunately, some tasks will never become inspiring and need discipline, conscientiousness, and hard work to complete them.

Considerations in Setting Priorities

Priorities are established by nurses using Maslow's Hierarchy of Needs while considering patients' immediate, short- and long-term goals, and the importance and urgency of each patient care activity.

Covey, Merrill, and Merrill (2002) have developed another way of setting priorities; activities are classified as:

- Urgent or not urgent
- Important or not important

If an activity is neither important nor urgent, then it becomes the lowest priority.

Some activities that are often thought of as important may not be. Sometimes laboratory data, vital signs, and intake and output reports are ordered more frequently than the status of the patient indicates. Frequent monitoring of these parameters when a patient is stable may make no significant difference in patient outcomes. When nurses begin their shifts, they should question the activities that make no difference in outcomes (Hansten & Jackson, 2009). If a practitioner orders these activities, a nurse should work to get the order changed. Similarly, if there is a nursing policy or procedure that does not make a difference in patient care, the nurse should work to change it. Nurses should give priority to the activities that they know are most likely to make a difference in patient outcomes.

CLINICAL PRACTICE GUIDELINES AND PATIENT CARE ROUTINES

The development and implementation of evidence-based clinical practice guidelines is one of the promising and effective tools for improving the quality of care. Nurses use clinical practice guidelines to standardize and improve patient care. Guideline sources include the Agency for Healthcare Research and Quality National Guideline Clearinghouse, (http://www.guideline.gov/), as well as many nursing and medical professional groups. Nurses also use unit routines to standardize and improve patient care. An example of a unit routine is seen in Case Study 12-2.

Shift Handoff Report and Making Assignments

Before a plan is made for a shift, the shift handoff report, at best, can lead to a smooth and effective start to the new shift. At worst, it can leave the oncoming shift members with inadequate or old data on which to base their plan. In 2005, the Joint Commission (JC) reported that communication breakdowns were correlated with adverse patient outcomes, and it included a standardized approach to shift handoff communication as one of its patient safety goals (Riesenberg, Leisch, & Cunningham, 2010). So the day of haphazard shift handoff reporting has ended. An effective shift hand off supports the transmission of critical patient information and provides continuity of care and treatment. There are various ways to conduct an end-of-shift handoff report, for example, a face-to-face meeting and walking rounds. Whichever way is used, the shift handoff report should be standardized, face to face, and should include the use of a consistent preprinted form with relevant patient information. With less reliance on verbal-only reports, communication is optimized (Friesen, White, & Byers, 2008).

Whether the report is relayed face to face or during walking rounds, information must be transmitted to allow for the effective and efficient implementation of care. If the outgoing nurse fails to cover all pertinent points, the oncoming shift must ask for the appropriate information. See Table 12-5 for a tool for taking and giving handoff reports.

During or after report, the oncoming nurse can complete an assignment sheet or a written or computerized action plan that sets the priorities for the shift and makes assignments to team members. Assignments should include specific reporting guidelines and deadlines for accomplishment of the tasks (Figures 12-4 and 12-5). When nurses make assignments, they plan patient care by reviewing several factors, for example, patient needs, agency organizational systems, and staffing. See Table 12-6.

Make Patient Care Rounds

If the end-of-shift handoff report does not include walking rounds, the oncoming nurse needs to

TABLE 12-5
Tool for Handoff Report

		Notes
Demographics	◆ Room number ◆ Patient name ◆ Sex ◆ Age ◆ Practitioner	
Diagnoses	◆ Primary ◆ Secondary ◆ Nursing and medical ◆ Admit date ◆ Surgery date	
Patient status	◆ Do Not Attempt Resuscitation (DNAR) status ◆ Current vital signs ◆ Problem with ABCs, level of consciousness, or safety ◆ Problem with comfort or healing ◆ Teaching needs ◆ Oxygen saturation ◆ Pain score ◆ Skin condition ◆ Ambulation, Fall risk ◆ Suicide risk ◆ Presence/absence of signs and symptoms of potential complications ◆ New orders/changes in treatment plan	
Fluids/tubes/ oxygen Laboratory tests and treatments	◆ IV fluid, rate, site ◆ Tube feedings—type of tube, solution, rate, and patient toleration ◆ Oxygen rate, route; other tubes, e.g., chest tube, nasogastric tube, Foley catheter (type and drainage) ◆ Abnormal laboratory and test values ◆ Laboratory and other tests to be done on oncoming shift ◆ Treatments done on your shift, include dressing changes (times, wound description) and other procedures ◆ Identify treatments to be done during next shift	

(Continues)

TABLE 12-5 (Continued)

Expected shift outcomes	◆ Priority outcomes for major nursing diagnoses ◆ Patient learning outcomes
Plans for discharge	◆ Expected date of discharge ◆ Referrals needed ◆ Progress toward self-care and readiness for home, teaching needs
Care support	◆ Availability of family or friends to assist in activities of daily living (ADL)
Priority Interventions	◆ Interventions that must be done this shift

© Cengage Learning 2014

make initial rounds on the patients at risk for life-threatening conditions or complications first. During rounds, the nurse performs rapid assessments. These assessments may vary from the information given during the shift handoff report, so the information gathered on rounds may change the shift plan. A patient with asthma who had been calm and without respiratory distress on the previous shift may have experienced a visitor who wore perfume and delivered bad news. As the oncoming nurse makes initial rounds and uses the quick ABC assessment, he or she may quickly determine that the patient has suddenly developed respiratory distress. The patient may have been initially prioritized as requiring only comfort activities directed at healing, but the patient is now experiencing a life-threatening reaction and requires appropriate nursing interventions as well as continuous monitoring. While assessing the patient, the nurse must check all the patient's IV lines to make sure that the correct fluid is infusing and the infusion site is without complication. The nurse must also check the patient's drains, tubes, and continuous treatments. The nurse should listen to the patient's concerns and desires. It is important to remember that plans are just that—plans—and have to be flexible based on ever-changing patient care needs. Times for treatments and medications may have to be changed. Often nurses believe that the times for administering medication are inflexible, yet practitioners usually write medication orders as daily, twice a day, three times a day, or four times a day. These kinds of orders give nurses flexibility in administration times. Although unit policy dictates when these medicines are given, unit policy is under nursing control.

Evaluate Outcome Achievement

At the end of the shift, the nurse must reexamine the shift action plan. Did he or she achieve the desired outcomes? If not, why? Were there staffing problems or patient crises? What was learned from this for future shifts?

If, at the end of a shift, the nurse did not accomplish the desired intended outcomes, the nurse might review the shift activities to see what time wasters interfered with outcome achievement. Marquis and Huston (2009) described time wasters as procrastination, inability to delegate, inability to say no, management by crisis, haste, and indecisiveness. Sullivan and Decker (2009) add interrupting telephone calls and socialization to the list. Reed and Pettigrew (2006) include complaining, perfectionism, and disorganization as well.

ASSIGNMENT SHEET EXCERPT Unit 2 South

Date October 2, 2013 Shift Days Charge nurse Mary RNs Break/Lunch Steve 0900 and 1100 Lakeisha 0930 and 1130 Colleen 1000 and 1200	Notify RN Ref immediately if: T <97 or >100 P <60 or >110 R <12 or >24 SBP <90 or >160 DBP <60 or >100 BS <70 or >200 Pulse oximetry <95% Urine output <30 cc/hour	
NAPs Break/Lunch Juan 0900 and 1100 Pat 0930 and 1130	Notify RN one hour prior to end of shift: I and O Patient goal achievement	Narcotic Count Steve Glucometer Check Colleen Stock Pyxis Lakeisha Pass Water Juan Stock Linen Pat Other Colleen attend in-service at 1300

Room and Initials	Patient	Staff	AM/PM Care	Weight I & O	IV	Activity	Accu-check	Tests	NPO	Comments
501, Mr. M. M.	27-year-old with newly diagnosed AIDS, left lower lobe pneumonia	Steve, RN	Complete care	0715 1400	KVO	Bedrest		Lab		Vitals Q4H
502, Mr. M. G.	61-year-old with acute congestive heart failure (CHF)	Lakeisha, RN	Partial care	0715 1400	KVO	BRP	1100	Lab	Yes	Vitals Q4H
503, Ms. S. C.	92-year-old with new right hip fracture, in Bucks traction	Juan, NAP	Complete care	I & O at 1400	KVO	Bedrest		Lab and X-ray	Yes	Vitals Q4H
504, Ms. N. J.	48-year-old, with new cholelithiasis	Pat, NAP	Self care		KVO	Up ad lib		Ultra-sound	Yes	
505, Ms. L. G.	89-year-old with new onset CVA with right side paralysis	Colleen, RN	Complete care	0715 1400	NS @ 125 cc/hr.	Bedrest	1100	Lab		Vitals Q4H

FIGURE 12-4

Assignment sheet excerpt.

© Cengage Learning 2014

ASSIGNMENT SHEET EXCERPT

Unit ______________________

Date ______ ______ Shift ______ Charge nurse ______ ______ RNs Breaks/Lunch ______ ______ ______ ______ ______	Notify RN immediately if: T <97 or >100 P <60 or >110 R <12 or > 24 SBP <90 or >160 DBP <60 or >100 BS <70 or >200 Pulse oximetry <95% Urine output <30 cc/hour	
NAPs Breaks/Lunch ______ ______	Notify RN one hour prior to end of shift: I and O Patient goal achievement	Narcotic count ______ Glucometer check ______ Stock pyxis ______ Pass water ______ Stock linen ______ Other ______

Room and Initials	Patient	Staff	AM/PM Care	Weight I & O	IV	Activity	Accu-check	Tests	NPO	Comments

FIGURE 12-5

Assignment sheet excerpt.

© Cengage Learning 2014

TABLE 12-6
Factors Considered in Making Assignments

- Priority of patient needs
- Geography of nursing unit
- Complexity of patient needs
- Other responsibilities of staff
- Attitude and dependability of staff
- Need for continuity of care by same staff
- Agency organizational system
- State laws, e.g., state nurse practice act
- In-service education programs
- Need for fair work distribution among staff
- Need for lunch/break times
- Need for isolation
- Need to protect staff and patients from injury
- Skill, education, and competency of staff, i.e., RN, LPN, NAP
- Hospital policy and procedure
- Patient care standards and routines for surgical, medical, maternal child, and/or mental health patients
- Environmental concerns
- Equipment checks, medication checks
- Accreditation regulations
- Needs of other units in hospital, number of staff, problems leftover from earlier shifts, etc.
- Desired patient outcomes

© Cengage Learning 2014

FIND PERSONAL TIME FOR LIFELONG LEARNING

Finding time for lifelong learning and maintaining a balance with family, school, and work is a struggle for recent graduates, and even for more-seasoned nurses. Returning to school is certainly a challenge, but with time management skills, the return to school can result in the accomplishment of personal outcomes, a degree, and new knowledge (Maloney, 2012).

Nurses can achieve their dreams, work, and have a personal life in many ways. Note the tips for balancing work and school at the University of Illinois at Chicago website, http://www.uic.edu/uic/studentlife/balance/index.shtml.

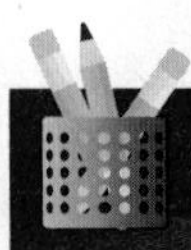

CASE STUDY 12-1

You are working the day shift on a medical-surgical unit. You are responsible for six patients with the assistance of NAP and an LPN. What are the outcomes you want to achieve? (Please use the criteria previously given for prioritizing, i.e., ABC, safety, etc.) Which patients will you give to each care provider? Make out an assignment sheet using Figure 12-5.

Patients-Group 1	Priority Nursing Assessments
Ms. J. D. is a 68-year-old patient who is post-op day 1 after a total shoulder replacement following a traumatic fall. She is confused and on multiple medications and has a history of hypertension and multiple falls. She is anxious and frightened by the "visiting spirits."	ABCs, level of consciousness, vital signs, safety, distal pulse, incision/dressing check, breath sounds. See this patient second during rounds.
Mr. D. B. is a 55-year-old patient with insulin-dependent diabetes mellitus, juvenile onset at age 12. He is post-op day 2 after a right below-the-knee amputation. He complains of severe right leg pain and is restless. Mr. D. B. has a history of noncompliance with diet and is on sliding-scale insulin administration.	ABCs, symptoms of hypoglycemia, glucoscan at 4 p.m. and 9 p.m., vital signs, safety, incision/dressing check, pain, DB teaching. See this patient third during rounds. You may need to check his glucose level STAT.
Mr. J. K. is a 35-year-old patient with a history of alcohol abuse, admitted for severe abdominal pain. He is throwing up coffee-ground-like emesis.	ABCs, level of consciousness, seizure and shock potential, hematemesis, DTs, safety, vital signs, CBC, hematocrit, type and cross-match, 16-gauge IV line for possible blood transfusion, oxygen, cardiac monitor. See this patient first during rounds.

Now, identify the priority nursing assessments for this group of patients below. Consider the factors in Table 12-6 in making your assignments.

Priority Patient Assessments, Group II

Patients, Group 2	Priority Nursing Assessments
Ms. H. M. is an 85-year-old patient who was transferred from a nursing home because of dehydration. She is vomiting and has abdominal pain of unknown etiology. Intravenous hydration continues and a workup is planned. Ms. H. M. is alert and oriented.	
Mr. A. B. is a 72-year-old patient who is status post cerebrovascular accident. He is to be transferred to rehabilitation. He needs his belongings gathered and a nursing summary written.	
Ms. V. G. is an 82-year-old patient who is post-op day 5 after an open reduction of a femur fracture. She has a history of congestive heart failure, hypertension, and takes multiple medications. Her temperature is elevated. She is confused.	

© Cengage Learning 2014

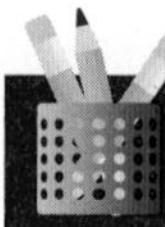

CASE STUDY 12-2

Throughout the day shift, nursing and unit staff communicate and work together to deliver quality patient care according to evidence-based patient care standards. These standards and routines that the nursing staff will apply to these patients reflect the American Nurses Association Standards of Nursing Practice and include routines of care such as:

Bedfast patients—Turn Q2H, intake and output, etc.

All patients—Q4H vital signs, hygiene, fresh water, etc.

Depending on the type of patient care unit, the day shift routine might go like this:

7:00 a.m. Charge nurse reviews patient care assignments with all nurses and unit staff. Day shift takes handoff shift report from night shift. Patient rounds and assessment begin and continue every hour; Monitor intravenous(IV) fluids throughout shift.

7:30 a.m. NAP obtain vital signs (VS). Patient breakfast is served.

7:45 a.m. Patient assessment, including ABCs, VS, lab work, medications, IV fluids; a.m. hygiene care begins following nursing care standards; turn and reposition patients Q2H.

8:00 a.m. Inter-professional team makes rounds; patients are sent for diagnostic tests; regular patient rounds and assessments are made hourly and as needed.

8:30 a.m. VS reassessment made as needed.

9:00 a.m. Medications are given; 15-minute breaks begin for all staff.

9:30 a.m. Documentation is begun.

10:00 a.m. Turn and reposition patients every two hours and as needed.

10:30 a.m.

11:00 a.m. Lunch breaks begin for all staff.

11:30 a.m. Reassessment made of VS of those patients with 7:30 a.m. abnormal VS.

12:00 p.m. Turn and reposition patients. Patient lunch is served.

12:30 p.m.

13:00 p.m. Medications are given.

13:30 p.m.

14:00 p.m. Intake and output reports are completed; documentation is completed. Turn and reposition patients.

15:00 p.m. Handoff shift report from day shift to evening shift is made.

Is this patient care routine similar to one you have seen on a patient care unit where you have worked? Make out a day shift routine for a unit you are familiar with. Make up an assignment sheet like the one in Figure 12-5 for the same unit.

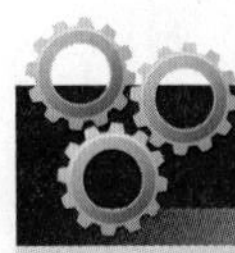

CRITICAL THINKING 12-2

Four of Jose's patients were discharged today by 10:00 a.m. The nursing supervisor asked Jose to help out in the emergency department. Jose agreed and was assigned to help the triage nurse. Identify the order in which the following patients should be seen in the ED.

Group I

- A 2-year-old boy with chest retractions
- A 1-year-old girl choking on a grape
- A 5-year-old boy with a knee laceration

How about Group II? Which patient would you see first?

Group II

- A 60-year-old female who is nonresponsive and drooling
- A 30-year-old male trauma patient who has absent breath sounds in the right side of his chest
- A 15-year-old female who cut her wrist in an attempted suicide

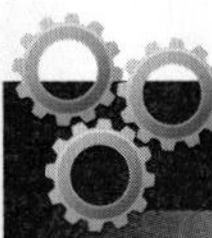

CRITICAL THINKING 12-3

Nurses set priorities fast when they "first look" at a patient. As you approach your patient, get in the habit of observing the following quickly (in less than a minute):

First Look

- Eye contact as you approach
- Speech
- Posture
- Level of consciousness

Airway

- Airway sounds or secretions
- Nasal flaring

Breathing

- Rate, symmetry, and depth
- Positioning
- Retractions

(Continues)

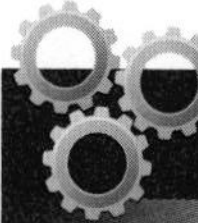

CRITICAL THINKING 12-3 (Continued)

Circulation

- Color
- Flushed
- Cyanotic
- Presence of IV or oxygen
- Pain
- Vital signs (TPR and BP)
- Pulse oximetry
- Cardiac monitor

Drainage

- Urine
- Blood
- Gastric
- Stool
- Sputum

Practice your "first look" the next time you approach a patient. Does this improve your assessment skills?

KEY CONCEPTS

- ✦ General time management concepts include having an outcomes and goal orientation, analyzing time cost and use, focusing on priority outcomes, and visualizing the big picture.
- ✦ Shift handoff reports may be given by different methods, for example, face-to-face meetings or walking rounds.
- ✦ The assignment sheet is evaluated at the end of the shift by determining whether priority outcomes have been achieved.
- ✦ Time management applies to one's personal life as well as one's job.
- ✦ Quality time can be achieved by analyzing time use and setting priorities.
- ✦ Time management strategies help balance work, family, and school for lifelong learning.
- ✦ Organize your patient care using these priorities: ABCs; safety; and comfort, healing, and teaching.

KEY TERMS

activity log

Pareto Principle

time management

REVIEW QUESTIONS

1. The nurse has just finished the shift handoff report. Which patient should the nurse assess first?
   A. A patient with asthma who had difficulty breathing during the prior shift
   B. A postoperative appendectomy patient who will be discharged in the next few hours
   C. A postoperative cholecystectomy patient who is complaining of pain but received an IM injection of morphine five minutes ago
   D. An elderly patient with diabetes who is on the bedpan

2. A new graduate RN organizing her assignment asks the charge nurse, "Of the list of patients assigned to me, whom do you think I should assess first?" What is the best response the charge nurse could make?
   A. "Assess the patients in order of their room number to stay organized."
   B. "Check the policy and procedure manual for whom to assess first."
   C. "I would assess the patient who is having respiratory distress first."
   D. "See the patient who takes the most time last."

3. On another day, which of the following patients would you assess first after shift handoff report?
   A. Patient who is concerned that he has had no bowel movement for two days
   B. Patient who has suffered several acute asthmatic attacks within the last 24 hours
   C. Patient who is now comfortable but has had several episodes of breakthrough pain since yesterday
   D. Patient who is severely allergic to peanuts who just ate potato chips fried in peanut oil

4. A nurse has begun to use an activity log to manage both her personal and professional time. When should she schedule her activities that require focus and creativity?
   A. During high-energy times
   B. During lunch
   C. In the morning
   D. As the last activity for the day

5. Assessing life-threatening emergencies is done by establishing priorities. By understanding how to prioritize patient care, the nurse knows that patients at risk for falls would be which of the following?
   A. First priority
   B. Second Priority
   C. Third priority
   D. Fourth priority

6. Prioritizing has several traps that nurses should avoid. Which of the following would be considered priority traps that may lead nurses to incorrectly prioritize tasks? Select all that apply.
   A. Assessing the patient who has airway compromise
   B. Documenting findings in the chart
   C. Responding to the patient's family that is complaining the loudest
   D. Taking on a task that could have been delegated to NAP
   E. Doing whatever the nurse thinks of first
   F. Responding to a confused patient who has recently pulled out his IV

7. The nurse has just completed the end of her shift and is ready to begin the shift handoff report to the oncoming nurse. Which types of data should the nurse include in her report to the next shift? Select all that apply.
   A. Birthday celebrations
   B. Patient demographics
   C. Patient diagnosis
   D. Patient status
   E. Plans for patient discharge
   F. Priority interventions for patient

8. When making shift assignments, the charge nurse must take patient objectives into consideration as well as tasks that require completion prior to the end of the shift. Which of the following considerations apply when completing shift assignments? Select all that apply.
   A. Complexity of patient needs
   B. Competency of staff
   C. Desired patient outcomes
   D. Fire drill times
   E. Number of licensed personnel available
   F. Scheduled time off of staff

9. The nurse has been assigned to a medical-surgical unit on a stormy day. Three of the staff cannot make it in to work, and no other staff is available. How should the nurse proceed? Select all that apply.
   A. Prioritize care so that all patients get safe care
   B. Provide nursing care only to those patients to whom the nurse is regularly assigned
   C. Have the patients' families and ambulatory patients take care of the other patients
   D. Refuse the nursing assignment, as the increased number of patients makes it unsafe
   E. Quickly make rounds on all assigned patients to assess needs
   F. Decide on desired outcomes

10. The nurse has just completed listening to the morning report. Which patient will the nurse see first?
   A. The patient with a sickle cell crisis and an infiltrated IV
   B. The patient who has a leaking colostomy bag
   C. The patient who is going for a bronchoscopy in two hours
   D. The patient who has been receiving a blood transfusion for the past two hours and had a recent hemoglobin of 7.2 g/dL

REVIEW ACTIVITIES

1. Make an assignment for a group of patients on your clinical unit using Figure 12-5. Consider all the factors in Table 12-5 in making your assignments.
2. For the next three days, complete an activity log for both your personal time and your work time.
   On what activities are you spending the majority of time?
   What are your biggest time wasters?
   How can you schedule your time more productively to ensure that 20 percent of your activities are designed to achieve 80 percent of your goals?

EXPLORING THE WEB

- Organizing Electronic-Filing Systems:
  http://www.computerorganizing.com
  http://www.livebinders.com
  http://www.smead.com/hot-topics/organizing-electronic-files-1413.asp
  http://www.officiency.com/electronic_file_organizing.html
  http://www.thepapertiger.com
- Systems to store/access calendars, contacts, documents, etc.:
  http://www.apple.com/icloud
  http://dropbox.com
  http://docs.google.com

- Other helpful software:
  http://www.apple.com/webapps//calendar
  http://www.microsoft.com/exchange
  http://www.calendar.yahoo.com
- Time management tools:
  http://www.mindtools.com Search for Time management.
  http://www.organizerswebring.com
- Mobile Learning or MLearning
  http://zelda23publishing.com/edci554/?p=342

REFERENCES

Abraham H. Maslow (1970). *Motivation and Personality,* (2nd ed.). New York, NY; Joanna Cotler Books.

Barrero, L. H., Katz, J. N., Perry, M. J., Krishnan, R., Ware, J. H., & Dennerlein, J. T. (2009). Work pattern causes bias in self-reported activity duration: A randomised study of mechanisms and implications for exposure assessment and epidemiology. *Occupational and Environmental Medicine, 66*(1), 38–44.

Covey, S. R., Merrill, A. R., & Merrill, R. R. (2002). *First things first: To love, to learn, to leave a legacy.* New York, NY: Simon & Schuster.

Friesen, M. A., White, S., & Byers, J. (2008). Handoffs: Implications for nurses. In R. G. Hughes (Ed.), *Patient safety and quality: An evidence-based handbook for nurses*, vol. 2. Rockville, MD: Agency for Healthcare Research and Quality (AHRQ Publication No. 08-0043, pp. 2-285–2-332). Retrieved September 20, 2011, from http://www.ahrq.gov/qual/nurseshdbk

Grohar-Murray, M. E., DiCroce, H. R., & Langan, J. C. (2010). *Leadership and management in nursing* (4th ed.). Upper Saddle River, NJ: Prentice Hall.

Hansten, R. I., & Jackson, M. (2009). *Clinical delegation skills: A handbook for professional practice* (4th ed.). Sudbury, MA: Jones and Bartlett Publications.

Hendrich, A., Chow, M.P., Skierczynski, B.A., & Lu, Z. (2008). A 36-Hospital Time and Motion Study: How Do Medical-Surgical Nurses Spend Their Time? *The Permanente Journal.* Summer; 12(3): 25-34.

Hendrich, A., Chow, M. P., Skierczynski, B. A., & Lu, Z. (2008). A 36-hospital time and motion study: How do medical-surgical nurses spend their time? *The Permanente Journal, 12*(3). Retrieved April 5, 2011, from http://xnet.kp.org/permanentejournal/sum08/time-study.html/clinicalTOC.html

Hummel, C.E. (1994). Tyranny of the Urgent! Inter-Varsity Press. Nottingham, England.

Jones, T. (2010). A holistic framework for nursing time: Implications for theory, practice, and research. *Nursing Forum, 45*(3), 185–196. doi:10.1111/j.1744-6198.2010.00180.x

Leadership and Management in Nursing (4th Edition) by Mary Ellen Grohar-Murray, Helen R. DiCroce and Joanne C. Langan Ph.D. RN (Mar 21, 2010).

Maloney, P. (2012). Time management and setting patient care priorities. In P. Kelly (Ed.), *Nursing leadership & management* (3rd ed.). Clifton Park, NY: Delmar Cengage Learning.

Marquis, B. L., & Huston, C. J. (2009). *Leadership roles and management functions in nursing: Theory and application.* Hagerstown, MD: Lippincott Williams & Wilkins.

Maslow, A. H. (1970). *Motivation and Personality,* (2nd ed.). New York, NY: Harper & Row.

Mind Tools. (2006). How to achieve more with your time. Retrieved February 27, 2006, from http://www.mindtools.com/tmintro.html

Pareto Principle—The 80–20 rule—complete information. (2008). Retrieved November 1, 2011, from http://www.gassner.co.il/pareto

Reed, F. C., & Pettigrew, A. C. (2006). Self-management: Stress and time. In P. S. Yoder-Wise (Ed.), *Leading and managing in nursing* (4th ed., pp. 413–430). St. Louis, MO: Mosby.

Riesenberg, L. A., Leisch, J., & Cunningham, J. (2010). Nursing handoffs: A systematic review of the literature. *American Journal of Nursing, 110*(4), 24–34.

Sullivan, E. J., & Decker, P. J. (2009). *Effective leadership and management in nursing* (7th ed.). Lebanon, IN: Pearson.

University of Illinois at Chicago. (2010). Balancing work and school. Retrieved January 8, 2013, from http://www.uic.edu/uic/studentlife/balance/index.shtml

Vaccaro, P. (2007). Five priority-setting traps: Taking control of your time. *BILLD Alumni Newsletter*: A publication of the Midwestern Office of the Council of State Governments, *8*(2), 1–2.

Vanhook, P. M. (2007). Cost-Utility analysis: A method of quantifying the value of registered nurses. The online journal of issues in nursing. Retrieved April 4, 2011, from http://www.nursingworld.org/MainMenu Categories/ANA Marketplace/ANAPeriodicals/OJIN/TableofContents/Volume122007/No3Sept07/CostUtilityAnalysis.aspx

SUGGESTED READINGS

Carrick, L., & Yurkow, J. (2007). A nurse leader's guide to managing priorities. *American Nurse Today, 2*(7), 40–41.

Childre, D. (2008). *De-stress kit for the changing times.* Boulder Creek, CA: Institute for Heartmath.

Hendry, C., & Walker, A. (2004). Priority setting in clinical practice: Literature review. *Journal of Advanced Nursing, 47*(4), 427–436.

Henrickson, M. (2009). Work life balance: Is there such a thing? *Nursing for Women's Health, 13*(2), 151–154.

MindTools. (2012). Retrieved November 23, 2012 from, http://www.mindtools.com/index.html

Vestal, K. (2009). Procrastination: Frustrating or fatal? *Nursing Leadership, 7*(2), 8–9.

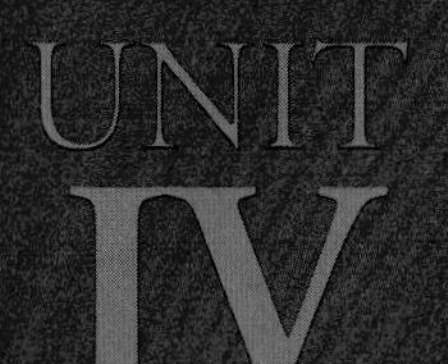

UNIT IV QUALITY IMPROVEMENT OF PATIENT OUTCOMES

CHAPTER 13

Quality Improvement and Evidence-Based Patient Care

KATHRYN L. WARD, RN, MS, MA; MARY ANNE JADLOS, MS, ACNP-BC, CWOCN; GLENDA B. KELMAN, PHD, ACNP-BC; MARY MCLAUGHLIN, RN, MBA; KAREN HOUSTON, RN, MS; AND EDNA HARDER MATTSON, RN, BN, BA (CRS), MDE

The best outcomes evaluation is likely to come from partnerships of technically proficient analysts and clinicians, each of whom is sensitive to and respectful of the contributions the other can bring.

—ROBERT L. KANE, PROFESSOR OF PUBLIC HEALTH, UNIVERSITY OF MINNESOTA, 1997

OBJECTIVES

Upon completion of this chapter, the reader should be able to:

1. Articulate major principles of quality improvement, including the need for customer identification, need for participation at all levels, need for improvement of the work process, and need for avoidance of criticism of individual performance.
2. Identify the importance of evidence-based practice.
3. Discuss the University of Colorado Model for Evidence-Based Practice.
4. Identify the PDSA Cycle, FOCUS, and other methods of quality improvement.
5. Discuss sentinel events, storyboards, benchmarking, and the use of quality data.
6. Identify how data are utilized for performance and quality improvement (time series data, Pareto charts).
7. Review an organizational structure for quality improvement.

During report, the staff nurse tells you about a 60-year-old woman, Miss Kelly, who was admitted to the unit today with left hip and sciatic pain after a recent fall at home. You immediately begin to think she has a hip fracture. The staff nurse interrupts your thoughts and says, "Wait, there is more. This woman has a new diagnosis of breast cancer and has also developed a pleural effusion, which necessitated the insertion of a chest tube this morning. Her dyspnea has improved since this morning, and her pulse oximetry on 2 liters of oxygen via nasal cannula is 99 percent."

Miss Kelly has lymphedema of her right hand and arm, and the right breast mass is a very large, open, foul-smelling lesion that bleeds intermittently. She appears anxious and has indicated that she is uncomfortable and afraid to move. She has Tylenol with codeine ordered orally every four hours as needed for pain, but has been very reluctant to take the medication because she believes it will alter her ability to think and make decisions regarding her care. Results of a bone scan and CT scan of the abdomen and pelvis indicate that she has further metastatic involvement of the left acetabulum. This could be the cause of her left hip pain—tumor replacing the bone. Although the CT scan does not reveal a fracture, Miss Kelly is at high risk for developing a pathological fracture.

Miss Kelly is single, has no children, and lives with her brother and five cats. She does not smoke or drink. She is a retired clerk for the state Department of Labor. She has been followed by a cardiologist for hypertension for several years. She has often called for prescription refills but canceled her appointments because she feared what the doctor would find or say.

What additional data do you need to develop a protocol of care to improve Miss Kelly's outcomes?

What priorities should be addressed to manage Miss Kelly's care?

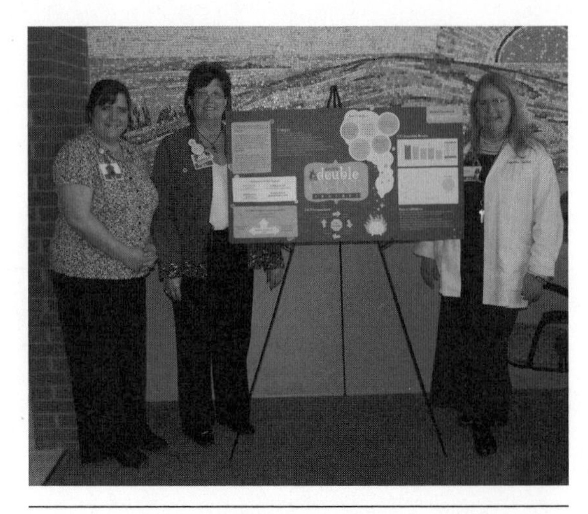

(*Source:* Courtesy Faxton-St. Luke's Infection Prevention Department: First Place Winners of the 2011 Safety First Poster Contest at Faxton-St. Luke's Healthcare.)

Quality improvement (QI) and evidence-based practice (EBP) have been shown to be powerful tools to make health care organizations more effective. Ransom, Joshi, and Nash (2005) stress the importance of management and leadership commitment to the success of quality improvement. The improvement philosophies of quality experts such as Deming (1986) and Crosby (1979) also emphasize the commitment of management, and without that commitment, successful quality improvement is jeopardized.

Nursing leaders and managers are particularly well placed to see that health care institutions have evidence-based practice and work processes in place that provide professional nurses with support to meet new challenges in the clinical delivery of care. Evidence-based practice integrates the best current evidence with clinical expertise and patient/family preferences and values for delivery of optimal health care (Quality and Safety Education for Nurses, 2012). All nurses have responsibility for promoting patient care based on the best scientific evidence available.

This chapter will discuss the importance of QI and EBP to patients and nursing. It will discuss the University of Colorado Model for Evidence-Based Practice, the PDSA Cycle, Focus, and other methods for quality improvement. The chapter will discuss sentinel events, storyboards, benchmarking, and the use of quality data, and will identify how data are utilized for performance and quality improvement. Nursing uses a scientific process driven by evidence-based standards and practice guidelines while also emphasizing continuous quality improvement.

QUALITY

Quality is defined by the Institute of Medicine (1990) as "the degree to which health services for individuals and populations increase the likelihood of health outcomes and are consistent with current professional knowledge" (p. 21). Quality assurance (QA) emerged in health care approximately in the 1950s. QA began as an inspection approach to quality used to ensure that health care institutions—mainly hospitals—maintained minimum standards of care. QA's methods consisted primarily of chart audits of various patient diagnoses and procedures. The method emphasized "doing it right," and did little to sustain change or proactively identify problems before they occurred. It did, however, encourage monitoring minimum standards of performance and improving performance when standards were not met. QA efforts also began to encourage hospitals to use Donabedian's (1966) structure, process, and outcome framework for looking at quality (see Table 2-2 in Chapter 2).

QUALITY IMPROVEMENT

Quality improvement is a management philosophy to improve the organizational structure and the level of performance of key processes in the organization to achieve high-quality outcomes. **Quality improvement** uses data to monitor the outcomes of care processes and uses improvement methods to design and test changes to continuously improve the quality and safety of health care systems (QSEN, 2012). QI notes that quality is an organizational issue, that is, that variation in quality is as much due to the way in which care is organized and coordinated as it is to the competence of the individual caregivers (Kimberly & Minvielle, 2003). QI was developed originally by several industrial quality experts and applied successfully in a variety of industries worldwide (Crosby, 1979; Deming, 1986; Juran, 1988). The principles espoused by these experts differ little, but are known by several terms, often used interchangeably with QI: total quality management (TQM), continuous quality improvement (CQI), and performance improvement (PI). Key philosophical concepts include the following:

- Productive work involves work processes. Most work implies a chain of processes whereby each worker receives input from suppliers (internal or external to the organization), adds value, and then passes it on to the customer. **Customers** are defined to include everyone internal or external to the organization who receives the product or service of the workers, for example, patients, nurses, physicians, community.
- The customer is central to every process. Look at improvement of all work processes to meet the customer's needs reliably and efficiently.
- There are two ways to improve quality: eliminate defects in the work process and add features that better meet customers' needs or preferences.
- The main sources of quality defects are problems in the work process. Workers basically want to succeed in carrying out the work process correctly. The problems derive from the work process being wrong.
- Quality defects are costly in terms of internal losses from lowered productivity and efficiency, increased requirements for inspection and monitoring, and dissatisfied customers. Preventing defects in the process by careful planning saves resources.
- Focus first on the most important work processes to improve. Use statistical thinking and tools to identify desired performance levels, measure current performance, interpret it, and take action when necessary.
- Involve every worker in QI and empower each worker to take action. Use new structures such as teams and quality councils to advise and plan QI strategies. Assure administrative support for QI.
- Set high standards for performance; go for being the best. Emphasize this until it becomes a work habit and part of the organization's daily operations.

QI logic suggests that high quality could lead to a higher volume of use of the organization by patients and providers who have the flexibility to make choices about where they seek health care. Higher volume generally leads to higher profits which, in turn, may be directed toward improving programs and services, thus achieving higher quality, a very positive spiral that can result in the organization's thriving.

Increased quality —> Increased volume —>
Increased profit —> Enhanced programs/services
—> Increased quality

The obverse spiral is more likely when quality is shoddy, a very negative and potentially fatal spiral.

Decreased quality —> Decreased volume —>
Decreased profit —> Cutting corners —>
Decreased quality

EVIDENCE-BASED PRACTICE (EBP)

Nursing, medicine, health care institutions, and health policy makers recognize EBP as care based on an approach to collecting, reviewing, interpreting, critiquing, and evaluating research and other relevant literature for direct application to patient care. EBP uses evidence from: research; performance data; quality improvement studies such as hospital or nursing report cards, program evaluations, and surveys; national and local consensus recommendations of experts; patient observation; and clinical experience. There are several levels of evidence (Table 13-1).

The EBP process further involves the integration of both clinician-observed evidence and research-directed evidence. This then leads to state-of-the-art integration of available knowledge and evidence in a particular area of clinical concern that can be evaluated and measured.

Joanna Briggs and AHRQ

One of the earlier proponents for EBP in nursing was the Joanna Briggs Institute for Evidence-Based Nursing (JBIEBN), established in 1996. Significant work has been done worldwide to implement EBP into Australian, Canadian, and United Kingdom (UK) institutions of care.

CRITICAL THINKING **13-1**

On an orthopedic unit, when the original data of lengths of stay by nursing unit were examined, one unit had a much shorter length of stay than the other. At first, there was discussion about this variance and the idea emerged of just going to the unit with the longer length of stay and fixing things there. The group members decided that rather than approach the task from this limited perspective, they would study the care delivery process as a whole and determine whether there were steps they could take to improve the work process before criticizing the staff on the floor with the longer length of stay. Several excellent opportunities for quality improvement were identified, for example, the need for preoperative home evaluation, increased physical therapy involvement, and shorter indwelling catheter use. All these areas contributed to the work process improvement, and the outcome was that both units ended up reducing their lengths of stay. These opportunities would have been lost had the group members used the data only to say that one unit was doing a bad job. They needed to review the process as a whole to improve the length of stay on both units.

Identify a problem or patient care work process on a patient care unit with which you are familiar.

What members of the interprofessional team could you ask to work on the improvements with you?

How can you develop an environment where members of the interprofessional team can suggest ideas for QI to other staff without making them feel that the quality of their care is being criticized?

TABLE 13-1
Levels of Evidence

LEVEL OF EVIDENCE
Level I: Evidence from a systematic review or meta-analysis of all relevant randomized controlled trials (RCTs), or evidence-based clinical practice guidelines based on systematic reviews of RCTs
Level II: Evidence obtained from at least one well-designed RCT
Level III: Evidence obtained from well-designed controlled trials without randomization
Level IV: Evidence from well-designed case-control and cohort studies
Level V: Evidence from systematic reviews of descriptive and qualitative studies
Level VI: Evidence from a single descriptive or qualitative study
Level VII: Evidence from the opinions of authorities and/or reports of expert committees

Source: Compiled with information from Melnyk & Fineout-Overholt, 2004.

In the United States, the Agency for Healthcare Research and Quality (AHRQ) has provided a stimulus for the EBP movement through recognition of a need for evidence to guide practice throughout the health care system. In 1997, the AHRQ launched its initiative establishing 12 evidence-based practice centers. This initiative partnered AHRQ with other private and public organizations in an effort to improve the quality, effectiveness, and appropriateness of care. Several EBP models are used in QI.

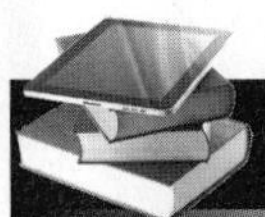

EVIDENCE FROM THE **LITERATURE**

Citation: Fineout-Overholt, E., Mazurek Melnyk, B., Stillwell, S. B., & Williamson, K. M. (2010, March). Evidence-Based practice step by step: Implementing an evidence-based practice change. *American Journal of Nursing. 111*(3): 54–60.

Discussion: This is the ninth article in a series of articles that began November 2009 from the Arizona State University College of Nursing and Health Innovation's Center for the Advancement of Evidence-Based Practice. Evidence-based practice (EBP) is a problem-solving approach to the delivery of health care that integrates the best evidence from studies and patient care data with clinician expertise and patient preferences and values. When delivered in a context of caring and in a supportive organizational culture, the highest quality of care and best patient outcomes can be achieved. The purpose of this series is to give nurses the knowledge and skills they need to implement EBP consistently, one step at a time. Articles appear every other month to allow time to incorporate information as readers work toward implementing EBP at their institution. Also, the authors have scheduled Chat with the Authors calls every few months to provide a direct line to the experts to help readers resolve questions.

Implications for Practice: Practicing nurses, nursing faculty, and students will want to review this series of articles. The articles in this series review various elements of EBP (e.g., use of PICO, and rapid critical appraisal of research). The articles can assist in planning continuing-education opportunities and in designing nursing curricula that prepare nurses for use of EBP and 21st-century professional practice.

EBP Models

There are several evidence-based practice models, e.g., The University of Colorado Hospital Model (Goode et al., 2000; Goode & Piedalue, 1999); the Iowa Model of Evidence-Based Practice to Promote Quality Care (Titler et al., 2001); Ace Star Model of Knowledge Transformation (Stevens, 2010); and the Johns Hopkins Nursing Evidence-Based Practice Model and Guidelines (Newhouse, Dearholt, Poe, & Pugh, 2007). Elements of the University of Colorado's EBP model can be applied to the case of Miss Kelly in the opening scenario of this chapter (see Table 13-2).

Benchmarking

Benchmarking is defined as the continuous process of measuring products, services, and practices against the toughest competitors or those customers recognized as industry leaders (Camp, 1994). Benchmarking against the best performers, for example, using the National Database of Nursing Quality Indicators (NDNQI) (https://www.nursingquality.org/), teaches us how to adapt the best practices to achieve breakthrough process improvement and build healthier communities. Benchmarking focuses on key services or work processes, for example, length of time from the patient entering the emergency department until the time of a treatment PCI procedure. A benchmark study will identify gaps in performance and provide options for selection of processes to improve, ideas for redesign of care delivery, and ideas for better ways to meet customer expectations. There are various types of benchmarking studies, such as clinical, financial,

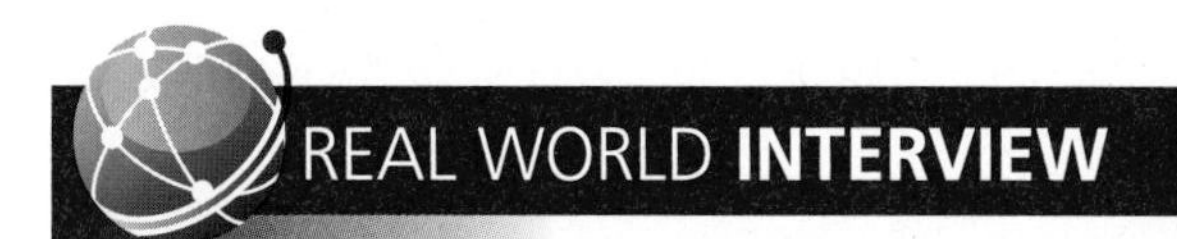

The first and most important tool in searching the literature for peer-reviewed, evidence-based journal articles is your institution's librarians. Speak to one of them and ask them to tell you about your library's key journals and databases for nursing. While many databases exist for health care literature, MEDLINE (http://www.nlm.nih.gov/databases/databases_medline.html) and the Cumulative Index to Nursing and Allied Health Literature (CINAHL) (http://www.ebscohost.com/cinahl/) are two of the most essential for nursing. MEDLINE is the National Library of Medicine's electronic journal database, indexing thousands of journal publications in the fields of medicine, nursing, dentistry, veterinary medicine, the health care system, and the preclinical sciences. MEDLINE provides a complete citation for each article within those journals, with an abstract of the article provided in most cases. PubMed (http://www.pubmed.gov) is the free search engine for MEDLINE, provided by the National Library of Medicine. Ovid Medline (http://www.ovid.com/site/catalog/DataBase/901.jsp) and its electronic access to full-text journal articles is available to you only if your parent institution's library subscribes to it. CINAHL is an electronic database that indexes the contents of nursing and allied health publications, including journals, dissertations, and other materials. As with MEDLINE, whether or not the full text of an article found in CINAHL can be accessed electronically depends on whether your parent institution's library subscribes to it. Other literature searching tools for nursing exist, such as the Cochrane Library (http://www.thecochranelibrary.com/view/0/index.html), PsycINFO (http://www.apa.org/pubs/databases/psycinfo/index.aspx), and Embase (www.elsevier.com/wps/product/cws_home/523328). These tools will get you started. When using electronic databases such as these, keep in mind that they often do not work like Internet search engines. There may be a few additional techniques to learn. Remember, if you have trouble, ask a librarian.

SCOTT THOMSON, MLIS
Reference and Education Librarian
Health Learning Centers
Northwestern Memorial Hospital
Chicago, Illinois

TABLE 13-2
EBP Hospital Model

Model Element	Application
Benchmarking data	Compare length of stay for Miss Kelly with that of other patients with breast cancer in this hospital and other hospitals nationally. Review the literature.
Cost-effective analysis	Analyze cost-effectiveness of wound care regimens, including nursing time and use of actual products (e.g., hydrogel vs. normal saline dressings). Benchmark with others.
Pathophysiology	Review biopsy results/findings of testing for metastatic disease and implications.
Retrospective/concurrent chart review	Assess changes in condition related to pressure ulcer development using the Braden Pressure Ulcer Risk Assessment Scale.
Quality improvement and risk data	Review and analyze documentation regarding patient progress and risk assessment (e.g., infection, bleeding, pressure ulcer development), and outcomes assessment (e.g., pain rating, falls, and dosage of narcotic administration).
International, national, and local standards	Assess effectiveness of care related to AHRQ guidelines for cancer pain and pressure ulcers.
Infection control data	Review wound culture results and institute appropriate precautions and treatment.
Patient preferences	Discuss, document, and implement patient's wishes regarding advance directives, pain management, and so forth.
Clinical expertise	Consult acute care nurse practitioner and other practitioners for wound, skin, and pain management.

Source: By permission of University of Colorado Hospital Research Council, Denver, CO.

and operational. A clinical benchmark study will review outcomes of patient care, for example, reviewing standards for managing the outcomes of care of patients with diabetes or a stroke. Financial benchmarking studies examine cost/case charges and length of stay. Operational benchmarking studies review systems that support care, for example, the case management system in an organization.

METHODOLOGIES FOR QUALITY IMPROVEMENT

Several models outline methodologies for quality improvement. Two are reviewed here: the PDSA Cycle (Figure 13-1) and the FOCUS method.

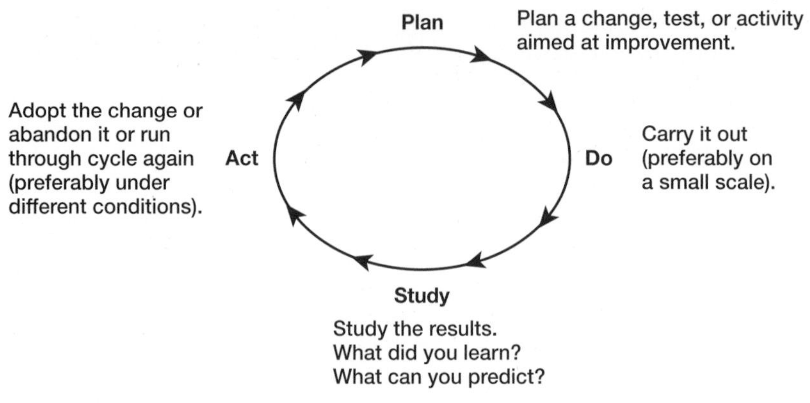

FIGURE 13-1

PDSA Cycle for improvement.
(*Source:* Courtesy of Albany Medical Center, Albany, NY.)

PDSA Cycle for improvement

Use of the PDSA Cycle (Figure 13-1) often is preceded by asking these questions (Langley et al., 1996) to define the problem and focus the quality improvement process:

1. What are we trying to accomplish?
2. How will we know that a change is an improvement?
3. What changes can we make that will result in improvement?

These three questions help focus the use PDSA Cycle for improvement (Ransom et al., 2005). We will apply the PDSA Cycle to Miss Kelly, the patient in the opening scenario presented at the beginning of this chapter, in relation to pain. This process can also be applied to the patient's pressure ulcers and wound management.

Application to Pain Management

Let us ask the three questions to improve the care of Miss Kelly, the patient in the opening scenario.

1. *What are we trying to accomplish?* The overall objective is to reduce or alleviate Miss Kelly's pain, which may be related to a variety of physiological, psychosocial, and spiritual issues.

   In conjunction with the other members of the health care team, the nurses will identify, implement, and document the best strategies for reducing Miss Kelly's pain.
2. *How will we know that a change is an improvement?* Miss Kelly will state that her pain is decreased or relieved. Behaviors that may indicate decreased pain include her verbal or nonverbal expression of pain relief or improved comfort, her ability to reposition herself, and statements such as "I feel more rested," along with an improved mood.
3. *What changes can we make that will result in improvement?* To standardize pain management for patients like Miss Kelly, the nursing staff will create a protocol that includes a plan to use a trial pain-management flow sheet to document the patient's reported pain status and pain interventions at various points in time.

Implementation of the PDSA Cycle for improvement

The PDSA Cycle can be individual or system focused. It can be used to solve a specific patient problem or to structure strategies for managing groups of patients with common problems. Based on our answers to the three questions, we will apply the PDSA Cycle as follows:

PLANNING PHASE: Once the three PDSA Cycle for improvement questions have helped staff identify what should be improved, the inter-professional staff (RN, MD, nurse practitioner, pharmacist, et al.) would develop a plan for improvement. The plan would have developed using the pain-management flow sheet and implementing evidence-based unit standards for assessing, managing, evaluating, and documenting patient comfort.

DOING PHASE: Nursing staff used the pain-management flow sheet to collect data on Miss Kelly during her hospital stay. All nurses assigned to care for Miss Kelly were asked to complete the documentation tool. Data to be collected would include the patient's pain rating, her nonverbal behaviors, level of consciousness, respiratory rate, side effects, activity, nonpharmacological therapies, pharmacological interventions, and patient response to interventions and teaching.

STUDYING PHASE: Data were collected for a period of two weeks. The nurses on the unit met and reviewed the documentation. Several improvements and issues were identified. Documentation of pain assessment and pain parameters had been completed 66 percent of the time during the two-week period. Staff nurses stated that they referred to the pain-management flow sheet when giving reports to the doctor or other nurses about Miss Kelly's pain status. As a result, Miss Kelly's pain management was central in discussions regarding her care, and decisions about changes in her pain medication regimen were made in a timely manner. The nursing and medical practitioners and pharmacists verbalized satisfaction with the flow sheet in terms of being able to see at a glance the amount and type of medication she was getting, how often, and her rating of pain. Within one week, Miss Kelly was reporting that her pain level improved to 2 or 3 on a scale of 0 to 10. She was receiving around-the-clock medication and bolus dosing three to four times a day as necessary. She remained alert and oriented and had no problems with constipation, urinary retention, or other medication side effects. Radiation therapy was started to her left leg in an effort to control her pain.

ACTING PHASE: After a meeting with the nurse manager, clinical nurse specialist, doctor, pharmacist, staff nurse, and other health care staff to discuss the findings, the staff agreed to continue to test the new pain-management interventions and flow sheet for four months on all patients admitted to the oncology unit. This next step in the improvement process reflects the use of additional, multiple PDSA cycles to improve not only Miss Kelly's outcomes, but also the total care delivery system.

Multiple Uses of the PDSA Cycle

Multiple PDSA cycles were used to improve care not just for Miss Kelly, but for all patients.

PLANNING PHASE: The inpatient oncology staff agreed to collect data for four months using the pain-management flow sheet on Miss Kelly and all new patients admitted to the oncology unit. The study also included a plan to orient the staff to the purpose, development, and procedures for using the tool and pain-management standards.

DOING PHASE: All nursing staff working on the inpatient oncology unit attended an inservice reviewing the pain standards and the purpose, development, and procedures for using the pain-management flow sheet. Once all the staff had completed the orientation, the data collection period was implemented.

STUDYING PHASE: Pain management was reviewed on an ongoing basis and documentation practices were reviewed after four months. Documentation of pain assessment was completed on 78 percent of all patients' charts on admission to the inpatient unit, 67 percent were completed 24 hours after admission, and 50 percent were completed 48 hours after admission. The majority of the unit's nurses agreed that they were using the pain-management flow sheet as a basis for their report to the practitioners regarding the patient's pain status. The pharmacist and the practitioners reported that they did review the pain-management flow sheet approximately 50 percent of the time, but they most often relied on the staff to verbally share with them information to improve the patient's pain status.

ACTING PHASE: A protocol for pain assessment, management, evaluation, and documentation was developed and integrated with the pain-management flow sheet. Eventually, this process was published in the oncology literature (Jadlos, Kelman, Marra, & Lanoue, 1996). This PDSA Cycle for improvement can also be used to focus on other aspects of Miss Kelly's care.

The FOCUS Methodology

The FOCUS methodology describes in a stepwise process how to move through the improvement process (Figure 13-2).

F: Focus on an opportunity for improvement. This step asks the question, What is the problem? During this phase, an improvement opportunity is articulated and data are obtained to support the hypothesis that an opportunity for improvement exists.

O: Organize a team that knows the process. This means identifying a group of staff members who are direct participants in the process to be examined—the point-of-service staff. A team leader is identified who will appoint team members.

C: Clarify what is happening in the current process. A flow diagram (see Figure 13-3) is very helpful for this.

U: Understand the degree of change needed. In this stage, the team reviews what it knows and enhances its knowledge by reviewing the literature, available data, and competitive benchmarks. How are other health care organizations doing the process?

S: Select a solution for improvement. The team can brainstorm and then choose the best solution. It can then use the PDSA Cycle for improvement to test this solution. An implementation plan should be used to track progress and the steps required. This implementation plan can be in the form of a work plan or Gantt chart (Figure 13-4). This is a chart in the form of a table that identifies what activity is to be completed, who is responsible for it, and when it is going to be done. It outlines the steps needed to implement the change.

OTHER QUALITY IMPROVEMENT STRATEGIES

Examples of other quality improvement tools are flowcharts and failure modes and effects analysis (FMEA). They are often used for work process management and improvement.

Flowcharts can be used to study a process for improvement. A flowchart is Za picture of each of the steps in a process in sequential order and subsequently can be applied to identify and understand how a process is done. A flowchart maps out each of the action steps and decisions within a process.

According to the Institute for Healthcare Improvement (IHI) (2011), **failure modes and effects analysis (FMEA)** is a systematic, proactive method for evaluating a work process to identify where and how it might fail and to assess the relative impact of different failures in order to identify the parts of the process that are most in need of change. FMEA includes review of the following:

- Steps in the process
- Failure modes (What could go wrong?)
- Failure causes (Why would the failure happen?)
- Failure effects (What would be the consequences of each failure?)

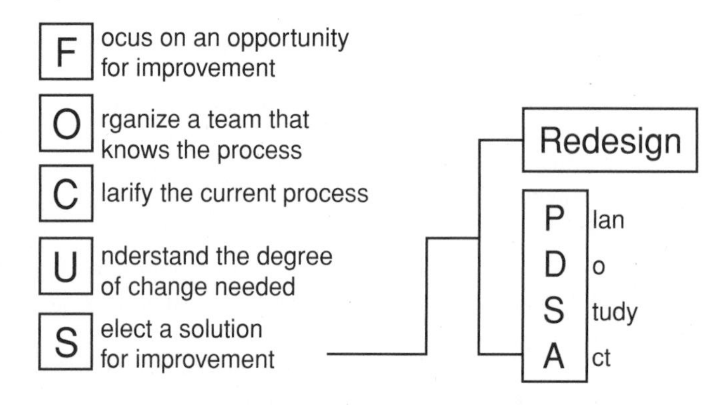

FIGURE 13-2
FOCUS method.
(*Source:* Courtesy of Albany Medical Center, Albany, NY.)

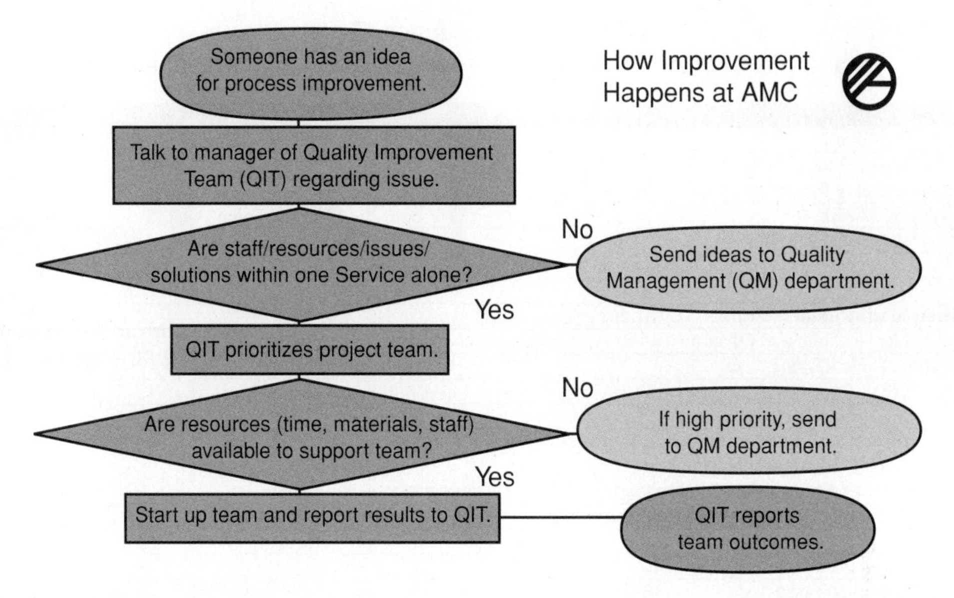

FIGURE 13-3

Flow diagram—How improvement happens.
(*Source:* Courtesy of Albany Medical Center, Albany, NY.)

Work teams use FMEA to evaluate work processes for possible failures. The FMEA teams work to prevent the failures by correcting the work processes proactively rather than reacting to adverse events and failures after they have occurred. This emphasis on prevention may reduce risk of harm to both patients and staff. FMEA is particularly useful in evaluating a new process prior to implementation and in assessing the impact of a proposed change to an existing work process.

Other improvement strategies identified at the organizational level involve the DMAIC Process Management Methodology (define, measure, analyze, improve, control) (Figure 13-5), as well as benchmarking, meeting regulatory requirements, identifying opportunities for system changes following sentinel event review, using visual measurements, and using a storyboard.

Regulatory Requirements

The Joint Commission (JC) has developed standards to guide critical activities performed by health care organizations. Preparation for an accreditation survey and the survey results will provide a wealth of information and data, which can be utilized as ideas for improvement strategies. In January 2003, the first six National Patient Safety Goals (NPSG) were approved by the JC. Recognizing that system design is intrinsic to the delivery of safe, high-quality health care, the goals focus on system-wide solutions wherever possible. Specific information regarding the history and ongoing requirements can be found at the JC website (www.jointcommission.org).

Det Norske Veritas (DNV) Healthcare, like the JC, has a hospital accreditation program approved by the CMS. However, DNV is the first and only CMS-approved accreditation program that surveys annually and employs International Organization for Standardization (ISO 9001) Quality Management System Standards. ISO 9001 provides a set of standardized requirements specific to quality management. DNV has been granted approval by the CMS for deeming authority for DNV's National Integrated Accreditation for Healthcare Organizations (NIAHO) accreditation program to determine hospital compliance with the Medicare Conditions of Participation. NIAHO integrates the Medicare Conditions of Participation and ISO 9001 quality management system requirements within one survey process. Under the ISO 9001 system, hospitals establish, document, and implement a quality management system and use the system to implement

Bed Access Improvement Team
Phase 2 Work Plan: Transition to Daily Management and Evaluation

Activity	Responsible Party	8/12	9/12	10/12	11/12	12/12
1.0 Modify the Team						
1.1 Identify Phase 2 tasks to be completed	Team	■				
1.2 Review & Modify Team Composition/membership	Team	■				
1.3 Develop Work Plan	Planning Team	■				
1.4 Review Work Plan with Team	Myers and Nolan		■			
2.0 Review/Modify Ideal Design						
2.1 Identify Modifications and Opportunities for Additional Change	Team			■		
2.2 Revise Ideal Flow Chart	Team			■		
3.0 Modify Structure & Supports: People/Forms Needed						
3.1 Revise Process Management Structure • Modify job descriptions—Triage Manager and Admitting Coordinator	Triage Management Subgroup				■	
3.2 Assess Communication Needed with Nursing Units	Team				■	
4.0 Draft/Standardize Tasks						
4.1 Draft/Standardize Tasks					■	
5.0 Transition to Daily Operations, Develop Data Collection Process, Evaluate, Monitor						
5.1 Evaluate Bed Access Simulation • Review ED & PACU data • Identify accomplishments and opportunities for structure and ideal work process	Team					■
5.2 Develop Plan to Transition Process and Structure to Daily Operations	Planning Team					■
5.3 Develop Data Collection Process	Planning Team					■
5.4 Evaluate Process & Structure (milestone meeting)	Team					■
5.5 Identify Subgroup of Pt Care Delivery System QIT to Monitor Progress	Team					■

FIGURE 13-4

Gantt chart/work plan.
(*Source:* Courtesy of Albany Medical Center, Albany, NY.)

The DMAIC Cycle:

Define - the process goals that are consistent with customer demands.

Measure - the current process and collect relevant data.

Analyze - to verify relationship of factors and determine root cause.

Improve - to optimize the process.

Control - to ensure sustainability.

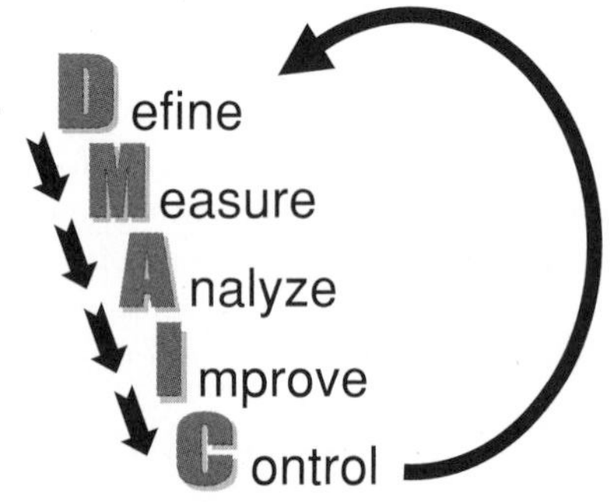

FIGURE 13-5

The DMAIC process management methodology.
(*Source:* Used with permission from Office of Performance Excellence, Faxton-St. Luke's Healthcare.)

work processes that support continuous quality improvement and enhanced patient outcomes. A component of ISO 9001 requires the hospital to monitor and measure its own performance and make improvements when necessary. DNV accreditation emphasizes both a continuous state of accreditation survey readiness each and every day, as well as continual improvement. Additional information on DNV accreditation can be found at http://dnvaccreditation.com.

Sentinel Event Review

A **sentinel event** is an unexpected occurrence involving death or serious physical or psychological injury to a patient, or the risk thereof. Events are called "sentinel" because they require immediate investigation. During analysis of these sentinel events, opportunities for improving the system will arise and should be taken advantage of. Linkage of sentinel event review to the organization's performance improvement system will identify strategies for prevention of future sentinel events. An example of a sentinel event is surgery performed on the wrong extremity of a patient. Reviewing the surgical process and developing a system to mark the appropriate site is an example of a performance improvement to prevent future sentinel events.

FINANCIAL INTEGRATION WITH HEALTH CARE QUALITY

The Institute of Medicine (IOM) acknowledged that as many as 98,000 people die each year due to preventable medical errors (1999). More than 10 years later, we have made little progress in reducing preventable medical errors. The response to inadequate quality of care and increased medical costs has been programs such as Pay-for-Performance (P4P) incentive programs and Core Measures.

P4P incentive programs align financial reward with improved patient outcomes. P4P programs differentiate payment among providers based on their performance on quality and efficiency measures. An early impetus in the progression of P4P was the IOM report *Crossing the Quality Chasm*, where the IOM strongly recommended that payment policies be aligned with quality improvement. The IOM report argued that current reimbursement methods provide little financial reward for improvements in the quality of health care delivery and may even inadvertently create barriers to improvement.

CORE MEASURES

In 2001, the JC along with CMS implemented a requirement that accredited hospitals collect and report data on standardized performance measures, called Core Measures. The CMS Core Measures are evidence-based performance measures that set national standards of care in distinct categories for targeted patient populations such as congestive heart failure, myocardial infarction, pneumonia, and surgical patients. Core Measure data is used for quality improvement and financial reimbursement and is also publicly reported on the Hospital Compare website (www.hospitalcompare.hhs.gov). Other reports are also available, e.g., the Leapfrog Group Hospital Safety Score (http://hospitalsafetyscore.org). While participation in Core Measure reporting is voluntary, those who choose *not* to participate will receive a reduction in their Medicare annual payment. An example of a Core Measure is: Patients with heart failure shall receive discharge instructions. Before the patient leaves the hospital, the staff at the hospital shall provide the patient or caregiver written information or educational material to help manage symptoms after they get home. The information shall address:

- Activity level
- Diet
- Medications
- Follow-up appointment
- Weight monitoring
- What to do if symptoms worsen

This Core Measure is designed to decrease hospital readmission of patients with congestive heart failure.

Measurements

To assess and monitor outcomes, heath care organizations collect and report quality measures at various levels in the organization. The terms "dashboard," "balanced scorecard," "report cards," and "clinical value compass" are often used to describe the concept of measuring performance at both a strategic and operational level in the organization. Measures may monitor patient clinical or functional status, patient satisfaction, cost, or organizational performance (Caldwell, 1998). Figure 13-6 illustrates these measures in the form of a clinical value compass.

Such an approach allows those reviewing data to examine a balanced approach to care (see Figure 13-7). Measures are selected based on what they have in common, so that if a change occurs in the cost-effectiveness category, it will affect the data in another category. From the control charts on the orthopedic unit in Figure 13-7, you can see that the total hip pathway length of stay increased and then decreased. The satisfaction scores remained at around 90 percent, so even though the length of stay decreased, satisfaction did not deteriorate. The ratio of complications went down; the average number of physical therapy visits varied and then went up. This reporting mechanism offers a balanced view.

The balanced scorecard guides the development of a unit-based performance improvement plan (see Figure 13-8), and provides a tool with which to present the outcomes of performance improvement in the succinct visual format of an executive summary.

Patient Satisfaction Data

Many health care facilities use the Hospital Consumer Assessment of Healthcare Providers and Systems (HCAHPS) Patient Satisfaction Survey on Communication with Nurses and Doctors, Responsiveness of Hospital Staff, Pain Management, Communication about Medicines, Cleanliness and Quietness of Hospital Environment. Data from the HCAHPS survey allows objective and meaningful comparisons between hospitals on information that is important to patients. Public reporting of the survey results is designed to create an incentive for hospitals to improve their quality of care and increases the transparency of the quality of hospital care.

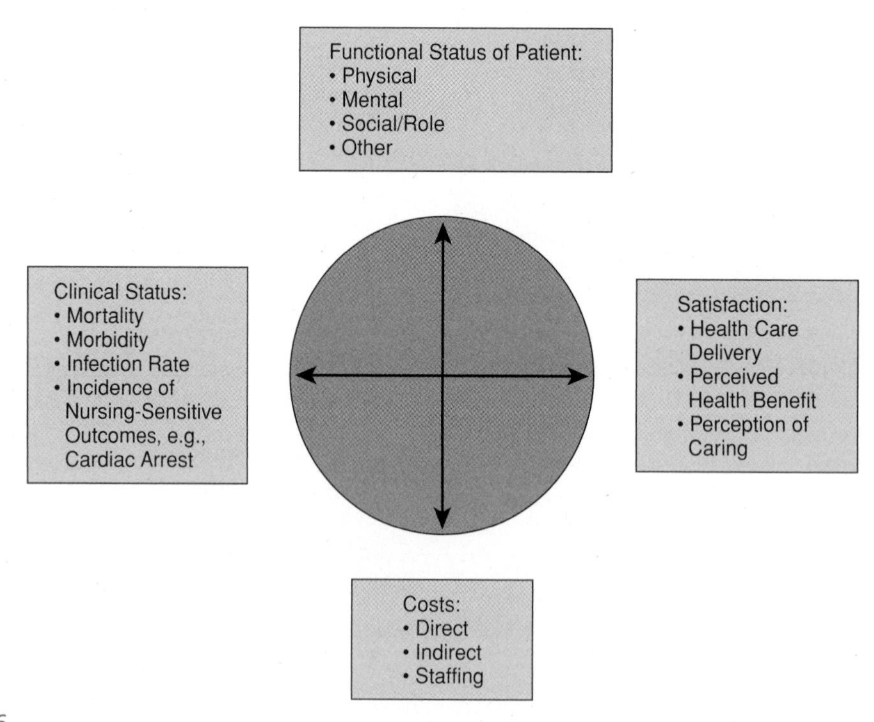

FIGURE 13-6

Clinical value compass.

(*Source:* Developed with information from Albany Medical Center, Albany, NY.)

Orthopedics Balanced Scorecard

Cost

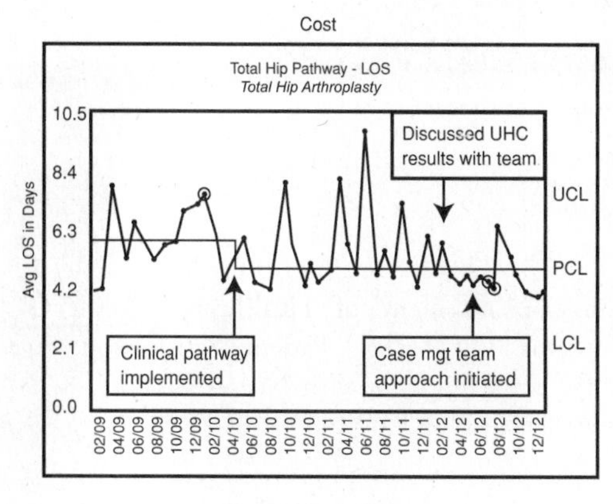

Satisfaction

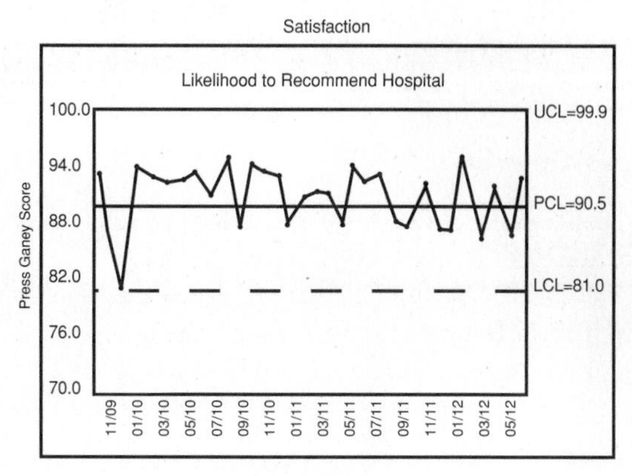

Clinical status: morbidity

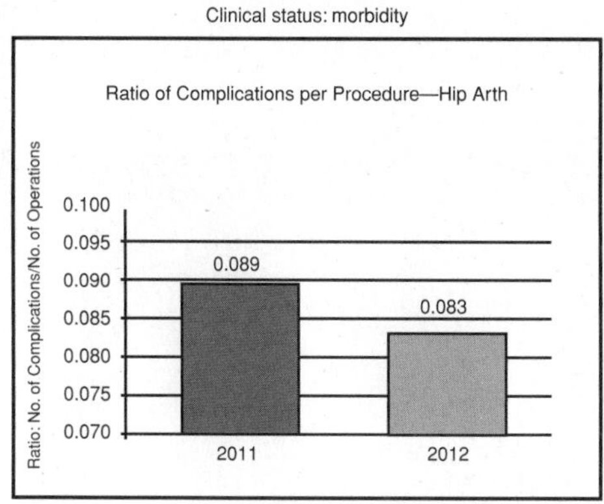

Functional outcome

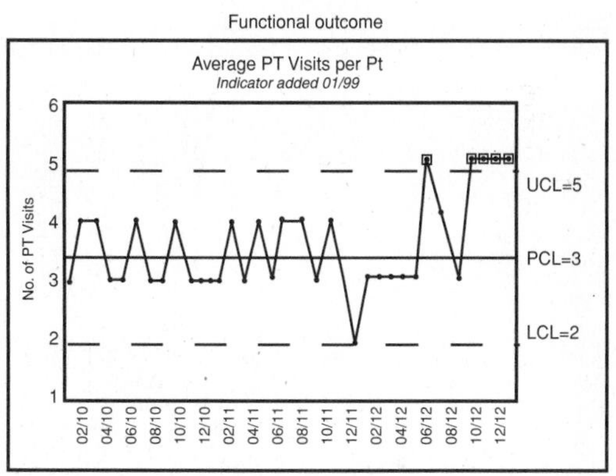

FIGURE 13-7

Orthopedic balanced scorecard.
(*Source:* Courtesy of Albany Medical Center, Albany, NY.)

Press-Ganey is another organization that assesses patient satisfaction (See http://www.pressganey.com/index.aspx). Other methods of patient data collection are a follow-up phone call or interview after patient discharge or a focus group. A focus group may involve talking with one or more patients after their discharge and getting feedback on their perceptions of their stay.

Storyboard: How to Share Your Story

Performance improvement teams share their work with others using a storyboard. The storyboard can be displayed in a high-traffic area of the organization to inform other staff of the QI efforts under way. Note the storyboard in the photo at the beginning of this chapter and again in Figure 13-9.

Storyboarding can be done when an improvement process is complete, or used during the process to communicate information, such as clinical outcomes or patient satisfaction.

QUALITY TOOLS

Several different types of tools are used to examine data in QI efforts. These include time series charts, Pareto charts, histograms, flowcharts, Ishikawa fishbone (root-cause or cause-and-effect) diagrams, pie charts, and check sheets. See Figures 13-10, 13-11, and 13-12.

INPATIENT SURGICAL UNIT

PERFORMANCE IMPROVEMENT PLAN

As part of Bassett's commitment to quality, the Surgical Unit will strive to improve performance through a cycle of planning, process design, performance measurement, assessment and improvement. There will be ongoing assessment of important aspects of care and service and correction of identified problems. Problem identification and solution will be carried out using a systematic intra- and interdepartmental approach organized around patient flow or other key functions, and in concert with the approved visions and strategies of the organization. Priorities for improvement will include high-risk, high-volume and problem-prone procedures.

The Surgical Unit will:

- promote the Plan-Do-Check-Act methodology for all performance improvement activities
- provide staff education and training on integrated quality and cost improvement
- collect data to support objective assessment of processes and contribute to problem resolution

In identifying important aspects of care and service, the Surgical Unit will select performance measures in the following operational categories:

A. Clinical Quality
1. Patient safety

- Patient falls
- Indicator: # of patient falls per month/# of patient days with upper control limits set by the research department based on statistical deviation

- Medication and IV errors
- Indicator: # of patient IV/medication errors per month/# of patient days with upper control limits set by the research department based on statistical deviation

- Restraint use
- Indicator: % of compliance with policy for use of restraints and overall rate of restraint use

2. Pressure ulcer prevention
- Indicator: Rates of occurrence—quarterly tracking report

3. Surveillance, prevention and control of infection
- Indicator: Infection-control statistical report of wound and catheter-associated infections
- Indicator: Quarterly monitoring of compliance with standards for Acid Fast Bacilli (AFB) room use; evidence of staff validation in AFB practice

4. Employee safety
- Injuries resulting from:
  - Back and lifting-related injuries
  - Morbidly obese patients
  - Orthopedic patients
- Indicators: # of injuries sustained by employees and any resultant workmen's compensation (Human Resources quarterly report)
- 100% competency validation in lifting techniques and back injury prevention
- Respiratory fit testing
- Indicator: competency record of each employee

5. Documentation by exception Indicators:
- 100% validation of RN/LPN staff
- Monthly chart audit (10% average daily census or 20 charts) meeting compliance with established standards

B. Access:
- Maintenance of the 30 minute standard for bed assignment of ED admissions
- Indicator: Quarterly review of ED tracking record

C. Service:
Patient Satisfaction
Indicator: Patient Satisfaction Survey: 90% or above response to, "Would return", and "Would recommend"

D. Cost:
- Nursing staff productivity will remain at 110% of target of 8.5 worked hours per adjusted patient day within a maximum variance range of 10%

For each of the above performance measures, this performance improvement plan will:

- address the highest priority improvement issues;
- require data collection according to the structure, procedure, and frequency defined;
- document a baseline for performance;
- demonstrate internal comparisons trended over time;
- demonstrate external benchmark comparisons trended over time;
- document areas identified for improvement;
- demonstrate that changes have been made to address improvement;
- demonstrate evaluation of these changes; document that improvement has occurred or, if not, that a different approach has been taken to address the issue.

The Inpatient Surgical Unit will submit biannual status reports to the Bassett Improvement Council (BIC) through the Medical Surgical Quality Improvement Council (MSQIC).
I

Approved by:_______________________________**Date:**____________________

(Chief or Vice President)

FIGURE 13-8

Inpatient surgical unit, performance improvement plan.
(*Source:* Courtesy Patricia Roesch, BS, RN, Bassett Healthcare.)

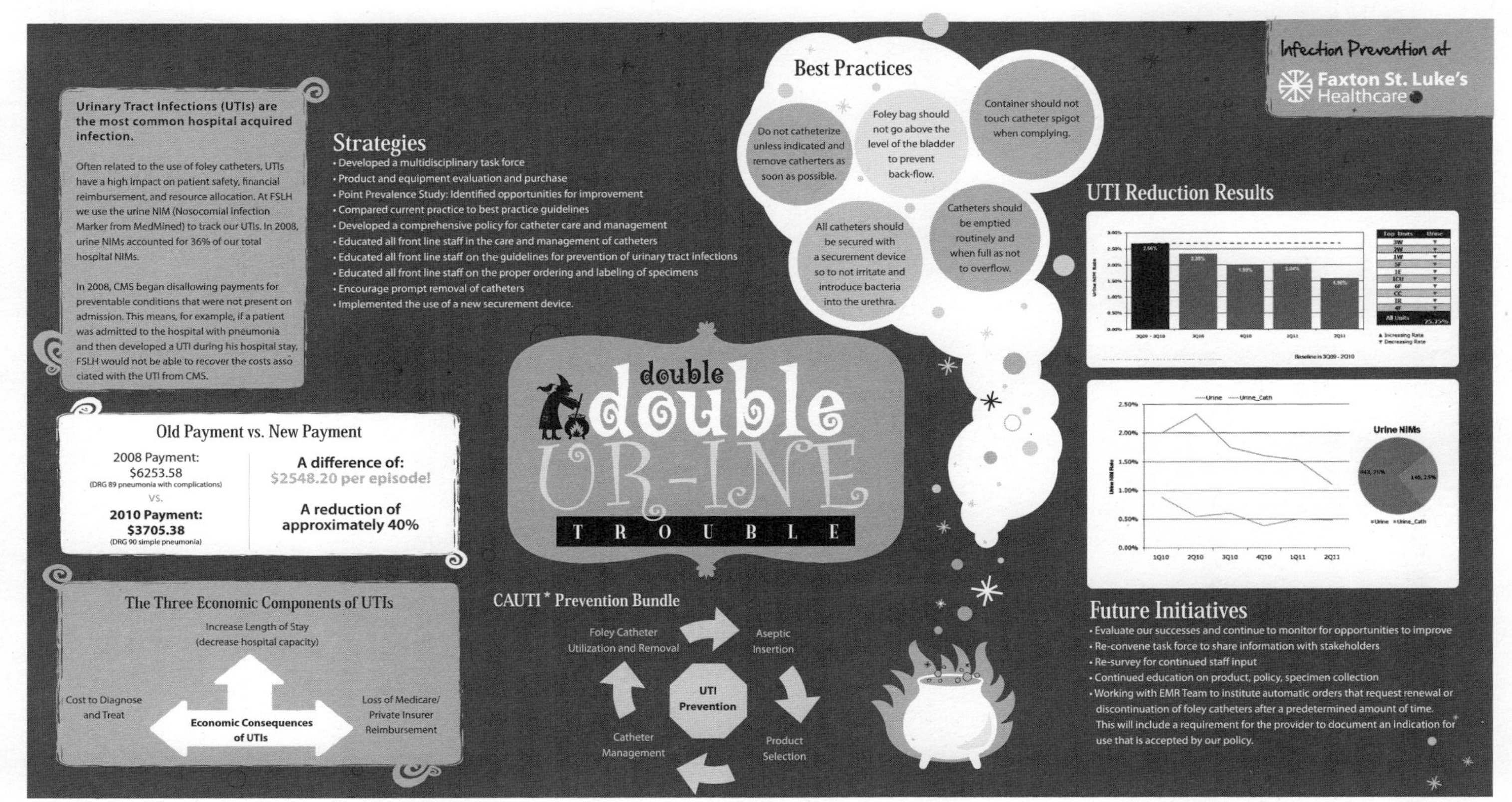

CAUTI* (Catheter-associated urinary tract infection)

FIGURE 13-9

Quality improvement storyboard.

(*Source:* UTI Reduction - First Place Winners of the 2011 Safety First Poster Contest at Faxton-St. Luke's Healthcare. Courtesy of Faxton-St. Luke's Healthcare Infection Prevention and Marketing Departments.)

REAL WORLD INTERVIEW

I work for the Utilization Management Service Line in the Veterans Integrated Service Network which includes Veterans' Affairs (VA) Medical Centers in Illinois, Wisconsin, and Upper Michigan. Utilization Management assesses 100 percent of all patients admitted to our Medical Centers using McKesson's standardized, evidence-based InterQual® Criteria to assure that patients are admitted to the correct level of care. Our goal is to assure that each veteran receives the right care, at the right time, and in the right setting. InterQual® Criteria are used in approximately 4,000 hospitals across the United States as well as in health care facilities internationally. There are different criteria for various levels of care; for example, patients cared for in an intensive care setting are evaluated against criteria specifically defined for this level of care. InterQual® Criteria are applied to review patients in acute as well as nonacute levels of care.

An example of using the InterQual® Criteria with an acutely ill, hospitalized patient with congestive heart failure (CHF) here at the VA is as follows: Each patient is reviewed by Utilization Management staff on admission and every day of their hospitalization to assure that the criteria are met for the designated level of care. A patient with CHF must meet one of the admission criteria such as elevated heart rate or low oxygen saturation, along with evidence of CHF treatments and interventions. Then, to stay in the hospital, the patient must meet criteria that include clinical findings related to CHF such as continued low oxygen saturation or an exacerbation of patient comorbidities (e.g., elevated blood sugar), along with the interventions to address the clinical findings. Finally, before we discharge the patient, the patient must meet the discharge criteria; for example, oxygen saturation and vital signs stability are within normal limits for the patient.

Most hospitals and insurance companies in the United States use InterQual® Criteria or similar criteria to assure that patients are admitted to the appropriate level of care, that they transition to the most appropriate level of care, and that they are discharged in a timely manner following the InterQual Transition Plan Guidelines to help prevent a readmission to the hospital.

A primary function of the Utilization Management review process is to identify and address system barriers to achieving the right care, at the right time, and in the right setting. Barriers are documented and analyzed to improve the efficiency and effectiveness of the care provided to veterans. The model used to accomplish this function consists of six processes:

- Team: A team of individuals who are involved in the improvement opportunity is formed.
- Aim: The team develops a specific, measurable aim that focuses on decreasing or eliminating the barrier.
- Map: The team develops a flow map of the current process as well as a map of the ideal state.
- Measure: The team measures the process both before and after improvements are made to assure that changes made result in improvement.
- Change: Improvements are made to the process. These changes or improvements may be in any of the following categories:
  - Balance supply and demand
  - Eliminate backlog
  - Reduce the number in queues
  - Develop contingency plans to manage variation in supply and demand
  - Use strategies to reduce demand

(*Continues*)

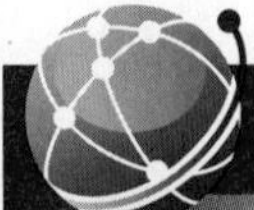

REAL WORLD INTERVIEW (Continued)

  - Use strategies to increase supply
  - Synchronize the work at each step
  - Predict and anticipate needs
  - Optimize space, equipment and staff
- Sustain: Actions are taken to assure that improvements are hard-wired into the work flow process to maintain the gains that have been achieved.

ANNA MARIE LIESKE, MS, RN
VISN 12 UM Manager
Milwaukee VA Medical Center
Milwaukee, Wisconsin

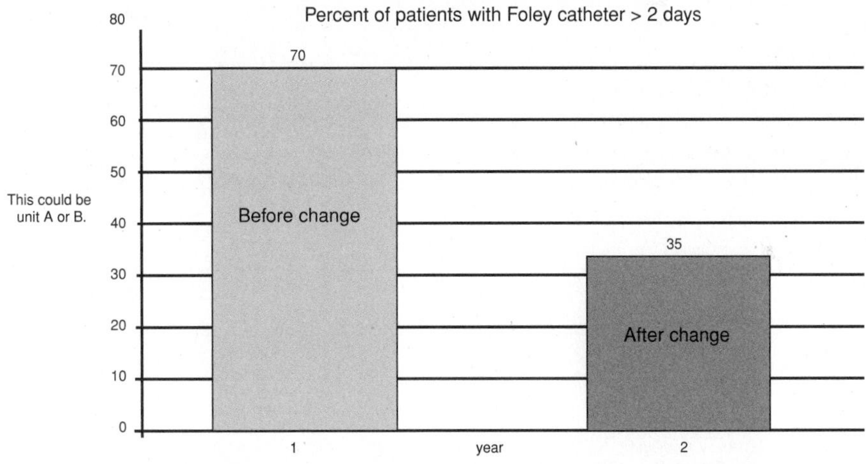

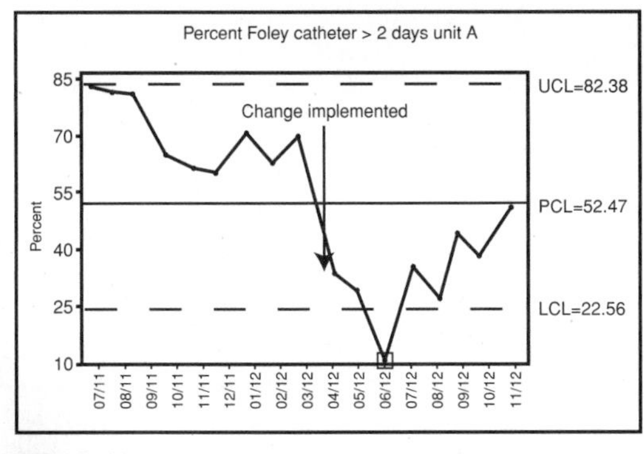

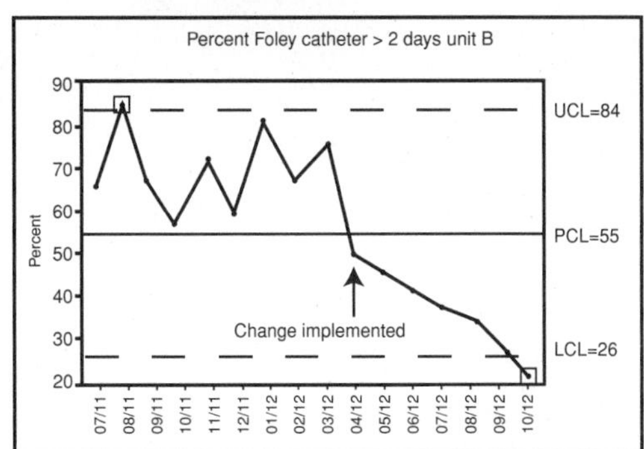

FIGURE 13-10

Time series versus bar charts.

(*Source:* Courtesy of Albany Medical Center, Albany, NY.)

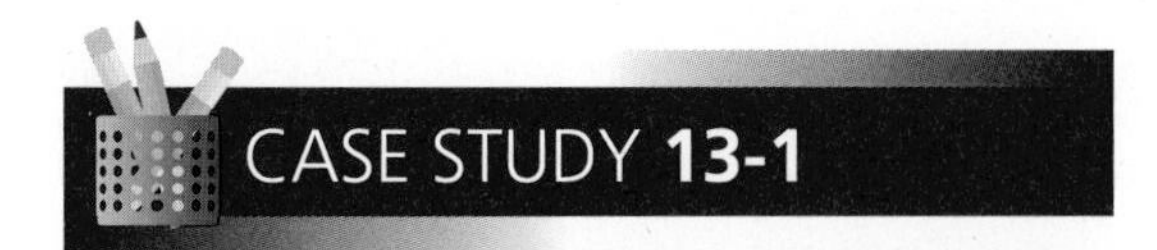

CASE STUDY 13-1

Identify one outcome to measure in each of the four areas of organizational quality improvement of patient outcomes—that is, clinical status, functional status, patient satisfaction, and cost.

ORGANIZATIONAL STRUCTURE FOR QI

Figure 13-13 is an organizational chart that shows a structure for quality improvement. Note that it includes staff at the board level to staff on individual quality improvement teams (QITs). Communicating priorities at all levels in the organization is key.

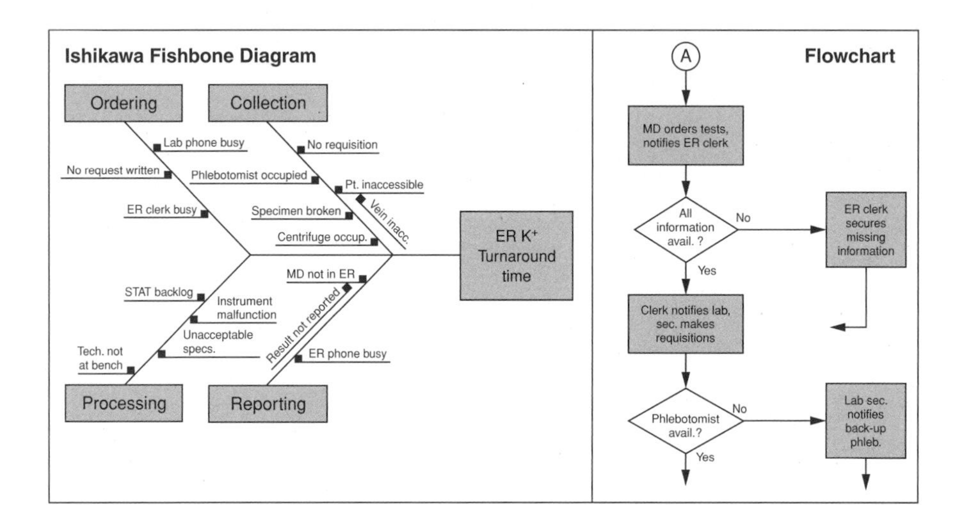

Check Sheet

Delays in production of Serum K^+ results from 1/1/91 to 1/7/91

Code/Delay Type		Mon	Tue	Wed	Thur	Fri	Sat	Sun	Total
A	Request not written by physician	I	I				I		3
B	Lab phone busy > 2 minutes	I		I		II		I	5
C	Phlebotomists unavailable	III	II	III	III	II	IIII	III	20
D	Requisition not ready	II	I	I	I	I	III	II	11
E	Patient inaccessible	I	I	II	I		II	I	8
F	Vein inaccessible	I		II		I	II		6
G	Centrifuge busy	II		I		I			4
H	Specimen broken	II		I				I	4
I	STAT backlog	III			I		II	I	7
J	Tech. not at bench	II		II		I	II	I	8
K	Unacceptable specimen	I	I		II		I	II	7
L	Lab. sec. unavailable to report	III		I		I	I		6
M	ER phone not answered			I			II		3
N	MD not in ER	II		I		II		I	5
O	MD not answer page	I	I	II		II		II	8
P	Results not reported by ER sec.	II	I	II	I	III	II	II	13

FIGURE 13-11

Ishikawa fishbone (root-cause or cause-and-effect) diagram, flowchart, and check sheet.

(*Source:* K. N. Simpson, A. D. Kaluzny, and C. P. McLaughlin, 1991, Clinical Laboratory Management Review, November/December 1991, 5[6]:448–462. ©Clinical Laboratory Management Association, Inc.)

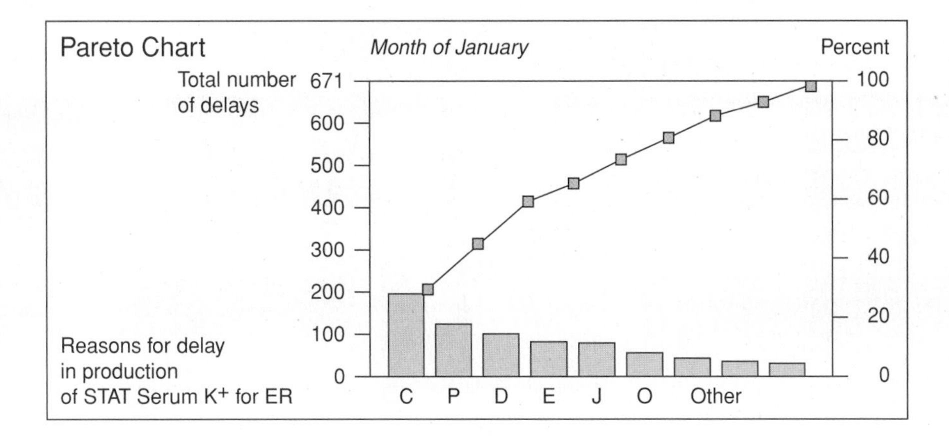

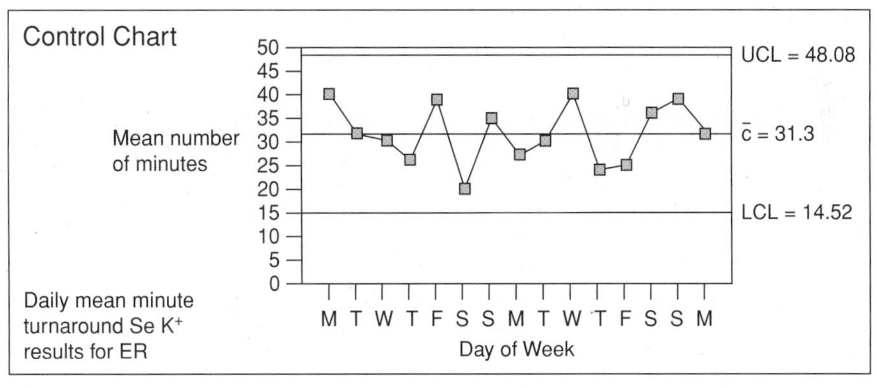

FIGURE 13-12

Pareto chart and control chart.

(*Source:* Total quality and the management of laboratories by K. N. Simpson, A. D. Kaluzny, and C. P. McLaughlin, 1991, Clinical Laboratory Management Review, 5(6), 448–449, 452–453, 456–458. © Clinical Laboratory Management Association, Inc.)

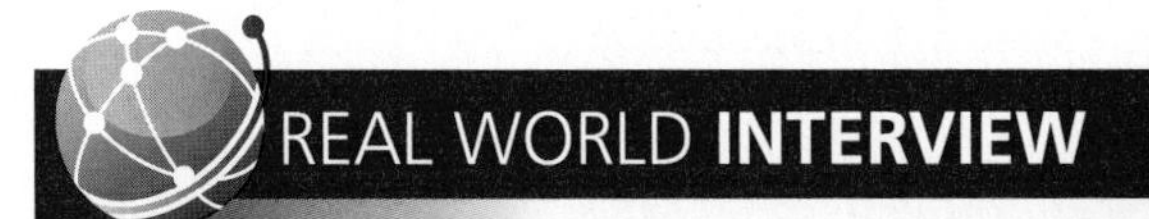

REAL WORLD **INTERVIEW**

In my job, I review a patient's chart and compare it to evidence-based guidelines from research and the literature to see if the patient's health care is being performed in the appropriate setting. I will review if the patient's care is medically necessary. If it is not, I assist the hospital case managers or physicians to move the patient to the appropriate level of care. For example, IV antibiotics can sometimes be administered at home or in another facility. When the situation at home is such that the family cannot manage it, the patient could move to a subacute facility, if available, or the patient could stay in the hospital with the hospital paid at a different rate. Documentation is critical in this type of review. An accurate clinical picture of the patient needs to be reflected in the documentation.

MARGUERITE MONTYSKO, RN

Case Manager, Albany Medical Center
Albany, New York

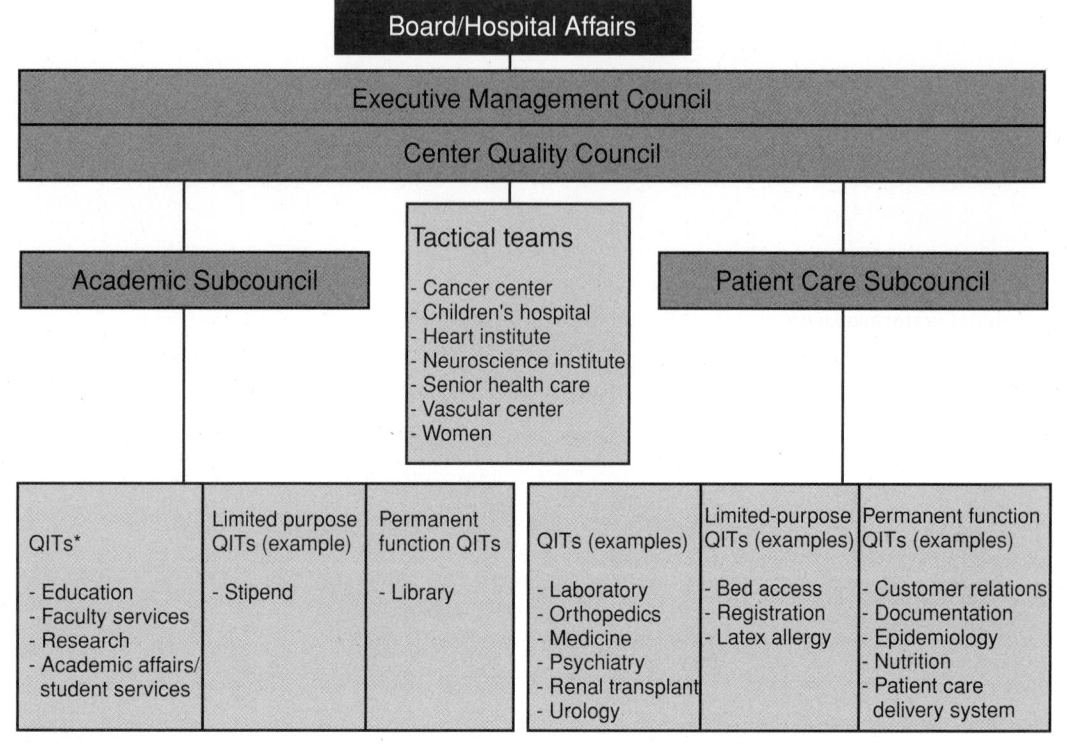

FIGURE 13-13

Structure for quality improvement.
(*Source:* Courtesy of Albany Medical Center, Albany, NY.)

Staff members must realize how their day-to-day work influences the accomplishment of strategic goals. Mission, vision, and value statements help accomplish this clarity of focus. This is discussed more in Chapter 11.

KEY CONCEPTS

- Quality improvement uses data to monitor the outcomes of care processes and uses improvement methods to design and test changes to continuously improve the quality and safety of health care systems (QSEN, 2012).
- Customers of health care are patients, nurses, doctors, the community, and so on.
- Patient care needs should drive improvement opportunities.
- Evidence-based practice decisions should be driven by data.

- Quality improvement initiatives should be linked to the organization's mission, vision, and values.
- Organizational goals and objectives should be communicated up and down the organization.
- There should be a balance in quality improvement goals focused on patient clinical and functional status, access, cost, and patient satisfaction outcomes.
- Many health care facilities use the Hospital Consumer Assessment of Healthcare Providers and Systems (HCAHPS) Patient Satisfaction Survey.
- A clinical value compass, dashboard, balanced scorecard, or report card can be used to identify key outcomes that are monitored for quality improvement.
- Hospital performance on core measures can be benchmarked at: http://hospitalcompare.hhs.gov
- The University of Colorado Hospital Model is one example of an inter-professional, evidence-based practice model for using different sources of information to change or support your practice.
- Note this website, Leapfrog Group Hospital Safety Score program, http://hospitalsafetyscore.org
- PDSA Cycle, the FOCUS and DMAIC methods, the FMEA method, and other methods can be used to improve quality.
- Several different types of tools are used to examine data in QI efforts. These include time series charts, Pareto charts, histograms, flowcharts, Ishikawa fishbone (root-cause or cause-and-effect) diagrams, pie charts, and check sheets.

KEY TERMS

customers
failure modes and effects analysis (FMEA)
quality
quality improvement
sentinel event

REVIEW QUESTIONS

1. Based on an understanding of the PDSA Cycle in health care, the first step a nurse would take in the quality improvement process is which of the following?
   A. Collect data to determine if standards are met
   B. Implement a plan to correct the problem
   C. Define the problem
   D. Determine the standard

2. A staff nurse has been assigned to a committee that has identified the lack of documentation of pain assessment and reassessment. As a result, the committee recommends a change in the facility's documentation form. The staff nurse is probably a member of which of the following committees?
   A. Medical Staff
   B. Performance Improvement
   C. Unit Council
   D. Ethics

3. A new nurse manager is trying to determine the best way to implement patient teaching to reduce falls in her Same Day Surgery Unit. She decides to gather data from other facilities' Same Day Surgery Units and compare their teaching methods and fall rates with her unit's methods and rates. Which quality improvement process is she using?
   A. Benchmarking
   B. Flowcharting
   C. FMEA
   D. DMAIC
4. Evidence-based practice has been established in nursing practice to do which of the following?
   A. Reduce health care costs
   B. Facilitate the highest quality of care and the best patient outcomes
   C. Communicate the values of the nursing profession
   D. Encourage increased research utilization
5. Which of the following is evidence that a work process change is effective?
   A. The desired work process improvement took place.
   B. Physicians do not complain.
   C. Employees are content.
   D. There is an increase in the customer satisfaction rate.
6. Identifying opportunities for quality improvement in the health care arena is the responsibility of which group?
   A. Administration
   B. Practitioners
   C. Patients
   D. Everyone
7. Following a sentinel event, which step would be initiated first?
   A. No action
   B. Corrective action of personnel
   C. Reporting to the health department and completing a root-cause analysis
   D. Immediate investigation
8. Nurses must do which of the following to implement the use of EBP?
   A. Benchmark
   B. Participate in root-cause analysis
   C. Use quality tools such as Pareto charts, check sheets, and histograms
   D. Participate in the development, use, and evaluation of practice guidelines
9. Which of the following are quality tools that can be used to analyze data in the quality improvement process? Select all that apply.
   A. DMAIC
   B. Pie charts
   C. Ishikawa diagram or root-cause analysis
   D. Pareto diagram
   E. Histogram
   F. Genogram

10. A hospital is trying to decrease hospital-acquired urinary tract infections. Which of the following would be the best method(s) of communicating information to the nurses during this quality improvement process? Select all that apply.

A. Fishbone diagram
B. FMEA
C. Storyboard
D. PDSA
E. Ishikawa diagram
F. Pie chart

REVIEW ACTIVITIES

1. Risk management, infection control practitioners, and a benchmark study have revealed that your unit's utilization of indwelling urinary catheters is above average. Brainstorm reasons why this may be occurring. Creating a fishbone diagram (i.e., root-cause or cause-and-effect diagram) may help identify any system causes for the problem.
2. Think about your last clinical rotation experience. Identify one work process that you believe could be improved and describe how you would begin improving the work process. Use the FOCUS or DMAIC methodology.

EXPLORING THE WEB

- Visit these sites for benchmark data: the University Health System Consortium (UHC): *http://www.uhc.edu; the Institute ...* for Healthcare Improvement (IHI), *http://www.ihi.org;* and the Leapfrog Group Hospital Safety Score program, *http://hospitalsafetyscore.org*
- These sites are recommended for a team that is looking for evidence-based guidelines or research studies for a particular diagnosis:
  - National Guideline Clearinghouse: *http://www.guideline.gov*
  - Cochrane Library: *http://www.cochrane.org*
  - PubMed's home page: *http://www.ncbi.nlm.nih.gov*
  - Joanna Briggs Institute for Evidence-Based Nursing & Midwifery: *http://www.joannabriggs.edu.au*
  - Evidence-based practice Internet resources: *http://www.hsl.lib.mcmaster.ca*
- The website for the Agency for Healthcare Research and Quality (AHRQ), formerly the Agency for Health Care Policy and Research (AHCPR), has a clinical information index page that lists evidence reports for topics such as swallowing disorders in stroke patients, therapies for stable angina, and provides access to agency-supported guidelines (e.g., cancer pain, cardiac rehabilitation, and pressure ulcers): *http://www.ahrq.gov*
- Go to *http://www.nursingworld.org.* Search for information about the Nursing Information and Data Set Evaluation Center. Note the ANA-Recognized Classification Systems listed.
- Check this source of quality information: *http://www.leapfroggroup.org*

REFERENCES

Anderson, J., Mokracek, M., & Lindy, C. (2009). A nursing quality program driven by evidence-based practice. *Nursing Clinics of North America, 44*(1), 83.

Caldwell, C. (1998). *Handbook for managing change in health care*. Milwaukee, WI: ASQ Quality Press.

Camp, R. (1994). Benchmarking applied to healthcare. *The Joint Commission on Quality Improvement, 20*, 229–238.

Crosby, P. B. (1979). *Quality is free*. New York, NY: New America Library.

Deming, W. E. (1986). *Out of the crisis*. Cambridge, MA: Center for Advanced Engineering Study.

Det Norske Veritas. (2011). DNV managing risk: Simply better accreditation. Retrieved October 29, 2011, from http://dnvaccreditation.com/pr/dnv/default.aspx

Donabedian, A. (1966). Evaluating the quality of medical care. *Milbank Memorial Fund Quarterly, 44*, 194–196.

Evidence-based Practice Centers Overview. Agency for Healthcare Research and Quality, Rockville, MD. Retrieved November 2012, from http://www.ahrq.gov/clinic/epc

Fineout-Overholt, E., Mazurek Melnyk, B., Stillwell, S. B., & Williamson, K. M. (2010, March). Evidence-Based practice step by step: Implementing an evidence-based practice change. *American Journal of Nursing. 111(3)*, 54 -60.

Goode, C. J., & Piedalue, F. (1999). Evidence-based clinical practice. *Journal of Nursing Administration, 29*, 15–21.

Goode, C. J., Tanaka, D. J., Krugman, M., O'Connor, P. A., Bailey, C., & Deutchman, M. (2000). Outcomes from use of an evidence-based practice guideline. *Nursing Economic$, 18*, 202–207.

Hospital Consumer Assessment of Healthcare Providers and Systems (HCAHPS) Patient Satisfaction Survey. 2012. Centers for Medicare & Medicaid Services, Baltimore, MD. Retrieved November 21, 2012, from http://www.hcahpsonline.org

Institute for Healthcare Improvement (IHI). (2011). Failure modes and effects analysis (FMEA) tool. Retrieved from http://www.ihi.org/knowledge/Pages/Tools/FailureModesandEffectsAnalysisTool.aspx

Institute of Medicine (IOM). (1990). *Medicare: A strategy for quality assurance*, vol. I. Washington, DC: National Academies Press.

Institute of Medicine (IOM). (1999). *To err is human: Building a safer health system*. Washington, DC: National Academies Press.

Institute of Medicine (2010). The future of nursing: leading, changing, advancing health. Retrieved from http://www.iom.edu/~/media/Files/Report%20Files/2010/The Future-of-Nursing/Future%20of%20Nursing%202010%20Recommendations.pdf

Jadlos, M. A., Kelman, G. B., Marra, K., & Lanoue, A. (1996). A pain management documentation tool. *Oncology Nursing Forum, 23*, 1451–1454.

Joint Commission. (July 2001). Core measure sets. Retrieved October 6, 2012, from http://www.jointcommission.org/core_measure_sets.aspx

Juran, J. M. (Ed.). (1988). *Quality control handbook*. (4th ed.). New York, NY: McGraw Hill.

Kane, R. L. (1997). *Understanding health care outcomes research* (1st ed.). Gaithersburg, MD: Aspen.

Kimberly, J. R., & Minvielle, E. (2003). Quality as an organizational problem. In S. S. Mick & M. Wyttenback (Eds.), *Advances in health care organization theory* (p.62). San Francisco, CA: Jossey-Bass.

Langley, G. J., Nolan, K. M., Nolan, T. W., Norman, C. L., & Provost, L. P. (1996). *The improvement guide: A practical approach to enhancing organizational performance.* San Francisco, CA: Jossey-Bass.

Melnyk, B. (Editor), & Fineout-Overholt, E. (Editors). (2004). Evidence-Based Practice in Nursing and Healthcare: A Guide to Best Practice. Lippincott.

Newhouse, R. P., Dearholt, S. L., Poe, S. S., & Pugh, L. C. (2007). *Johns Hopkins nursing evidence-based practice model and guidelines*. Indianapolis, IN: Sigma Theta Tau International.

Quality and Safety Education for Nurses (QSEN). (2012). Retrieved October 6, 2012, from http://www.qsen.org/definition .php?id=3

Ransom, S. B., Joshi, M. S., & Nash, D. B. (2005). *The healthcare quality book: Vision, strategy, and tools.* Chicago, IL: Health Administration Press.

Simpson, K. N., Kaluzny, A. D., & McLaughlin, C. P. (1991). Total quality and the management of laboratories. *Clinical laboratory management review, 5*(6), 448–449, 452–453, 456–458.

Stevens, K. R. (2010). Ace star model of knowledge transformation: Model for evidence-based practice of the Academic Center for Evidence-Based Nursing at the University of Texas Health Sciences Center. San Antonio, TX. Retrieved from http://www.acestar.uthscsa.edu/acestar-model.asp" \o "Open this link" \t "_blank

Titler, M., Kleiber, C., Steelman, V., Rakel, B., Budreau, G., Everett, L., Buckwalter, K., Tripp-Reimer, T., Goode, C. (2001). The Iowa model of evidence-based practice to promote quality care. *Critical Care Clinics of North America, 13*(4), 497–509.

U.S. Department of Health & Human Services (HHS). (2011). Hospital compare. Retrieved October 6, 2012, from http://www.hospitalcompare.hhs.gov

U.S. Department of Health & Human Services (HHS). (2012). Hospital Compare. Retrieved November 21, 2012, from http://www.hospitalcompare.hhs.gov

SUGGESTED READINGS

Allen, D. E., Bockenhauer, B., Egan, C., & Kinnaird, L. S. (2006). Relating outcomes to excellent nursing practice. *The Journal of Nursing Administration (JONA), 36*(3), 140–147.

Anderson, J., Mokracek, M., & Lindy, C. (2009). A nursing quality program driven by evidence-based practice. *Nursing Clinics of North America, 44*(1), 83.

Arnold, L., Campbell, A., Dubree, M., Fuchs, M. A., Davis, N., Hertzler, B., et al. (2006). Priorities and challenges of health system chief nursing executives: Insights for nursing educators. *Journal of Professional Nursing, 22*(4), 213–220.

Berwick, D. M., Calkins, D. R., McCannon, B. A., & Hackbarth, A. D. (2006). The 100,000 lives campaign: Setting a goal and a deadline for improving health care quality. *Journal of the American Medical Association, 295*(3), 324–327.

Chassim, M., Loeb, J., Schmaltz, S., & Walchter, R. (2011). Accountability measures: Using measurement to promote quality improvement. *The New England Journal of Medicine. 343*(7), 683–688.

Cochrane Library at McMaster University. Retrieved October 6, 2012, from http://www.cochrane.org

Engelke, M. K., & Marshburn, D. M. (2006). Collaborative strategies to enhance research and evidence-based practice. *The Journal of Nursing Administration, 36*(3), 131–135.

Glaser, J. (2012). The variability of patient care: Hospitals & health networks. American Hospital Association. Retrieved September 20, 2012, from http://www.hhnmag.com/hhnmag/jsp/articledisplay.jsp?dcrpath=HHNMAG/Article/data/05MAY2010/100510HHN_Weekly_Glaser&domain=HHNMAG

Goetz, K., Janney, M., & Ramsey, K. (2011). When nursing takes ownership of financial outcomes: Achieving exceptional financial performance through leadership, strategy, and execution. *Nursing Economic$, 29*(4), 173–182.

Guyatt, G. H., Haynes, R. B., Jaeschke, R. Z., Cook, D. J., Green, L., Naylor, C. D., et al. (2000). Users' guides to the medical literature: XXV. Evidence-based medicine: Principles for applying the users' guides to patient care. *Journal of the American Medical Association, 284,* 1290–1296.

Institute of Medicine (IOM). (2001). *Crossing the quality chasm: A new health system for the 21st century.* Washington, DC: National Academies Press.

Joanna Briggs Institute. Retrieved October 6, 2012, from http://www.joannabriggs.edu.au

Joint Commission. (2011). Cost of accreditation. Retrieved July 2012 from http://www.jointcommissioninternational.org/Cost-of-Accreditation

Kahn, C. N., Ault, T., Isenstein, H., Potetz, L., & Van Gelder, S. (2006). Snapshot of hospital quality reporting and pay-for-performance under Medicare. *Health Affairs, 25* (1), 148–162.

Majid, S., Foo, S., Luyt, B., Zhang, X., Theng, Y., Chang, Y., & Mokhtar, I. (2011). Adopting evidence-based practice in clinical decision making: Nurses' perceptions, knowledge, and barriers. *Journal of the Medical Library Association, 99*(3), 229–236.

National Institute of Standards and Technology (NIST). (2010, February.) Baldrige performance in excellence program: Why take the Baldrige journey? Retrieved from http://www.nist.gov/baldrige/enter/index.cfm#

National Quality Forum (NQF). (2008, October). Serious reportable events. Retrieved from http://www.qualityforum.org/Publications/2008/10/Serious_Reportable_Events.aspx

Quality and Safety Education for Nurses (QSEN). (2012). An introduction to the competencies and the knowledge, skills, and attitudes. Retrieved from http://www.qsen.org/search_strategies.php?id=148

Ring, N., Coull, A., Howie, C., Murphy-Black, T., & Watterson, A. (2006). Analysis of the impact of a national initiative to promote evidence-based nursing practice. *International Journal of Nursing Practice, 12*(4), 232–240.

Stillwell, S., Fineout-Overholt, E., Mazurek Melnyk, B., & Williamson, K. (2010). Asking the clinical question: A key step in evidence-based practice. *American Journal of Nursing, 10*(3), 58–61.

Wennberg, J., & Fisher, E. (2006). *The care of patients with severe chronic illness: A report on the Medicare program by the Dartmouth Atlas Project.* Hanover, NH: Center for the Evaluative Clinical Sciences, Dartmouth Medical School.

Wolf, Z. R., & Hughes, R. G. (2009). Error reporting and disclosure. In R. G. Hughes (Ed.), *Patient safety and quality: An evidence-based handbook for nurses* (Chapter 35). Retrieved from http://www.ncbi.nlm.nih.gov/books/NBK2652

CHAPTER 14

Legal Aspects of Health Care

JANICE TAZBIR, RN, MS, CCRN, CS, CNE;
JUDITH W. MARTIN, RN, JD; SISTER KATHLEEN CAIN,
OSF, JD; CHAD S. PRIEST, RN, BSN, JD; AND
SARA ANNE HOOK, MLS, MBA, JD

The role of the nurse in medical malpractice litigation has experienced a paradigm shift over the last several years. In the past, nurses were considered to be mere . . . 'custodians' who played a limited role in the care and treatment of patients . . . now the focus is on the nurse as a clinician, responsible for using professional judgment in the course of treatment.

–CNA FINANCIAL CORPORATION, 2009

OBJECTIVES

Upon completion of this chapter, the reader should be able to:

1. Discuss the sources of law.
2. Name the most common areas of nursing practice cited in malpractice actions.
3. List some protections in nursing practice to decrease liability.

You are working on a postsurgical unit and have been given an order to discharge a 72-year-old male who has just had a total hip replacement. Per hospital policy, you obtain a set of vital signs before discharging him home and note his temperature to be 100.9°F (38.3°C). Upon assessing the patient, he tells you that he feels a bit "chilled." You notify the practitioner of the elevated temperature and the patient's comments, but you are told to continue with the discharge.

After notifying the practitioner about the elevated temperature, do you need to gather additional information about the patient's condition before you discharge him?

What do you do if the patient appears to be too ill for discharge? Is there anyone else you can contact?

If you discharge the patient and he develops sepsis or a serious illness, are you responsible or is the health care practitioner responsible?

Law that affects the relationship between individuals is called "civil law." Law that specifies the relationship between citizens and the state is called "public law." This chapter reviews how various types of law affect nursing practice and actions nurses can take to minimize risks to their professional practice. Additionally, common types of nursing malpractice and ways to decrease professional liability will be discussed.

SOURCES OF LAW

The authority to make, implement, and interpret laws is generally granted in a constitution. A **constitution** is a set of basic laws that specifies the powers of the various segments of the government and how these segments relate to each other.

Generally, it is the role of a legislative body, both on the federal and state levels, to enact laws. Agencies under the authority of the administrative branch of the government draft the rules that implement the law. Finally, the judicial branch interprets the law as it rules in court cases. Table 14-1 gives examples of these relationships.

Also, a judicial decision may set a precedent that is used by other courts and, over time, has the force of law. This type of law is referred to as **common law**.

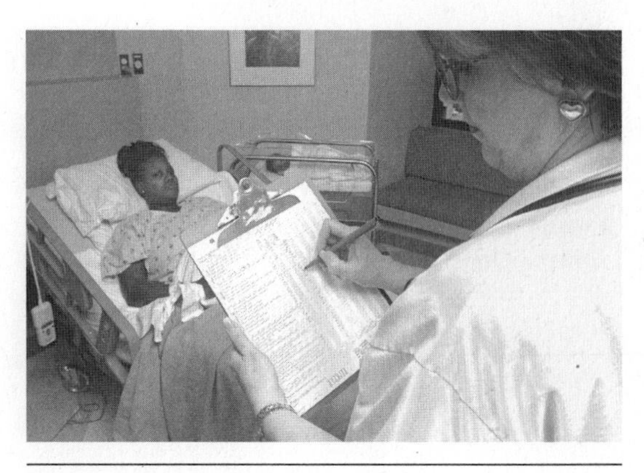

© Cengage Learning 2014

Public Law

Public law consists of constitutional law, criminal law, and administrative law and defines a citizen's relationship with government.

Constitutional Law

Several categories of public law affect the practice of nursing and patient-centered care. For example, the nurse accommodates patients' constitutional right to practice their religion every time the nurse calls a patient's clergy as requested, follows a specific religious custom for preparation of meals, or prepares a deceased person's remains for burial.

Nurses may not believe in a right personally and may refuse to work in areas where they would have to assist a patient in exercising a right. Nurses may not, however, interfere with another person's ability to exercise his constitutional right.

Criminal Law

Criminal law focuses on the actions of individuals that can intentionally do harm to others. Often the victims of such abusive actions are the very young or the very old. These two categories of people generally cannot defend themselves against physical or emotional abuse. The nurse, in caring for patients, may notice that a vulnerable patient has unexplained bruises, fractures, or other injuries. Most states have mandatory statutes that require the nurse to report unexplained or suspicious injuries to the appropriate child or elderly protective agency. Generally, the institution in which the nurse is employed will have clear guidelines and policies to

TABLE 14-1
The Three Branches of Government in the United States

	Legislative Branch	Administrative Branch	Judicial Branch
Example at Federal Level	Americans with Disabilities Act (ADA) (1990)	The Equal Employment Opportunity Commission (EEOC) publishes rules specifying what employers must do to help a disabled employee.	In 1999, the U.S. Supreme Court interpreted the law to require that to be protected by this law, the individual must have an impairment that limits a major life activity and that is not corrected by medicine or appliances (e.g., blood pressure medicine, glasses). (Sutton *v.* United Airlines 1999; Murphy v. United Parcel Service, Inc., 1999).
Example at State Level	Nurse Practice Act	The state board of nursing develops rules specifying the duties of a registered nurse in that state.	Courts and juries determine whether a nurse's actions comply with the law governing the practice of nursing in a state.

© Cengage Learning 2014

follow in such a situation. Failure to report the problem as required by law can result in criminal penalties.

Another aspect of criminal law affecting nursing practice is the state and federal requirement that criminal background checks be performed on specified categories of prospective employees who will work with the very young or the elderly in institutions such as schools and nursing homes. Again, this is an attempt to protect the most vulnerable citizens from mistreatment or abuse. Failure to conduct the mandated background checks can result in the institution having to defend itself for any harm done by an employee with a past criminal conviction. One assisted-living facility was found negligent for failing to conduct a criminal background check or investigate complaints against an employee who later sexually abused a patient. The facility owner failed to exercise reasonable care when hiring a certified nurses' assistant with a criminal background (Rosenfeld, 2008).

The third area in which criminal law concerns affect nursing practice is the prohibition against substance abuse. Both federal and state laws require health care agencies to keep a strict accounting of the use and distribution of regulated drugs. Nurses routinely are expected to keep narcotic records accurate and current.

Nurses' behavior when off duty can also affect their employment status. Abusing alcohol or drugs on one's own time, if discovered, can result in nurses being terminated from employment and their license to practice nursing being restricted or revoked. Frequently, boards of nursing have programs for the nurse with a drug or alcohol problem, and completion of such a program may be required before the nurse can resume practice. Additionally, health care facilities may do random drug screens on their employees to identify those who may be using illegal substances.

Administrative Law

Both the federal government and state governments have administrative laws that affect nursing practice. The laws pertaining to Social Security and, more

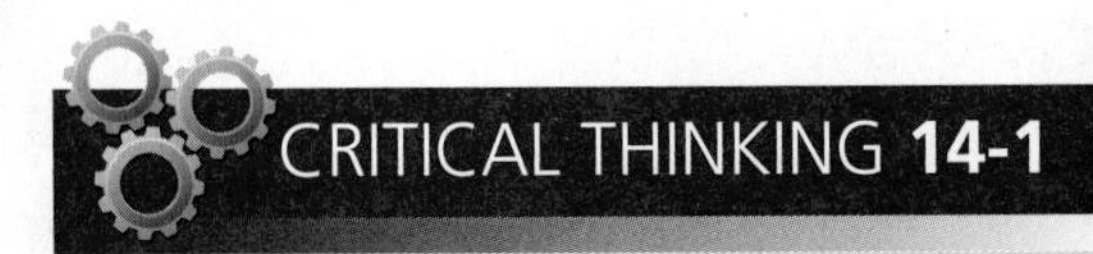

CRITICAL THINKING 14-1

You are a new nurse working on the OB unit of your local hospital. Your close friend also got a job on this unit. He has a reputation as a smart, likeable, and hard-working nurse, who also knows how to let loose and have a good time outside of work. However, recently your friend has been coming to work late and appears "out of it." You spoke with him and he told you that he was having a difficult time at home, and had not been as focused at work as he needed to be. Your friend promised that he would try to leave his personal life at home.

For a month after your discussion with your friend, everything seemed fine. However, in the past two weeks, you have noticed that he has had bloodshot eyes and his speech seems slurred at times. He looks unkempt and unclean, and the narcotic count for Vicodin was off for three separate shifts that he worked. You are concerned that your friend may be using drugs or alcohol and that it may be impacting patient safety and his nursing care.

What action do you take? Whom can you go to for help in this situation?

specifically, Medicare, are interpreted in the Code of Federal Regulations, which contains the administrative rules for the federal government. These rules have specific requirements that hospitals, nursing homes, and other health care providers must adhere to if they are to qualify for payment from federal funds. Likewise, state laws are interpreted in administrative rules that specify licensing requirements for health care providers in the state.

Federal Law: Administrative law deals with protection of the rights of citizens. It extends some rights and protections beyond those granted in the federal and state constitutions.

As with most federal laws, the agency responsible for implementing the law has a great deal of power to draft specific rules and regulations. For example, the Occupational Safety & Health Administration (OSHA), an administrative agency, works to establish a safe workplace for employees. This includes enacting regulations concerning storage of hazardous substances, protection of employees from infection, and protection of employees from violence in the workplace. Hospitals are subject to numerous OSHA regulations designed to protect the health and safety of nurses and other health care workers. From the minute new nurses join the hospital staff, they will come into contact with OSHA-mandated products or programs every day. For example, any unvaccinated nurse joining the staff of a hospital will be offered Hepatitis B vaccination pursuant to OSHA regulations. Additionally, nurses working with patients who may have tuberculosis will be issued special OSHA-approved particulate respirators to prevent them from becoming infected. Every day, nurses will utilize OSHA-mandated and approved sharps containers that hold used needles and personal protective equipment such as gloves, gowns, and surgical face masks. New nurses should review hospital policies and procedures to ensure they are using these safety devices properly. Another federal law that affects nursing practice is the Health Insurance Portability and Accountability Act (HIPAA), which was enacted to, among other things, safeguard certain private medical information (Martin, Cain, Priest & Hook, 2012). Under the law, disclosure of certain protected health information, such as a patient's medical diagnosis or plan of care, can result in criminal penalties. HIPAA is implicated anytime a patient's private medical information may be shared with another, whether intentionally or accidentally. Numerous provisions of HIPAA were expanded, clarified, and even strengthened by the American Recovery and Reinvestment Act of 2009 through Title XIII, named the Health Information Technology for Economic and Clinical Health (HITECH) Act, because of the use of informatics and potential for privacy invasion (Committees on Energy and Commerce, Ways and Means, and Science and Technology, 2009).

State Law: An example of a state's administrative law is its nurse practice act. Under nurse practice acts, state boards of nursing are given the authority to define the practice of nursing within certain broad parameters specified by the legislature, mandate the requisite preparation for the practice of nursing, and discipline members of the profession who deviate from the rules governing the practice of nursing. Other professions such as medicine and dentistry have similar practice acts established in state law.

Currently, an issue that is affecting licensure of nursing is the Multistate Licensure Compact, which affords mutual state recognition of nursing licenses.

Multistate Licensure Compact

An important issue to nurses is the transferability of their nursing license from one state to another. A license to practice nursing is generally valid only in the state where it is issued. In most cases, nurses wanting to practice in a state other than where their license was issued must apply for a license in that state. For nurses who frequently move from one state to another, this can be a burdensome process. There is an ongoing movement to allow nurses licensed in one state to automatically receive licensure to practice in another state. The Nurse Licensure Compact, a project of the National Council of State Boards of Nursing (NCSBN), is an agreement among states to allow nurses licensed in other states who are parties to the agreement to practice without applying for a new license (NCSBN, 2011). As of the date of this writing, only 25 states had joined this agreement, meaning that most states still require nurses to apply for a license in the state where they want to practice. You may check the Internet to determine if your state is a member of the compact by pointing your browser to http://www.ncsbn.org. Of course, nurses should always contact the board of nursing in any state where they intend to practice to determine eligibility and licensure requirements.

Civil Law

Civil law governs how individuals relate to each other in everyday matters. It encompasses both contract and tort law.

Contract Law

Contract law regulates certain transactions between individuals and/or legal entities such as businesses. It also governs transactions between businesses. An agreement between two or more parties must contain the following elements to be recognized as a legal contract:

- Agreement between two or more legally competent individuals or parties stating what each must or must not do
- Mutual understanding of the terms and obligations that the contract imposes on each party to the contract
- Payment or consideration given for actions taken or not taken pursuant to the agreement

The terms of the contract may be oral or written; however, a written contract may not be legally modified by an oral agreement. Another way this is often expressed is by the phrase "all of the terms of the contract are contained within the four corners of the document," that is, if it is not written, it is not part of the agreement or contract. A contract may be express or implied. In an express contract, the terms of the contract are specified, usually in writing. In an implied contract, a relationship between parties is recognized, although the terms of the agreement are not clearly defined, such as the expectations one has for services from the dry cleaner or the grocer.

The nurse is usually a party to an employment contract. The employed nurse agrees to do the following:

- Adhere to the policies and procedures of the employing entity
- Fulfill the agreed-upon duties of the employer
- Respect the rights and responsibilities of other health care providers in the workplace

In return, the employer agrees to provide the nurse with the following:

- A specified amount of pay for services rendered
- Adequate assistance in providing patient-centered care
- The supplies and equipment needed to fulfill the nurse's responsibilities

- A safe environment in which to work
- Reasonable treatment and behavior from the interprofessional health care team with whom the nurse must interact

This contract may be express or implied, depending on the practices of the employing entity. Sometimes, what is determined to be "reasonable" by the employer is not considered "reasonable" by the nurse. For instance, after 20 years of working as a nurse on the orthopedic unit, a nurse may not view it as reasonable to be pulled to the labor and delivery unit for duty as a nurse there. It would be prudent for this nurse to express any misgivings to the supervisor and then to cooperate but take only assignments that are in keeping with the responsibilities the nurse can safely complete. In this instance, it is reasonable to give nursing assistance on the labor and delivery unit that the nurse can competently deliver, although it may not be reasonable to assume total responsibility for these patients without additional education and experience.

Tort Law

A **tort** is a negligent or intentional civil wrong not arising out of a contract or statute that injures someone in some way, and for which the injured person may sue the wrongdoer for damages ('Lectric Law Library's Lexicon on Tort, 2011).

A tort can be any of the following:

- The denial of a person's legal right
- The failure to comply with a public duty
- The failure to perform a private duty that results in harm to another

A tort can be unintentional, as occurs in malpractice or neglect, or it can be the intentional infliction of harm, such as assault and battery. In a tort suit, the nurse can be named as a defendant because of something the nurse did incorrectly or because the nurse failed to do something that was required. In either case, the suit is usually classified as a tort suit. Other tort charges that a nurse may face include false imprisonment, invasion of privacy, defamation, and fraud. See Table 14-2.

TABLE 14-2
Selected Torts

Tort	Definition	Example
Assault	Threat to touch another person in an offensive manner without that person's permission.	Nurse who threatens to give a patient a treatment against his or her will.
Battery	Touching of another person without that person's consent.	Nurse who forces a treatment against a patient's will.
Invasion of privacy	All patients have the right to privacy and may bring charges against any person who violates this right.	Nurse who discloses confidential information about a patient or photographs a patient without consent.
False imprisonment	This occurs when individuals are physically prevented, or incorrectly led to believe they are prevented, from leaving a place.	Nurse who restrains a patient who is of sound mind and is not in danger of injuring self or others.
Defamation, including libel and slander	Intentionally false communication or publication, including written (libel) or verbal (slander) remarks that may cause damage to a person's reputation.	Nurse who makes a statement that could either ruin the patient's reputation or cause the patient to lose his job.

© Cengage Learning 2014

Negligence and Malpractice in Nursing

If a nurse fails to meet the legal expectations for care, usually defined by the state's nurse practice act, the patient, if harmed by this failure, can initiate an action against the nurse for damages. The term **malpractice** refers to a professional's wrongful conduct in the discharge of his or her professional duties, or failure to meet standards of care for the profession, which results in harm to another individual entrusted to the professional's care. **Negligence** is the failure to provide the care a reasonable person would ordinarily provide in a similar situation.

Simply proving malpractice or negligence is not sufficient to recover damages. Proof of liability or fault requires proof of the following four elements:

1. A duty or obligation created by law, contract, or standard practice that is owed to the complainant by the professional
2. A breach of this duty, either by omission or commission
3. Harm, which can be physical, emotional, or financial, to the complainant (patient)
4. Proof that the breach of duty caused the harm being complained of

A Louisiana appellate court described the plaintiff's (patient's) specific burden of proof in a negligence or malpractice case against a nurse as follows:

> [T]he three requirements which a plaintiff must satisfy to meet plaintiff's burden of proving the negligence of a nurse are (1) the nurse must exercise the degree of skill ordinarily employed, under similar circumstances, by the members of the nursing or health care profession in good standing in the same community or locality; (2) the nurse either lacked this degree of knowledge or skill or failed to use reasonable care and diligence, along with her best judgment in the application of that skill; and (3) as a proximate result of this lack of knowledge or skill or the failure to exercise this degree of care, the plaintiff suffered injuries that would not otherwise have occurred (Odom *v.* State Dept. of Health & Hospitals, 1999).

Once a plaintiff presents his or her case, the defendant nurse must refute the claims either by showing that, if a duty was owed, it was fulfilled, or by demonstrating that the breach of that duty was not the cause of the plaintiff's harm.

Proving that a duty was owed is not difficult. The person need only show that the nurse was working on the day in question and was responsible for the plaintiff's care. This can usually be accomplished by producing staffing schedules and assignment sheets.

To demonstrate a breach of duty, the courts employ a "reasonable man" standard by asking what a reasonable nurse would do in a like situation. This is accomplished by reviewing the employing institution's policies and procedures and the state's nursing and medical practice acts and hearing testimony from nurses who are accepted as expert witnesses to the standard of nursing practice in the community. Other sources that may be reviewed include evidence-based interprofessional health care research, nursing and medical literature, standards of professional associations such as the American Nurses Association Standards, equipment manufacturers' manuals, health care accreditation agency criteria, and/or medication books.

The defendant nurse would employ the same methodology to refute the plaintiff's charges. The nurse would present evidence that the institution's policies and procedures were followed and that the care rendered adhered to accepted nursing standards. To present the nurse's case, the nurse's attorney would also use expert witnesses to document that the care given fulfilled the duty owed, was the kind that would be given by a reasonable nurse in such a circumstance, and that it was not the cause of the plaintiff's harm.

It is not sufficient for patient plaintiffs to show a breach of duty to prevail in a tort suit. They must also show that the breach of the duty caused them harm. Even if it is proved that a nurse made an error, if the error was not the cause of the plaintiffs' harm, they will not win in recovering damages from the nurse. A recent case awarded $23.1 million in the case of a patient, a licensed practical nurse, who had to have both of her legs and a finger amputated because of an infection that went septic and gangrenous (Elliot-Engel, 2011). A registered nurse whose employer specified procedures for the insertion of catheters into the bloodstreams of patients, including watching out for and reporting redness at the site of catheters, failed to report catheter redness. After visiting the patient, the registered nurse planned to see the patient one week later. The patient called the agency two days later with shortness of breath, had to be airlifted, and was in septic shock. The pretrial memorandum stated, "Even though nurse Yurchak RN knew that infection can spread quickly and cause catastrophic injuries quickly, in violation of the standard of care, nurse Yurchak failed to report Ms. Smoyer's clinical presentation to any of her physicians or take any other steps to have Ms. Smoyer promptly evaluated for eight days." The patient, a licensed practical nurse (LPN), was not considered negligent in her own care because, even though she had trained as a nurse, the training of LPNs is not as high as the skilled nursing training that RNs go through (Elliot-Engel, 2011).

Note that "the role of the nurse in medical malpractice litigation has experienced a paradigm shift over the last several years. In the past, nurses were considered by many plaintiffs' lawyers and some judges to be mere 'functionaries' or 'custodians' who played a limited role in the care and treatment of patients." (CNA Financial Corporation, 2009, p. 35). "While nurse as custodian claims continue to be asserted, plaintiffs' lawyers have now begun to pursue claims that focus on the nurse as clinician, responsible for using professional judgment in the course of treatment." (p. 36)

> "The following are examples of the new paradigm of nursing claims:
>
> - Following a fall by a geriatric patient, the nurse is sued for failure to change the service plan despite increasing patient problems with gait and behavior.
> - A child is born with profound brain damage and the nurse is alleged to have failed to properly interpret fetal monitoring strips.
> - A lawsuit charges the nurse with failure to appreciate a patient's risk for skin breakdown and to take appropriate preventive measures.
> - After a patient experiences adverse drug reactions, the family alleges that the nurse failed to properly administer and provide the correct dosage.
> - A patient in the emergency department has a cardiac arrest, and a lawsuit is filed alleging that the triage nurse failed to appreciate acute cardiac symptomatology" (p. 36).

In the preceding cases, plantiffs were able to successfully prove a breach of duty, the breach was found to be the cause of the patient's injuries, and the nurse was found to be guilty of negligence. Table 14-3 reviews types of nursing actions that are common causes of malpractice. The clinical settings of these malpractice cases included hospitals (medical-surgical, maternity, emergency room, pediatrics, nursery, and recovery room units), nursing homes, home health care, clinics, and urgent care facilities. Table 14-4 identifies the most common and costly liabilities by location, allegation, and injury.

When a nurse is listed as a party in a medical malpractice lawsuit, the nurse's liability is reviewed. If state laws mandate that a nurse must have a nursing or medical practitioner's order before doing something, then that practitioner's order must be present. Problems arise when the orders are verbal, and later

TABLE 14-3
Nursing Malpractice Cases

Treatment
◆ Failure to timely treat symptoms/illness/disease in accordance with established standards/protocols/pathways
◆ Failure to timely implement established treatment protocols or established critical pathways
◆ Delay in implementing ordered, appropriate treatment
◆ Improper/untimely nursing technique or negligent performance of treatment resulting in injury
◆ Premature cessation of treatment

(Continues)

TABLE 14-3 (Continued)

Communication

- Failure to timely report complications of pregnancy, labor, or delivery to physician/licensed independent practitioner
- Failure to timely respond to patient's concerns related to the treatment plan
- Failure to timely notify physician/licensed independent practitioner of patient's condition and/or lack of response to treatment
- Failure to timely report complications of postoperative care to physician/licensed independent practitioner
- Failure to timely obtain physician/licensed independent practitioner orders to perform necessary additional treatment(s)

Medication

- Wrong route
- Wrong medication
- Wrong rate
- Infiltration of intravenous medication into tissue and/or sensory injury
- Wrong dose
- Medication not covered under state scope of practice
- Failure to immediately report and record the incorrect or improper administration of medication/prescription
- Wrong patient
- Wrong/delayed time of medication administration
- Missed dose

Monitoring/Observing/Supervising

- Abandonment of patient, including checking patient's status at appropriate intervals
- Improper/untimely nursing management of patient or medical complication
- Improper/untimely nursing management of preoperative, perioperative, or postoperative treatment or complication
- Improper/untimely application of restraints, or ordering or management of physical or chemical restraints, and/or failure to remove restraints at proper increments of time
- Improper/untimely nursing management of behavioral health/mental health patient or behavioral health complication
- Improper/untimely nursing management of patients in need of physical restraints, including 1:1 supervision, timed release of restraints, comfort breaks, fluids, and nourishment

© Cengage Learning 2014

it is claimed that the nurse misunderstood and acted in error. Another pitfall is illegible writing, which is then misinterpreted and the result causes harm to the patient. Many nurses who have been in practice for a long time have encountered practitioners who write orders that are contrary to accepted practice. In these situations, the nurse must exercise professional judgment and follow the policies and procedures of the institution. Usually these require the nurse to notify the nursing supervisor and the medical director for the area where the nurse works. Illegible writing and incorrect orders are being minimized, even eliminated, with the use of the electronic health record and computerized order-entry systems. The institution's policies and procedures describe the performance expected of nurses in its employ, and a nurse deviating from them can be liable for negligence or malpractice. Failure to adhere to institutional protocol can result in the employer denying the nurse a defense in a lawsuit.

Practicing nurses must also adhere to the standards of practice for the nursing profession in the community. These standards include such things as checking the "rights" in medication administration or repositioning the patient at regular intervals. It is not uncommon for nurses to encounter conflicts between an employer's expectations and the nursing standards of care, resulting in problems such as having insufficient time or staffing to adhere to the standards taught in nursing school, or receiving poor evaluations for taking too long to render care. In all situations, nurses must prioritize and evaluate what standards they must follow to preserve their professional practice, protect patients, and protect themselves from liability.

TABLE 14-4
The Most Common and Costly Liabilities by Location, Allegation, and Injury

The Most Common and Costly Liabilities
Location
◆ Hospital—inpatient
◆ Prison
◆ Aging services long-term care facility
◆ Hospital—emergency department
◆ Patient's home
◆ Hospital—inpatient perinatal services
Allegation
◆ Treatment and care management
◆ Assessment
◆ Medication administration
◆ Abuse/patient's rights/professional misconduct
◆ Monitoring
Injury
◆ Death
◆ Infection/abscess/sepsis
◆ Fracture
◆ Birth-related brain damage
◆ Brain damage other than birth-related
◆ Pain and suffering

Source: CNA healthpro nurse claims study: An analysis of claims with risk management recommendations 1997-2007. CNA Financial Corporation.

Assault and Battery

Assault is a threat to touch another in an offensive manner without that person's permission. **Battery** is the touching of another person without that person's consent. In the health care arena, lawsuits of this nature usually question whether the individual consented to the treatment administered by the health care professional. Most states have laws that require patients to make informed decisions about their treatment.

Informed consent laws protect the patient's right to practice self-determination. The patient has the right to receive sufficient information to make an informed decision about whether to consent to or refuse a procedure. The individual performing the procedure is responsible for explaining to the patient the nature of the procedure, benefits, alternatives, and the risks and potential complications. The signed consent form is used to document that this was done, and it creates a presumption that the patient had been advised of the appropriate risks.

Often the nurse is asked to witness a patient signing a consent form for treatment. When you witness a patient's signature, you are vouching for two things: that the patient signed the paper and that the patient knows that they are signing a consent form. For a consent form to be legal, a patient, in most states, must: be at least 18 years old; be mentally competent; have the procedures, with their risks and benefits, explained in a manner the patient can understand; be aware of the available alternatives to the proposed treatment; and consent voluntarily. The nurse must also be familiar with who is allowed by state law to consent to medical treatment for another when that person cannot personally consent. Frequently, these include the person possessing medical power of attorney, a spouse, adult children, or other relatives if no one is available in one of the other categories listed.

A nurse may also face a charge of battery for failing to honor an advance directive, such as a medical power of attorney, durable power of attorney, or living will.

Federal law requires that a hospital ask upon admission whether the patient has a living will; if the answer is negative, the hospital must ask whether the patient would like to enact one. A **living will** is a written advance directive voluntarily signed by the patient that specifies the type of care desired if and when the patient is in a terminal state and cannot sign a consent form or convey this information verbally. It can be a general statement, such as "no life-sustaining measures," or specific, such as "no tube feedings or respirator." Often, the patient's family has difficulty allowing health care personnel to follow the wishes expressed in a living will, and conflicts arise. These should be communicated to the hospital ethics committee, pastoral care department, risk management, or whichever hospital department is responsible for handling such issues. If the patient verbalizes wishes regarding end-of-life care to the family, such difficult situations can sometimes be avoided, and the patient should be encouraged to do this, if possible.

Invasion of Privacy and Confidentiality

The nurse is required to respect the privacy of all patients. As a health care practitioner, the nurse may be privy to very personal information and must make every effort to keep it confidential. Only authorized individuals can access patient information, although patients have the right to access their own records. This is particularly important with computers on wheels where nurses document on patient care by logging in under their username. If another member of the interprofessional team accesses another patient's information under the nurse's login, the nurse can be held accountable for a breach in confidentiality. Only by obtaining the patient's permission can information be given to others. It is often necessary to monitor conversations with coworkers that have the potential of being overheard by others so that no patient information is accidentally revealed. Sometimes the protection of a patient's privacy conflicts with the state's mandatory reporting laws for the occurrence of specified infectious diseases such as syphilis or human immunodeficiency virus (HIV). The need to protect an individual's privacy may also conflict with the state's mandatory reporting laws on suspected patient abuse, discussed previously. Other information that state or federal law may require to be revealed include a patient's blood alcohol level, incidences of rape, gunshot wounds, and adverse reactions to certain drugs.

Failing to strictly follow reporting laws could lead to: criminal, civil, or disciplinary action; termination of employment; or all of these. Nurses must consult the institution's policies and confer with its risk management department to ascertain their responsibilities and course of action. The ANA Code of Ethics for Nurses states that nurses must protect the patient and the public when incompetence or unethical or illegal practice compromise health care and safety (2001). Many states have adopted this concept in their nurse practice acts, thereby creating a legal obligation to report. If nurses observe unethical behavior in a hospital, they should report this as directed in the institution's policies and procedures manual or by the laws of the state.

Defamation

Defamation is defined as false or unjustified injury of the good reputation of another, as by slander or libel (Dictionary.com, 2011). "Slander" is the term for verbal communication. "Libel" is the term for false written communication.

Two essential elements must be proved in a charge of defamation:

1. The information conveyed must be untrue.
2. The false information must be published or communicated to another party.

Note that publication or communication may mean simply telling one other person or writing a friend a letter containing the false information. The nurse may face such an accusation if the nurse communicates inaccurate information to another or if it is claimed that the information charted was untrue. However, several courts have ruled that charting information in a medical record, whether accurate or not, does not constitute publication as required for a charge of defamation.

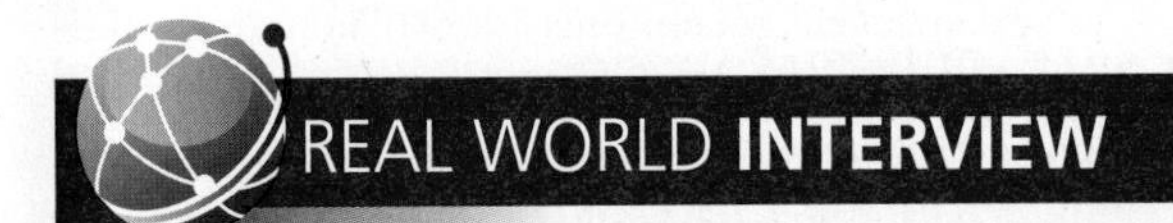

Nursing practice in today's health care environment is multifaceted and complex. Our patients and our communities expect quality care from nurses at all levels of practice. Responsibility to keep abreast of current practices is an integral component of a nurse's licensure requirements. Nursing professionals must understand their scope of practice and the legal requirements necessary to maintain their license in good standing. As a former member of a state board of nursing, I can assure you that this is important for all nurses, novice or experienced.

Increased emphasis is being placed on patient safety through regulatory agencies, the Joint Commission, and other national initiatives. Commitments to reducing medication errors and surgical infections and improving patient outcomes are just a couple of the ongoing issues that have become fundamental components of nursing practice.

As a sustained focus is placed on improvement of care and patient safety, evidence-based practice must be integrated into the daily practice patterns of patient-centered care. Proven methods and research-based policies and procedures need to dictate how patient care is administered, rather than "this is how we have always done it." Failure to adhere to best practices within your scope of practice can result in negative patient outcomes, safety breaches, and ultimately lead to licensure problems or legal action.

Above all, staying current in skills, knowledge, and education helps nurses to meet the practice standards that are expected in today's health care environment.

MARSHA KING, RN, MS, MBA, CNAA
Chief Nursing Officer
St. Joseph Regional Medical Center
South Bend/Mishawaka Campuses

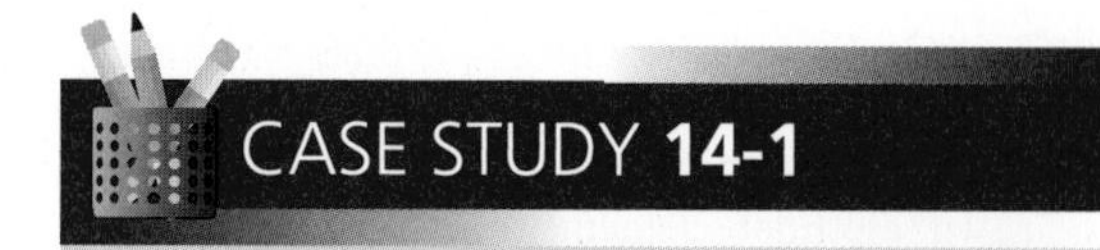

CASE STUDY 14-1

You are working the night shift. One of your patient's practitioners has prescribed a dose of a medication to be given that you know is too high for this patient. You are unable to locate the practitioner to check the order. What would you do to ensure safe care for your patient?

Following Orders, Including "Do Not Attempt Resuscitation" (DNAR)

The attending medical practitioner may write a "do not attempt resuscitation" (DNAR) order on an inpatient, which directs the staff not to perform the usual cardiopulmonary resuscitation (CPR) in the event of a sudden cardiopulmonary arrest. The practitioner may write such an order without evidence of a living will on the medical record, and the nurse should be familiar with the organization's policies and state law regarding when and how a practitioner can write such an order in the absence of a living will. Often, a DNAR order is considered a medical decision that the doctor can make, preferably in consultation with the family, even without a living will executed by the patient.

If the nurse feels that a DNAR order or any order is contrary to the patient's good, the nurse should consult the policies and procedures of the institution. These may include going up the chain of command until the nurse is satisfied with the course of action. This may entail notifying the nursing supervisor, the medical director, the institution's chief operating officer, the risk manager, the state regulators, and/or the accreditation agency (e.g., the Joint Commission). Organizations have an ethics committee that examines such issues and makes a determination of the appropriateness of the order. Because of the opportunity for misunderstanding, verbal orders are not encouraged and the use of electronic order entry is encouraged. When a nurse has a problem with a practitioner's order, it is often prudent to discuss it first with the practitioner involved before reporting the problem up the chain of command. Often problems can be resolved at this first step. However, if the problem is not resolved by discussing it with the practitioner, the nurse should report the problem to her supervisor and follow the state law and the agency's policies.

False Imprisonment

False imprisonment occurs when individuals are incorrectly led to believe they cannot leave a place. A claim of false imprisonment may be based on the inappropriate use of physical or chemical restraints. Federal law mandates that health care institutions employ the least restrictive method of ensuring patient safety. Physical or chemical restraints are to be used only if necessary to protect the patient from harm when all other methods have failed. If the nurse uses restraints on a competent person who is refusing to follow the practitioner's orders, the nurse can be charged with false imprisonment or battery. If restraints are used in an emergency situation, the nurse is to contact the practitioner immediately after application to secure an order for the restraints. Also, the nurse must check the institution's policies regarding the type and frequency of assessments required for a patient in restraints and how often it is necessary to secure a reorder for the restraints. These policies ensure the patient's safety and must be consistent with state law.

A charge of false imprisonment may occur because the nurse misinterprets the rights granted to others by legal documents such as powers of attorney and does not allow a patient to leave a facility because the person with the power of attorney (agent) says the patient cannot leave. A **power of attorney** is a legal document executed by an individual (principal) granting another person (agent) the right to perform certain activities in the principal's name. It can be specific, such as "sell my house," or general, such as "make all decisions for me, including health care decisions." In most states, a power of attorney is voluntarily granted by the individual and does not take away his right to exercise his own choices. Thus, if the principal (patient) disagrees with his agent's decisions, the patient's wishes are the ones that prevail.

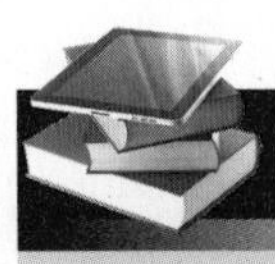

EVIDENCE FROM THE **LITERATURE**

Citation: Reising, D. L., & Allen, P. N. (2007). Protecting yourself from malpractice claims: Greater nursing autonomy comes at the price of increased legal exposure. *American Nurse Today, 2*(2), 39–43.

Discussion: This article provides a wealth of practical information on how to reduce your risk of being sued for malpractice and what to do if you are named in a malpractice lawsuit. The article defines the elements of a malpractice suit, which are based on the traditional four-factor test for negligence. According to the article, the most common malpractice claims against nurses are for failure to follow standards of care, failure to use equipment in a responsible manner, failure to communicate, failure to document, failure to assess and monitor, and failure to act as a patient advocate. The article suggests that nurses take a proactive approach, including performing only those skills that are within your practice scope, staying current in your field or specialty area, knowing your strengths and weaknesses, documenting all patient care activities and communications, and knowing how to invoke the chain of command in your facility.

Implications for Practice: The expansion of the nurse's responsibilities, along with the public recognition that a nurse's role has evolved from a custodian to a full member of the clinical treatment team, means that a nurse is more likely to be faced with a lawsuit for malpractice.

PROTECTIONS IN NURSING PRACTICE

As discussed earlier in this chapter, nursing practice is guided by states' nurse practice acts and agency policies and procedures. Other resources for the nurse include Good Samaritan laws, useful health records, risk management, and professional liability insurance.

Good Samaritan Laws

Good Samaritan laws are laws that have been enacted to protect the health care professional from legal liability. The essential elements of commonly enacted Good Samaritan laws are as follows:

- The care is rendered in an emergency situation.
- The health care worker is rendering care without pay.
- The care provided did not recklessly or intentionally cause injury or harm to the injured party.

Note that these laws are intended to protect the volunteer who stops to render care at the scene of an accident. They would not protect a nurse, an emergency medical technician (EMT), or other health care professional rendering care at the scene of an accident as part of their assigned duties and for which they receive pay. In doing their duties, paid emergency personnel are evaluated according to the standards of their professions (Martin et al., 2012).

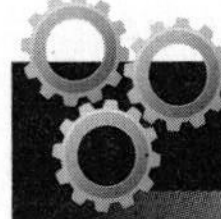

CRITICAL THINKING **14-2**

A physician writes a DNAR order for a patient with end-stage lung cancer. You carry out the order and put a DNAR bracelet on the patient. The patient's son visits and comes to the nursing station. He asks you, "What does the new bracelet mean?" You explain the meaning of "do not attempt resuscitation." The son becomes visibly upset and states, "No one talked to me about this; don't I have any say so on my own parent's life?" What will you do? Whom will you contact? What will you do if the patient has a cardiopulmonary arrest right now?

Useful Health Records

The nurse must communicate accurately and completely, verbally, in writing, and electronically. Often a case involving patient care takes several years to come to trial; by that time, the nurse may have no memory of the incident in question and must rely on the record done at the time of the incident. This record is frequently in the courtroom, blown up to billboard size for all to see. All errors are apparent and omissions stand out by their absence, especially if it is data that should have been recorded per organizational policy. The old adage that "if it isn't written, it wasn't done" will be repeated to the jury numerous times.

Documentation

Professional responsibility and accountability are two primary reasons that nurses document. Other reasons to document include communication, education, research, meeting legal and practice standards, and reimbursement. Documentation is the professional responsibility of all health care practitioners. Thorough documentation provides:

- accurate data needed to plan the patient's care in order to ensure the continuity of care;
- a method of communication among the health care team members responsible for the patient's care;
- written evidence of what was done for the patient, the patient's response, and any revisions made in the plan of care;
- evidence of compliance with professional practice standards, e.g., American Nurses Association Standards;
- compliance with accreditation criteria, e.g., Joint Commission (JC), Healthcare Facilities Accreditation Program (HFAP);
- a resource for review, quality improvement, reimbursement, education, and research;
- a documented legal record to protect the patient, organization, and nursing and medical practitioners.

For protection when charting, the nurse should use the CLEAR (contemporaneous, logical, explicit, accurate, and readable) acronym (Miller, 2011).

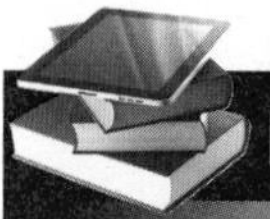

EVIDENCE FROM THE **LITERATURE**

Citation: Jha, A. K., Doolan, D., Grandt, D., Scott, T., & Bates, D. W. (2008). The use of health information technology in seven nations. *International Journal of Medical Informatics, 77*(12)–262.

Discussion: The authors assessed the state of health information technology (HIT) adoption and use in seven industrialized nations. They used a combination of literature review and interviews with experts in individual nations to determine the use of key information technologies. They examined the rate of electronic health record (EHR) use in ambulatory care and some hospital settings, along with current activities in health information exchange (HIE) in seven countries: the United States, Canada, United Kingdom, Germany, the Netherlands, Australia, and New Zealand. Four nations (United Kingdom, the Netherlands, Australia, and New Zealand) had nearly universal use of EHRs among general practitioners (each >90%) and Germany also exhibited widespread use (40–80%). The United States and Canada had a minority of ambulatory care physicians who used EHRs consistently (10–30%). Although there are no high-quality data for the hospital setting from any of the nations the authors examined, evidence suggests that only a small fraction of hospitals (<10%) in any single country had the key components of an EHR. HIE efforts were a high priority in all seven nations, but early efforts have demonstrated varying degrees of active clinical data exchange.

Implications for Practice: Increased efforts will be needed if interoperable EHRs are soon to become universally available and used in these seven nations. Nurses and other practitioners in these nations must be part of the solution to making the EHR universally used and available.

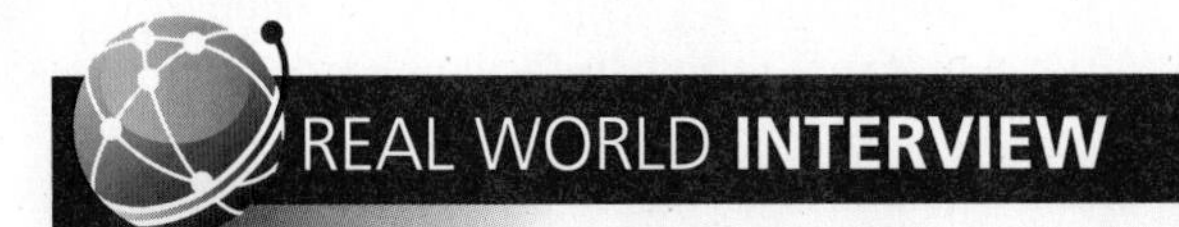

Most nurses are familiar with the phrase, "If it was not documented, it was not done." Insofar as this phrase is used to encourage thorough documentation, it reflects good nursing practice. Timely, accurate, and complete documentation is an excellent way to protect oneself from litigation. However, lawyers who represent plaintiffs in medical malpractice cases are aware of this "rule" and often attempt to use it against nurses in health care liability claims.

Imagine the following scenario: A patient is admitted to the hospital, and Nurse A performs an initial assessment of the patient. Nurse A notes in the patient's chart that the patient has good capillary refill. Nurse A proceeds to take the patient's vital signs, including capillary refill, hourly throughout Nurse A's eight-hour shift. The patient's capillary refill remains reassuring and the nurse makes no further documentation in the chart relating to the patient's capillary refill. After Nurse A's shift, Nurse B takes over the patient's care. One hour into Nurse B's shift, the patient codes and expires. The patient's family sues Nurse A. The plaintiffs' lawyer is cross-examining Nurse A.

Lawyer: "Nurse A, are you familiar with the phrase, 'If it wasn't charted, it wasn't done'?"

Nurse A: "Yes."

Lawyer: "That's a common rule in nursing practice, isn't it?"

Nurse A: "Yes."

Lawyer: "You were taught that in nursing school, weren't you?"

Nurse A: "Yes, I was."

Lawyer: "And after you documented that the patient had good capillary refill upon admission, you did not document anything relating to the patient's capillary refill for the next eight hours, did you?"

Nurse A: "Well, no."

Lawyer: "So if we use the rule, 'If it wasn't documented, it wasn't done,' we can assume you never checked the patient's capillary refills during your shift after the initial assessment, right?"

Nurse A: "No. I checked, but it hadn't changed, so I didn't chart anything."

Do you see what just happened? Nurse A provided competent nursing care, but the lawyer made it appear as if Nurse A was negligent. A nurse involved in litigation should not blindly agree with this documentation rule. The rule ignores the concept of charting by exception. You simply cannot document everything noted in an assessment of a patient. Moreover, most nurses would agree that patient care takes priority over charting. This rule ignores that. Bad charting looks bad. Good charting protects you. However, charting by exception does not correlate with providing bad nursing care. Even lapses in charting do not correlate with bad nursing care. Nurses should not lose sight of that when faced with litigation.

ROBYN D. POZZA-DOLLAR, JD
Austin, Texas

Electronic Health Records

Most hospitals have adopted electronic health records (EHR). The EHR uses informatics to eliminate paper-record storage, improve access to patient records, control legibility, and facilitate timely capture of data. The EHR can also be used to gather data about patient care and outcomes, staff activities, and other data for clinical, administrative, and financial decision making.

By 2015, use of a certified EHR is mandated under the Health Information Technology for

Economic and Clinical Health (HITECH) Act (CMS, 2010). HITECH created new Medicare and Medicaid incentive payment programs totaling as much as $27 billion to help eligible physicians, other professionals, and hospitals as they transition from paper-based medical records to EHRs. The Veterans Affairs Department is currently using Veterans Health Information Systems and Technology Architecture (VistA) supporting more than 150 hospitals and 887 ambulatory care facilities (Lipowicz, 2011). VistA is considered a world-class EHR system, yet the Veterans Affairs Department is currently in the process to update and modernize the system.

The Healthcare Information and Management Systems Society (HIMSS, 2008) published information about the use of EHRs in Germany, the Netherlands, Greece, England, Wales, Denmark, Norway, India, New Zealand and Malaysia, Hong Kong, Singapore, Israel, Canada, and the United States. It appears that all countries are aware of the importance to move to EHRs and the potential of global EHR integration. Problems that arise include the differences in each country's health care system, the national EHR status, the approach, the type of government, and the technology resources (HIMSS, 2008). Some countries, like Canada, are clearly ahead of the United States. Approximately 50 percent of Canadians have EHRs available to authorized professionals who provide care, while other countries, such as India, though technically savvy, do not have a mandatory, comprehensive EHR plan in place yet.

Risk-Management Programs

Risk-management programs in health care organizations are designed to identify and correct system problems that contribute to errors in patient care or to employee injury. The emphasis in risk management is on quality improvement and protection of the institution from financial liability. Institutions usually have reporting and tracking forms for recording incidents that may lead to financial liability for the institution. Risk management will assist in identifying and correcting the underlying problem that may have led to an incident, such as faulty equipment, staffing concerns, or the need for better orientation for employees. After a system problem is identified, the risk-management department may develop educational programs to address the problem.

The risk-management department may also investigate and record information surrounding a patient or employee incident that may result in a lawsuit. This helps personnel remember critical factors if called to testify at a later time. The nurse should notify the risk-management department of all reportable incidents and complete all risk-management and/or incident report forms as mandated by institutional policies and procedures. Note also that employee complaints of harassment or discrimination can expose the institution to significant liability and should promptly be reported to supervisors and the risk-management department, human resources, or whichever department is specified in the institution's policies. See Table 14-5 for a checklist of actions to decrease the risk of nursing liability.

Professional Liability Insurance

Nurses may need to carry their own liability insurance. Nurses often think their actions are adequately covered by the employer's liability insurance, but this is not necessarily so. Although the hospital's insurance company almost always pays malpractice awards, insurance contracts often have provisions that allow them to refuse repayment if the insured intentionally injures another party. Also, if in giving care, the nurse fails to comply with the institution's policies and procedures, the institution may deny the nurse a defense, claiming that because of the nurse's failure to follow institutional policy, or because of the nurse working

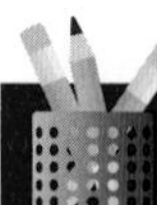

CASE STUDY **14-2**

A patient is admitted from the emergency department after a minor motor vehicle accident. The blood alcohol level is four times the legal limit and the patient is very combative. The physician prescribes soft wrist restraints. Once you apply the restraints, the patient starts screaming, "I'm going to sue you; you can't tie me up!" Is the patient right? What should you do? Whom will you contact?

TABLE 14-5
Nursing Checklist of Actions to Decrease Liability

- Delegate patient care based on patients' needs, staff competency and skill, and the documented education, skill, and experience of licensed and unlicensed personnel. Monitor the outcomes.
- Develop a professional, assertive communication style with nursing and medical practitioners to assist you with meeting patient care goals. Use SBARR as a guide.
- Communicate with your patients and keep them informed. Treat them with kindness and respect.
- Acknowledge unfortunate incidents and express concern about these events without either taking the blame, blaming others, or reacting defensively.
- Avoid taking telephone and verbal orders. If necessary to maintain patient safety, however, repeat the order back to the practitioner to assure clarity. Document that you did this, for example, telephone order repeated back (TORB) or verbal order repeated back (VORB).
- Follow professional standards for education, licensure, and competency in all hiring and promotion decisions, orientation, and ongoing continuing-education programs.
- Provide access to professional evidence-based health care standards, policies, procedures, library, and medication information with unit availability and efficient Internet access.
- Have clear policies and procedures for delegation, supervision, and chain-of-command reporting lines for all staff from RN to charge nurse to nurse manager to nurse executive and, as appropriate, to risk management, the hospital ethics committee, the hospital administrator, medical practitioners, the chief of the medical staff, the board of directors, the State Licensing Board for Nursing and Medicine, and the accreditation agency, (e.g., the JC).
- Note that the RN always has an independent responsibility to protect patient safety. Blindly relying on another nursing or medical practitioner is not permissible for the RN.
- Provide standards for regular RN evaluation of NAP and LPN/LVN and reinforce the need for NAP and LPN/LVN accountability to the RN. RNs must delegate and supervise. They cannot abdicate this professional responsibility.
- Develop physical, mental, and verbal "No Abuse" policies to be followed by all professional and nonprofessional health care staff.
- Consider applying for Magnet status for your facility. This status is awarded by the American Nurses Credentialing Center to hospitals that have worked to improve nursing care, including the empowering of nursing delegation and nursing decision making.
- Develop EHRs and monitor patient outcomes, including nurse-sensitive outcomes, staffing ratios, and other clinical, financial, and organizational quality indicators. Develop ongoing clinical quality improvement practices.
- Maintain ongoing monitoring of incident reports, medication errors, equipment maintenance, patient, family, and staff complaints, sentinel events, and other elements of risk management and quality improvement of the process and outcome of patient-centered care.
- Attain Joint Commission Patient Safety Goals, 2011.
- Monitor Medicare's "Do Not Pay" list; for example, note that Medicare will not pay for transfusions gone wrong due to human error.

© Cengage Learning 2014

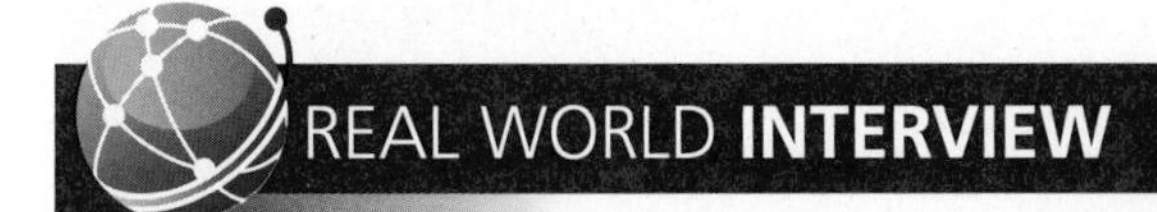

Patient safety and risk management are synonymous terms. Health care delivery processes are inherently complex, high risk, and problem prone. In order to create an environment that promotes safety and optimal patient outcomes, basic nursing and patient care processes and procedures must be properly designed. Well-designed nursing care processes possess the following characteristics:

- Staff-level nursing policies and procedures should be designed with input and participation by those closest to the process—that is, staff level nurses.
- Nursing care policies, processes, and procedures should be simple, practical, and written in universally understandable terms.

During a shadowing experience, I was once asked by a BSN student, "What can bedside nurses do to protect themselves and the organization from liability?" My answer was multifaceted. The single most important risk-management tool is well-documented nursing care. It is a challenge in today's nursing environment to ensure that an accurate record is made that includes all of the details of a patient's care. Many hospitals utilize "charting by exception," which is designed for efficiency and to capture the essence of nursing care delivery under "normal" circumstances without variation. However, in-depth narrative must be documented, with changes in patient condition or care needs, along with the patient response to our interventions.

The medical record is the only document we will have several years out if a patient care incident results in litigation. For this reason, it must tell a vivid story in complete detail about what the patient looked like, smelled like, felt like, and sounded like at accurate points in time during our care, as well as everything we did for the patient and how the patient responded to what we did. It is the nurse's responsibility to supplement any standard form to provide this type of information.

Communication between nurses, physicians, and other health care team members is another critical element of safe patient care and effective risk management. Patient safety and risk management are every individual's responsibility, and everyone has a role to play.

TAMARA L. AWALD, RN, BSN, MS, HSA
Vice President of Patient Care Services
St. Joseph Regional Medical Center
Plymouth, Indiana

outside the scope of nursing employment, the nurse was not acting as an employee at that time. Also, nurses are being named individually as defendants in malpractice suits more frequently than in the past. In some cases, nurses will be the first to pay in lawsuits. In a case where parents filed a lawsuit against the hospital where their baby was born with cerebral palsy, allegedly caused by the negligence of the physician and the labor and delivery nurses who were present for the mother's labor, the insurance companies for the hospital and for one of the nurses agreed to pay the parents a settlement of $900,000, then went back to court to argue how exactly that sum would be paid out.

The U.S. District Court for the District of New Jersey ruled the hospital's insurance had a valid $100,000 self-insured retention, and the nurse's own insurance policy was intended to pay and would contribute that amount on her behalf (General Hospital of Passaic *v.* American Casualty Company, 2007).

It is advantageous for nurses to be assured of a defense independent of that of their employer. Professional liability insurance provides that assurance and pays for an attorney to defend nurses in a malpractice lawsuit. When purchasing malpractice insurance, nurses should clarify whether the insurance covers liability just as long as the premiums are being paid or if the insurance covers a prescribed time period.

Note that in the event that unaffiliated nurses (e.g., agency per diem nurses) are held individually liable for a judgment, their personal insurance carrier will be responsible for paying the verdict rendered against them. Unaffiliated, uninsured nurses could be forced to pay for their own defense and be financially responsible for any judgments rendered against them.

In making the decision of whether to obtain separate insurance, nurses should consider the value of their personal assets. Nurses should also consider the laws of the state where they practice regarding those assets that are exempt from being seized to satisfy civil monetary judgments. Generally, one home and one automobile are exempt from seizure.

Nurses Involved in Litigation

Nurses may be sued individually for damages resulting from their negligent acts. However, a plaintiff will often name the nurse's employer as a defendant instead of or in addition to suing the nurse individually. It is a well-established law throughout the United States that "a master is subject to liability for the torts of his servants committed while acting in the scope of employment" (American Law Institute, 1958). This law is called *Respondeat Superior*. In other words, a hospital, nursing home, clinic, and so on is legally responsible for the damages caused by the negligence of its nurses.

Customarily, plaintiffs in medical malpractice cases name a combination of health care providers as defendants. It is common for some or all of the defendants to settle the cases before they reach the trial phase. However, in the event that a case proceeds to trial, a jury may find that none, some, or all of the defendants were negligent in their care and treatment of the plaintiff. A jury may determine that the nursing care was appropriate, but that the medical treatment was substandard. Likewise, a jury could hold that the medical practitioner rendered appropriate care but that the nurses' conduct fell below the standard of care. The new paradigm in legal matters makes nurses more accountable for independent thinking and judgment. The CNA Financial Corporation (2009) gives the following example of the recent claims against nurses: A child is born with profound brain damage, and the nurse is alleged to have failed to properly

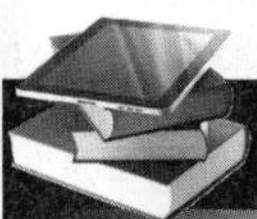

EVIDENCE FROM THE **LITERATURE**

Citation: Campos, N. K. (2010). The legalities of nursing documentation. *Men in Nursing, (40)*1, 7–9.

Discussion: The author discusses the duties associated with nursing practice and documentation set forth by governing bodies such as state and federal laws and institutional policies. Nurses need to understand the state practice act of the state in which they are practicing to ensure their documentation meets these standards. The purpose of documentation is to provide a clear and accurate picture of the patient while under the care of the nurse and the rest of the health care team. To provide this clear and accurate picture, the nurse must be aware of the state's practice act, the policy and procedure of the institution, and specialty organization standards (e.g., the American Association of Critical-Care Nurses). When providing and documenting care, always keep in mind: What would a reasonable and prudent nurse have done in the same situation? To avoid legal pitfalls, the nurse should keep in mind the audience who would be reading the documentation—lawyers, judges, juries, and other members of the health care team. The nurse should document to assist remembering a situation. Considering that most legal cases take years to go to court, nurses will have to rely on their charting to refresh their memories on what happened with patients and the surrounding circumstances.

Implications for Practice: Charting in the electronic format does not change requirements of providing a clear and accurate picture of the patient while under the care of the nurse. Always document on abnormal findings and responses to interventions, and do not become complacent with check-box systems.

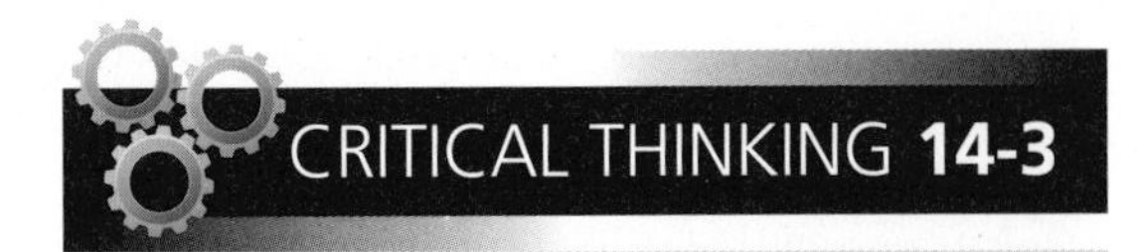

You are assigned to a medical-surgical unit, working the night shift. Your supervisor calls and says that one of the RNs assigned to the critical care unit has called in sick and you must work that unit instead of your usual assignment. You have never worked in the critical care setting before and have received no orientation to this unit. You are now asked to work there when it is short of staff.

What should you do?

interpret fetal monitoring strips. This shift in nurse accountability has afforded increasing opportunities for plaintiffs' attorneys to name nurses as defendants in medical malpractice cases.

Common Monetary Awards

Many malpractice cases are dismissed or settled prior to trial. In those cases that do reach the trial stage, jury verdicts are unpredictable and awards can vary dramatically. Cady (2011) reports these monetary awards:

- $150,000 for medical errors leading to two patients' deaths
- $125,000 for leaving a malleable retractor in a patient's abdomen during surgery
- $25,000 for an overdose of intravenous medication causing a patient's death
- $6.2 million for a nurse practitioner failing to diagnose a child with cancer

A jury may award the plaintiff both compensatory and punitive damages. Compensatory damages are awarded to compensate the plaintiff for injuries. Compensatory damages include damages for both economic losses (medical expenses, lost wages, lost earning capacity) and noneconomic losses (pain and suffering). Punitive damages are not intended to compensate the plaintiff for any loss. Rather, punitive damages are intended to punish the defendant for acting with "recklessness, malice, or deceit" (*Black's Law Dictionary*, 2005). Punitive damage awards are particularly common in cases involving nursing homes. For example, a Texas jury awarded the family of a nursing-home resident $90 million in punitive damages for gross negligence that caused the resident to develop pressure ulcers and contractures (Horizon/CMS Healthcare Corp. *v.* Auld, 2000; Pozza, 2003).

Monetary Liability Limits in Some States

Since 1970, at least 30 states have enacted legislation capping the damages plaintiffs can recover in a lawsuit (Babcock & Pogarsky, 1999). Currently, there exist as many different cap schemes as states that employ them (Pozza, 2003).

A plaintiff may claim that he or she is entitled to damages in excess of the applicable cap. Jurors are customarily not informed of the caps applicable in their states. Therefore, it is common for a jury's award to exceed the state's cap on damages. In the event that a jury awards a plaintiff damages in excess of a statutory cap, the judge will reduce the jury's award to the cap (Pozza, 2003).

Other Legal Risks for the Nurse, Doctor, or Hospital

Other than increased insurance premiums, health care providers have plenty at stake when named as defendants in medical malpractice cases. Medical practitioners are required to report adverse verdicts and settlements to the National Practitioner Data Bank. The National Practitioner Data Bank was established through the Health Care Quality Improvement Act of 1986. The federal regulations regarding the data

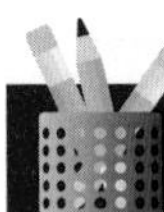

CASE STUDY 14-3

While working as a nurse in a medical-surgical unit, you get a phone call from the medical-legal department of the hospital. They tell you a patient whom you cared for six months ago is suing the hospital for a pressure ulcer that developed during the hospital stay. You are named in the suit and have no memory of the patient.

What will you do? How do you prepare yourself? Are you covered legally?

bank can be found in 45 CFR Part 60 (National Practitioner Data Bank, 2011). Significant awards against a practitioner or numerous malpractice payments by a practitioner can affect the practitioner's licensure or ability to gain privileges to practice at certain hospitals and health care entities. Failure to report malpractice payments to the data bank can result in civil monetary penalties. The U.S. Department of Health and Human Services, Office of the Inspector General, may impose a civil money penalty of up to $11,000 for each violation.

Federal and state statutes and regulations prescribe nursing standards of care. See the Code of Federal Regulations, Title 42—Public Health and Title 45—Public Welfare. Every jurisdiction that licenses nurses has a nurse practice act. In addition to instructing nurses on the definition of the standard of care for that jurisdiction, the nurse practice act mandates strict rules for reporting and disciplining nurses who violate the standard. Likewise, state boards of nursing and administrative agencies may take action to suspend or revoke the licenses of nurses who they determine have violated the standard of care. Private entities, such as the Joint Commission, and nursing organizations, such as the American Nurses Association, promulgate their own rules of conduct that serve as guidelines for acceptable nursing care. National and international evidence-based practice guidelines for nursing care and practice are the highest standards of care because of the thorough and rigorous process in which they are created.

Nurse/Attorney Relationship

Despite the nurse's best intentions, a nurse may be named as a defendant in a lawsuit and need to retain the services of an attorney. LaDuke (2000) made the following suggestions for consulting and collaborating with an attorney:

1. Retain a specialist. Generalists are competent to handle many matters, but professional malpractice, professional disciplinary proceedings, and employment disputes are best handled by specialists in those areas.
2. Be attentive. Read the documents the attorney produces and travel to court proceedings to observe the attorney's performance.
3. Notify your insurance carrier as soon as you are aware of any real or potential liability issue. Inform your agent about the status of your case every few months, even if it is unchanged.
4. Keep costs sensible. Your attorney should explain initially how the fee will be computed and how you will be billed. The attorney may require you to pay a retainer fee.
5. Keep informed. The attorney should address your questions and concerns promptly. You are entitled to be kept informed about the status of your case. You are entitled to copies of all correspondence, legal briefs, and other documents.
6. Weed through writing. Your attorney needs to explain all facts and options. Examine all relevant documents and do not hesitate to make corrections in the same way you would correct a medical record by drawing a line through the incorrect or misleading information, writing in the correction, and signing your initials after it.
7. Set your own course. Insist on a collaborative relationship with your attorney for the duration of your case.

KEY CONCEPTS

- Nursing practice is governed by civil, public, and administrative laws.
- Nurses need to be familiar with their institution's policies and procedures in giving care and in reporting variances, illegal activities, or unexpected events.
- Nurses must have good oral, written, and electronic communication skills.
- Common torts include negligence and malpractice, assault and battery, false imprisonment, invasion of privacy, and defamation.
- Nurses need to be familiar with their state's Nurse Practices Act.
- The Multistate Licensure Compact allows nurses to practice in more than one state.

- Many sources of evidence are used to identify the standard of care.
- Nursing malpractice examples include treatment problems, communication problems, medication problems, and monitoring/observing/supervising problems.
- Legal protections in nursing practice include Good Samaritan laws, useful health records, risk-management programs, and professional liability insurance.

KEY TERMS

administrative law
assault
battery
civil law
common law
constitution
contract law
criminal law
defamation
false imprisonment
Good Samaritan laws
living will
malpractice
negligence
power of attorney
public law
tort

REVIEW QUESTIONS

1. You are given a written order by a provider to administer an unusually large dose of pain medicine to your patient. In this situation, which is an appropriate nursing action?
   A. Administer the medication because it was ordered by a provider.
   B. Refuse to administer the medication, and move on to another patient.
   C. Speak with the provider about your concerns, and clarify whether the medication dose is accurate.
   D. Select a dose that you feel comfortable with, and administer that dose.

2. A practitioner has ordered you to discharge Mr. Jones from the hospital, despite a new temperature of 102.0°F (38.8°C). The practitioner refuses to talk with you about the patient. In this situation, which is an appropriate nursing action?
   A. Administer an antipyretic medication, and discharge the patient.
   B. Discharge the patient with instructions to call 911 if he has any problems.
   C. Do not discharge the patient until you have discussed the matter with your nursing manager and are satisfied regarding patient safety.
   D. Discharge the patient, and tell the patient to take Tylenol when he gets home.

3. A practitioner has issued a Do Not Resuscitate (DNR) order for a patient, a 55-year-old man with cancer. While you are speaking with the patient one morning, he clearly states he wishes to be resuscitated in the event that he stops breathing. What is the most appropriate course of action?
   A. Ignore the patient's wishes because the practitioner ordered the DNR.
   B. Consult your hospital's policies and procedures, speak to the practitioner, and discuss the matter with your nurse manager.
   C. Attempt to talk the patient into agreeing to the DNR.
   D. Contact the medical licensing board to complain about the practitioner.

4. While explaining the concept of negligence to a new nurse, the manager gives an example. Which is an example of negligence?
   A. A comatose patient was not turned every two hours and subsequently developed a stage 3 decubitus ulcer, sepsis, and died.
   B. A patient was given Tylenol without an order and the headache was resolved.
   C. An alert patient fell getting out of the shower and broke an arm.
   D. A depressed patient began crying when the nurse said the medication had been changed.

5. Which of the following elements is NOT necessary or required for a nurse to be found negligent in a court of law?
   A. A duty or obligation for the nurse to act in a particular way
   B. A breach of that duty or obligation
   C. The nurse's intention to be negligent
   D. Physical, emotional, or financial harm to the patient

6. A patient has a sudden change in condition and is emergently intubated. Where does the nurse document this change in the EHR? Select all that apply.
   A. The respiratory assessment flow sheet
   B. Narrative nurse note
   C. The ventilator flow sheet
   D. Nursing care plan
   E. The initial assessment
   F. The medication administration record

7. You are a new nurse working on a medical-surgical unit. One of your patients, an elderly woman, has an advance directive that requests that no CPR be done in the event that she stops breathing. One day she stops breathing, and someone on your unit calls a "code" and begins resuscitative efforts. You go along with the team and help to resuscitate the patient. She regains a pulse but never regains consciousness. She is now ventilator dependent, and her family is very angry with you and the staff. Which of the following is a potential legal action you will face?
   A. Violation of patient privacy
   B. Battery
   C. Criminal recklessness
   D. Revoked nursing license

8. Which of the following is NOT an essential element of a Good Samaritan law?
   A. The care is rendered in an emergency situation.
   B. The health care worker is rendering care without pay.
   C. The health care worker is concerned about the safety of the victims.
   D. The care provided did not recklessly or intentionally cause injury or harm to the injured party.

9. In which of the following situations could a nurse be accused of false imprisonment? Select all that apply.
   A. Inappropriate use of chemical restraints
   B. Inappropriate use of physical restraints
   C. Restraining a competent person
   D. Failure to follow the institution's policies regarding the type and frequency of restraints
   E. Using restraints in an emergency situation to protect the patient from harm

10. Which of the following are goals of a risk-management program in an institution? Select all that apply.
    A. Identify and correct systemic problems in the facility
    B. Identify when better orientation is needed for staff
    C. Identify issues with equipment and staffing
    D. Punish the person responsible for the error
    E. Reduce legal and financial liability for the institution
    F. Reduce the number of errors made in patient care

REVIEW ACTIVITIES

1. Identify a common practice in your clinical setting such as a central line dressing change. How do you know if you are performing this the way "a reasonable nurse" would? What is the evidence and what standard of care are you held accountable to?
2. Research the various companies that offer nursing malpractice insurance and determine the cost and coverage associated with a nursing malpractice policy. Go to an Internet search engine, such as www.google.com. Search for "nursing malpractice insurance." What did you find? Note the Nursing Service Organization (NSO) website at http://www.nso.com. Recent legal cases are reported there.
3. Discuss how nurses' off-duty behaviors can affect their nursing practice. Note if your state lists any actions in its nurse practice act that you might take outside of work that might cause your license to practice nursing to be revoked by your state nursing licensure board (e.g., a driving while intoxicated conviction). Check your state's nurse practice act. Go to http://www.ncsbn.org and click on Boards of Nursing. Click on Member Boards, and then click on the map for the state you want to access for information.

EXPLORING THE WEB

- You have a patient who is to be transferred to a nursing home for recuperation. Where can you tell the family to look to evaluate the local nursing homes regarding their adherence to the federal regulations for nursing homes? *http://www.medicare.gov*
  Search for "long-term care" and "nursing homes compare."
- Where can you find a copy of the ANA Code of Ethics? *http://www.nursingworld.org*
  Search for Code of Ethics.
- Where can you find state and federal laws regulating hospitals? *http://www.findlaw.com*
- Note the Medical Liability Monitor at: *http://www.medicalliabilitymonitor.com*
  Go to this site to find out about the impact of the HITECH Act on the privacy of health information: *http://www.hhs.gov*

REFERENCES

American Law Institute. (1958). Restatement of the Law of Agency (Second). American Law Institute.

American Nurses Association (ANA). (2001). The Code of Ethics for Nurses with Interpretive Statements. American Nurses Association. Retrieved October 25, 2011, from http://www.nursingworld.org/codeofethics

Babcock, L., & Pogarsky, G. (1999). Damages caps and settlement: A behavior approach. *Journal of Legal Studies, 28*, 341.

Cady, R. F. (2011). Legal briefs. *JONA's Healthcare Law, Ethics, and Regulation, 13*(3), 62–78.

Campos, N. K. (2010). The legalities of nursing documentation. *Men in Nursing, 40*(1), 7–9.

Centers for Medicare & Medicaid Services (CMS). (2010). Meaningful use. Retrieved October 29, 2011, from https://www.cms.gov/EHRIncentivePrograms/30_Meaningful_Use

CNA Financial Corporation. (2009). CNA healthpro nurse claims study: An analysis of claims with risk management recommendations 1997–2007. CNA Financial Corporation. Hatboro, PA. Retrieved October 17, 2011, from https://www.nso.com/pdfs/db/rnclaimstudy.pdf? fileName=rnclaimstudy.pdf&folder=pdfs/db&isLiveStr=Y&refID=rnstudynsna

Code of Federal Regulations. Retrieved October 29, 2011, from http://www.gpoaccess.gov/cfr/"www.gpoaccess.gov/cfr

Committees on Energy and Commerce, Ways and Means, and Science and Technology. (2009). Health Information Technology for Economic and Clinical Health (HITECH) Act. Retrieved October 16, 2011 from http://waysandmeans.house.gov/media/pdf/110/hit2.pdf

Dictionary.com. Retrieved November 20, 2011, from http://dictionary.reference.com/browse/defamation

Elliot-Engel, A. (2011). Lehigh county jury awards $23 million in medical malpractice case: Smoyer *v.* St. Luke's. *The Legal Intelligencer*. Retrieved October 19, 2011, from http://www.law.com/jsp/pa/PubArticlePA.jsp?id=1202516817108&slreturn=1

General Hospital of Passaic *v.* American Casualty Company, 2007 WL 2814655 (D.N.J., September 24, 2007).

Healthcare Information and Management Systems Society (HIMSS). (2008). Electronic health records: A global perspective. *The Healthcare Information and Management Systems Society*. Retrieved September 27, 2011, from http://himss.org/content/files/200808_EHRGlobalPerspective_whitepaper.pdf?src= winews2009114

Horizon/CMS Healthcare Corp. *v.* Auld, 34 S.W.3d 887(Tex. 2000).

Jha, A. K., Doolan, D., Grandt, D., Scott, T., & Bates, D. W. (2008). The use of health information technology in seven nations. *International Journal of Medical Informatics*, 254–262.

LaDuke, S. (2000). What should you expect from your attorney? *Nursing Management, 31*(10), 10.

'Lectric Law Library's Lexicon on Tort. (2011). Retrieved October 29, 2011, from http://www.lectlaw.com/def2/t032.htm

Lipowicz, A. (2011). VA wants help modernizing health care records system. *Washington Technology*. Retrieved September 27, 2011, from https://owa.purduecal.edu/exchweb/bin/redir.asp?URL=http://washingtontechnology.com/articles/2011/01/28/va-looking-for-help-to-set-up-governance-for-open-source-vista.aspx" t "_blank".

Martin, J. W., Cain, S. K., Priest, C. S., & Hook, S. A. (2012). Legal aspects of health care. In P. Kelly (Ed.), *Nursing leadership and management* (3rd ed.). Clifton Park, NY: Delmar Cengage Learning.

Medicare's Do Not Pay List. (2011). Retrieved October 29, 2011, from http://www.hhs.gov/ash/initiatives/hai/appendices.html

Miller, L. (2011). Intrapartum fetal monitoring: Liability and documentation. *Clinical Obstetrics and Gynecology, 54*(1), 50–55.

National Council of State Boards of Nursing (NCSBN). (2011). Nurses licensure compact. Retrieved October 29, 2011, from https://www.ncsbn.org/ncl.htm

National Practitioner Data Bank. Healthcare integrity and protection data bank. Retrieved October 29, 2011, from http://www.npdb-hipdb.hrsa.gov

Occupational Safety & Health Administration, U.S. Department of Labor. Retrieved October 28, 2011, from http://www.osha.gov

Odom *v.* State Department of Health & Hospitals, 322 So. 2d 91 (La. 1999).

Pozza, R. (2003). Nursing malpractice cases. Unpublished manuscript.

Reising, D. L., & Allen, P. N. (2007). Protecting yourself from malpractice claims: Greater nursing autonomy comes at the price of increased legal exposure. *American Nurse Today, 2*(2), 39–43.

Rosenfeld, J. (2008). Failure to properly screen CNA could cost facility $3.5 million. Retrieved October 16, 2011, from http://www.jdsupra.com/post/documentViewer.aspx?fid=12f6e5eb-d672-4d77-89bf-f435c461b08b

Sutton v. United Airlines 1999; Murphy v. United Parcel Service, Inc., 1999.

U.S. Department of Health and Human Services. (n.d.). The data bank. The National Practitioner Data Bank (NPDB) and Healthcare Integrity and Protection Data Bank (HIPDB). Retrieved October 18, 2011, from http://www.npdbhipdb.hrsa.gov/topNavigation/aboutUs.jsp

SUGGESTED READINGS

Austin, S. (2010). 7 legal tips for safe nursing practice. *Nursing 2010 Critical Care, 5*(2), 15–20.

Morris, S. (2011). Health care reform and electronic health records. *Contact Lens Spectrum*, 32–54.

Sanchez, A. P., & Cava, A. (2008). Health privacy in a techno-social world: A cyber-patient's bill of rights. *Northwestern Journal of Technology and Intellectual Property, 6*(3), 244–276.

Smith, M. H. (2009). Legal basics for professional nursing: Nurse practice acts. Continuing Education, American Nurses Association. Retrieved October 17, 2011, from http://nursingworld.org/mods/mod995/canlegalnrsfull.htm

Weld, K. K., & Garmon Bibb, S. C. (2009). Concept analysis: Malpractice and modern-day nursing practice. *Nursing Forum, 44*(1), 2–10.

Worel, M. A., & Wirtes, D. G., Jr. (2007). Don't neglect the nurse's duty of care. *Trial, 43*(11), 50–57.

Young, A. (2009). Review: The legal duty of care for nurses and other health professionals. *Journal of Clinical Nursing, 18*(22), 3071–3078.

Zalon, M. L., Constantino, R. E., & Andrews, K. L. (2008). The right to pain treatment: A reminder for nurses.

CHAPTER 15

Ethical Aspects of Health Care

JOAN DORMAN, RN, MS, CEN; AND
CAMILLE B. LITTLE, RN, BSN, MS

Moral excellence comes about as a result of habit. We become just by doing just acts, temperate by doing temperate acts, brave by doing brave acts.

—ARISTOTLE

OBJECTIVES

Upon completion of this chapter, the reader should be able to:

1. Define ethics.
2. Review the use of ethical theories and principles in professional nursing practice.
3. Discuss a nursing philosophy.
4. Discuss values and values clarification.
5. Identify a guide for ethical decision making.
6. Promote ethical leadership and management in health care organizations.
7. Review ethical codes for nurses.

In a large teaching hospital, a patient you are caring for says he does not want to go on living. He has had cancer for several years and states he is tired of being sick. He has discussed this with his health care practitioner and has been declared Do Not Attempt Resuscitation (DNAR). One of your nursing assistive personnel (NAP) says to you, "I don't know why he is giving up. I think we should call a code if he arrests."

Where are your thoughts on this?

Where can you turn for guidance in this situation?

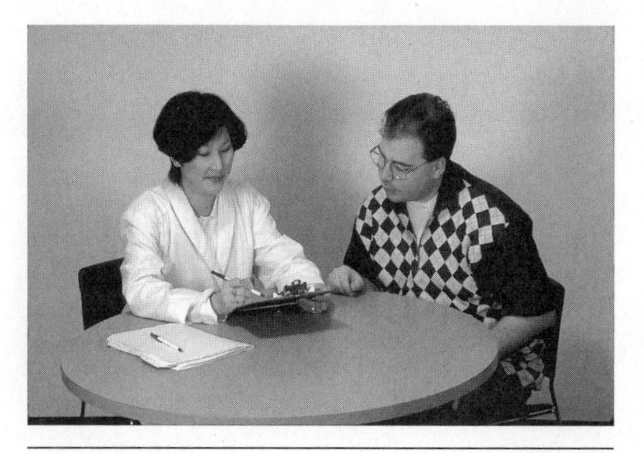

© Cengage Learning 2014

Throughout its history, nursing has relied on ethical principles to serve as guidelines in determining patient care. Nurses are confronted with ethical dilemmas in all types of practice settings. This chapter provides an overview of ethics, ethical theories, and the increased ethical challenges faced by nurses in leadership and management roles in today's health care environment.

There will be discussion of the importance of an individual philosophy of nursing as well as awareness of one's own values and those of the profession. Finally, this chapter introduces a guide for making ethical decisions that relies heavily on the importance of a code of ethics.

ETHICS

Ethics is the branch of philosophy that concerns the distinction of right from wrong on the basis of a body of knowledge, not just on the basis of opinions. **Morality** is behavior in accordance with custom or tradition and usually reflects personal or religious beliefs (DeLaune & Ladner, 2011). Ethics governs professional groups and provides a framework for determining the right course of action in a particular situation. For nurses, the actions they take in practice are primarily governed by the ethical principles of the profession. These principles influence practice, conduct, and relationships that nurses are held accountable for in the delivery of care. An **ethical dilemma** occurs when two or more ethical principles are in conflict and there is no obviously "correct" decision.

Laws, in contrast, are state and federal government rules that govern all of society. Laws mandate behavior. In some health care situations, the distinctions between law and ethics may not be clear. Ethics and law may be similar in some cases. In other cases, ethics and law may differ more dramatically.

Moral Development

Lawrence Kohlberg (1971) identified a moral development process that progresses through various levels. At the first level, the Preconventional Level, morals are all about rules imposed by some authority. Moral decisions made at this level are done in response to some threat of punishment. Labels of good and bad or right and wrong have meaning only in reference to a reward and punishment system. People at this Preconventional Level have no concept of the underlying moral code guiding the decision about what is good or bad or right or wrong. They act because an authority tells them to do so.

At the next level, the Conventional Level, people begin to internalize their view of themselves in response to something more meaningful and interpersonal. A desire to be viewed as a good person develops when the person wants to find approval from others. He or she may want to please, help others, be dutiful, and show respect for authority. Conformity to expected social and religious mores and a sense of loyalty often emerge at the Conventional Level. Not all people develop beyond this level.

A morally mature Postconventional Level person is an independent thinker who strives for a moral code beyond that dictated merely by respect for authority. The morally mature Postconventional Level person's actions are based on broader principles of respect for the dignity of all humankind, and not just on principles of respect for authority, duty, or loyalty to others (Kohlberg, 1971).

Ethical Theories

A standard way of making ethical decisions is to refer to ethical theories. Some of these theories are identified in Table 15-1.

Philosophy

Philosophy is the rational investigation of the truths and principles of knowledge, reality, and human conduct. Personal philosophies stem from an individual's beliefs and values. These beliefs and values, in turn, develop based upon a person's experiences in life, cultural influences, and education.

Philosophy of Nursing

A professional nurse's personal philosophy affects that nurse's philosophy of nursing. Throughout the nursing educational process, students begin forming their philosophy of nursing. This philosophy is influenced significantly by a student's personal philosophy and experiences. One's personal philosophy should be compatible with the philosophy of the nursing department where he or she works.

This helps the nurse to be an effective leader and practitioner. An example of a personal nursing philosophy is:

> I believe professional nursing care promotes an optimal level of wellness in body, mind, and spirit to those being served. I believe professional nurses must hold themselves to the highest standards of the profession and honor the profession's code of ethics in all aspects of practice.

Values and Virtues

Values

Values are personal beliefs about the truth of ideals, standards, principles, objects, and behaviors that give meaning and direction to life. If you were told that you must pack a bag for a special trip but you may bring only three items from your belongings, what items would you choose? The ones selected are what you value.

It is important to clarify your personal values. Personal values provide a baseline for identifying your professional nursing values. The professional nursing values of altruism, autonomy, human dignity, integrity, and social justice guide the nurse in providing

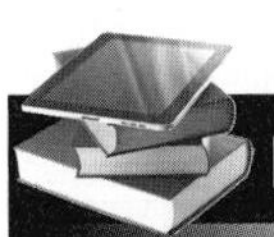

EVIDENCE FROM THE **LITERATURE**

Citation: Hernandez, A. H. (2009). Student articulation of a nursing philosophical statement: An assignment to enhance critical thinking skills and promote learning. *Journal of Nursing Education, 48*(6), 343–349.

Discussion: This article discusses a graduate or undergraduate nursing school assignment that focuses on the development of a personal philosophical statement of nursing. The finished product is a 5- to 10-page paper, but the process involves class discussion and group work. The students discuss their beliefs, assumptions, and values as they relate to the four metaparadigm concepts of nursing, person, health, and environment. Although the grading criteria for the final paper is firm, students are able to express their personal thoughts and are encouraged to think critically.

Implications for Practice: The self-discovery process that is integral in this assignment would be beneficial for all nurses. The assignment itself could be adapted and incorporated to fit in any type of nursing program.

TABLE 15-1
Selected Ethical Theories

Ethical Theory	Interpretation
Deontology	Actions are based on moral rules and unchanging principles, such as, "do unto others as you would have them do unto you." An ethical person must always follow the rules, even if doing so causes a less desirable outcome. This theory states that the motives of the actor determine the goodness or value of the act. Thus, a bad outcome may be acceptable if the intent of the actor was good.
Teleology	A person must take those actions that lead to good outcomes. This theory states that the outcome of an act determines whether the act is good or of value and that achievement of a good outcome justifies using a less desirable means to attain the end.
Virtue ethics	Virtues such as truthfulness and trustworthiness are developed over time. A person's character must be developed so that by nature and habit, the person will be predisposed to behave virtuously. Living a virtuous life contributes both to one's own well-being and to the well-being of society.
Justice and equity	A "veil of ignorance" regarding who is affected by a decision should be used by decision makers because it allows for unbiased decision making. An ethical person chooses the action that is fair to all, including both the advantaged and the disadvantaged groups in society.
Relativism	There are no universal ethical standards, such as "murder is always wrong." Ethical standards are relative to person, place, time, and culture. Whatever a person thinks is right, is right. This theory has been largely rejected.

© Cengage Learning 2014

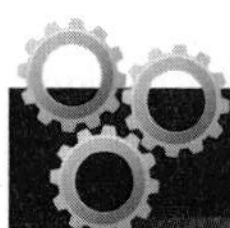

CRITICAL THINKING **15-1**

New graduates formulate a philosophy of nursing based on personal beliefs and on values. Reflections on the following questions can assist in the development of a philosophy:

How can nurses influence patient care based on their nursing philosophy?

Are compassion, discernment, trustworthiness, and integrity essential both personally and professionally?

Do nurses have an ethical responsibility to demonstrate caring and maintain current competency?

ethical care to patients (American Association of Colleges of Nursing, 2008).

Values clarification is the process of analyzing one's own values to better understand what is truly important. In their classic work *Values and Teaching*, Raths, Harmin, and Simon (1978) formulated a theory of values clarification and proposed a three-step process for valuing, as follows:

Choosing

1. Analysis of alternative beliefs and their consequences
2. Free choice of your beliefs from alternatives

Prizing

3. Feeling satisfied with your choice
4. Being willing to share your choice with others

Acting

5. Making your choice a part of your behavior
6. Repeating the choice

Virtues

Burkhardt and Nathaniel (2008) list four virtues that are more significant than others and that are illustrative of a virtuous person: compassion, discernment, trustworthiness, and integrity. **Compassion** is a deep awareness of the suffering of another along with the desire to relieve it. **Discernment** is possession of acuteness of judgment. **Trustworthiness** is present when trust is well founded or deserving. **Integrity** may be considered to be firm adherence to a code of conduct or an ethical value. These virtues form the foundation for an ethically principled discipline and have been endorsed throughout the nursing profession's history. Nurses who subscribe to these four virtues are inclined to recall and value that patients also have their own personal values.

Ethical Principles

In addition to the theories, ethical principles and values provide a basis for nurses to determine the appropriate action when faced with an ethical dilemma in the practice setting. See Table 15-2 for a summary of the major ethical principles and rules. Principle-based ethics has, for centuries, been viewed as the foundation for ethical behavior. There are, of course, differences in the stature of the various principles among societies. **Autonomy**, or the freedom to determine one's own actions, is valued in some societies, but not in others. In the U.S., beginning in the 1960s, the civil rights movement, women's rights, and, later, patients' rights, have added an additional component to ethical thought. This might be termed "the ethic of care." It refers to the caring in a health care professional–patient relationship. It helps increase awareness that an ethical problem exists. Caring is the foundation of the ANA Code of Ethics (2001) and is central to most nursing interventions. Because patient-perceived nurse caring is a predictor of patient satisfaction, several tools have been developed to measure nurse-caring behaviors. Some of the items addressed include attentive listening, showing concern, responding quickly, spending time, and demonstrating knowledge and skill.

Guides for Ethical Decision Making

Nurses have long sought guidance in the face of ethical dilemmas. The differences in knowledge and skill between novice and seasoned nurses might be measurable, but the ease, or torment, with which these same nurses make ethical decisions might be virtually the same. For that reason, it seemed that a specific ethical decision-making tool was called for. Just as most of us rely on some sort of GPS device when traveling into unfamiliar places, nurses find themselves looking for the route that might lead them to an ethical decision. Several authors have proposed guides for ethical decisions.

Burkhardt and Nathaniel (2008) propose a five-step decision-making process to guide nurses in making ethical decisions. The five steps are as follows:

1. Articulate the problem
2. Gather data and articulate conflicting moral claims
3. Explore strategies
4. Implement the strategy
5. Evaluate the outcome

Husted and Husted (2007) discuss an ethical decision-making approach based on a Symphonological Model. Central in this model is the professional/patient agreement. This agreement is linked to the ethical principles of autonomy, freedom, self-assertion, beneficence, objectivity, and fidelity, and

TABLE 15-2
Ethical Principles and Rules

Ethical Principles/Rules	Definition	Example
Beneficence	The duty to do good to others and to maintain a balance between benefits and harms.	◆ Provide all persons, including patients and the terminally ill, with caring attention and information.
Nonmaleficence	The principle of doing no harm.	◆ Keep your knowledge and skills up to date.
Justice	The principle of fairness that is served when an individual is given that which he or she is due, owed, deserves, or can legitimately claim.	◆ Treat all patients fairly, regardless of economic or social background.
Confidentiality	Ensuring that information is accessible only to those authorized to have access.	◆ Become familiar with federal and state laws and facility policies dealing with privacy, e. g., HIPAA legislation.
Fidelity	The principle of promise keeping; the duty to keep one's promise or word.	◆ Be sure that you keep your promises.
Autonomy	The right of people to make their own decisions; self-determination.	◆ Provide all persons with information for decision making. Avoid making paternalistic decisions for others.
Veracity	The obligation to tell the truth.	◆ Refuse to participate in any form of fraud. Give an "honest day's work" every day.
Advocacy	The obligation to look out or speak up for the rights of others.	◆ Provide patients with high-quality, evidence-based care.

© Cengage Learning 2014

surrounded by the context of the situation and the context of knowledge.

Jonsen, Siegler, and Winslade (2006) have published a practical approach to ethical decision making in clinical medicine. Their model is directed to not only physicians and medical students, but to hospital administrators, ethics committees, and other health care workers. Their model consists of four topics:

1. Medical indications: How might this patient benefit?
2. Patient preferences: Is the patient's right to choose being respected?
3. Quality of life: What are the prospects for a meaningful life?
4. Contextual features: What other issues need to be considered?

In examining each of these four areas, the authors ask that we consider the ethical principles inherent in the decision we ultimately make.

It is apparent, when examining these ethical decision-making tools, that nurses, physicians, and other health care workers might well find themselves looking for guidance when faced with an ethical dilemma. The question arises of whether there could be a single tool for all situations, and, if so, which tool might that be.

In 2009, Dorman wrote a paper and made a presentation at Oxford University, at a round table titled Ethics: The Convolution of Contemporary Values. At that time, the Ethical Positioning System was introduced by Dorman to an audience of doctors, lawyers, theologians, journalists, philosophers, and ethicists. It was well received, and representatives from specialties other than nursing thought they might easily adapt the tool.

The EPS follows the nursing process and is a framework for ethical decision making, the steps include: (see Figure 15-1)

1. Assessment: In this step the nurse gathers all available data. This includes all the people involved in the decision-making process and everything pertinent to the context of the situation.
2. Nursing Dilemma: This is a simple statement of the problem. What should the nurse do in this case?
3. Planning: In this step, the nurse examines all possible choices of actions. For each choice, the pros and cons are listed. Then the ethical principles that need to be considered in making this decision, along with the provisions of the ANA Code of Ethics that are pertinent, are applied to make a diagram.
4. Diagram: This is a visual image of the planning process that facilitates making a decision. You can see which choices need to be eliminated (see Figure 15-2).
5. Implementation: Once a decision has been reached, that choice is implemented.
6. Evaluation: How well did your chosen decision work? What was the outcome?

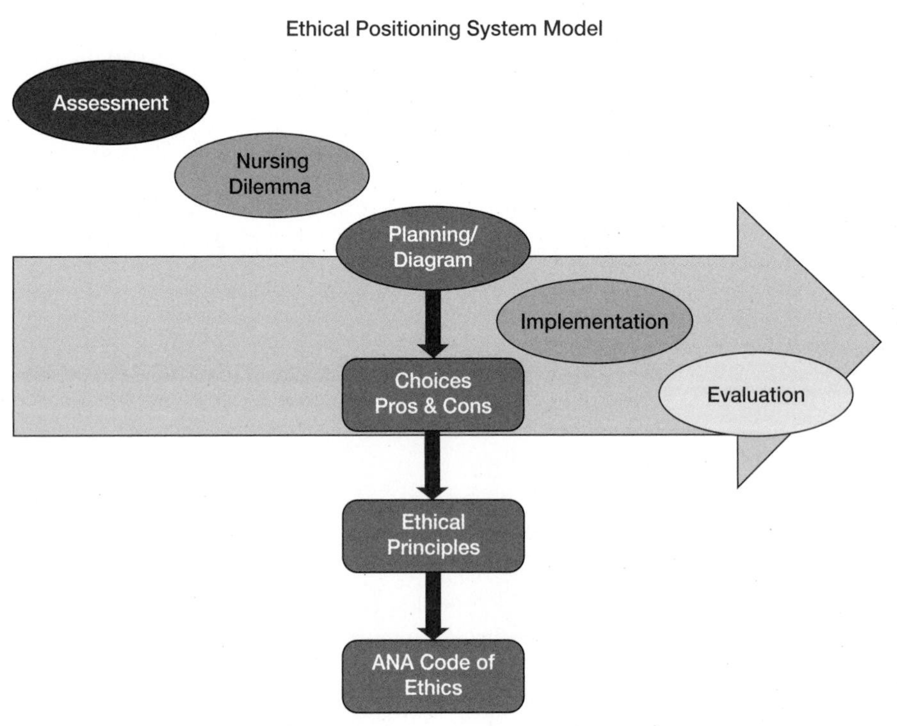

FIGURE 15-1

The ethical positioning system model.
(*Source:* P. Kelly (2012), *Nursing Leadership and Management* (3rd ed.), p. 572.)

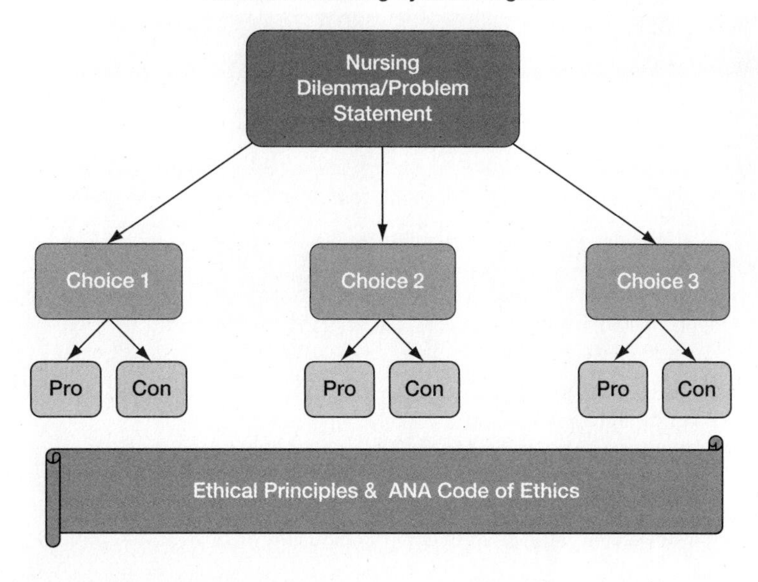

FIGURE 15–2

The ethical positioning system diagram.

(*Source:* Kelly, P. (2012). *Nursing Leadership & Management* (3rd ed.). Clifton Park, NY. Cengage Learning. p. 573.)

Patient Rights

A Patient's Bill of Rights was first adopted by the American Hospital Association (AHA) in 1973, and was revised in 1982 and 1992. The Bill of Rights was intended to ensure the health care system would be fair and meet patients' needs. It provides patients a means of addressing problems with their care and encourages them to participate in staying healthy and getting well. In 2003, The American Hospital Association replaced the Bill of Rights with the Patient Care Partnership. This is a booklet informing patients of what to expect during their hospital stay. It discusses their right to high-quality hospital care, a clean and safe environment, involvement in their care, protection of their privacy, help when leaving the hospital, and help with billing claims (AHA, 2003).

Ethical Leadership and Management

Health care leaders are charged with the responsibility of creating an environment that is ethically principled and that supports upholding the standards of conduct set by the health care professions.

Research conducted by the Ethics Research Center concluded the following:

- If positive outcomes are desired, an ethical culture is what makes the difference.
- Leadership, especially senior leadership, is the most critical factor in promoting an ethical culture.
- In organizations that are trying to strengthen their culture, formal program elements can help to do that (Harned, 2005).

Organizational Benefits Derived from Ethics

Health care institutions are increasingly faced with making decisions that, based on the financial bottom line, might ultimately affect the quality of patient-centered care provided. Ethically and socially responsible decisions often come with a price tag. Problems in the Enron Corporation and the banking industry represent a few recent examples of this. Hospitals have also suffered financial losses when ethics were cast aside. There have been countless medical errors and subsequent malpractice suits that can be traced back to cutbacks in staff or other resources.

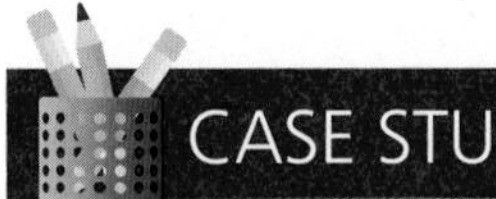

CASE STUDY 15-1

A Guide for Decision Making

The following case study illustrates the Ethical Positioning System. This particular case focuses on the experience of a nursing student. However, it could just as easily apply to a new nurse or a nurse who was new to a facility.

A student was assigned to spend a clinical day in the emergency department of a hospital. This student, Tom, was sitting at the nurses' station when a patient with schizophrenia was brought into the department, shouting loudly and struggling to leave. The patient was placed in full leather restraints, for her own safety and the safety of the staff. By this time, she was yelling obscenities, crying, and begging to be released. The nursing staff was laughing and joking about her behavior.

Tom had assessed the situation, and he knew that this nursing behavior was unethical, as well as, nontherapeutic. But he was only a nursing student, and he was not sure what he could do. That was the nursing dilemma. Next, in the planning step, he considered all the possible solutions. First, he could do nothing, a commonly selected possibility. The pro to this choice is that Tom would not have to confront the nurses, and would not be looked on as a busybody and a know-it-all. The cons to this choice are that he will feel guilty for not acting as a patient advocate, the patient will remain distressed, and the other patients in the department will suffer.

Another solution would be to confront the nurses about their nontherapeutic handling of this patient and their unprofessional behavior. The pro to this would be that Tom would feel he was actively being a patient advocate. The cons would be that they might ignore him, they might condemn his interference, and the situation would not change.

Tom could approach the manager, who in turn could arrange for some kind of educational program to deal with this lack of sensitivity. The pro would be that Tom would feel he was at least addressing the problem; however, this choice would do nothing for the immediate situation.

Tom also considered that he could go sit with the patient, calm her down, and give emotional support. The pro would be that he would be proactive and therapeutic. The con would be that there would be no lasting effect in the staff nurses' view of, or approach to, patients with schizophrenia.

The Code of Ethics discusses several provisions that are applicable to this case. Some of these are respect for human dignity (1.1), primacy of the patient's interests (2.1), professional boundaries (2.4), responsibility for nursing judgment and action (4.2), moral self-respect (5.1), influence of the environment on moral virtues and values (6.1), and responsibilities to the public (8.2). There are also several ethical principles that apply to this case. Tom considered respect, justice, beneficence, nonmaleficence, and fidelity.

Tom addressed step four in the Ethical Positioning System by making a diagram of his choices. This allowed him to conceptualize his choices. As he analyzed the diagram, Tom selected the fourth alternative. He then took step five, implementation: He entered the room and spent considerable time with the patient. She calmed down, and appreciated his concern. The other patients no longer had to listen to her scream. Tom felt he made the most effective choice at the time.

In the Ethical Positioning System's final step, Tom evaluated the process, and his choice; he found he was not completely satisfied. He felt he could have made a point of being sure all the nurses knew what he was doing, and that he was responding in a professional and therapeutic manner. Perhaps at some point, the other nurses might model his behavior and act accordingly. Then, his choice would have had a more lasting effect. Thus, this final step provided an opportunity to reevaluate and learn from the situation.

CRITICAL THINKING 15-2

Mr. Davis is a 76-year-old retired professor who lives by himself in a small apartment. He is admitted to the medical-surgical unit of the community hospital with a diagnosis of weakness, dehydration, electrolyte imbalance, and malnutrition. He has no close family, but a neighbor who accompanied Mr. Davis to the hospital informed the nurse that she felt he had a preoccupation with his bowel movements and took large quantities of over-the-counter laxatives. During the admission interview, Mr. Davis was mildly disoriented to place and time but denied taking any over-the-counter medications. He was started on IV fluid and electrolyte replacement and placed on a high calorie diet and bed rest. He was very compliant with the treatments, except that he frequently visited the bathroom for bowel movements.

On entering the room, one of the nurses noted that Mr. Davis was hurriedly returning a bottle of what appeared to be laxative pills to his shaving kit. The nurse asked him about it but was told "It's none of your business—just stay out of my stuff!" by a very irate M. Davis. The nurse later informed the physician of the episode. The physician ordered the nurse to obtain the shaving kit and to see if there were any laxatives in it. He reasoned that if the patient was taking large doses of laxatives and having diarrhea, all treatments would be without benefit.

Initially the nurse agreed with the physician, but after thinking about the situation and remembering some basic ethical and legal principles, she felt uncomfortable searching a patient's belongings without permission.

You are the nurse. Use the Ethical Positioning System to analyze this case.

Quality and safety issues in health care have increasingly come under scrutiny. The American Hospital Association, the National League of Nursing, the National Institutes of Health, and the American Association of Colleges of Nursing have all designated quality and safety initiatives as the highest priority. Additional information is available on each of their websites.

Creating an Ethical Workplace

Quality and Safety Education for Nurses (QSEN, 2011) makes creating an ethical workplace for nurses a necessity. In order for that workplace to be ethical, it must be dedicated to the well-being of the patients. Safety is the foundation of the workplace, enabling the nurse to be beneficent, to do good, to be nonmaleficent, and to prevent harm. Considerations of quality and safety help us design a work environment dedicated to caring for patients in every sense of the word. The following suggestions might be useful.

- Establish a formal mechanism for monitoring ethically responsible behavior and attitudes.
- Have written organizational codes of conduct as well as standards, policies, and procedures.
- Have mentors to role model ethical behavior and training programs in ethical awareness and social responsibility.
- Support the development of a strong ethics committee that is available to all staff and that is composed of interprofessional persons including nursing, medicine, administration, clergy, consumers, psychiatry, social work, nutritional services, and pharmacy, as well as an ethicist.
- Have clear policies of scope of practice for delegation and chain of command.
- Share the Joint Commission's Safety Goals for the current year. Available at: http://www.jointcommission.org/standards_information/npsgs.aspx
- Consider applying for Magnet Status, awarded by the American Nurses Credentialing Center.
- Encourage discussion about ethical deviations as well as errors or incidents.
- Perform a root-cause analysis to see how to prevent these incidents in the future.

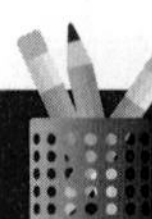

CASE STUDY 15-2

To better relate the study of ethics to yourself, take the self-quiz below. Do you agree or disagree with the following statements?

1. I would report a nursing coworker's drug abuse.
2. I see no harm in taking home a few nursing supplies.
3. I would tell the truth to a patient who asked if he was dying.
4. I would tell a patient who asked what narcotic pain medicine he was receiving.
5. It is unacceptable to call in sick to take a day off, even if only done once or twice a year.
6. I would accept a permanent, full-time job even if I knew I wanted the job for only six months.
7. If I received $100 for doing some odd jobs, I would report it on my income tax returns.
8. When applying for a nursing position, I would cover up the fact that I had been fired from a recent job.
9. I would report the family of a child who has findings not consistent with the reported story.
10. I would give ordered drugs on a temporary basis to a drug-addicted patient who is out of narcotics and who presents to the emergency department.

Source: C. S. Faircloth, RN, Personal Communication, March 13, 2003.

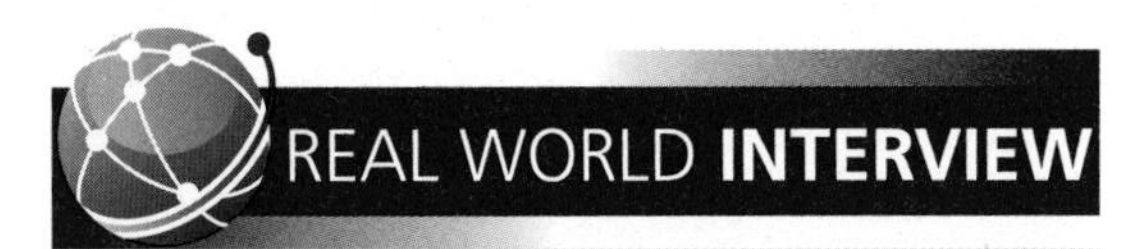

One of my most difficult cases involved a man in his early 40s who was in a coma, ventilator dependent, and declared brain dead. The patient was from a different culture, and when the family arrived six weeks later from abroad, they refused to allow him to be removed from the ventilator. His parents said they were told by the gods that their son would be well several months in the future. After two months in the hospital, the administration began to put pressure on the family to transfer the patient.

EMILY DAVISON, RN
Case Manager
Pleasant Hill, Missouri

Nurse-Physician Ethics and Relationships

In this time of incredible technological advancement, hospitals find themselves increasingly faced with ethical dilemmas. These dilemmas span the age continuum from prebirth and birth to death and postdeath. For that reason, most health care institutions have ethics committees to help deal with these dilemmas. An ethics committee is comprised of an interdisciplinary group representing medicine, nursing, pastoral care, pharmacy, nutritional services, social services, quality management, legal services, and the community. On any given occasion, there may also be guest members from a specialty area, such as OB or oncology. Family members may also be invited to an ethics committee meeting (Figure 15-3).

The mission of an ethics committee is to provide a timely response when an ethical issue arises. This might involve an emergency meeting of some or all of the members. There is generally a written policy guiding this consultation process. Appropriate committee members, as well as family representatives, patient physicians, and other caregivers may be invited. In most cases there is a process for consultations. The committee needs to know the background of the case and all pertinent information. Members of the committee need to know the options, along with the risks and benefits, as well as the values and principles involved.

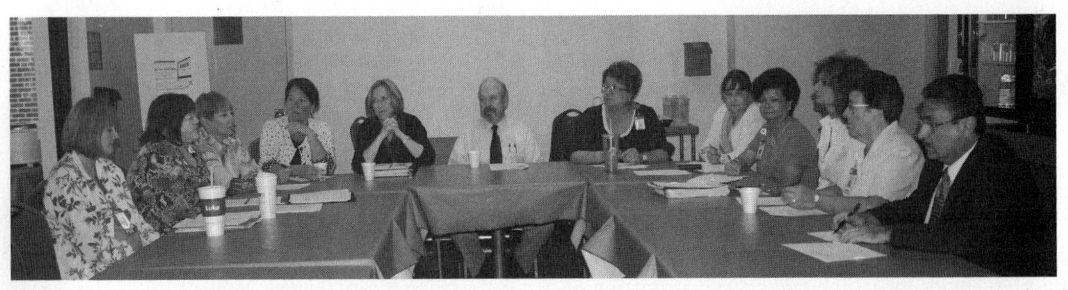

FIGURE 15-3

Bio-Ethics committee meeting in progress.
(*Source:* Courtesy St. Catherine's Hospital Ethics Committee, July 2010.)

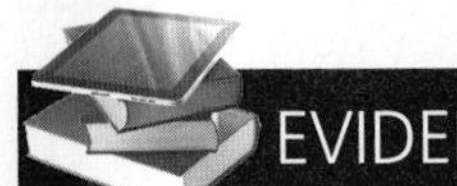

EVIDENCE FROM THE **LITERATURE**

Citation: Nelson, W. (2009, July/August). Ethical uncertainty and staff stress. *Healthcare Management Ethics,* 38–40.

Discussion: Ethical conflicts and concerns have a significant negative impact on health care organizations. Everyone is affected, from the executives to the clinicians. For staff members, managers, and even executives, moral distress greatly diminishes job satisfaction.

This article discusses how recognizing moral distress can be the first step in managing its negative impact. In this step, staff members develop self-awareness and seek assistance. Second, an open environment is developed in which ethical concerns can be shared and discussed. Third, the ethics committee needs to be available and easily accessible for consultation. Finally, health care organizations need to have an accessible employee-assistance program to offer confidential, emotional support.

Implications for Practice: With these four approaches in place, nurses would be better equipped to deal with ethical dilemmas and would have some support when faced with ethical distress.

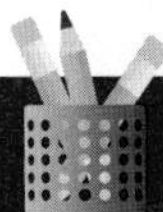

CASE STUDY **15-3**

You are caring for a 67-year-old male with chronic obstructive pulmonary disease (COPD) at a free clinic. This patient, Joe F., smokes heavily and does not want to quit smoking. He has tried numerous times in years past, but now feels smoking is his one pleasure in life. Joe has had numerous exacerbations of his COPD, and will probably need home oxygen before long.

1. Does Joe still have a right to free treatment?
2. Are limits to his treatment justified?
3. What ethical principles come into this situation?

Divide the class into two groups and select a moderator. One group will argue for giving treatment and the other group will argue that treatment is not justified in this case.

They need to examine the possibilities of a resolution and the potential outcome. The committee does not make a decision. The committee lends guidance and provides resources, so that ethically sound decisions might be made.

Ethical Codes

One mark of a profession is the determination of ethical behavior for its members. Several nursing organizations have developed codes for ethical behavior.

The International Council of Nurses Code of Ethics for Nurses 2006 is available at www.icn.ch/icncode.pdf.

The American Nurses Association has also developed a Code of Ethics for Nurses (2006). See www.nursingworld.org. Click on Code of Ethics.

The Canadian Nurses Association (CNA, 2002) has also developed a Code of Ethics.

The first Code, adopted in 1954, was the International Council of Nursing Code for Nurses. The CNA Code of Ethics for Registered Nurses was adopted in 1997. In 2002, the CNA Code of Ethics for Registered Nurses was expanded and revised. The code may be obtained from the CNA website, www.cna-nurses.ca. Search for Code of Ethics.

The Gallup Organization's 2010 annual poll on professional honesty and ethical standards ranked nurses number one. Of the 22 professions tested, five had high ethical ratings: nurses (81%), military officers (73%), pharmacists (71%), grade school teachers (67%), and medical doctors (66%). For more information, see poll.gallup.com. Search for Ethical Standards.

KEY CONCEPTS

- Ethics is the branch of philosophy that concerns the distinction of right from wrong on the basis of a body of knowledge, not just on the basis of opinions.
- A personal philosophy stems from an individual's beliefs and values. This personal philosophy will influence an individual's philosophy of nursing.
- Values clarification is an important step in helping one understand what is truly important.
- Ethical principles include autonomy and confidentiality, beneficence, nonmaleficence, fidelity, autonomy, respect for others, veracity, and advocacy.
- The Ethical Positioning System is a helpful tool.
- The Patient Care Partnership encourages more effective patient care.
- Organizations have a responsibility to society to practice ethically, with a focus on quality and safety.
- Ethics committees provide guidance for decision making about ethical dilemmas that arise in health care settings.
- The International Council of Nurses' Code of Ethics for Nurses influences patient care.
- Various nursing ethical codes influence patient care.

KEY TERMS

autonomy
beneficence
compassion
confidentiality
discernment
ethical dilemma
ethics
fidelity
integrity
justice
morality
nonmaleficence
philosophy
trustworthiness
values
values clarification
veracity

REVIEW QUESTIONS

1. The nurse caring for a relatively immobile patient demonstrates Kohlberg's Preconventional Level of Development by following the hospital turning protocol, for which of the following reasons?
   A. The nurse is following the cultural beliefs of the patient.
   B. The nurse fears punishment for breaking the rules.
   C. The nurse is following a personal value.
   D. The nurse is focusing on the needs of the patient.

2. A new nurse asks the manager about the hospital ethics committee. Which of the following statements by the manager is correct about an ethics committee?
   A. Ethics committees are consulted only for life and death situations.
   B. Ethics committees can prevent ethical dilemmas from occurring.
   C. The ethics committee provides guidance to patients, their families, and the health care team.
   D. A nurse would have no need to seek guidance from an ethics committee.

3. As the nurse prepares the patient for surgery, the patient confides that the physician did not give information about the risks for surgery. Which is the best action for the nurse to take in this situation?
   A. Tell the patient the risks.
   B. Tell the patient not to worry, that the patient is in good hands.
   C. Report the surgeon to the unit manager.
   D. Inform the surgeon that the patient has questions about the risks of surgery.

4. A nurse is dedicated to furthering her education, taking continuing-education classes whenever possible, and keeping up with new advances as reported in nursing journals. This dedication reflects which ethical principle?
   A. Justice
   B. Beneficence
   C. Veracity
   D. Confidentiality

5. The nurse realizes that neglecting to inform the patient about the plan of care is a violation of which of the following?
   A. The Patient Care Partnership
   B. The patient's right to privacy
   C. The patient's right to confidentiality
   D. The Ffth Amendment of the Constitution

6. Which idea statement by the nurse reflects a teleological theory?
   A. The goodness of an action is based on the intent.
   B. There are no universal ethical standards.
   C. Do unto others as you would have others do unto you.
   D. The end justifies the means.

7. Mrs. Jones rides the elevator to the fifth floor where her husband is a patient. While on the elevator, she hears two nurses talking about Mr. Jones. They are discussing the potential prognosis and whether Mrs. Jones should be told. Which ethical principle is being violated by the nurses?
   A. Autonomy
   B. Confidentiality
   C. Beneficence
   D. Justice

8. During morning report, the night nurse tells the day nurse that a patient who was admitted for pancreatitis is a drug addict and an alcoholic and causes all his own problems. As the day nurse, you realize that the night nurse is exhibiting a lack of which of the following?
   A. Autonomy
   B. Compassion
   C. Veracity
   D. Discernment

9. The nurse demonstrates nonmaleficence by doing which of the following actions? Select all that apply.
   A. Observing the six rights of medication administration
   B. Reviewing practitioner orders for accuracy and completeness
   C. Keeping knowledge and skills up to date
   D. Dressing professionally, with hair tied back and nails short.
   E. Identifying herself/himself as an RN, with name badge clearly visible
   F. Washing hands at least before and between each patient contact

10. The nurse notices that a coworker is slurring speech, has an unsteady gait, and appears unable to practice safely. Which is the best action for the nurse to take?
   A. Inform the manager or shift director immediately
   B. Give the coworker some black coffee
   C. Discuss the situation with the other nurses working
   D. Do nothing, but keep an eye on the nurse

REVIEW ACTIVITIES

1. An elderly woman, age 88, is admitted to the emergency department in acute respiratory distress. She does not have a living will, but her daughter has power of attorney (POA) for health care and is a health care professional. The patient has end-stage renal disease, end-stage Alzheimer's disease, and congestive heart failure. Her condition is grave. The doctors want to intubate her and place her on a ventilator. The sons agree. The daughter states that their mother would not want to be on a machine just to prolong her life.

   Divide into groups. Discuss the ethical theories that can be applied to this situation.

2. As a hospice nurse, you are involved with pain control on a regular basis. Many of the medications prescribed for the management of pain also depress respirations.

   Divide into groups and determine a protocol for the use of these medications, keeping in mind that the purpose of hospice is to promote comfort. Support your decision with ethical theories and principles.

3. You have been caring for Mr. Adams, on and off, for several months. He has been terminally ill with colon cancer and has been in and out of the hospital. You have developed a caring relationship with Mr. Adams, his wife, and several of his grown children and their families.

   Shortly after your shift begins, you enter the room to find Mr. Adams dead. He did have DNR orders. Even though he was terminally ill, his death on this day seemed unexpected. You phone his wife and, rather than telling her he has taken a turn for the worse, you decide to tell her he is dead. She says she will call the family and they will be in.

   You greet the family in a quiet room, and offer your condolences. The family wants to know how he died and if he was alone. You tell them, you entered the room to find him taking very slow shallow breaths. You sat with him for what was less than a minute and held his hand. So, no, he was not alone, and it was very peaceful.

1. Is it ethical to tell lies from benevolent motives?
2. What ethical principles come into this situation?
3. Did the nurse do the right thing?
   Divide into groups and support the divergent positions on this question.

EXPLORING THE WEB

- Nursing ethics: *http://www.ana.org*
  Click on Code of Ethics.
- Use the International Council of Nurses website to find the ICN Code of Ethics for Nurses: *http://www.icn.ch*
  Click on the ICN Code of Ethics.
- Visit: *http://www.aha.org*
  Search for Patient Care Partnership to view the American Health Association's Patient Care Partnership.
- ANA Center for Ethics and Human Rights: *http://www.nursingworld.org/ethics*
  Search for ANA Center for Ethics and Human Rights.
  Search for About the Center.
- National Center for Ethics in Health Care home: *http://www.ethics.va.gov*
- Visit Quality and Safety Education for Nurses (QSEN): *http://www.qsen.org*
- The Center for Bioethics and Human Dignity: *http://www.cbhd.org*
- Nursing ethics network: *http://www.bc.edu*
  Search for Nursing Ethics Network.

REFERENCES

American Association of Colleges of Nursing (AACN). (2008). Essentials of baccalaureate education for professional nursing practice. Retrieved from http://www.aacn.nche.edu/Education/pdf/BaccEssentials08.pdf

American Hospital Association (AHA). (2003). Patient care partnership. Retrieved from http://www.aha.org/aha/issues/Communicating-With-Patients/pt-care-partnership.html

American Nurses Association (ANA). (2001). *Code of ethics for nurses with interpretive statements.* Washington, DC: American Nurses Publishing.

Burkhardt, M. A., & Nathaniel, A. K. (2008). *Ethics & issues in contemporary nursing* (2nd ed.). Clifton Park, NY: Delmar Cengage Learning.

Canadian Nurses Association (CNA). (2002). Code of ethics for RN. Retrieved from http://www.cna-nurses.ca. Search for "code of ethics."

DeLaune, S. C., & Ladner, P. K. (2011). *Fundamentals of nursing* (4th ed.). Clifton Park, NY: Delmar Cengage Learning.

Dorman, J. (2009). The convolution of contemporary values. Oral presentation at the Ethical Roundtable at Oxford University, Oxford, United Kingdom.

Faircloth, C. S. (2003). Personal communication with Patricia Kelly.

Harned, P. (2005). National business ethics survey. *Ethics Today Online, 4*(2). Retrieved from http://www.ethics.org/research/2005-press-release.asp

Hernandez, A. H. (2009). Student articulation of a nursing philosophical statement: An assignment to enhance critical thinking skills and promote learning. *Journal of Nursing Education, 48*(6), 343–349.

Husted, G. L., & Husted, J. H. (2007). *Ethical decision making in nursing and healthcare* (4th ed.). New York, NY: Springer Publishing Co.

International Council of Nurses (ICN). (2006). *Code of ethics for nurses.* Geneva, Switzerland: Author.

Joint Commission. (2011). National patient safety goals. Retrieved November 20, 2011, from http://www.jointcomission.org

Jone, J. M. (2010). Nurses top honesty and ethics list for the 11th year. Gallup Poll. Retrieved from http://poll.gallup.com

Jonsen, A. R., Siegler, M., & Winslade, W. J. (2006). *Clinical ethics* (6th ed.). New York, NY: McGraw Hill.

Kelly, P. (2012). *Nursing Leadership & Management* (3rd ed.). Clifton Park, NY: Cengage Learning.

Kohlberg, L. (1971). Stages of moral development as a basis for moral development. In C. M. Beck, B. S. Crittenden, & E. V. Sullivan (Eds.). *Moral interdisciplinary approaches.* Paramus, NJ: Newman.

Nelson, W. (2009, July/August). Ethical uncertainty and staff stress. *Healthcare Management Ethics*, 38–40.

Quality & Safety in Nursing. (2011). Retrieved from http://www.qsen.org

Raths, L. E., Harmin, M., & Simon, S. B. (1978). *Values and teaching* (2nd ed.). Columbus, OH: Merrill Publishing.

SUGGESTED READINGS

Beard, E. L., Jr., Johnson, L. W. (2007, October–December). Conversations in ethics. *JONAS Healthcare Law Ethics Regulation, 9*(4), 117–118.

Bowditch, J. L., & Buono, A. F. (1997). *A primer on organizational behavior* (4th ed.). New York, NY: Wiley.

Greene J. (2002, March). The medical workplace: No abuse zone. *Hospitals and Health Networks, 76*(3), 26, 28.

Milton, C. L. (2008, January). Boundaries: Ethical implications for what it means to be therapeutic in the nurse-person relationship. *Nursing Science Quarterly, 21*(1), 18–21.

Nursing Ethics conference on the globalisation of nursing: Ethical, legal and political issues. (2007, January) *Nursing Ethics, 14*(1), 3–4.

Pauly, B., Goldstone, I., McCall J., Gold, F., & Payne, S. (2007, October). The ethical, legal and social context of harm reduction. *Canadian Nurse, 103*(8), 19–23.

Pendry, P. S. (2007, July–August). Moral distress: Recognizing it to retain nurses. *Nursing Economics, 25*(4), 217–221.

Tschudin, V. January (2006). How nursing ethics as a subject changes: An analysis of the first eleven years of publication of the journal *Nursing Ethics. Nursing Ethics, 13*(1), 65–85.

Tschudin, V. (2007, November). How is the nursing profession perceived from outside the profession itself . . . ? *Nursing Ethics, 14*(6), 709–710.

CHAPTER 16

Culture, Generational Differences, and Spirituality

CAROLYN CHRISTIE-MCAULIFFE, RN, PHD, FNP; KAREN LUTHER WIKOFF, RN, PHD; AND SARA SWETT, RN, BSN, MSN

> *The behavior of leaders must exemplify their commitment to sustain their own journey and to coordinate and facilitate the efforts of others to build a desired future.*
>
> —PORTER-O'GRADY & MALLOCH, 2011

OBJECTIVES

Upon completion of this chapter, the reader should be able to:

1. Define culture.
2. Discuss cultural competence.
3. Identify key cultural nursing theories.
4. Discuss organizational culture.
5. Review strategies for working with a multicultural team.
6. Discuss generational differences.
7. Integrate understanding of spiritual beliefs into patient care.

Mr. Wu is brought into the emergency department with diaphoresis, nausea, and vomiting, and he is clutching his left chest. He is speaking with his wife in Chinese and says he understands only a little English. His wife understands none. Fortunately, Charles Lin, a new nurse, is working this shift and is able to communicate in Chinese with the Wu family. How can Charles most effectively communicate Mr. Wu's concerns to the health care staff? If Charles was not working, how could the other staff communicate with Mr. Wu?

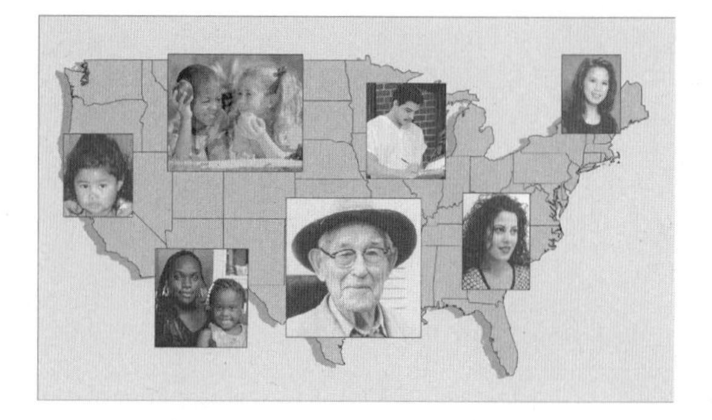

© Cengage Learning 2014

We live in a global society rich with different and ever-changing cultures, traditions, religions, spiritual beliefs, and generations, all of which influence the delivery of patient-centered care. New immigrants arrive daily. Consideration of all of these differences and sensitivity to patient and health care staff diversity are necessary in all nursing roles as situations arise that call for evaluating patient and staff behavior. Though each person is first and foremost an individual, each is also a member of a cultural group. Clues to people's behaviors come from understanding the cultural, generational, and spiritual focus of the individual or group. Nurses and other health care professionals need to recognize, respect, and be able to work and care for all in a culturally and spiritually competent manner. This chapter will enable the nurse to begin to prepare for cultural, organizational, generational, and spiritual aspects of leadership and management with patients and the inter-professional health care staff.

CULTURE

Culture can be defined as "the integrated lifestyle, the learned and shared beliefs, values, world views, knowledge, artifacts, rules, and symbols that guide behavior of a particular group of people" (Racher & Annis, 2007, p. 256). Although people from all cultures share most human characteristics, the study of culture highlights both the way individuals differ and are similar to individuals in other cultures. Individuals from different cultures may think, solve problems, and perceive and structure the world differently from individuals of another culture. Cultural beliefs serve as a conscious and unconscious point of reference that guides the outlook and decisions of people. Culture incorporates the experience of the past and influences the present. It transmits traditions to future members of a culture. Culture "explains patterns of thought and action, and it contributes to the group's social and physical survival" (Racher & Annis, 2007, p. 256).

Normally, children learn about their culture while growing up. However, when people emigrate from their native cultures into a new culture, they often experience culture shock. **Culture shock** is when the values and beliefs upheld by a person's new culture are radically different from the person's native culture. For successful assimilation into a new culture, immigrants may want to learn that culture's important values.

In addition to belonging to a major cultural group, people also belong to a variety of subcultures, or smaller groups within a culture. Each culture has its own value system and related expectations. Subcultures may be based on the following:

- Professional and occupational affiliations (RNs)
- Nationality or race (a shared historical and political past)
- Age groups (adolescents, senior citizens)
- Gender (women's, men's groups)
- Socioeconomic factors (working class, middle class, upper class)
- Political viewpoints (Democrat, Republican)
- Sexual orientation (gay and lesbian groups)

Upon admission to a hospital, home health care agency, or even a private medical practice, patients also become members of a culture. In this world filled with strange health care sights, unfamiliar sounds, and strangers, many patients experience culture shock. The unknowns related to being a consumer of health care become even more complex and stressful when a person is not originally from the United States and does not speak English as a first language (Munoz & Luckmann, 2005; Racher & Annis, 2007).

Race and Ethnicity

Race describes a geographical or global human population distinguished by genetic traits and physical characteristics such as skin color or facial features. Major U.S. Census classifications of race are American Indian, Asian, Black or African American, Pacific Islander/Hawaiian, or White, as shown in Figure 16-1. Cultural ethnicity identifies a person or group based on a racial, tribal, linguistic, religious, national, or cultural group, for example, Jewish or Irish. In years past, when new immigrants arrived in the United States, they sought to become acculturated to their new country by adopting the conditions, language, and customs of the United States. Acculturation has taken a generation or two in the past and often resulted in the loss of a separate cultural identity. Today's immigrant population is more likely to maintain a strong tradition of valuing their historical cultural identity.

Health Care Disparity

Because of differences in cultural beliefs, there is often the **marginalization** or separation of some cultural groups away from the mainstream. According to the Office of Minority Health and Health Disparities (OMHD, 2010), correlations can be made between race and/or ethnicity and increased mortality and morbidity. Differences in health risks and health status measures that reflect the poorer health status that is found disproportionately in certain population groups are referred to as "health disparities." OMHD notes that race and ethnicity correlate with continual, and often escalating, health disparities among residents of the United States (2010). Although there has been significant improvement in the general health of the United States, ongoing disparities in morbidity and mortality are experienced by African Americans, Hispanics, American Indians, Alaska Natives, Native Hawaiians, and other Pacific Islanders compared to the entire U.S. population (2010). For example:

- The death rate in 2006 for the black population surpassed that of the white population by 48 percent for cerebrovascular disease, 31 percent for heart disease, 21 percent for malignant

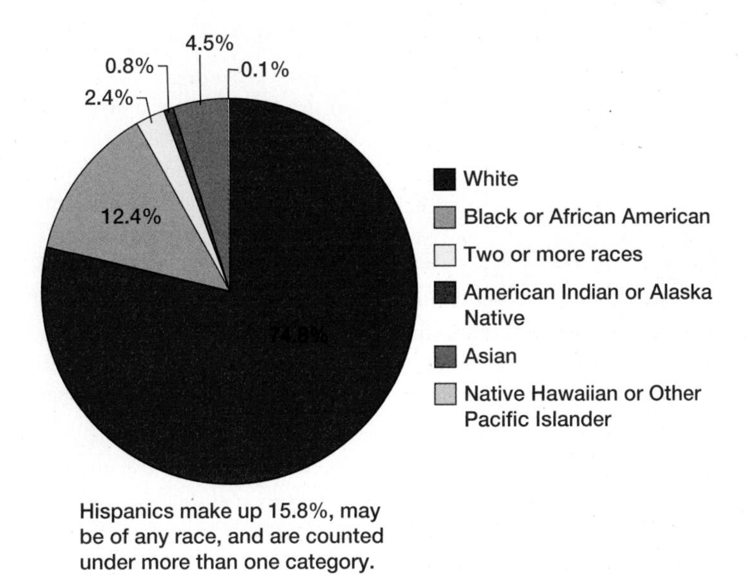

FIGURE 16-1

2007 Estimate of the U.S. Population by race.

(*Source:* U.S. Census Bureau, 2009 American Community survey.)

neoplasms, 113 percent for diabetes, and 786 percent for HIV disease (Centers for Disease Control (CDC), 2009).
- The infant mortality rates in 2005 were highest among babies born to non-Hispanic black mothers (13.63 deaths per 1,000 live births), American Indian or Alaska Native mothers (8.06 per 1,000), and Puerto Rican mothers (8.30 per 1,000) (CDC, 2009). These increased rates may be due to a lack of health care access, inadequate financial resources, immigrant resident status, or a lack of knowledge of how to seek help.

According to the U.S. Census Bureau (2011), 30 percent of Native Americans live below the poverty line, compared with 29.5 percent of Blacks, 25.3 percent of Hispanics, 14.1 percent of Asian/Pacific Islanders, and 9.8 percent of Whites. Also, Native Americans have the lowest life expectancy of any ethnic group in the United States. Native Americans can expect to live only two-thirds as long as other people in the United States (Wikoff, 2008).

The life expectancy gap between African Americans and Caucasians is 5.6 years, with the average life expectancy being 75.2 years for Caucasians and 69.6 years for African Americans. The infant death rate for African Americans is twice that of Caucasians (Nies & McEwen, 2007).

Note that concern for quality care must focus not only on ethnic minorities and populations that have a different heritage than Euro-Americans, but also on the needs of other marginalized populations. Examples of other marginalized populations may include gays and lesbians, older adults, recently arrived immigrants (e.g., from South America or Rwanda), as well as groups that have been in this country for some time (e.g., people from China and the Middle East). These populations are often less visible than federally defined minorities (Lenburg et al., 1995).

Diversity in Nursing

While most nurses are Caucasian women, increasing numbers of minority students are graduating from nursing programs. The American Association of Colleges of Nursing (AACN) has collected data on the race/ethnicity of students enrolled in baccalaureate programs since 2001 (2010). During the preceding nine-year period, Black or African Americans represented the largest minority group, with percentages ranging from 8.5 percent in 2001 to 10.9 percent in 2010. American Indians or Alaska Natives made up the lowest percentage with relatively no change in numbers during the nine-year span (0.5% in 2001 and 0.6% in 2010).

Males are also considered a minority population in nursing. According to AACN (2011), "though men only comprise 6.2 percent of the nation's nursing workforce, this percentage has steadily climbed since the National Sample Survey of Registered Nurses (NSSRN) was first conducted in 1980. The number of men in nursing has increased steadily from 45,060 in 1980 to 189,916 nurses in 2008" (AACN Fact Sheet, 2011, p.1).

Enrollment in undergraduate and graduate nursing programs reflects similar statistics relative to minority ethnic and gender groups. It is interesting to note, however, that African-American, Hispanic, and Asian nurses are much more likely to pursue baccalaureate and graduate degrees compared to nurses who are Caucasian.

Cultural Competence

Nurses providing patient-centered care need to ensure that the cultural needs of their patients are considered. **Culturally competent care** is a complex integration of knowledge, attitudes, and skills that enhances cross-cultural communication and appropriate and effective interactions (American Academy of Nursing, 1992). The goal of culturally competent nursing care is to provide care that is consistent with the patient's cultural needs. The AAN expert panel report (1992) on culturally competent nursing care suggested the following four principles:

- Care is designed for the specific patient.
- Care is based on the uniqueness of the person's culture and includes cultural norms and values.
- Care includes empowerment strategies to facilitate patient decision making in their personal health behavior.
- Care is provided with sensitivity to the cultural uniqueness of the patient.

Since the 1960s, a united effort has been underway to include concepts sensitive to cultural diversity in nursing education. The National League for Nursing (NLN) has made this requirement mandatory for accreditation. Additionally, the Transcultural Nursing Society has been certifying nurses in transcultural nursing since 1988.

A new nurse leader is often asked to work with people from different cultures. To manage and understand these cultures, cultural nursing theories and conceptual models offer direction, for example, Leininger's Transcultural Nursing (1978, 1997), Purnell's Model for Cultural Competence (2005), Campinha-Bacote's Process of Cultural Competence in the Delivery of Health Care Service (2003), Spector's Cultural Heritage Model (2005), and Giger and Davidhizar's Transcultural Assessment Model (2004). Purnell's Model for Cultural Competence is represented by a circle with rims moving from the global society to the community, to the family, and to the individual. The inner circle has 12 pie slices representing 12 domains of culture, that is, overview/heritage, communication, family roles and organization, workforce issues, biocultural ecology, high-risk behaviors, nutrition, pregnancy, death rituals, spirituality, health care practices, and health care practitioners. Analyzing the patient belief system in each of the 12 domains gives direction to the nursing process.

Nurses have opportunities to participate in continuing education to increase cultural competence. For example, the Office of Minority Health, U.S. Department of Health and Human Services, offers a free, online, continuing-education program entitled Culturally Competent Nursing Care: A Cornerstone of Caring, available at: https://ccnm.thinkculturalhealth.hhs.gov/.

These nursing journals will also assist with building your cultural competence:

- *The Journal of Transcultural Nursing*
- *Journal of Cultural Diversity*
- *International Journal of Nursing Studies*
- *International Nursing Review*
- *Journal of Holistic Nursing*

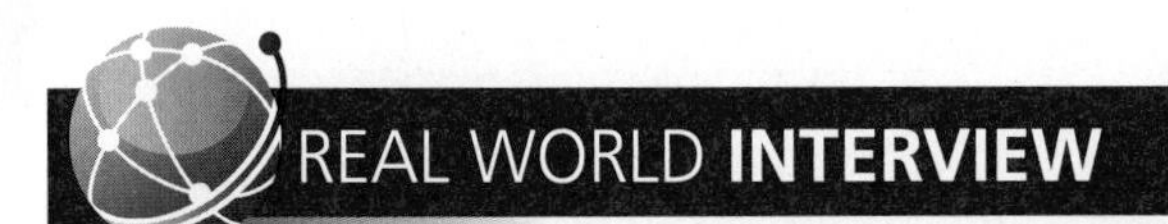

In the southern part of California, we have an under-representation of Hispanic nurses in our hospitals. To encourage and promote nursing enrollment, we have brought Hispanic nurses from Mexico to experience our health care system. They are provided with a hospital orientation of key programs in their areas of interest. They also spend time in the clinical area.

At the high school level, we have brought a group of about 30 high school students, the majority Hispanics, to the hospital. We talk to them about health care, nursing opportunities, and the need for Hispanic nursing staff.

As a nursing executive, I feel that it is important to be a role model for minority students. Recently, I participated in mock interviews for high school students. The majority of these students were Hispanic, Black, and Asian. We wanted to mentor and coach them on how to successfully interview for jobs. These are students without role models in their lives. Just seeing what other people have done creates a high sense of inspiration and desire to do better because they see that it is possible.

PABLO VELEZ, RN, PHD,
Chief Nursing Officer
Sharp Chula Vista Medical Center
Chula Vista, California

Language

As you work with patients, you will encounter a great diversity in both body language and spoken language. According to the U.S. Census Bureau American Community Survey (2007), 80 percent of the population over 5 years of age spoke only English at home. Of the 20 percent who spoke a language other than English, a total of 381 languages were counted. Sixty-two percent of those 55 million people spoke Spanish; 19 percent spoke another Indo-European language; 15 percent spoke an Asian/Pacific Island language; and 4 percent spoke another language.

Linguistically Appropriate Services

Any individual who is seeking health care services and who has limited English proficiency (LEP) has the right, based on Title VI of the Civil Rights Act of 1964, to have an interpreter available to facilitate communication within the health care system. Open and clear communication is essential to develop appropriate diagnosis, treatments, and to ensure safety.

Unfortunately, use of family members or friends as interpreters is convenient and continues to be common practice in some health care settings. This practice is discouraged and can be acceptable only when the patient expresses the preference to have a family member or friend be the interpreter. Clearly, situations may arise in which a formally trained interpreter is unavailable and the use of a telephone interpretation service is not practical; family members may then be used with permission from the patient. Although telephone interpreter services are permissible, the use of a face-to-face in-person interpretation is desirable, acceptable, and appropriate.

Health care organizations are expected to make known to all their patients and families the availability of interpreter services at no cost to the patient. Information about available bilingual staff can also help patients access these services. For more information, see the National Standards for Culturally and Linguistically Appropriate Service in Health Care, 2007, available at http://minorityhealth.hhs.gov/templates/browse.aspx?lvl=2&lvlID=15.

The Institute of Medicine describes "patient-centered care" as providing health care in a manner that creates and maintains a partnership between inter-professional health care practitioners and their

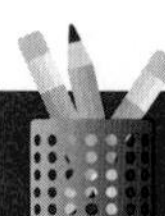

CASE STUDY 16-1

Following are different levels of response you might have toward a person.

Levels of Response:

- *Greet:* I feel I can greet this person warmly and welcome him or her sincerely.
- *Accept:* I feel I can honestly accept this person as he or she is and be comfortable enough to listen to his or her problems.
- *Help:* I feel I would genuinely try to help this person with his or her problems as they might be related to or arise from the label or stereotype given to him or her.
- *Background:* I feel I have the background of knowledge and experience to be able to help this person.
- *Advocate:* I feel I could honestly be an advocate for this person.

The following is a list of individuals. Read down the list and place a check mark by anyone you would not greet or would hesitate to greet. Then move to response level 2, Accept; follow the same procedure for all five response levels. Try to respond honestly, not as you think might be socially or professionally desirable. Your answers are only for your personal use in clarifying your initial reactions to different people. How did you do?

(*Continues*)

CASE STUDY 16-1 (Continued)

Individual	1 Greet	2 Accept	3 Help	4 Background	5 Advocate
1. White Anglo-Saxon American					
2. Hispanic American					
3. Black African American					
4. Native American					
5. Asian American					
6. Filipino American					
7. Chinese American					
8. Pacific Islander American					
9. Jewish American					
10. Iranian American					
11. Muslim American					
12. Amish American					
13. Gay/Lesbian American					
14. Catholic American					
15. Jehovah's Witness American					
16. Protestant American					
17. Male Nurse					
18. Female Nurse					
19. Older Nurse					
20. Young Nurse					
21. Elderly American					
22. American with AIDS					
23. Unmarried Expectant Teen					
24. Obese American					
25. Alcoholic					

Source: Compiled with information from Munoz, C., & Luckmann, J. (2005). *Transcultural Communication.* Clifton Park, NY: Delmar Cengage Learning.

patients as well as the patient's families and others involved in that person's care (2001). This sense of teamwork is created to help ensure that patients' values and preferences are not only respected but also based on relevant support to aid the patients in, as fully as possible, participating in their own care. Patient-centered care becomes particularly relevant when addressing the needs of patients from backgrounds differing from those of the health care professional providing care (Table 16-1). Many professions, including nursing, have responded to this need by heeding the call of the Institute of Medicine

TABLE 16-1
Cultural Norms, Health Care Beliefs, and Religious Beliefs*

Cultural Group	Cultural Norms	Health Care Beliefs	Religious Beliefs
Hispanics	◆ Maintaining eye contact is valued. ◆ A pat on the back or arm is considered friendly. ◆ Treating others with respect is valued. ◆ Cakes and sweets may be a regular part of the diet. ◆ Children are highly valued and loved. ◆ May have different perception of time; e.g., may have a problem being on time for appointments.	◆ Fatalistic and may view illness as a punishment from God. ◆ View health as the ability to rise in the morning and go to work. ◆ May or may not follow medical advice. ◆ May consult a folk healer, e.g., *curandero*. ◆ Will use Western medications but may stop when they feel they can no longer afford it.	◆ Are often Roman Catholic but may be member of other Christian group; may light candles, attend Mass, pray to God, Jesus, the Virgin Mary, and saints. ◆ Traditional men view religion as a preoccupation of women. ◆ May have statues of saints at home.
Muslims	◆ Have modest lifestyles for both men and women. Women wear loose-fitting clothing that includes a head covering such as a *hijab*. ◆ Immediate and extended family needs are very important, often above the needs of the individual.	◆ Often have a fatalistic view of health. ◆ Disease is often viewed as "God's will," a test of an individual's conviction, or as retribution for transgressions. ◆ Due to issues of modesty, having a health care provider and interpreter of the same sex is generally preferred.	◆ Pray daily. While praying, often face southeast towards Mecca. ◆ Have a restrictive diet similar to that of Orthodox Judaism. ◆ Believe the Koran to be the book of divine guidance and direction for humanity and consider the text in its original Arabic to be the literal word of God (Rahman, 2009).
Black and African Americans	◆ Have tradition of involving many in raising children. ◆ Many households are headed by women. ◆ May be frank and direct in speech. ◆ Unrelated persons often live in the home.	◆ Often distrust or have discomfort with majority group and health care system. ◆ May be private about their health and may not want family members present during care or treatment.	◆ Are heavily involved in church religious groups. ◆ Black minister is strong influence in community. ◆ May use faith healers or herbalists.

TABLE 16-1 (Continued)

Cultural Group	Cultural Norms	Health Care Beliefs	Religious Beliefs
Black and African Americans	◆ High incidence of poverty. ◆ Oriented to the present.	◆ May try self-care first and use all forms of pharmacological and some nonpharmacological alternatives and complementary medicines prior to seeking care. ◆ May view health as being in harmony with nature, and view illness as disharmony. ◆ Some have fatalistic attitude about illness.	◆ Are active in singing and praying. ◆ Illness is between the individual and God; illness may be viewed as punishment from God. May see illness as the will of God.
Asians	◆ Work hard, have respect for elders and nature, have esteem for self-control and loyalty to all family and extended family. ◆ Are traditionally patriarchal. ◆ Have respect for elders.	◆ Prefer a same-sex health care practitioner. ◆ Often expect health care to include an injection or prescription. ◆ May not make important decisions without checking with an astrologer or almanac for a lucky day. ◆ May not consider shaking hands to be polite. ◆ Submissive to authority. ◆ Pride and honor are extremely important.	◆ Have broad group of practices from Christianity to Buddhism, Taoism, ancestor worship, Muslim, and many others, depending on the geographic area. ◆ Prayer and offerings are dominant in many groups. ◆ May use faith healers or herbalists.
Pacific Islanders	◆ May ascribe to a holistic world view—interconnectedness of family, environment, self, and spiritual world. ◆ Family and community play an important role and often live in close proximity or tightly knit communities.	◆ Often distrust Western style of health care. Rarely respond positively to health education and treatment based on scare tactics. ◆ Stoic; do not complain.	◆ Have deeply rooted spiritual connections. ◆ Hold belief in unity, balance, and harmony. ◆ Use traditional healers. ◆ Some may be Christian.

(Continues)

TABLE 16-1 (Continued)

Cultural Group	Cultural Norms	Health Care Beliefs	Religious Beliefs
Pacific Islanders	◆ Interpersonal and social behavior is based on mutual respect and sharing.	◆ May use Western medication but choose over-the-counter drugs for minor ailments. ◆ Massage is a method to achieve harmony.	
Native Americans	◆ Family and tribal affiliations are part of daily life. ◆ May have extended family structure and live with relatives from both sides of the family. ◆ Have a holistic view of life and health. ◆ Often suffer from poverty, poor nutrition, and inadequate access to health care. ◆ May avoid eye contact. ◆ Elders often assume leadership role. ◆ Share goods with others. ◆ Cooperate with others. ◆ Work for good of the group.	◆ Physical illness may be due to violation of a taboo or being out of harmony. ◆ Skeptical regarding the benefit and habit-forming properties of medications. ◆ Holistic orientation to health. ◆ May wait to see Western practitioner until seen by a healer. ◆ Oriented to the present. ◆ Accept nature rather than try to control nature.	◆ Religion or spiritual affiliation is based on personal choice. ◆ May have Christian beliefs and traditional beliefs. ◆ Have spiritual orientation. ◆ May fear witchcraft as cause of illness and use a medicine bag received from a healer, which should be kept with the patient at all times. ◆ May carry object at all times to guard against witchcraft.

* The information presented is from multiple sources and is meant to serve as a starting point to understanding. All people are individuals and these norms and beliefs may not be valid for all within a cultural group identified in the table.

Source: Compiled with information from: The Provider's Guide to Quality and Culture. Retrieved October 11, 2012, from http://erc.msh.org/mainpage.cfm?file=1.0.htm&module=provider&language=English; Lipson, J. G., & Dibble, S. L. (2005). *Culture and Clinical Care.* San Francisco, CA: UCSF Nursing Press; and Muñoz, C., & Luckmann, J. (2005). *Transcultural Communication in Nursing* (2nd ed.). Clifton, NY: Delmar Cengage Learning.

and other organizations to collaborate from an interdisciplinary focus in order to capitalize on multiple perspectives and expertise when addressing the potentially complex issues of patients and/or their families. The goal of this collaboration is to prevent disease but also to function as holistically, effectively, and efficiently as possible (Interprofessional Education Collaborative Expert Panel, 2011).

Organizational Culture

Organizational culture is the system of shared values and beliefs that actively influences the behavior of organization members. The term "shared values" is important because it implies that many people are guided by the same values and that they interpret them in the same way. Values develop over time and reflect an organization's history and traditions. Culture consists of the culture of an organization, such as being helpful and supportive toward new members.

Five dimensions of organizational culture are of major significance in influencing organizational culture (Ott, 1989):

- *Values:* Values are the foundation of any organizational culture. The organization's philosophy is expressed through values, and values guide behavior on a day-to-day basis.
- *Relative diversity:* The existence of an organizational culture assumes some degree of similarity. Nevertheless, organizations differ in how much deviation can be tolerated.
- *Resource allocation and reward:* The allocation of money and other resources has a critical influence on culture. The investment of resources sends a message to people about what is valued in the organization.
- *Degree of change:* A fast-paced, dynamic organization has a culture different from that of a slow-paced, stable one. Top-level managers, by the energy or lethargy of their stance, send messages about how much they welcome innovation.
- *Strength of the culture:* The strength of a culture, or how much influence it exerts, is partially a by-product of the other dimensions. A strong culture guides employees in many everyday actions. It determines, for example, whether employees will

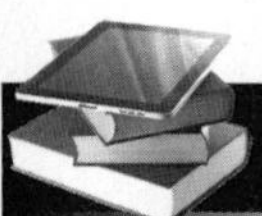

EVIDENCE FROM THE **LITERATURE**

Citation: DeRosa, N., & Kochurka, K. (2006, October). Implement culturally competent health care in your workplace. *Nursing Management, 37*(10), 18–26.

Discussion: This article discusses selected verbal and nonverbal communication patterns of culture. Even when two people speak the same language, communication may be hindered by different values or beliefs. Nonverbal differences or ethnic dialects can also block mutual understanding. Communication differences include the following:

- *Conversational style:* Silence may show respect or acknowledgment. In some cultures, a direct "no" is considered rude, and silence may mean "no." A loud voice or repeating a statement may mean anger or simply emphasis, enthusiasm, or a request for help.
- *Personal space:* Beliefs about personal space vary. Someone may be viewed as aggressive for standing "too close" or as "distant" for backing off when approached.
- *Eye contact:* In some cultures, direct eye contact may be a sign of respect. In other cultures, direct eye contact may be seen as a sign of disrespect.
- *Subject matter and conversation length:* Even what constitutes an appropriate subject matter, when it's appropriate to discuss certain ideas, and how long the discussion should last may vary from culture to culture. Some cultures value communication that's subtle and circumspect; forthright discussion is considered rude. In some cultures, it's acceptable to discuss topics such as sexuality and death, whereas in other cultures, these topics are taboo.

The article also discusses elements of a cultural assessment, including nutrition, medications, pain, and psychological and primary language assessment. It also explores how to approach the patient with educational needs.

Implications for Practice: Be aware of these cultural differences when working with patients and staff from other cultures. Remember that not everyone sees things the way that you do.

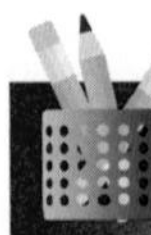

CASE STUDY 16-2

Mrs. P was recently admitted with exacerbated chronic obstructive pulmonary disease (COPD); she recently turned 81. Her prognosis is good; however, it is likely she will return home with the need for oxygen. Because all her family lives out of town, she is often alone in her room for extended periods of time. She lives alone in an apartment she has had since her husband passed away 25 years ago. She has volunteered in a nearby elementary school for years, but assumes she will not be able to continue with this once on continuous oxygen therapy. She is pleasant and likes to talk with staff about her career as a nurse during World War II. This is her first hospitalization since having a hysterectomy 30 years ago and she reflects often on how much things have changed since then. She is scheduled to be discharged in three days but is becoming increasingly anxious. The social worker who is helping coordinate her discharge has stated in her notes that Mrs. P is reluctant to share the cause of her emotional distress. The majority of nurses as well as the social work team caring for Mrs. P are from Generation Y and X. Is it possible for any of them to adequately address the concerns Mrs. P might have?

If the cause of Mrs. P's increasing anxiety is related to returning home alone, are there options for her to consider as an alternative?

In light of the generation from which Mrs. P was born, what are the potential causes of her increasing anxiety that would specifically come from her being 81?

inconvenience themselves to satisfy a patient. If the culture is not so strong, employees are more likely to follow their own whims, that is, they may decide to please patients only when convenient for them.

Each organization will have embedded in its environment the dos and don'ts that are specific to its workplace. When beginning in a new organization, observe and ask questions to learn about the organization and culture and how decisions are made (Table 16-2).

TABLE 16-2
Questions to Ask When Assessing Organizational Culture

- Are the organization's values consistent with your values?
- What cultures, ages, and genders are represented on the work team? How are members of these cultures similar? How are they different?
- Is the organization or the department centralized or decentralized?
- What is the formal chain of command?
- What is the informal chain of command?
- Do individuals participate in changing policies or procedures?
- What are the rules about how things should be done?
- Where does one take new ideas or suggestions?
- Are risk and change encouraged?
- How are individuals rewarded for quality improvement, or are all rewards oriented primarily toward the total group?
- Does the team work well together?

© Cengage Learning 2014

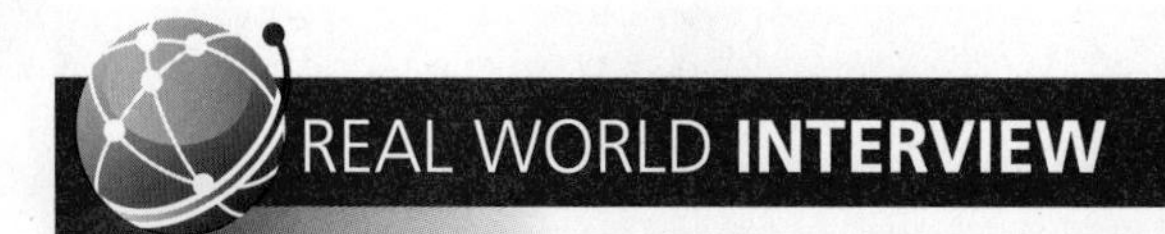

The culture of an organization is crucial to its adaptability that the ever-changing regulatory health care system demands. I have discovered working with a variety of institutions, that the clearer and more cohesive the values are among the members of the organization, the stronger they are as a culture. With that, they are also more able to adapt to needed and/or desired change.

CHRIS JOHNS, RHIT
Consultant
Quality Health Services

Organizational Socialization

As a new member of a team or a collaborative workgroup, it is important to be socialized into the organization. Socialization is beneficial to the organization when employees are a good fit, that is, employees have a high commitment to the organization, little intention to leave, high levels of job satisfaction, and little work-related stress. Things to consider when entering a new work environment in any culture are the organizational behavior style for greetings, titles, punctuality, body language, and dress (Table 16-3).

Most organizations have a workplace culture that has a strong mission and vision, and members work tirelessly to ensure the organization's success. However, some organizations can only be described as toxic. In these organizations, the staff and/or leadership are dysfunctional. Instead of problem solving, the goal of these organizations is finding fault and placing blame. This dysfunctional, toxic environment may be a unit within a hospital or the entire organization. Choosing your workplace environment wisely will make your work life more satisfying.

Working with Staff from Different Cultures

Staff nurses from different cultures may have different perceptions of staff and nursing roles in patient care, a different perception of their own locus of control, a different time orientation, and may speak a different language.

Different Perceptions of Staff Responsibilities

Cultural values deeply influence whether a person values the rights of the individual more or values the rights of the collective group more. Individualism emphasizes the importance of individual rights and rewards. Collectivism emphasizes the importance of the group's rights and rewards. Staff educated in Western culture may place more value on individualism and independence. These staff may complain to their supervisor if they feel assignments are unfair or involve menial work. Assertive behavior that is consistent with values of equitable work distribution and respect for education and professionalism usually defines the American work style. Staff members from other cultures that emphasize collective group rights tend to accept such assignments without complaint. Ensuring harmony, teamwork, and commitment to group loyalty may be more important to them.

American-educated nurses tend to value individuality and personal achievement as well as to demonstrate much more assertive behavior, particularly in relation to fair work conditions, compared to nurses educated, for example, in Europe or Eastern cultures (Andrews, 2008).

Different Perceptions of the Nurse's Role

Nurses from other cultures have different perceptions of the nurse's role and nursing care values, which American nurses may not appreciate. For example, in a study of Filipino American nurses, the most important

TABLE 16-3
United States Organizational Behavioral Styles

Concepts	Things to Consider
Greetings	◆ Americans usually acknowledge each other with a smile, nod of the head, and/or verbal greeting, such as "Hello," or "Hi." ◆ When greeting someone in a business situation, a firm handshake is appropriate, such as when greeting a manager of nursing or a recruiter from human resources.
Titles	◆ When introducing yourself, give your first name and your last name, e.g., "I am Susan Clover, a registered nurse, and I will be caring for you until 7 P.M." ◆ Use the appropriate title the first time you address an individual, such as Mrs., Dr., Ms., or Mr. Wear a badge with your full name and title of RN prominently displayed. ◆ Wait to be directed to call a person by his or her first name. Expect the same respect for yourself.
Time	◆ Punctuality is highly respected in nursing. Be on time to interview appointments and work.
Body language	◆ Use of direct eye contact is expected in all work situations and when working with patients. However, some people may not respond to direct eye contact, depending on their culture. ◆ In conversation, it is important to keep approximately one arm's length of distance from the speaker; closer proximity is considered rude in some cultures.
Dress	◆ When in doubt, wear business attire for interviews, that is, a professional suit. For your work environment, ask what the traditional dress is for a particular work area or nursing unit before starting a new job or purchasing new uniforms. ◆ Even in areas where daily dress is more casual, business situations and clinical work settings require professional dress. Avoid uniforms that cover you in cartoons if you expect professional respect.

© Cengage Learning 2014

finding was the theme of obligation to care that prevailed in all aspects of their work (Spangler, 1992). This theme reflected the Filipino American nurses' strong belief that bedside nursing is truly the core of nursing. This value conflicted with the attitude of some American nurses that the physical care of patients is devalued work with low prestige and should therefore be delegated to ancillary personnel (Spangler, 1992).

Differences in Locus of Control: Locus of control refers to the degree of control that individuals feel that they have over events. People who feel in control of their environment have an internal locus of control. People who believe that luck, fate, or chance control their lives have an external locus of control.

Health care providers who are trained in the United States often have an internal locus of control. American medical and nursing practitioners often feel that it is their duty to diagnose disorders, plan interventions, carry out procedures, and do everything possible to save the patient's life.

Conversely, health care providers from other cultures that promote an external locus of control (e.g., some Mexican Americans, Appalachians, and Puerto

CRITICAL THINKING 16-1

In today's diverse workplace, you will work closely with various nursing and medical practitioners and ancillary personnel who are from different cultures and who speak English as a second language. How do you feel about working with practitioners who are from foreign countries, or from different racial or ethnic groups? Take a minute to answer the following questions. You do not need to share your answers with anyone, so be honest with yourself. Self-awareness is an important step in building cultural competence.

	Agree	Neutral	Disagree
I would rather work with an American nurse than a foreign nurse.			
I find it frustrating to work with medical and nursing practitioners who are not proficient in English.			
If I thought that a medical or nursing practitioner was not fulfilling duties because of cultural or language problems, I would hesitate to report the person for fear that I would be considered prejudiced.			
I enjoy working with a skilled foreign nurse. I feel that I can learn a lot from this person.			
I like to attend classes and informal meetings where I can learn more about how nurses from other countries are educated.			
I do not feel prepared to work with or supervise a nursing assistive worker who has some problems with understanding English.			
Responsible adults prepare for the future and strive to influence events in their lives.			
Intelligent people use their time wisely and are punctual.			
It is disrespectful to address people by their first name unless they give you permission to do so.			
It is rude and intrusive to obtain information by asking direct questions.			

Source: Compiled with information from Munoz, C., & Luckmann, J. (2005). *Transcultural Communication.* Clifton Park, NY: Delmar Cengage Learning.

Ricans) may have a more fatalistic attitude toward their patients and thus feel that they cannot control matters of life and death. For example, when a patient who is expected to die does die on the operating room table, care providers with an external locus of control may be puzzled when hospital administration asks for a quality indicator review of the case (Giger & Davidhizar, 1996). Finally, some American Indians, Chinese Americans, and Japanese Americans believe themselves to be in harmony with nature rather than being controlled by nature or in control of nature (Giger & Davidhizar, 1996).

Differences in Time Orientation: Cultural groups are either past, present, or future oriented. Americans generally value the future over the present. The differences in time values are often related to differences in values, religious beliefs, and variation in the perception and meaning of work (Andrews, 2008). Southern Blacks and Puerto Ricans value the present over the future. Southern Appalachians, traditional Chinese Americans, and Mexican Americans value the present (Munoz & Luckmann, 2005). Many Asian cultures value the past (Munoz, 2009).

The ways in which different cultural groups value time can create challenges in the health care workplace. For example, staff meetings are influenced by the time orientation of staff members (Figure 16-2). Staff members who are meeting to plan for the future may become annoyed with members who want to spend all of the time on present-day problems and issues.

Educational and Language Differences: Foreign nurses are educated differently from American nurses. Generally, nursing education outside of the United States is less theory oriented, focusing primarily on the development of clinical skills. Also, there is less emphasis on meeting the psychosocial needs of patients.

Language differences also raise the potential for serious miscommunications between health care providers and patients. Today, large medical centers in the United States may be primarily staffed by nurses and practitioners for whom English is a second language. For example, in urban medical centers on the East Coast, it is not unusual to hear a Filipino nurse and a Haitian nurse attempting to communicate with a resident practitioner who has been educated in India. Unless these caregivers take the time to clarify their communications, serious errors may result. The potential for miscommunication exists (especially over the telephone) unless careful and specific attention is paid to ensuring respectful, culturally competent, and verified communication (Munoz & Luckmann, 2005; Andrews, 2008) (Figure 16-2).

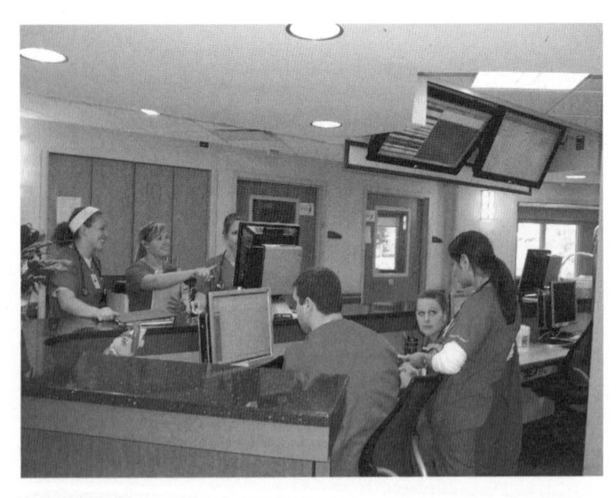

FIGURE 16-2

Appreciating the background of fellow employees can enhance the work environment.

© Cengage Learning 2014

Improving Communication on the Team

If you are working with a coworker from a different culture who speaks English as a second language, try these techniques to facilitate communication:

- Recognize that your coworker probably has an educational background in nursing that is very different from your own.
- Acknowledge that the coworker's value system and perception of what constitutes good patient care may differ from your own.
- Clarify your coworker's level of understanding of verbal and written communication.
- Avoid the use of slang terms and regional expressions. For example, Chinese, Japanese, and Filipino nurses may not understand such terms as "piggybacking," "doing a double," or "rigging" something to work.
- Provide your coworker with resources such as written procedures and protocols that may help to reinforce your verbal communication.
- Remember to praise your coworker's competency in technical skills. Inspiring self-confidence in a foreign nurse will make it easier for that person to ask for assistance when needed.
- Appreciate the knowledge that you can gain by working alongside a skilled nurse from another culture. Observe how foreign nurses relate to patients who are from their culture. If you have an open mind, working with foreign coworkers can increase your knowledge of other cultures, enrich your work as a nurse, and foster personal growth.
- When offering constructive criticism, try to use "I" statements instead of "you" statements. For

example: "I think that it's very important to address the patient's emotional state when you chart" is better than "You never seem to chart anything about the patient's emotional state."

- If you feel you cannot achieve effective communication with a coworker, request to work with another person. You do not want to be held accountable for the actions of a nurse with whom you cannot communicate.
- Delegate only appropriate tasks to an unlicensed worker. Match assignments to the worker's level of understanding and skill.
- Do not stop at just delegating an assignment or giving instructions. Instead, make sure that the worker understands your instructions.
- To reduce miscommunication, check for understanding by asking the worker to repeat instructions or do a return demonstration.
- Report to your supervisor if you feel that a nurse or a practitioner is endangering patients because of language difficulties or different cultural values. Record any problems that occur, and keep a copy of the notes you provide to your supervisor.
- Do not take verbal orders, particularly over the telephone. Even when an order is written, take the time to clarify the order with the practitioner. Because patients may also find it difficult to understand a foreign practitioner, you may need to listen carefully and then explain the practitioner's remarks to the patient.

Managerial Responsibility

Nurse managers may use the following approaches to improve communication:

- Plan informal meetings for nurses to discuss their cultural values. For example, it may benefit Asian nurses to share with American-born nurses their cultural values concerning respect for authority.
- Provide cultural workshops, and ask knowledgeable individuals to present information about the values, behaviors, and communication patterns of the different cultural groups that are represented on staff.
- Provide classes in English as a second language for foreign nurses who do not speak fluent English or who have difficulty pronouncing words.
- Establish a program for orienting foreign nurses to the hospital or agency. The orientation program should be designed to help newcomers adjust to the new work environment. It is helpful to assign each new nurse to a preceptor who is a member of the nurse's cultural group. For maximum benefits, the nurse manager should interview each new nurse every week to find out how that person is adapting to the new hospital culture (Williams & Rodgers, 1993).
- Plan events at which nurses, practitioners, and other staff members can socialize and discuss cultural differences informally, in a relaxed environment. For example, each unit in the hospital might plan one potluck event for each shift on a monthly basis. Potluck meals could be planned around a cultural theme, for instance, a traditional Vietnamese dinner one month and a traditional Costa Rican meal the next month (Burner, Cunningham, & Hattar, 1990).
- Confer with specialists in transcultural communication; also hire experts to identify potential areas of conflict and resolve conflicts peacefully before they erupt into legal battles (Munoz & Luckmann, 2005).

GENERATIONAL PERCEPTIONS

Different perceptions and values are created as each generation deals with the experiences of their lives as they are altered by the changing times. A **generation** is a group that shares birth years, age, location, and significant life events (Kupperschmidt, 2000). A generation is approximately 15 to 20 years in length and has a different value system from the preceding generation and later generations. Like culture, we take our generational differences with us into patient care and the work environment. We often assume that those around us are like us and think like us. This is not always true.

Four distinct generations make up the current patient and workforce population. These generations are the Traditional Generation, born before 1940; the Baby Boomers, born between 1940 and 1960; Generation X, born between 1960 and 1980; and the newest generation to hit the workforce, Generation Y (Echo Boomers or Millennials), those born after 1980.

The Traditional Generation came of age after the Great Depression and were raised to be disciplined and obey their elders. They feel obligated to conform and believe that work is one's duty. The Traditional Generation was followed by the Baby Boomers, who came of age during a time of much available education and economic expansion. They work for the challenge of work and career advancement (Calhoun & Strasser, 2005). Baby Boomers have been characterized as workaholic, strong-willed individuals who are working for material gain, promotions, recognition, job security, and corner offices. Baby Boomers are the largest generation. They have had a dramatic financial impact on the present and will continue to impact the future dramatically, as they began to retire in 2006.

The Generation Xers are often called "latchkey kids," as their parents were often away working.

Generation Yers are primarily the children of the Baby Boomers. They grew up with the end of the Cold War, the Internet, and a speak-your-mind philosophy. This generation is just beginning to make its mark on the workforce. What is known is that they are focusing on early retirement. Change is their mantra, and they expect countless options.

In the workplace, these generations all have different goals and needs.

Nursing leadership for this diverse group of workers requires a different management style and increased flexibility. The ACORN Model discussed by Kupperschmidt (2000) illustrates how a new leader can use opportunities to **A**ccommodate employee differences; **C**reate workplace choices; **O**perate from a theoretically sound, sophisticated management style; and nourish **R**etention of **N**urses. For example, when creating workplace choices, a nurse leader might devise multiple scheduling options and provide multiple opportunities for cross-training and lateral and upward movement through the organization. Each generation has different needs for orientation, training, and opportunities for advancement and benefits. An effective nurse leader draws from the skills and positive attributes of each of these different groups to function as a team.

SPIRITUALITY

Spirituality is an important area of assessment during hospitalization. The national health care accrediting body, the Joint Commission (JC), requires an assessment of spirituality, requiring nurses to ask patients some questions regarding their spiritual needs (Hodge, 2001). However, asking the questions, What is your religion? or What religious needs can we meet during your hospitalization? leaves the nurse with only descriptive labels. To meet the spiritual needs of patients, nurses need to understand more than these labels. The JC provides examples of spiritual assessment components that may be utilized by health care providers, including: the use of prayer, philosophy of life, the meaning of dying to the patient, and how faith has helped with the coping abilities of the patient (JC, 2008). Patients may be asked if they would like to see their spiritual leader or advisor, with the understanding that not all patients will want to meet with a clergy member. Nurses can use various resources available for providing spiritual support to patients. Many inpatient facilities have pastoral care departments that conduct formal services, visit and pray with patients and their families, conduct support groups (e.g., bereavement), and provide information regarding organ donation, living wills, and other end-of-life services (Duldt, 2002). Kuepfer, as cited in Ray (2004), addresses a shift in the duties of hospital chaplains from focusing mainly on providing religious rites to empowering the hospital staff members to serve the community.

Several research tools are used for measuring spirituality:

- *Spiritual Well-Being:* This tool measures the psychological dimension of spiritual wellness (Ellison & Paloutzain, 1999).

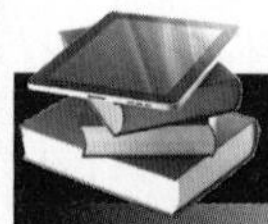

EVIDENCE FROM THE **LITERATURE**

Citation: Grossman, C. L. (2006, September 12). View of God can reveal your values and politics. *USA Today,* 1A.

Discussion: This article reports on the Baylor University religion survey of 1,721 Americans. The survey found that 91.8 percent of those surveyed say they believe in God, a higher power, or a cosmic force. The other respondents said they were atheists, did not answer, or were not sure. Respondents had four distinct views of God's personality, namely, Authoritarian, Benevolent, Critical, and Distant. The article discusses how these four views of God affect political issues, such as gay marriage, stem cell research, war, abortion, and federal government involvement in life and world affairs.

Implications for Practice: Many Americans believe in God, a higher power, or a cosmic force and may want assistance with their spiritual needs during times of illness and stress. Nurses can help patients obtain the assistance they need.

- *JAREL Spiritual Well-Being Scale:* This tool measures harmony as a function of interconnectedness (Hungelmann, Kenkel-Rossi, Klassen, & Stollenwerk, 1989).
- *Spiritual Perspective Scale:* This tool measures the extent to which one holds spiritual views during spirituality-related interactions (Reed, 1986).

For the nurse looking to understand spirituality in an effort to provide comfort to patients during illness or crisis, these tools provide some guidance.

Spiritual Distress

Spiritual distress is a North American Nursing Diagnosis Association (NANDA) term used to identify a condition in which an individual has an impaired ability to integrate meaning and purpose in life through the individual's connectedness with self, others, art, music, literature, nature, or a power greater than oneself (Ackley & Ladwig, 2006). To decrease or eliminate spiritual distress, it is expected that an individual will connect with the elements he or she considers important to arrive at meaning and purpose in life. These elements may include: meditation; prayer; participating in religious services or rituals; communing with nature, plants, and animals; sharing of self; and caring for self and others. The Wikoff (2003) Spiritual Focus Questionnaire (Table 16-4) is designed to ascertain what is spiritually important to the individual. It assesses the concepts of relationships with a higher power, self, others, nature, and religion. Each question can be scored on a 0–4 scale, arriving at a total score for each area of the questionnaire.

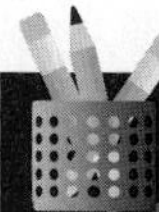

CASE STUDY **16-3**

Sally M. is a 28-year-old RN who has worked on the same critical care unit for five years. During the past three months, the unit has lost four staff who have yet to be replaced, resulting in significant overtime for everyone including Sally. In addition, acuity of the unit has remained high with an unusual number of admissions of young adults as well as deaths. It has been necessary for Sally to work three weekends in a row. She is feeling physically tired but is aware she is feeling emotionally tired as well and is worried she might be depressed.

Could Sally be spiritually distressed? Please discuss.

If this is spiritual distress, what are a few things Sally could do to help herself? What could Sally's manager do to help her as well as her colleagues best attend to their spiritual needs?

The tool is not designed to measure the strength or amount of spirituality; rather, the higher score(s) suggest(s) the concepts most important to the patient.

Reviewing the Spiritual Focus Questionnaire helps a nurse develop interventions to help patients. Nursing interventions for spiritual needs could include the nurse requesting a visit from a patient's spiritual leader or helping a patient obtain spiritual or religious tapes or music. The nurse can also offer the patient uninterrupted quiet time to allow him or her time for personal prayer, reading of spiritual and religious material, or meditation.

Championing Spirituality

The nurse leader who champions spirituality for all ensures that this component of holistic nursing is not forgotten or marginalized. Spirituality uses compassion, caring, and nurturing to create an environment that reflects the values and beliefs of the leaders, patients, staff, and organization. For example, an employee may request a Saturday or Sunday off every week to attend religious services. When nurses are needed to work every other weekend, this can pose a problem for the nurse leader. A possible solution is to pair two nurses, where one works every Saturday and the other works every Sunday. Both nurses are then able to meet their spiritual needs without a negative impact on staffing. The incorporation of spirituality and compassionate caring allows leaders and staff to acknowledge one's differences and function from a place of acting justly and professionally (Guglielmi, 2010).

Religious holidays or celebrations also have spiritual and cultural significance. An understanding and empathetic approach to vacation requests will help ensure contented staff and minimize turnover. It is also important to consider significant markers of life such as weddings, births, and deaths. There are many cultural and spiritual overtones to these life events that need to be respected by nursing leadership practices. Sensitivity to the spiritual practices of the staff will enable the nurse manager to provide compassionate and caring leadership.

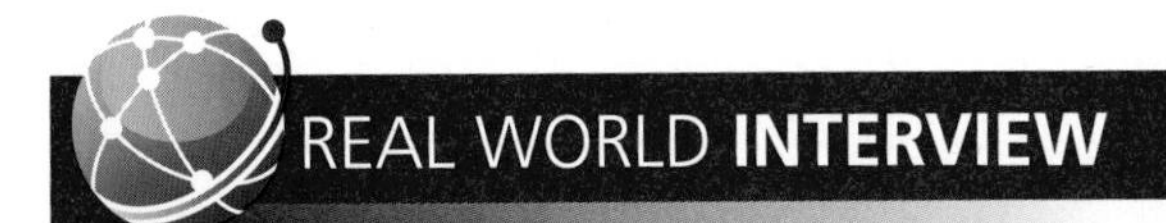

I believe spirituality is a part of everyone which influences how one sees oneself, others, and the world around them. It involves a knowing that leads to a sense of meaning and purpose. As such, the spiritual "health" of nurses and other health care professionals becomes an important factor in the ability to listen and communicate effectively as well as handle stress.

In my department, my nurses interact with patients, families, physicians, regulatory authorities, other nurses, as well as with me and the rest of our research staff. They witness the extremes of human emotion while needing to meet only the highest standards of nursing care and research. I believe I can make a difference with my nursing staff in their ability to cope with the stressors of their job by reinforcing the values of our department and practice as well as supporting each of them in their ability to balance their lives and find time to do the things which reinforce their personal purpose.

KAREN CALLAHAN, RN, BS
Manager, Department of Research
Hematology/Oncology Associates of Central New York

TABLE 16-4
Wikoff Spiritual Focus Questionnaire

Spiritual Focus Questionnaire Instructions: The following questions assess your expressions of spirituality. Please rate each question by checking the box indicating importance to you as 4=very important, 3=somewhat important, 2=not important, 1=very unimportant, 0=neither important nor unimportant.

Question	4	3	2	1	0
1. My strongest relationship is with a Higher Power.					
2. The time I spend in connection with a Higher Power is essential.					
3. In my personal life, I feel close to a Higher Power/Supreme Being.					
4. I spend time daily talking to a Higher Power.					
Higher Power Total Score					
5. I count on myself as my spiritual center.					
6. I feel an internal calmness when I am at peace with myself.					
7. My spirituality comes from within me.					
8. To find spiritual peace, I look inside myself.					
Self Total Score					
9. I renew my spirit with my family/friends.					
10. Special people within my life are my spiritual focus.					
11. When spiritually discouraged, I seek help from my family/ friends.					
12. Others around me help quiet my spirit.					
Others Total Score					
13. I make an effort to spend time in the quiet solitude of nature.					
14. In nature, I reflect on its magnitude and importance to me.					
15. My connection with natural things helps me find inner peace.					
16. When in nature, I feel thankful for my blessings.					
Nature Total Score					
17. Through my religion, I find inner calmness.					
18. My religion gives my life spiritual focus.					
19. The time I spend in religious activities renews my spirit.					
20. My religion helps me keep my life in perspective.					
Religion Total Score					
Overall Total					

Source: Wikoff, K. L. (2003). Development and psychometric evaluation of the Wikoff Spiritual Focus Questionnaire. Dissertation Abstracts International, 64 (04),1691. (UMI No. AAT 3088678).

KEY CONCEPTS

- Culture affects both the nursing staff and the patient.
- Cultural competence is an important component of nursing.
- Working on a multicultural team requires an understanding of culture.
- Some nursing theorists on culture include Leininger, Giger and Davidhizar, Campinha-Bacote, Purnell, and Spector.
- Organizations that nurses work in have distinct cultures.
- Each generation has different values, goals, and expected outcomes from its work and life experiences.
- Spirituality may include religion and reflects one's values and beliefs.
- Spiritual Assessment is a requisite of holistic nursing.
- Nurses need to be aware of their own spirituality and beliefs to feel comfortable in addressing the spiritual needs of others.

KEY TERMS

culture
culture shock
culturally competent care
generation
marginalization
race
spiritual distress

REVIEW QUESTIONS

1. Which of the following statements must be true for a multicultural team to work together successfully?
   A. Everyone should be focused on the same goals and objectives.
   B. All nurses should be from the same professional background.
   C. Everyone should have the same values about health care.
   D. Everyone in the United States should have the same beliefs because they all are living in the United States.
2. The Gen-X night-shift charge nurse is requesting more time off than any other charge nurse. What reason for this best represents this generation?
   A. Prefers to work the day shift and is hoping for a schedule change
   B. Believes that other nurses are just as capable of performing her role
   C. Wants to increase her leisure time to balance with work
   D. Seeks to be rewarded for time spent at work
3. During orientation to work on a new unit, a nurse experiences a sense of isolation from the preceptors. Which of the following actions will best increase the nurse's socialization into the preceptor group?
   A. Ask as many questions as possible
   B. Request that the orientation be increased for two more weeks
   C. Study the differences between the nurse's values and the preceptor group's values
   D. Arrive late for duty frequently
4. A nurse manager is discussing why she feels traditional generation nurses make good employees. Which statement by the nurse manager reflects those values?
   A. Value working as one's duty
   B. Reflect a speak-your-mind philosophy
   C. Value working primarily for the challenge
   D. Use the Internet daily as a part of one's life

5. The nurse is teaching an outpatient session on cultural awareness at a local church. As part of the assessment of the program, the nurse asks, "Can anyone give examples of subcultures?" Replies include age, socioeconomic status, sexual orientation, and first names. Which response shows additional teaching is necessary?
   A. Age
   B. Socioeconomic status
   C. Sexual orientation
   D. First names

6. A nurse manager is explaining to the staff the significance of discharge instructions and stressing the importance of identifying the patient's native language. A nurse asks why this is important because the hospital patient population is mostly Caucasian and speaks English. Which response by the nurse manager is most correct?
   A. "It is a policy, therefore important. Questioning policy may lead to corrective action."
   B. "Approximately 20 percent of the population does not speak English at home and Spanish is the second most common language."
   C. "Questioning patients on their language of origin may lead to meaningful conversation."
   D. "Our printed information is at the sixth-grade level and most people who do not speak English read at a lower level."

7. In a patient care conference, members of many disciplines are discussing why patient-centered care is important to their institution. Which responses by the team members describe why patient-centered care helps ensure quality and safety? Select all that apply.
   A. "It's a means of engaging patients in their own care."
   B. "It includes coordination between all relevant health care providers for that patient."
   C. "It can include families when appropriate in the decision-making process."
   D. "It has been supported and influenced by Institute of Medicine's recommendation for increased interdisciplinary collaborations."
   E. "It means the patient is the only individual making decisions about their care."
   F. "It incurs more costs to patients and their insurance companies."

8. A nurse has a patient who speaks only Polish and the nurse requires a surgical consent to be signed. Which is the best alternative for the nurse to take?
   A. Have the family interpret the form to the patient.
   B. Ask the Polish housekeeper to interpret the form to the patient.
   C. Explain the form to the patient in English and have them sign.
   D. Use a certified translation service to interpret the form to the patient.

9. A nurse tells the manager, "My patient says they have spiritual distress and I don't think spiritual distress exists." The nurse manager politely disagrees and reminds the nurse that spiritual distress is recognized and defined by NANDA and is a nursing diagnosis. Which definition of spiritual distress by the manager is most correct? Select all that apply.
   A. Sadness preventing one from praying
   B. Inability to acknowledge a higher power
   C. Impaired ability to integrate meaning and purpose in one's life
   D. Dislike for communion
   E. Anger at nursing leadership
   F. Inability to see beauty of nature

10. As a new nurse you are asked to be part of the Cultural Competence Committee. While bringing back to your unit the committee's recommendations for providing culturally competent care to patients, which principles listed should be included? Select all that apply.

A. Care is designed for the specific patient.
B. Care is based on the uniqueness of the person's culture and includes cultural norms and values.
C. Care includes empowerment strategies to facilitate patients' decision making in their personal health behavior.
D. Cost containment of care should be a priority.
E. A high school degree or higher is a prerequisite for any patients to make a decision for themselves.
F. Care is provided with sensitivity to the cultural uniqueness of the patient.

REVIEW ACTIVITIES

1. The hospital where you work is in a predominantly white, non-Hispanic area. Lately, there has been an influx of migrant farmworkers from Mexico because local farms cannot find local workers. What do you perceive as some of the health needs of the migrant farmworkers? How would you facilitate the provision of care for these workers and their families?
2. You are taking care of a trauma patient in the ER. The patient has burns over 70 percent of his body. The likelihood of the patient's survival is unknown. There is a lot of noise and distraction in the ER, as well as many family members within earshot. The patient asks you to pray for him and his family. How will you respond?
3. You work with a variety of nurses from many educational backgrounds, cultures, and age groups. You want to be a helpful part of the team. What are some ways in which you can support the variety of values and perspectives of your colleagues?

EXPLORING THE WEB

- Language and cultural effects on health care delivery are the focus of this site:
  http://www.diversityrx.org
- Search for statistics:
  http://www.census.gov
  Click on Latest Race, Ethnic, and Age Estimates, or click on Poverty.
- The International Sigma Theta Tau (nursing honor society) site contains a position paper on diversity. What does the nursing honor society believe about diversity?
  http://www.nursingsociety.org
  Search for Diversity.
- This site contains information about cultural beliefs pertinent to the health care of recent immigrants to the United States:
  http://www.ethnomed.org
  Click on Cultural Competency.
- The U.S. Department of Health and Human Services–Office of Minority Health:
  http://minorityhealth.hhs.gov
  Click on Cultural Competency.
- Canadian Nurses Association:
  http://www.cna-aiic.ca/cna
- National Alaska Native American Indian Nurses Association (NANAINA):
  http://www.nanainanurses.org

- National Black Nurses Association, Inc.:
  http://www.nbna.org
- Transcultural Nursing Society:
  http://www.tcns.org
- Islamic Information Center of American (IICA):
  http://www.iica.org
- U.S. Citizenship and Immigration Services:
  http://www.uscis.gov/
- American Civil Liberties Union (ACLU):
  http://www.aclu.org
- American Indian Heritage Foundation:
  http://www.indians.org
- American Jewish Community:
  http://www.ajc.org
- Anti-Defamation League:
  http://www.adl.org
- Asia Society:
  http://www.asiasociety.org
- National Association for the Advancement of Colored People:
  http://www.naacp.org
- International Council of Nurses:
  http://www.icn.ch
- Global Health Council:
  http://www.globalhealth.org
- World Health Organization:
  http://www.who.org
- Quality and Safety Education for Nurses:
  http://www.qsen.org

REFERENCES

Ackley, B. J., & Ladwig, G. B. (2006). *Nursing diagnosis handbook: A guide to planning care* (7th ed.). St. Louis, MO: Mosby.

American Academy of Colleges of Nursing (AACN). (2010). Race/Ethnicity of students enrolled in generic (entry-level) baccalaureate, master's, and doctoral (research-focused) programs in nursing, 2001–2010. Retrieved October 30, 2011, from http://www.aacn.nche.edu/research-data/EthnicityTbl.pdf

American Academy of Colleges of Nursing (AACN). (2011). Fact sheet: Enhancing diversity in the workforce. Retrieved October 30, 2011, from http://www.aacn.nche.edu/media-relations/fact-sheets/enhancing-diversity

American Academy of Nursing (AAN). (1992). AAN expert panel report: Culturally competent health care. *Nursing Outlook, 40*(6), 277–283.

Andrews, M. (2008). Cultural diversity in the health care workforce. In M. Andrews & J. Boyle (Eds.), *Transcultural concepts in nursing care* (5th ed., pp. 297–354). Philadelphia, PA: Lippincott Williams and Wilkins.

Burner, O. Y., Cunningham, P., & Hattar, H. S. (1990). Managing a multicultural nurse staff in a multicultural environment. *Journal of Nursing Administration, 20*(6), 30–34.

Calhoun, S. K., & Strasser, P. B. (2005). Generations at work. *American Association of Occupational Health Nurses, 53*(11), 469–471.

Campinha-Bacote, J. (2003, January 31). Many faces: Addressing diversity in health care. *Online Journal of Issues in Nursing, 8*(1), manuscript2. Retrieved April 18, 2006, from nursingworld.org/ojin/topic20/tpc20_2.htm

Centers for Disease Control and Prevention (CDC). (2009). Healthy United States, 2009. Retrieved October 30, 2011, from http://www.cdc.gov/nchs/data/hus/hus9.pdf#highlights

DeRosa, N., & Kochurka, K. (2006, October). Implement culturally competent health care in your workplace. *Nursing Management, 37*(10), 18–26.

Duldt, B. (2002). The spiritual dimension of holistic care. *Journal of Nursing Administration, 32*(1), 20–24.

Ellison, C. W., & Paloutzain, R. F. (1999). *Measures of religiosity.* Birmingham, AL: Religious Education Press.

Giger, J., & Davidhizar, R. J. (2004). *Transcultural nursing: Assessment and intervention* (4th ed.). St. Louis, MO: Mosby Year Book.

Giger, J., & Davidhizar, R. J. (1996). When the operating room has a multicultural team. *Today's Surgical Nurse, 18*(5), 26–32.

Grossman, C. L. (2006, September 12). View of God can reveal your values and politics. *USA Today,* 1A.

Guglielmi, C. L. (2010). The freedom to embrace the spirituality of leadership. *Association of Perioperative Registered Nurses, 91,* 645–646.

Hodge, D. R. (2001). A template for spiritual assessment: A review of the JCAHO requirements and guidelines for implementation. (Joint Commission on Accreditation of Healthcare Organizations). *Social Work,* 51, 317-326. Available at www.accessmylibrary.com/coms2/summary_0286-28917948_ITM

Hungelmann, J., Kenkel-Rossi, E., Klassen, L., & Stollenwerk, R. (1989). Development of the JAREL spiritual well-being scale. In R. M. Carroll-Johnson (Ed.), *Classification of nursing diagnoses: Proceedings of the eighth conference, North American Nursing Diagnosis Association* (393–398). Philadelphia, PA: Lippincott.

Institute of Medicine (IOM). (2001). Hurtado, M. P., Swift, E. K., & Corrigan, J. *Envisioning a national health care quality report.* Washington, DC: National Academies Press.

Interprofessional Education Collaborative Expert Panel. (2011). *Core competencies for interprofessional collaborative practice: Report of an expert panel.* Washington, DC: Interprofessional Education Collaboration.

Joint Commission (JC). (2008). Provision of care, treatment, and services: Spiritual assessment. Retrieved December 29, 2011, from http://www.jointcommission.org/AccreditationPrograms/HomeCare/Standards

Kupperschmidt, B. R. (2000). Multigeneration employees: Strategies for effective management. *Heath Care Management, 19*(1), 65–76.

Leininger, M. (1978). *Transcultural nursing: Concepts, theories and practice.* New York, NY: Wiley.

Leininger, M. (1997). Transcultural nursing research to nursing education and practice: 40 years. *Image Journal of Nursing Scholarship, 29*(4).

Lenburg, C., Lipson, J., Demi, A., Baney, D., Stem, P., & Gage, I. (1995). *Promoting cultural competence in and through nursing education: A critical review and comprehensive plan for action.* Washington, DC: American Academy of Nursing.

Lipson, J. G., & Dibble, S. L. (2005). *Culture and clinical care.* San Francisco, CA: UCSF Nursing Press.

Munoz, C. (2009). Personal Communication, January 8, 2009.

Munoz, C., & Luckmann, J. (2005). *Transcultural communication.* Clifton Park, NY: Delmar Cengage Learning.

NLNAC accreditation manual. (2008). National League for Nursing Accrediting Commission, Inc. Available at www.nlnac.org/manuals/NLNACManual2008.pdf

Nies, M., & McEwen, M. (2007). *Community/public health nursing* (4th ed.). Philadelphia, PA: W. B. Saunders.

Office of Minority Health and Health Disparities (OMHD). (2010). About minority health. Retrieved October 30, 2011, from http://cdc.gov/omhd/AMH/AMH.htm

Ott, J. (1989). *The organizational culture perspective.* Chicago, IL: Dorsey Press.

Porter-O'Grady, T., & Malloch, K. (2011). *Quantum leadership: Advancing innovation, transforming health care.* p. 10. Sudbury, MA: Jones and Bartlett Learning.

Provider's Guide to Quality and Culture. Retrieved October 11, 2012, from http://erc.msh.org/mainpage.cfm?file=1.0.htm&module=provider&language=English

Purnell, L. (2005). The Purnell model for cultural competence. *The Journal of Multicultural Nursing and Health, 11*(2), 7–15.

Racher, R. E., & Annis, R. C. (2007). Respecting culture and diversity in community practice. *Research and Theory for Nursing Practice: An International Journal, 21,* 255–270.

Rahman, F. (2009). *Major themes of the Qur'an,* (2nd ed.). Chicago, IL: University of Chicago Press.

Ray, R. (2004). The faith connection. *NurseWeek, A Nursing Spectrum Publication, 11*(9), 17–20.

Reed, P. G. (1986). Spirituality and well-being in terminally ill hospitalized adults. *Research in Nursing and Health, 35,* 368–374.

Spangler, A. (1992). Transcultural care values and practices of Philippine-American nurses. *Journal of Transcultural Nursing, 4*(2), 28–31.

Spector, R. E. (2004). *Cultural diversity in health and illness* (6th ed.). Upper Saddle River, NJ: Pearson-Prentice Hall.

Transcultural Nursing Society. (2011). Standards of practice. Retrieved from http://tcns.org

U.S. Census Bureau. (2007). American community survey. Retrieved November 26, 2012 from http://www.census.gov/acs/www

U.S. Census Bureau. (2011). 2010 census data. Retrieved October 11, 2012, from http://2010.census.gov/2010census/data/

Wikoff, K. L. (2003). Development and psychometric evaluation of the Wikoff Spiritual Focus Questionnaire. *Dissertation Abstracts International, 64*(04), 1691. (UMI No. AAT 3088678).

Wikoff, K. L. (2008). Culture, generational differences, and spirituality. In P. L. Kelly, (Ed.). *Nursing leadership & management* (2nd ed.). Clifton Park, NY: Delmar Cengage Learning.

Williams, J., & Rodgers, S. (1993). The multicultural workplace: Preparing preceptors. *Journal of Continuing Education in Nursing, 24*(3), 101–104.

SUGGESTED READINGS

Buerhaus, P. I., Auerbach, D. I., & Staiger, D. O. (2007, March–April). Recent trends in the registered nurse labor market in the U.S.: Short-run swings on top of long-term trends. *Nursing Economics, 25*(2), 59–66, quiz 67.

Casida, J., & Pinto-Zipp, G. (2008, January–February). Leadership–organizational culture relationship in nursing units of acute care hospitals. *Nursing Economics, 26*(1), 7–15; quiz 16.

Christmas, K. (2007, November–December) Workplace abuse: Finding solutions. *Nursing Economics, 25*(6), 365–367.

D'Avanzo, C. (2008). *Pocket guide to cultural health assessment* (4th ed.). St. Louis, MO: Mosby.

Dossey, B. M., & Keegan, L. (2009). *Holistic nursing: A handbook for practice* (5th ed.). Boston, MA: Jones & Bartlett.

Gaston-Johansson, F., Hill-Briggs, F., Oguntomilade, L., Bradley, V., & Mason, P. (2007, December). Patient perspectives on disparities in health care from African American, Hispanic, and Native American samples including a secondary analysis of the Institute of Medicine focus group data. *Journal of the National Black Nurses Association, 18*(2), 43–52.

Hall, J., Stevens, P., & Meleis, A. (1994). Marginalization: A guiding concept for valuing diversity in nursing knowledge development. *Advances in Nursing Science, 16*(4), 23–24.

Hobbs, F., & Stoops, N. (2000). U.S. Census Bureau. Census 2000 special reports. Series CENSR-4. *Demographic trends in the 20th century*. Washington, DC: U.S. Government Printing Office. 2002. Available at www.census.gov/prod/2002pubs/censr-4.pdf

Hu, J., Herrick, C., & Hodgin, K. A. (2004). Managing the multigenerational nursing team. *The Health Care Manager, 23*(4), 334–340.

Irwin, W. (2008, January 24). Nursing: A reality check for diversity. *Health Services Journal*: 40–41.

Jein, R. F., & Harris, B. L. (1989). Cross-cultural conflict: The American nurse manager and a culturally mixed staff. *Journal of the New York State Nurses Association, 20*(2), 16–19.

Keltner, B., Kelley, F., & Smith, D. (2004). Leadership to reduce health disparities: A model for nursing leadership in American Indian communities. *Nursing Administration Quarterly, 28*(3), 181–190.

Newman, M. A. (2008). *Transforming presence: The difference that nursing makes*. Philadelphia, PA: F.A. Davis.

Racher, F. E., & Annis, R. C. (2007). Respecting culture and honoring diversity in community practice. *Research and Theory of Nursing Practice, 21*(4), 255–270.

Roenkoetter, M. M., & Nardi, D. A. (2007, October). American Academy of Nursing expert panel on global nursing and health: White paper on global nursing and health. *Journal of Transcultural Nursing, 18*(4), 305–315.

Scott, D. E. (2008, January–February). The multicultural health care work environment. *American Nurse, 40*(1), 7.

Shin, H. B., & Kominski, R. A. (2010). *American community survey reports: Language use in the United States: 2007, ACS-12*. Washington, DC: U.S. Census Bureau.

Taylor, R. A., & Alfred, M.V. (2010). Nurses' perceptions of the organizational supports needed for the delivery of culturally competent care. *Western Journal of Nursing Research, 32*, 591–609.

Tracey, C., & Nicholl, H. (2007, October). The multifaceted influence of gender in career progress in nursing. *Nursing Management, 15*(7), 677–682.

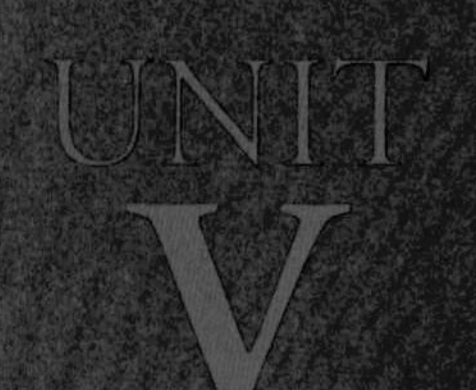

LEADERSHIP AND MANAGEMENT OF SELF AND THE FUTURE

CHAPTER 17

NCLEX-RN Preparation and Your First Job

DONNA BOWLES, MSN, CNE, EDD; PATRICIA KELLY, RN, MSN;
EDNA HARDER MATTSON, RN, BN, BA(CRS), MDE;
KARIN POLIFKO-HARRIS, RN, PHD, CNAA; AND
STEPHEN JONES, RN, MS, CPNP, ET

Luck is a matter of preparation meeting opportunity.

—OPRAH WINFREY

OBJECTIVES

Upon completion of this chapter, the reader should be able to:

1. Discuss preparation for the National Council of State Boards of Nursing Licensure Examination for Registered Nurses (NCLEX-RN).
2. Detail the process of beginning a successful nursing job search.
3. Develop a résumé and cover letter.
4. Identify appropriate preparation for a successful job interview.
5. Discuss potential interview questions and identify acceptable answers.
6. Describe typical components of health care orientation.
7. Discuss elements of performance feedback.

Mary will be graduating from her nursing education program in two months. She plans to focus her current efforts on preparing to take the NCLEX-RN Licensure Examination. She knows that three important areas of examination preparation are having the knowledge, being adept at testing, and controlling test anxiety.

How should she prepare for the examination?

Where should she focus?

How can she decrease her test anxiety?

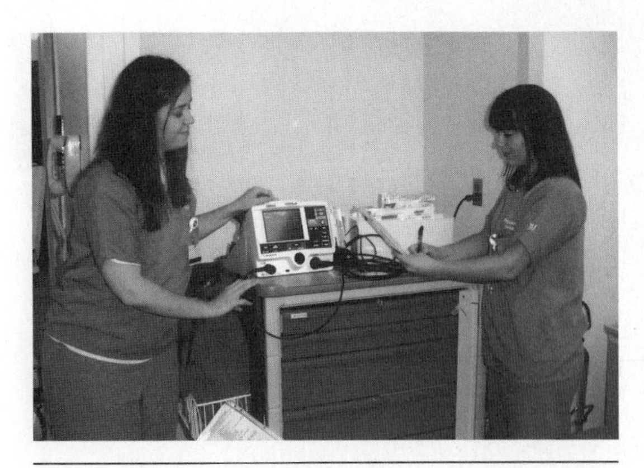

© Cengage Learning 2014

A new graduate from an educational program that prepares RNs will take the National Council of State Boards of Nursing Licensure Examination for Registered Nurses (NCLEX-RN). The NCLEX is taken after graduation and prior to practice as an RN. NCLEX examinations are developed by the National Council of State Boards of Nursing. (NCSBN). NCSBN administers these examinations on behalf of its member boards that consist of the boards of nursing in the 50 U.S. states, the District of Columbia, and four U.S. territories: American Samoa, Guam, Northern Mariana Islands, and the Virgin Islands.

To ensure protection of the public, each board of nursing requires a candidate for licensure to pass the NCLEX examination. NCLEX examinations are designed to test the knowledge, skills, and abilities essential to the safe and effective practice of nursing at the entry level.

NCLEX examinations are provided in a computerized adaptive testing (CAT) format and are presently administered by Pearson VUE in their network of Pearson Professional Centers (PPC). Information about the exam as well as an online tutorial are available at http://www.vue.com/nclex/.

Note also the NCSBN Learning Extension website http://learningext.com/ where you can see and answer the NCSBN Question of the Week and sign up for NCSBN's online NCLEX-RN review course.

It is wise to schedule your exam date soon after your graduation. Graduates submit their credentials to the state board of nursing in the state in which licensure is desired. After the state board accepts the graduate's credentials, he or she can schedule the examination. The NCLEX-RN examination ensures a basic level of safe nursing practice to the public and is essential to working as a professional RN. The examination follows a test plan formulated on four categories of client needs that RNs commonly encounter. Integrated processes include: the nursing process; caring; communication and documentation; and teaching/learning. These are integrated throughout the four major categories of client needs (NCSBN, 2013). See Table 17-1.

The focus of this chapter is to give new nursing graduates the tools to pass NCLEX and to seek and obtain a nursing position. Included in this chapter are tips on NCLEX preparation, writing a résumé, cover letter, and thank you letter, sample interview questions and answers, preparation for the interview, and hints on how and where to search for a job. Finally, orientation at a health care facility and staff nurse performance feedback are discussed.

PREPARATION FOR NCLEX-RN

Graduates may receive anywhere from 75 to 265 questions on the NCLEX examination during their testing session. Fifteen of the questions are questions that are being piloted to determine their psychometric value and validity for use in future NCLEX examinations. Students cannot determine whether they passed or failed the NCLEX examination from the number of questions they receive during their session.

TABLE 17-1
NCLEX Test Plan

Client Needs Tested	Percent of Test Questions
Safe and Effective Care Environment	
◆ Management of Care	17–23%
◆ Safety and Infection Control	9–15%
Heath Promotion and Maintenance	6–12%
Psychosocial Integrity	6–12%
Physiological Integrity	
◆ Basic Care and Comfort	6–12%
◆ Pharmacological and Parenteral Therapies	12–18%
◆ Reduction of Risk Potential	9–15%
◆ Physiological Adaptation	11–17%

Source: NCLEX-RN® Examination Test Plan for the National Council Licensure Examination for Registered Nurses NCLEX-RN® TEST PLAN. Effective April 2013. Retrieved November 26, 2012 from https://www.ncsbn.org/2013_NCLEX_RN_Test_Plan.pdf

Test Question Formats and Samples

Questions are presented in alternate item formats. Alternate item formats may include the following:

- Multiple-response items that require a candidate to select one or more than one response
- Fill-in-the-blank items that require a candidate to type in number(s) in a calculation item
- Hot spot items that ask a candidate to identify one or more area(s) on a picture or graphic
- Chart/exhibit format where the candidate will be presented with a problem and will need to read the information in the chart/exhibit to answer the problem
- Ordered response items that require a candidate to rank order or move options to provide the correct answer
- Audio item format where the candidate is presented an audio clip and uses headphones to listen to and select the option that applies
- Graphic option that presents the candidate with graphics instead of text for the answer options and the candidate will be required to select the appropriate graphic answer

Note that any item formats, including standard multiple-choice items, may include multimedia, charts, tables or graphic images. Multiple-choice questions may be four-option, single-answer items, or multiple-option items that require more than one response.

Sample Questions

Some of the various formats for test questions are illustrated here. See other examples at https://www.ncsbn.org/2334.htm# What_ is_an_alternate_item_format.

Test Question 1—Fill in the blanks

A man underwent an exploratory laparoscopy yesterday. He is on strict intake and output. Calculate his intake for an 8-hour period.

Intake
0.9% NS at 125 mL per hour
Ranitidine (Zantac) 50 mg/50 mL D5W IVPB Q8H

Test Answer 1

Intake = 1050 mL
0.9% NS 125 mL × 8 hours is 1000 mL
IVPB is 50 mL

Test Question 2—Question that requires more than one response

The nurse is aware that certain occupations put an individual at risk for developing carpal tunnel syndrome. Of the following, select all occupations that apply.

A. Sports announcer
B. Assembly line worker
C. Computer programmer
D. Professional bowler
E. Barber

Test Answer 2

Answer is B, C, D, and E
The area in the wrist where the nerve enters the hand is called the carpal tunnel. This tunnel is normally narrow, so any swelling can pinch the nerve and cause pain, numbness, tingling, or weakness resulting in carpal tunnel syndrome. It is common in people who perform repetitive motions of the hand and wrist such as the assembly line worker, computer programmer, professional bowler, and barber.

Test Question 3—Single answer, multiple-choice question

A nurse is working in a long-term care facility and has an 85-year-old resident with dehydration secondary to diarrhea. The health care provider has ordered the infusion of potassium chloride 10 mEq intravenously over one hour for this patient. Prior to infusing the potassium chloride, the nurse's plan should include which of the following?

A. Validating that the patient has adequate urine output
B. Obtaining an accurate height and weight
C. Arranging for a central line IV catheter placement
D. Assessing possible causes for the diarrhea

Test Answer 3

A is the correct choice. Potassium is excreted through the kidneys. When patients are dehydrated, urine output may be affected. If the resident receives the drug and is unable to void, it could be life threatening as the potassium level rises in the patient's system. The patient's height and weight will have little bearing on administering this drug dose. A central line is not necessary for potassium administration. Giving the medication through a peripheral venous access is acceptable. Assessing the cause for the diarrhea is not the first priority when giving the medication. The patient's low potassium level should be reversed or hypokalemia can result in cardiac failure. Determining the cause of the diarrhea may take a while.

Test Question 4—Fill in the blanks

Identify the height of the fundus at 22 weeks on this picture. Mark the site with an X.

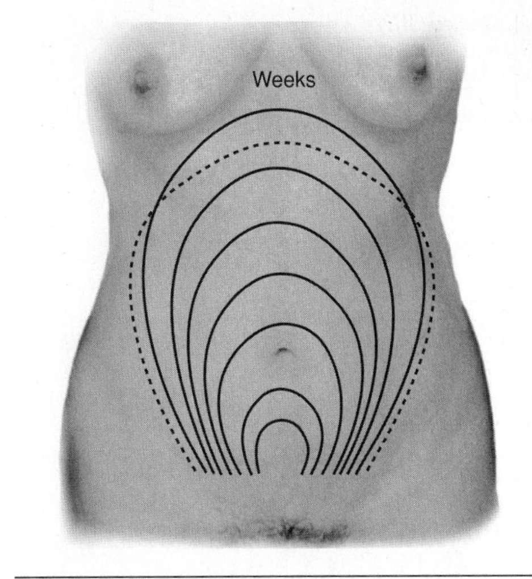

© Cengage Learning 2014

Test Answer 4

The fundus is located at this site at 22 weeks.

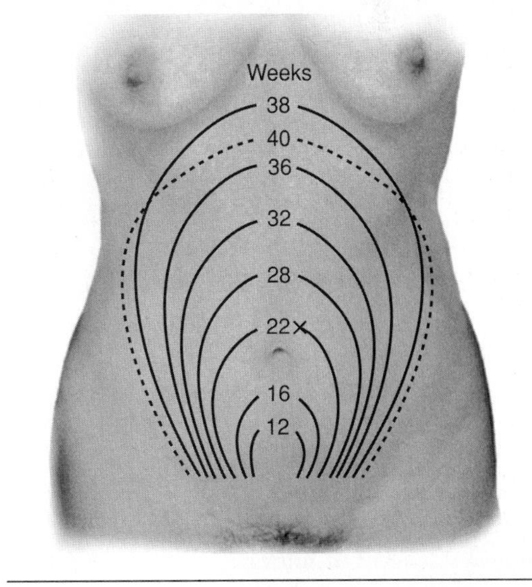

© Cengage Learning 2014

Test Question 5—Fill in the blanks

A physician prescribes lorazepam (Ativan) 0.5 milligrams (mg) intravenously for a patient with a history of seizure disorder. The medication vial reads lorazepam 2 mg/1 mL. The nurse plans to prepare how many milliliters (mL) to administer the correct dose?

Test Answer 0.25 mL

$$\frac{0.5 \text{ mg} \times \text{mL}}{2 \text{ mg}} = 0.25 \text{ mL}$$

Test Question 6—Put items in correct order

Put these steps in the correct order to insert a Foley catheter.

1. Check integrity of Foley balloon.
2. Attach drainage bag to bed.
3. Send urine specimen to laboratory.
4. Cleanse meatus.
5. Spread the labia.
6. Insert the Foley.

Test Answer 6

1. Check integrity of Foley balloon.
2. Attach drainage bag to bed.
3. Send urine specimen to laboratory.
4. Cleanse meatus.
5. Spread the labia.
6. Insert the Foley.

Factors Affecting NCLEX-RN Performance

Several factors have been identified as being associated with performance on the NCLEX examination. Some of these factors are listed in Table 17–2.

Review Books and Courses

In preparing to take the NCLEX, the new graduate may find it useful to focus his or her preparation on three areas: NCLEX knowledge review, NCLEX test question practice, and test anxiety control. Review books often include nursing content, sample test questions, or both. They frequently include CDs or online sites with test questions. The test questions in the review books and software may be arranged by clinical content area, or they may be presented in one or more comprehensive examinations covering all areas of the NCLEX.

Try to answer as many questions correctly as you can. As you study, be sure to actually practice taking the examinations. Do not jump ahead to the answer section before you have completed an examination. Completing the examinations in this way may improve your performance on the NCLEX.

It is helpful to use several of these NCLEX-RN review books and the computer software that comes with many of them when preparing for the NCLEX. Listings of NCLEX review books are available at www.amazon.com.

Prioritize your review by focusing on content in NCLEX-RN in your weak areas.

NCLEX review courses are also available. Brochures advertising these courses are often sent to schools and are available in many sites nationwide. The quality of these review courses can vary, and you may want to ask faculty and former nursing graduates for recommendations. You may also find it helpful to note the excellent NCSBN review course and test question of the week at www.learningext.com.

Nursing Exit Exams

Many nursing programs administer an examination to students at the completion of their nursing program, (e.g., the HESI Evolve or Assessment Technologies Institute Exit Exam). New graduates who examine their feedback from such an examination have important information regarding their strengths and weaknesses that can help them focus their review for the NCLEX.

A strategy for organizing this Self Needs Analysis for NCLEX Review is identified in Table 17-3.

Knowledge, Anxiety Management, and Test-Taking Skills

Successful test performance requires nursing knowledge, anxiety management, and test-taking skills. Knowledge of the test content is the first critical element. Students gain knowledge of nursing as the result of a course of nursing study. Nursing students attend either a two-year associate degree nursing

TABLE 17-2
Factors Associated with NCLEX-RN Performance

- Exit exam performance, i.e., HESI Evolve*or ATI**
- Verbal SAT score
- ACT score
- High school rank and GPA
- Undergraduate nursing program GPA
- GPA in science and nursing theory courses
- Competency in American English language
- Reasonable family responsibilities or demands
- Absence of emotional distress
- Critical-thinking competency

*HESI Evolve Learning System. (2011). HESI Frequently Asked Questions. Retrieved April 20, 2011, from https://evolve.elsevier.com/staticPages/hesi-faq.html

** Assessment Technologies Institute. (2011). About ATI. Retrieved April 20, 2011, from http://www.atitesting.com/About.aspx

Source: Table developed with information from McGahee, T.W., Gramling, L. & Reid, T.L. (2010). NCLEX-RN® Success: Are There Predictors. Southern Online Journal of Nursing Research. Volume 10. No. 4. Retrieved November 26, 2012 from, http://www.resourcenter.net/images/SNRS/Files/SOJNR_articles2/Vol10Num04Art13.html.

TABLE 17-3
Self-Needs Analysis for NCLEX-RN

Anxiety level (circle) 1 2 3 4 5 6 7 8 9 10

Weak content areas identified on NCLEX Test Plan in Table 17-1, exit exam, or comprehensive exam, etc.: ______________________________

____

Nursing courses below a grade of B: ______________________________

Factors identified from Table 17–2: ______________________________

____

Weak content areas identified in common U.S. patient conditions and causes of death:

- Mental Health, e.g., schizophrenia, bipolar disorder, anxiety, personality disorders, suicide, eating disorders, abuse ______________________________
- Women's Health, e.g., antepartum care, intrapartum care, postpartum care, newborn care ______________________________
- Adult Health, e.g., cancer, myocardial infarction, diabetes, pneumonia, HIV, hepatitis, cholecystectomy, lobectomy, nephrectomy, cardiac arrest, major cardiac arrhythmias, thyroidectomy, shock, CVA, appendectomy ______________________________
- Children's Health, e.g., leukemia, cardiovascular surgery, fractures, cancer, diabetes, tonsillectomy, asthma, Wilms' tumor, cleft palate ______________________________

Weak content areas identified in any of the following:

- Therapeutic communication
- Growth and development (developmental milestones and toys used by each pediatric age group)

(Continues)

TABLE 17-3 (Continued)

- Management, delegation, referrals, and priority setting
- Medications
- Defense mechanisms
- Immunization schedules
- Diagnostic tests and laboratory data
- Nutrition

Organize your review. Practice many test questions. Note that many students who are successful on the NCLEX-RN have prepared for the exam by completing 3,000 NCLEX-RN style exam questions. Study when you are fresh. Are you a day person? Are you a night person?

Your study schedule could look like the following, depending on the results of your self-analysis above:

Day 1: Practice 60 Adult Health test questions. Score the test; analyze your performance; and review test question rationales and content weaknesses. Practice deep breathing, relaxation exercises, and positive thinking.

Day 2: Practice 60 Women's Health test questions. Repeat the above process.

Day 3: Practice 60 Children's Health test questions. Repeat the above process.

Day 4: Practice 60 Mental Health test questions. Repeat the above process.

Day 5: Continue with content review and test question practice in all weak content areas. Practice deep breathing, relaxation exercises, and positive thinking. Continue this process of practicing 60 test questions daily until you are doing well in all areas and are scheduled to take your NCLEX-RN. Note that many students find it useful to complete 3,000 NCLEX questions in 50 days, doing 60 questions per day ($50 \times 60 = 3{,}000$).

© Cengage Learning 2014

program, a three-year diploma nursing program, a four-year baccalaureate nursing program, or a baccalaureate or master's second-degree nursing program to gain the knowledge needed to satisfactorily complete the NCLEX-RN.

Anxiety management through visualization and relaxation techniques before and during the test is the second element of successful test performance. Plan to use any or all of the following to control your anxiety level:

- Positive thinking, that is, I can do it!!!
- Guided imagery, which requires using your imagination to create a relaxing sensory scene on which to concentrate
- Reward yourself after the test
- Once you have adequately prepared for a test, do something relaxing
- Avoid classmates who generate anxiety and tend to upset others; anxiety is contagious
- Take several deep, slow breaths regularly (Schultz, 2010)
- Relaxation audio tapes (Idris, 2011)

Additional resources for reducing test anxiety include *Conquering Test Anxiety* (Pescar, 2009), and *Insider's Guide to Beating Test Anxiety* (Bedford-St. Martin's, 2010).

Test-taking skills are the final, critical element needed for successful test completion. Strategies to improve test-taking skills include practicing 60 test questions daily from different NCLEX-RN review books, CDs, and online NCLEX review sites (e.g., www.cengage.com/delmar/). Search for NCLEX.

Practice test-taking skills with exam questions until performance is satisfactory in all areas covered

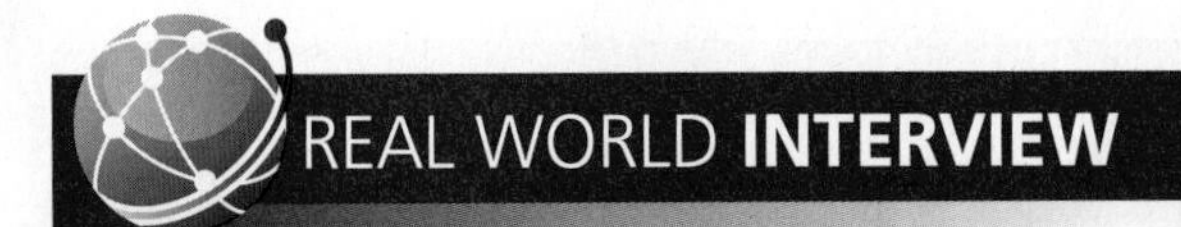

My best advice to anyone preparing for the NCLEX is to take lots of practice tests. I answered close to 1,500 questions in preparation and I feel it did me a world of good. I kept my nursing textbooks handy and when I ran into something I didn't know, I looked it up.

AMANDA MEADOWS, RN, BSN
Huntington, West Virginia

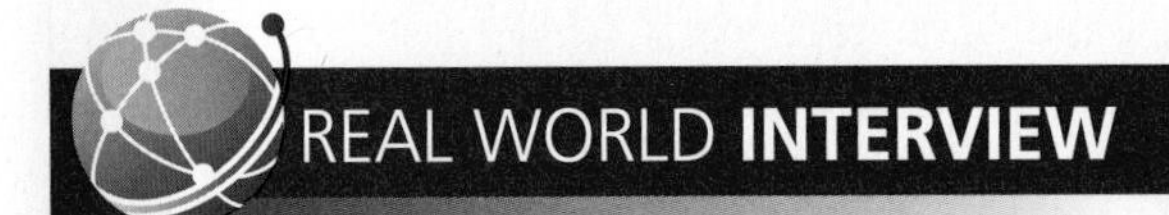

Just as location, location, location is important to businesses, preparation, preparation, preparation is crucial to NCLEX success. Many nursing programs require students to take some variety of exit examination. This provides the soon-to-graduate nurse with an opportunity to evaluate personal readiness for the licensure examination. My personal experience demonstrates that some students, despite achieving the benchmark required by a nursing program, may be unsuccessful first-time test takers. One reason may be that some think the licensure examination is a nursing knowledge test. The NCLEX does not test mere nursing knowledge. The NCLEX tests nursing judgment and discretion. To prevent becoming an NCLEX casualty, I recommend the following:

Actively participate in any NCLEX preparation activities provided by your nursing program.

Pay close attention to any test-taking strategies in your exit exam preparation book.

Approach an exit exam as a challenge, not a chore.

Embrace the opportunity to learn about NCLEX-style test questions.

Use any remediation services offered by your nursing program to review content that is unfamiliar or difficult.

Once the benchmark score is achieved on your program's exit examination, *do not* decrease your NCLEX preparation activities. Anecdotal evidence from graduates who were successful first-time NCLEX takers indicates that answering in the neighborhood of 3,000 NCLEX-style questions from a book or computer program that includes the rationale for the answer and explains why the distractors are incorrect is associated with success on the NCLEX.

DR. JAQUELYN REID
Professor of Nursing
Indiana University SE
New Albany, Indiana

by the NCLEX exam. Note that successful students often practice 60 questions daily in their weak content areas until their performance improves. Sixty questions daily for 50 days expose students to 3,000 questions ($60 \times 50 = 3{,}000$). Use the results of an exit exam or comprehensive exam to guide you in your selection of test questions. Practice using the ARKO and ABC-Safe-Comfort methods discussed in the critical-thinking exercise later in this chapter as you review the test questions.

Tips and Medication Guide

Table 17-4 offers some final tips on reviewing for NCLEX. Table 17-5 is a Medication Study Guide Starter to aid you in your NCLEX preparation. Use these tables as starting points in your review for NCLEX.

TABLE 17-4
Selected NCLEX Tips

- Remember Maslow's Hierarchy of Needs. Physical needs are met first, e.g., airway, breathing, circulation (ABCs) threats.
  - Airway threats
    - Altered level of consciousness (LOC)
    - Foreign object in airway
  - Breathing threats
    - Asthma
    - Suicide threat
    - Sedation
  - Circulation threats
    - Cardiac arrest
    - Shock
- Safety needs are met second, for example, safety and infection control threats.
  - Confusion
  - Tuberculosis
  - The RN uses patient care data such as vital signs, collected either by the nurse or others, to make clinical judgments. The RN continuously monitors and evaluates patient care and delegates care involving standard, unchanging procedures to LPNs and NAPs.
  - The RN makes appropriate referrals to community resources.
  - The RN never delegates patient Assessment, Teaching, Evaluation (ATE), or judgment.
  - Review Chapter 8, especially Tables 8-1 through 8-7 and Figures 8-1 through 8-3, for information on nursing delegation.
  - When delegating care, do not mix the care of a patient with an infection with the care of a patient who has decreased immunity, e.g., a patient with AIDS, diabetes, steroids, the very young, the very old.
- Comfort needs and teaching needs are met after physical and safety needs are met. Do not choose a test question answer that gives the patient comfort or meets teaching needs before the patient's ABC and safety needs have been met.
  - Remember the nursing process—assess your patient first; then plan, implement, and evaluate.
  - Keep all your patients safe, e.g., airway open, side rails up, IV access line in place on unstable patient; monitor vital signs, pulse oximeter, cardiac rhythm, and urine output as needed.
  - Know delegation guidelines for RNs, LPNs, and NAP. Observe the five rights of delegation, i.e., the right task, the right circumstance, the right person, the right direction/communication, and the right supervision. See Chapter 8.
    - The RN assures quality care of all patients, especially complex patients. RNs delegate care of stable patients with predictable outcomes.
  - Know the most common adult, maternal-child, and psychological health care disorders. For each disorder, know the medications, laboratory and diagnostic tests, procedures, and treatments commonly used.
  - Know common medications (see Table 17-5).
  - Know common laboratory norms, e.g., sodium, potassium, blood sugar, complete blood count, hematocrit, prothrombin time, partial thromboplastin time, international normalized ratio (INR), arterial blood gas (ABG), cardiac enzymes, digoxin level, dilantin level, lithium level, blood urea nitrogen (BUN), creatinine, uric acid, and specific gravity of urine.

(Continues)

TABLE 17-4 (Continued)

- When delegating care, note the following:
  - LPNs can perform medication administration (includes IV meds in some states), sterile dressings, Foley insertions, etc.
  - NAP can perform basic care—e.g., vital signs measurement, bathing, transferring, ambulating, communicating with patients, and stocking supplies.
  - In some states, with documented competency, LPNs can insert IVs, pass nasogastric tubes, etc.
  - In some states, with documented competency, NAP can perform venipuncture, do blood glucose tests, insert Foley catheters, etc.
- In answering test questions, do the following:
  - When choosing priorities, select the first action you would take if you were alone and could do only one thing at a time. Do not think that one RN will do one task, and another RN will do another task.
  - Assume you have the nursing or medical practitioner's order for any possible choices.
  - Assume you have perfect staffing, plenty of time, and all the necessary equipment for any possible test question choices. Choose the answer that indicates the best nursing care possible.
  - Assume you are able to give perfect care "by the book." Do not let your personal clinical experience direct you to choose a test answer that is less than high-quality care.
  - Remember to safeguard the patient ABCs and safety first and then check the equipment.
- Know communication techniques—look for answers that give patients support and allow them to keep talking and verbalize their concerns and problems. Be their comforting nurse, not their therapist. Avoid giving advice.
- Know common food choices included in special diets, e.g., low sodium diet, diabetic diet.
- Know common food choices for potassium, sodium, vitamin K, calcium replacement, etc. (Table 17-6).
- Know the defense mechanisms.
- Know growth and development, such as the developmental tasks for each childhood stage, toys for each childhood stage, and so on.
- Know immunization schedules (see Centers for Disease Control and Prevention, 2012).
- Prepare mentally with the following:
  - Anxiety control and relaxation techniques.
  - Regular exercise.
  - Thinking positively and avoiding negative people and negative thoughts.
  - Visualizing your name with "RN" next to it on your name badge.
- Remember—you graduated from an accredited nursing program. You can do it!

© Cengage Learning 2014

TABLE 17-5
Medication Study Guide Starter

Complete/Add to this as you study for NCLEX*

General Tips

1. Drowsiness and changes in vital signs (VS) are side effects of many medications given for their analgesic, antiemetic, antiseizure, tranquilizer, sedative/hypnotic, antihistamine, antianxiety, cardiac, or blood pressure effects.
2. Note that if the medication listed in Table 17-5 below is a cardiac or BP medication or can cause drowsiness or changes in vital signs, consider the need to monitor level of consciousness (LOC), airway, blood pressure (BP), temperature (T), pulse (P), respirations (R), pulse oximetry, and the cardiac monitor.
3. Consider the need to insert an IV line to safeguard at-risk patients. Consider the use of side rails and fall precautions and the need to have high-risk patients avoid driving. You may also need to monitor for postural hypotension.
4. Many meds cause renal, liver, heart, neurological, and bone marrow side effects. Monitor labs that reflect these organs' functions. Check allergies.

Category	Prefix or Suffix	Examples	Nursing Implications
Phenothiazine Antiemetic Antipsychotic Antianxiety	-zine	Promethazine (Phenergan); Fluphenazine (Prolixin)-IM	Drowsiness Guidelines
Benzodiazepines Tranquilizer Hypnotic Antianxiety Antiseizure Anesthetic	-azepam -azolam	Diazepam (Valium); Lorazepam (Ativan); Clonazepam (Klonopin); Alprazolam (Xanax); Midazolam (Versed)	Drowsiness Guidelines Check for habituation; taper dose when discontinued. Versed used for short-term sedation—monitor closely. Romazicon (Flumazenil) reverses sedative effect of benzodiazepines.
Anticoagulant	-arin	Heparin (antidote is protamine sulfate) Enoxaparin (Lovenox)	Monitor bleeding, e.g., stool, gums, urine, bruising. For Heparin, check ptt level. Give Heparin IV to get ptt level to 1.5–2 times the control time.

(Continues)

TABLE 17-5 (Continued)

Category	Prefix or Suffix	Examples	Nursing Implications
Anticoagulant	-arin	Coumadin (Warfarin) (Antidote is Vitamin K)	Monitor bleeding, e.g., stool, gums, urine, bruising. Check PT/INR (Desirable INR range is 2.0–3.0 for many conditions).
Angiotensin Converting Agent (ACE Inhibitor) Anti-hypertensive	-pril	Lisinopril (Zestril) Enalapril (Vasotec) Captopril (Capoten)	Monitor cough.
Angiotensin Receptor Blocking Agents Anti-hypertensive	-sartan	Telmisartan (Micardis) Irbesartan (Avapro) Losartan (Cozaar)	
Beta adrenergic blockers Anti-hypertensive Anti-anginal	-olol	Metoprolol (Lopressor) Propranolol (Inderal) Atenolol (Tenormin)	Monitor for broncho-spasm, bradycardia.
Anti-hypertensive	-pres	(Catapres) Clonidine (Apresoline) Hydralazine	
Calcium channel blockers Anti-hypertensive	-pine	Nifedipine (Procardia) Amlodipine (Norvasc)	
Anti-hyperlipidemic	-vastatin	Lovastatin (Mevacor) Atorvastatin (Lipitor)	
Diuretic	-ide	(Furosemide) Lasix	Monitor intake and output. Check potassium.
Potassium		Potassium electrolyte	Give IV slowly—use IV pump for infusions. Potassium can kill if given quickly. Maintain adequate urine output.
Anti-infectives	-mycin -cin	Gentamycin (Garamycin) Vancocin (Vancomycin)	
Anti-infective	ceph- cef-	Cephalexin (Keflex) Ceftriaxone (Rocephin)	
Antiviral	-vir	Zidovudine (Retrovir) Acyclovir (Zovirax)	Antivirals are given in combination with other antivirals to increase therapeutic effect. Check liver and renal lab tests.

(Continues)

TABLE 17-5 (Continued)

Category	Prefix or Suffix	Examples	Nursing Implications
NSAID	-cox	Celecoxib (Celebrex)	Tinnitus/GI bleed. Check platelets. Check renal function, BUN, and creatinine.
Steroids Anti-inflammatory Many anti-inflammatory uses for conditions such as CVA, asthma, arthritis, etc.	-one	(Dexamethasone) Decadron Prednisone (Deltasone) Methylprednisolone (Solu-Cortef, Depo-Medrol)	Monitor "S"s—sad, stress, sight, susceptibility, sugar, sodium. Decreases stress (inflammatory response), sight (cataracts), and potassium. Increases sad (mood), susceptibility (infection, ulcers), sugar (hyperglycemia), sodium (edema), and osteoporosis. Wean off steroids to avoid adrenal crisis and shock.
Histamine H2-Receptor Antagonists	-tidine	Ranitidine (Zantac) Famotidine (Pepcid)	
Proton Pump Inhibitors	-prazole	Esomeprazole (Nexium) Pantoprazole (Protonix) Lansoprazole (Prevacid)	
Miotic eye drops		Pilocarpine	Constrict the pupil—reduce intraocular pressure.
Mydriatic eye drops		Atropine	Dilate the pupil.
Thrombolytic	-ase	Streptokinase (Streptase)	
Anti-fungal	-azole	Fluconazole (Diflucan) Micronazole (Monistat)	
Antiarrhythmic	-caine	Lidocaine	
Calcium	cal-	Calcium gluconate	
Anti-infective	-cillin	Amoxicillin, Penicillin	
Antibiotic	-cycline	Tetracycline (Sumycin) Doxycycline (Vibramycin)	

(Continues)

TABLE 17-5 (Continued)

Category	Prefix or Suffix	Examples	Nursing Implications
Bone resorption inhibitor	-dronate	Olendronate (Fosamax) Ibandronate (Boniva)	
Antibiotic	-floxacin	Ciprofloxacin (Cipro) Levofloxacin (Levaquin)	
Bronchodilator	-phylline	Aminophylline	
Other Medications			
Antipsychotics	Cardiac drugs	Antidepressants	Mood Stabilizers
Zyprexa Seroquel Haldol Prolixin Abilify Resperidal (Resperidal M melts in the mouth for patients who are med avoiders)	Digoxin Diltiazem Epinephrine Nitroglycerin Norpace Amiodarone (Cordarone)	Celexa Cymbalta Effexor Lexapro Zoloft Prozac Paxil Prozac Remeron (older patient)	Lithium (Know medication levels) Depakote (Hair loss) Tegretol

–Other important drugs include Acetaminopen, Albuterol, Aspirin, Atropine, Diphenhydramine, Codeine, Benztropine, Insulin, Lactulose, Magnesium Sulfate, Morphine, Gabapentin, Oxycodone, Oxytocin, Levothyroxine, Isoniazid, Rifampin, Ethambutol, Pyrazinamide, Rhogam, Synthroid, Terbutaline, Allopurinol, Alteplase, etc. Review chemotherapy guidelines.
–Learn the generic and trade names, action, nursing implications, and side effects of all the medications in this table. Add to the table as you study.

Source: Kelly, P., & Hernandez, G. (2012). Medication Study Guide Starter. Unpublished manuscript.

TABLE 17-6
Guidelines for Various Nutrients and Diets

Nutrient	Common Sources
Iron	Iron in animal foods (heme iron) is best absorbed when eaten in a meal containing Vitamin C: Liver/liver sausage, beef, chicken, eggs, pork Non-heme iron sources (less efficiently absorbed than heme iron): Dark green leafy vegetables, fortified breakfast cereals, kidney beans and other legumes, whole grain breads/cereals

(Continues)

TABLE 17-6 (Continued)

Nutrient	Common Sources
Potassium	Bananas, cantaloupe, oranges/orange juice, potatoes, prune juice
Vitamin C (antioxidant)	Citrus fruits (e.g., oranges, grapefruit), strawberries, sweet peppers, tomatoes
Vitamin D	Exposure to sunshine! Cod liver oil, fatty fish (e.g., tuna, salmon/canned salmon with bones), most milk, cheese, yogurt (check label)
Vitamin E (antioxidant)	Nuts, salad dressings, vegetable oils, wheat germ, whole grain breads/cereals/starches
Calcium	Milk, cheese, yogurt, dark leafy green vegetables, fortified cereal, fortified orange juice
Therapeutic Diets:	**Foods to limit/restrict on diet:**
Bland/Soft	Caffeine, fatty/fried foods, fresh fruit, raw vegetables, spicy foods, whole grain breads/cereals/pasta Eat smaller, more frequent meals.
Diabetic	Foods/beverages containing regular sugar (e.g., cakes, candy, cookies, ice cream, pies, soda, jams/jellies, syrup) Plan meals in advance for consistent carbohydrate intake daily.
Gluten Free	Foods containing white flour, wheat flour (e.g., breads, cereals, noodles/pasta), barley, oats, rye Look for "Gluten Free" on the package label.
Low Fat/Low Cholesterol	Bacon, fried foods, gravies/sauces made with butter, whole milk/whole-milk cheese/cream, sausage Remove visible fat from meat; remove skin from poultry.
Low Sodium	Bacon, corned beef, ham, hot dogs, sausage, canned soups, snack foods (e.g., potato chips, pretzels), canned vegetables Do not add salt in cooking or at table.
Low Protein	Beef, chicken, eggs, fish, pork, turkey, dairy products, legumes Restriction varies. In general, 1 oz. meat = 7 grams protein. Plan meals in advance and monitor correct portion sizes.
Selected Diet needs:	*Food choices:*
High Calorie	Avocados, butter, cheese, cream, mayonnaise, oil-based salad dressings, olives, peanut butter
High Fiber	Fresh fruit (with peel or skin, when applicable), legumes, nuts, peas, raw vegetables, whole grain breads/cereals/starches
High Protein	Beef, chicken, dairy products, eggs, fish, legumes, pork, turkey

Source: Developed by: Georgia Hammerli, RD, LDN, Registered Dietitian, Arlington Heights, Illinois.

CRITICAL THINKING **17-1**

When you are presented with a difficult test question, use these test-taking ARKO Strategies and ABC-Safe-Comfort Tips to help you answer it correctly. Use ARKO Strategies as follows:

- **A** Is the question stem asking for you to take **A**ction or take no **A**ction?
- **R** **R**eword the question.
- **K** Identify any **K**ey words in the question stem.
- **O** Review and eliminate **O**ptions.

Apply this ARKO Strategy to the test question below:

What should the nurse do first for a patient with a spinal cord injury who complains of a headache?

A. Insert a new Foley catheter.
B. Assess the patient's pupils.
C. Take the patient's blood pressure.
D. Administer a beta adrenergic blocker.

Apply the ARKO strategy:

A Stem asks for the nurse to take **A**ction.

R **R**eword the question as follows: What is a priority nursing action for a patient with a spinal cord injury who has a headache?

K **K**ey words are "first," "spinal cord injury," and "headache."

O Note the following as you eliminate **O**ptions:

Option A may be useful if the patient's blood pressure is elevated, as a plugged catheter can trigger autonomic dysreflexia.

Option B would not give us useful information about this patient.

Option C would be useful to assess blood pressure for autonomic dysreflexia.

Option D would reduce the patient's blood pressure, but the stem does not say his or her blood pressure is elevated.

The correct answer is C.

As you review a test question, it is also helpful to review Maslow's Hierarchy of Needs and use the ABC-Safe-Comfort Tips. Assess your patient's ABCs, then assess his or her Safety, and finally, after these are secured, assess his or her Comfort and then any Teaching needs. Remember this sequence when prioritizing your nursing actions:

A – Airway
B – Breathing
C – Circulation
Safety
Comfort
Teaching

(Continues)

CRITICAL THINKING 17-1 (Continued)

Apply these Tips to this test question:

The nurse is unable to obtain a pedal pulse on doppler examination of the cold, painful leg of a patient who has just been admitted with a fractured femur. What is the priority intervention for this patient?

A. Give morphine, as ordered.

B. Teach the patient cast care.

C. Notify the health care practitioner.

D. Comfort the patient and keep the leg elevated.

Apply ABC-Safe-Comfort Tips to the question's options.

A. Comfort can be given with pain medication, but this is an emergency. Call the health care practitioner. Comfort care is done after ABC and Safety are assured.

B. Teaching is done after ABC-Safe-Comfort is assured.

C. Patient has absent pulse on doppler and cold, painful leg—this is an emergency! Patient's arterial circulation cannot be occluded long before there is permanent damage to tissues.

D. Patient is not safe or comforted if there is no arterial circulation to leg. Comfort care is done after ABC and Safety are assured.

The correct answer is C.

Recall that NCLEX often wants you to take all nursing actions before calling the health care practitioner. In an emergency, however, the health care practitioner should be called without hesitation when needed. Always recall that Maslow's Hierarchy of Needs directs us to monitor our patients' ABCs and then keep them Safe. After this is done, we can Comfort and Teach our patients. Now practice the test questions at the end of this chapter using these strategies. How did you do?

BEGINNING A JOB SEARCH

The critical first step in your job search is preparation. Know what clinical area you are interested in and what skills you have that may fit that area. Consider what type of hospital you want to work in, for example, a large university teaching hospital, a small private community hospital, or other.

Magnet Hospitals

In 1993, the American Nurses Credentialing Center (ANCC) established the Magnet Services Recognition Program. A Magnet hospital is a health care organization that has met the rigorous nursing excellence requirements of the ANCC, a division of the American Nurses Association (ANA). As a testament to the increasing recognition given to magnet hospitals, *U.S. News & World Report* recently included magnet designation in its criteria for its annual "100 Best Hospitals of America" list (U.S. News & World Report, 2011). Of the 5,795 hospitals in the United States (AHA, 2011), 391 (or 6.75%) are Magnet-designated facilities (ANCC, 2011). Many nurses choose to work in magnet hospitals. See Chapter 11.

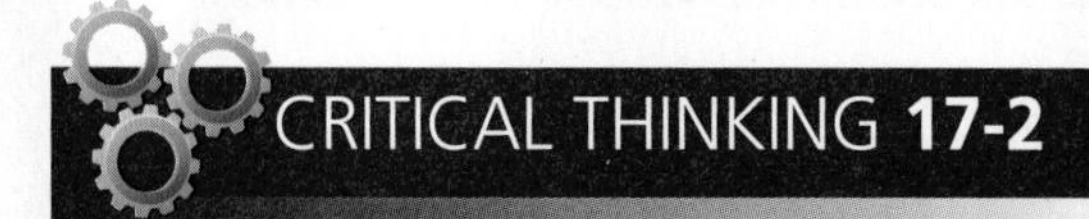

CRITICAL THINKING 17-2

You are responsible for being the nurse you want to be. To do this, set your goals. Monitor and self-evaluate those goals regularly. Gather data on the following indicators of being a professional nurse and add to the list of indicators, as appropriate.

How did you do on this self-evaluation?

What other goals have you added?

- Pass NCLEX-RN.
- Monitor literature so that I am up to date on evidence-based practice for my patients.
- Monitor data that show that my patient care is patient-centered and that my patients are safe, satisfied, pain-free, and feel cared about.
- Monitor data that show that my patients are complication-free and have no nurse-sensitive outcomes.
- Offer high-quality professional nursing service to my patients and my community.
- Give and receive professional respect to and from the interprofessional health care team.
- Speak up about the important role that nurses play in preventing patient complications.
- Develop rapport with and network with other health care professionals.
- Participate in interprofessional committees at work to improve the quality of care delivered to patients. Communicate assertively with the interprofessional health care team.
- Receive professional salary and benefits.
- Take good care of myself and strive for professional and personal balance.
- Continue my education, for example, certification, formal education, continuing education.
- Join my professional organization.
- Dress like a professional.
- Communicate pride in being a nurse.
- Improve my use of the computer in nursing documentation, decision making, and literature searches.

Nursing Residency Programs

Nursing residency programs have been developed to recruit and retain nurses and to reduce nursing turnover. Generally lasting one year, these structured programs facilitate transition to practice that goes beyond a typical hospital orientation process. After obtaining licensure, the nurse residents have a focused program designed to learn about new equipment, policies, procedures, and competencies along with professional socialization. The nurse residents demonstrate improvement in their skills and abilities, including their ability to organize and prioritize their work, be comfortable communicating with the care team, patients, and families, and in providing clinical leadership on the unit where they work. The nurse residents' stress scores decrease and staff turnover decreases (Goode, Lynn, Krsek, Bednash & Janetti, 2009).

Multistate Licensure Compact

The multistate licensure compact allows a nurse to have one license (in his or her state of residency) and to practice in other states (both physically and electronically), subject to each state's practice law and

Agency and Referral Source	Telephone Number	Contact Name	Resume Sent/Date	Thank-You Letter	Follow-Up

FIGURE 17-1

Tracker for job leads.
(*Source:* Courtesy of Polifko-Harris, K. (2012). Career Planning. In P. Kelly . (Ed.). *Nursing Leadership and Management* (3rd ed.). Clifton Park, NY: Delmar Cengage Learning.)

regulation. Under mutual recognition, a nurse may practice across state lines unless otherwise restricted. View guidelines of the multistate licensure compact at www.ncsbn.org. Click on Nursing Education, Licensure, and Practice. Then, click on Nurse License Compact to view the map. As of this writing, in 2012, 24 states participate in the Nurse License Compact.

Where to Look for a Job

One place many nurses think to begin a job search is the local newspaper. Other places include employment bulletin boards, telephone lines, and job fairs. Many health care employers have an employment bulletin board, telephone line, or website that identifies job openings on a weekly basis. It is often helpful to begin a job-tracking file (see Figure 17-1). Be sure to look closely at the requirements for the position. If the position requirements state that a skill or educational element is a *required* element, recruiters will call first only those candidates who meet the minimum *required* qualifications. If the position requirements state that a skill or educational element is a *preferred* element, recruiters will call candidates first who have the *preferred* element.

Electronic Media and the Internet

There are several sources of online application for employment. These sources include search engines, job boards, and agency and company sites such as those for a specific hospital, health care agency, or health care company. Electronic media sites can also include health care journals. Following are some examples of search engines:

- Dogpile (allows you to search multiple search engines at one time; this site is known as a metasearch engine): *http://www.dogpile.com*
- Excite: *http://www.excite.com*
- WebCrawler: *http://www.webcrawler.com*
- Infoseek: *http://www.infoseek.com*
- Google: *http://www.google.com*

Some examples of job boards specific to health care include the following:

- *http://www.healthcareerweb.com*
- *http://www.healthcarejobs.org/resource.htm*
- *http://www.rn.com*
- *http://www.aone.org* (This site requires membership to use.)

A few examples of other sites with job openings include the following:

- *http://health-care.careerbuilder.com*
- *http://www.careercity.com*

DEVELOPING A RÉSUMÉ

Résumés are generally the first opportunity a prospective employer has to see who you are and what your qualifications are for a given position. A **résumé** is a brief summary of your background, training, and experience, as well as your qualifications for a position (see Figure 17-2). It should be viewed as a marketing tool to sell yourself to a prospective employer. Generally, a résumé should be no longer than two pages on good quality white or ivory paper. It needs to contain concise information that clearly identifies your specific skills, strengths, and experiences. A résumé should be honest, neat, easy to read, and have no errors. In companies that are highly desirable to work for, the résumé is also often used as a screening tool so that a recruiter's time can best be spent wisely with potential employees who are seen as welcome team members.

There is no one perfect résumé style. It is agreed that an effective résumé (1) catches the employer's interest; (2) identifies critical areas such as education, work experience, and special qualifications; (3) should be tailored to the employer's needs; (4) creates a favorable first impression about you and your abilities; (5) communicates that you are someone who is a good fit for the position; and (6) is visually appealing. If sending a hard copy of your résumé, send a copy that is crisp in appearance and easy to read, not a photocopy. If you must fax it, use the fine setting. Use plain white 8.5- by 11-inch paper with no folds or staples. A good résumé takes time to prepare. You should ensure that what is presented on paper is truthful and presents you as a capable person who is able to make immediate and sustained contributions to an organization.

The statement "References available upon request" can be placed on the last line of a résumé. You can either provide a listing of references on the application, or bring a separate reference list to a job interview. Include at least three professional references, with names, titles, addresses, and phone numbers—but only after receiving permission from these persons to use them as references. Do not use family, friends, or neighbors as professional references. Notify your references before you interview to let them know they may be contacted.

Writing a Cover Letter

A résumé should always be accompanied by a letter of introduction, known as the "cover letter." This is a one-page letter designed to entice the prospective employer to become interested enough to read the résumé. It does not reiterate the entire résumé, but presents highlights and a summary of the essential points found on the résumé. Figure 17-3 is an example of a cover letter. Your cover letter should highlight your strengths that well suit you to a job opportunity for which the recruiter is actively seeking applicants. Be sure to follow up sending your résumé and cover letter with a phone call to the recruiter. Be professional in your phone call. Consider it part of your interview. If you get the recruiter's answering machine when you call, leave your phone number very slowly twice. Do not abuse the recruiter's time. Do not assume he or she has your phone number handy even though it is on the résumé. Be brief in leaving any phone messages. Do not repeat your whole professional history and goals. The recruiter will see this on your résumé.

Developing an Electronic Résumé

Sending cover letters and résumés via the Internet is an acceptable practice. It does require some additional considerations in terms of both safeguards and catching the attention of the reader. It is safest to initially send the e-mail to yourself or to a mentor to determine how it will appear to the reader. Send the résumé as an attachment to your cover letter. The human resources personnel or nurse manager can then reproduce it readily and circulate it to other managers or members of the interviewing committee. Catching the attention of human resources personnel is vital. Many employers use automated applicant-tracking systems to sort and track résumés. These systems are databases that allow prospective employers to use keywords to search for applicants who meet certain criteria. For example, instead of entering "Résumé" in the subject line of your e-mail, enter "Résumé for pediatric registered nurse with 9 years EMT experience."

James Mattern
214 Christie Avenue
Gladstone, OH 43523
(604) 775-3424 (home)
(604) 725-7356 (cell)
James123@school.edu

KEYWORD SUMMARY: Registered Nurse. RN. Emergency Room. Nurse Aide. Ambulance. Advanced Cardiac Life Support. Volunteer.

OBJECTIVE: An entry-level position as an emergency room registered nurse

EDUCATION: Associate of Science in Nursing, June, 2012
Freedom Community College, Gladstone, OH

Highlights:
* Maintained 3.66 GPA, Dean's List
* Class President
* Clinical Rotation, Emergency Department, Concordia Hospital, March, 2012.

EXPERIENCE: Patient Care Assistant, Medical-Surgical Unit
St. Mary's Medical Center, Gladstone, OH
(August 2010–present)

Duties:
* Provide basic patient care and monitoring
* Prepare and stock patient rooms

Ambulance Attendant
Mayfair Ambulance Service, Gladstone, OH
(2003–2012)

Duties:
* Answer emergency calls, including mass disasters

CERTIFICATION: Certified in Advanced Cardiac Life Support, 2003–present
Certified in Cardiopulmonary Resuscitation, 2003–present

PROFESSIONAL ORGANIZATIONS: National Student Nurses Association
American Red Cross, Blood Drive Volunteer
Gladstone Free Clinic, Registration Volunteer

References available upon request.

FIGURE 17-2

Résumé.

© Cengage Learning 2014.

James Mattern
214 Christie Avenue
Gladstone, OH 43523
(604) 775-3424

April 11, 2012

Ms. Eileen Carter, BSN, RN
Director of Human Resources
Concordia Hospital
200 Jones Drive
Austin, OH 43524

Dear Ms. Carter:

I am requesting the opportunity to discuss my career plans with you. I will be graduating on June 30, 2012 from Freedom Community College with an Associate of Science Degree in Nursing. I will take my NCLEX-RN on July 30, 2012.

I have served as an ambulance attendant for nine years. This service provided me with the skills to handle emergency calls, including mass disasters such as airline crashes and hotel and apartment fires. I also performed many tasks of varying priorities within many Fire and Police Departments. I also recently completed a five-week clinical rotation in your emergency department. I feel that these skills, combined with my newly acquired nursing skills, will be an asset to your Emergency Department.

I would appreciate the opportunity to discuss my career plans with you. I will call you next week to schedule an appointment to discuss employment possibilities. In the meantime, I can be contacted at (604) 775-3424 or at James123@school.edu. I am willing to rotate shifts.

Thank you for your time and consideration of my resume.

Sincerely,

James Mattern

James Mattern

FIGURE 17-3

Cover letter.

© Cengage Learning 2014.

Human resources personnel enter the words "pediatric" and "registered nurse" as required keywords that résumés must include to come up in the search results. The human resources personnel may add other keywords, for example, things that are helpful for the job but not mandatory. The tracking system then searches all résumés in the system and retrieves those with keywords the employer specified. These résumé databases may be in-house or they may be available on the Internet.

Those résumés containing the most key word nouns are selected and then ranked. Many electronic résumés contain a key word summary section toward the top of the résumé, listing the standard phrases that describe the applicant's skills, area of expertise, job titles, and credentials. It is good to put key words in the order of importance to your job search. Also use common abbreviations for words used in the body of the résumé to increase your odds of matching the employer's key word specifications. For example, if you list "registered nurse" in the body of your résumé, use "RN" in the key word summary. In constructing your résumé, ensure that any formatting you use is readable to any computer system. Be sure to do the following:

- Keep it simple. Use a plain font, such as Helvetica for headings and Times Roman for body text, and a font size of 12.
- Avoid fancy highlighting. Do use boldface or ALL CAPS for emphasis. Avoid fancy fonts, italics, graphics, shading, italics, underlining, slashes, dashes, parentheses, and ruled lines.
- Avoid a two-column format. Multiple columns can be jumbled by scanners that read across the page.

One way to ensure that your résumé can be read is to check whether there are formatting specifications you must meet. Some databases require that you meet certain margins or not use tabs. Many databases require that résumés be sent in plain text or ASCII format (Becze, 2008).

A SUCCESSFUL INTERVIEW

In preparation for an interview, learn more about the agency and the possible questions you may be asked or that you should ask (Emery, 2011). You would be wise to obtain a copy of the job description beforehand. Familiarize yourself with it, as this will further demonstrate your interest in the position. It will also give you an opportunity to prepare appropriate interview questions. For example, if the job description requires the nurse to demonstrate the use of computer equipment, you can clarify what type of computer equipment is used in the unit. Go online and find the agency's website. Review what you find there. Search for the agency by name and location by using a search engine (e.g., www.google.com).

Arrive shortly before the interview to demonstrate your time management skills. The interviewer will note this. Prepare a folder that contains a description of the organization and its services, extra copies of your résumé, questions you have researched and are prepared to ask, and blank paper as well as a pen and any other documents that may be helpful. The nurse manager or representatives of the human resources department will verify your license, assess your competency, review your employment references, and complete background and criminal checks, as appropriate. They will assess your ability to meet any health requirements or any other job requirements of a nursing position. Your ability to fit in with the agency's culture as well as the patient care unit's culture will be assessed. Your communication skills, maturity, dependability, and learning and nursing skills, as well as your ability to delegate, take initiative, use judgment, and be loyal and dedicated to your work are all items that may be assessed. The nursing representatives and the human resources representatives will often offer you a competitive salary or hourly rate within approved budget guidelines, and they will assure the completion of any required organizational and governmental paperwork. Some organizations may require a group interview with multiple persons interviewing you to assess such things as your ability to work on a team. For entry-level position interviews, it is customary to have only the nurse manager or the nurse manager and a nurse recruiter or human resources person present during the interview. In some situations, other staff nurses are included in interviews for new unit staff.

You will also want to assess such items as whether the organization offers a nurse internship program for new graduates, what the program consists of, who serves as preceptors for the program, their backgrounds, and the salary during the internship. Note that internship programs may vary from organization to organization in content, length, preceptor requirements, salary, and so on.

Rehearse an interview scenario with a trusted colleague or by video. Types of interviews can vary from one-to-one interviews, panel interviews, telephone interviews, and follow-up interviews with varying types of questions involving hypothetical case scenarios. You are applying for an entry-level position, and therefore the questions will be directed at your nursing care knowledge. For example, if you are applying for a nursing position on a general medical unit, be ready to give the nursing interventions for a patient experiencing chest pain or hypoglycemia. You may also be asked to recall a difficult nursing situation and describe your behavior in that situation. For example, you may be asked, "If you are faced with a demanding patient who has been waiting for a long time to have his dressing changed, what would you do?" To respond, use the STAR acronym and include each component. Describe Specifically (S) what happened; the Task (T), problem, or issue; the Action (A) you took; and the Result (R) of the action. The interviewer is looking for what you learned from the difficult nursing situation and how you would handle a similar situation in the future (Table 17-7).

Interviews that ask about your behavior are designed to provide the employer with information about how you have handled both negative and positive experiences in the past. Employers are seeking employees who are able to reflect on their past performance and learn from the experience. In this information age, nursing employers are recognizing the need to transform work sites into learning sites (Holden, 2006).

During the introductory phase of the interview, the employer should outline the job and the conditions of employment. If the job and conditions do not reflect your understanding of the position, be sure to clarify by asking questions at this time. The employer is looking for the traits that successful registered nurses demonstrate, such as flexibility, willingness to work in various areas, organizational skills, the ability to complete work assignments, and the ability to remain calm and collected during times of crisis.

The employer may ask, "Tell me about a time when you had to work in an area of the hospital in which you had very little orientation." Or "Tell me about a time when you had to complete an unusually large amount of work." Or "Tell me about a time when you had to deal with a stressful crisis at work."

The employer may ask you to job shadow. This job shadow is in effect a second interview. Often, the prospective employee will show a very different side of his or her personality while shadowing. Input from current employees who spent time with a prospective employee during a job shadow will likely be sought. Valuable information about the prospective employee's personality fit with the department may be gained during a job shadow (Olmstead, 2007).

Another phase of the interview will begin with the employer asking you questions about your cover letter and résumé. All the questions during the interview will usually reflect the job description. Familiarize yourself with the legal and illegal questions that may be asked. Legally acceptable questions include your reason for applying, your career goals, any problems you foresee, and your strengths and weaknesses.

TABLE 17-7
STAR Interviews

Specifics	A patient was overdue for his dressing change. He became angry and demanded that I come now to change his dressing.
Task	I was busy with other high-priority patients. I was having trouble getting to this dressing change.
Action	I called my charge nurse and asked for help. The charge nurse was able to change the patient's dressing, talk with him, and help him to relax. I stopped in to tell the patient I was sorry for the delay.
Result	I asked the charge nurse to review assignments for future care of this type of patient who has extensive dressing-change needs. I also resolved to examine the way I prioritize my patients at the beginning of a shift to determine the best way to meet patient care needs. I resolved to change my future patients' dressings early in the shift before it gets busy.

© Cengage Learning 2014

While it is not possible to predict every question you will be asked during an interview, certain questions are generally avoided by all employers. The following personal questions are not allowed (Gaddis, 2009).

- Are you married? Divorced?
- If you are single, are you living with anyone?
- How old are you?
- What is your family situation like?
- Do you have children? If so, how many and how old are they?
- Do you plan on having a baby within the next few years?
- Do you own or rent your home?
- What church do you attend?
- Do you have any debt?
- Do you belong to any social or political groups?
- How much and what kinds of insurance do you have?
- Do you suffer from an illness or disability?
- Have you been hospitalized? What for?
- Have you ever been treated by a psychiatrist or psychologist?
- Have you had a major illness recently?
- How many days of work did you miss last year because of illness?
- Do you have any disabilities or impairments that might affect your performance in this job?
- Are you taking any prescribed drugs?
- Have you ever been treated for drug addiction or alcoholism?

Rather than refusing to answer an illegal question, which may be seen as being uncooperative or confrontational, respond as if it is a legally acceptable question. For example, should the interviewer ask how many children you are caring for at home, respond by indicating that you are able to handle the demands and hours of the job for which you are applying. Responding in this manner may signal to the interviewer your ability to serve as a team player without compromising the legal or ethical issues of the job requirements.

Highlight specific personal and professional accomplishments that reflect your ability; however, be careful not to inflate them as this can raise doubts concerning your truthfulness and accuracy. If you give the interviewers reason to question your veracity, you may lose the job opportunity. Respond in a calm, problem-solving fashion to all questions. See Table 17-8 for other interview questions you may be asked.

Avoid any discussion of how bad your last employer or faculty was or how incompetent you think that your coworkers or classmates are. Keep the entire interview process as positive as possible. Avoid any discussions of any personal problems. If an employer has a choice between you and the person who lost their last job because they kept calling in sick over child care or personal problems, they are going to pick you every time.

Dressing for the Interview

Dress appropriately for the position by wearing professionally acceptable, comfortable, and neatly pressed clothing. For women, this may be a solid-color conservative suit with a coordinated blouse, medium-heeled polished shoes, limited jewelry, neat professional hairstyle, and neutral hosiery. Skirt length should be long enough so you can sit down comfortably. Choose a soft color that complements your skin tone and hair color such as brown, tan, beige, black, blue, navy, or gray. Use light makeup and perfume and have neat, manicured nails.

For men, appropriate dress may be a solid-color dark blue, gray, muted pinstripe, or very muted brown conservative suit with a white, long-sleeved shirt and conservative tie. Wear a conservative stripe or paisley tie that complements your suit, in silk or good quality blends only. Wear dark socks with professional polished leather dress shoes, brown, cordovan, or black only. Wear limited or no jewelry and have a neat, professional hairstyle. Limit aftershave lotion and have neatly trimmed nails. Both women and men should avoid body piercing jewelry and cover tattoos. Don't chew gum, eat, or use a cell phone or iPod during the interview. Use a breath mint before you enter the building for the interview.

Termination

Terminating an interview is important. The employer will close an interview by asking if you have any questions (Table 17-9).

TABLE 17-8
Interview Questions and Suggested Answers

What made you choose nursing as a career?

- I am seeking a career which is challenging, mentally stimulating, and has a daily potential for making a difference in someone's life.
- There are two nurses in my family who specialize in totally different areas, yet they have always expressed a positive image and satisfaction with their career choice.

How has your training prepared you for a nursing career?

- I had a summer externship position at an oncology center prior to beginning my senior year. This experience allowed me hands-on experience with patients, and showed me the importance of palliative and end-of-life care which I hope to specialize in.
- My nursing program included many community-based clinical sites. Working with disadvantaged patients is a rewarding experience that I approach with passion.

What interests you about working here?

- Your facility has one of the top-rated diabetic-patient units in the country. I am interested in utilizing my experience with patients with this disease in a hospital engaging in the latest research and techniques.
- I really enjoy working with geriatric patients, and your facility has a vibrant and innovative reputation for its programs and population.
- I have worked in large teaching hospitals, where I gained valuable experience, but I enjoy working in a small community-focused hospital, where you can get to know your patients well.

How do you handle stress on the job?

- By focusing on the most important thing, the care of the patient. I have witnessed and believe in the importance of staying calm and focused.
- I take good care of my own physical and mental health and I do not allow on-the-job stress to interfere with my work.

How would you deal with a doctor who was rude?

- In general, I would try to avoid this situation by building good rapport from my first day with the doctors and other interprofessional health team members. If the doctor was dissatisfied with me in some way or any way, I would attempt to find out why so I could take action to rectify the situation.
- If it was a one-time occurrence, I would try to realize he was probably just having a bad day. If it happened repeatedly, I would notify my supervisor.

What do you feel you contribute to your patients?

- I offer my patients the very best patient-centered care and serve as their advocate.
- I offer my patients comfort from a holistic approach.
- My patients know that I am there to keep them safe, deliver high-quality nursing care, work well with the other members of the interprofessional team, and that I will listen to their concerns. They also know that I am committed to evidence-based practice and will work hard to maintain this .

(Continues)

TABLE 17-8 (Continued)

What would you do if your replacement did not arrive?

- I would wait until the nurse arrived, or until someone else was called in.
- I would notify the supervisor, and offer to stay until my replacement arrived.

Source: Compiled with information from A. Doyle, A.(2012). Answers to Nursing Interview Questions.Retrieved on November 27, 2012, from http://jobsearch.about.com/od/interviewquestionsanswers/a/nurse-interview-answers.htm.

TABLE 17-9
Sample Questions to Ask During an Interview

1. How can I prepare myself to work on this unit and do a good job?
2. May I have a copy of the job description (Figure 17-4) and performance appraisal form?
3. How often will I be evaluated?
4. Is there a clinical ladder program that identifies clinical, managerial, and educational levels for promotion?
5. Who will be my preceptor?
6. What shift will I be scheduled to work?
7. Will I rotate shifts?
8. Are special requests for time off honored?
9. What holidays and weekends will I be scheduled to work?
10. What types of benefits are offered with this position? (Health, dental, retirement, holiday time, sick time, continuing-education opportunities, educational reimbursement)
11. What type of orientation or nursing residency program will I receive?
12. How long is it?
13. Does it address how to develop rapport and work well with patients and other health care practitioners?
14. What is the salary?
15. When do raises occur?
16. Is there a shift differential?
17. Is there a differential for advanced nursing degrees?
18. Is this a Magnet hospital?
19. Do you monitor nurse-sensitive outcomes?

© Cengage Learning 2014

Expect to be quite tired by the end of the interview. However, take time to review your notes, seek clarification regarding any concerns, and conclude the interview by asking when you can expect to hear from the employer. Asking this indicates that you are actively seeking employment and suggests that if the employer is serious about hiring you, he may want to offer you a position. Many sources recommend waiting to ask questions such as the following until after a position has been offered: What is the salary? When do raises occur? Is there a shift differential? Is there a differential for advanced nursing degrees? What type of health, dental, retirement, vacation, holiday time, sick time, continuing education, and educational

ALBANY MEDICAL CENTER HOSPITAL PATIENT CARE SERVICES
Job Description—REGISTERED PROFESSIONAL NURSE

SUMMARY: The Registered Professional Nurse utilizes the nursing process to diagnose and treat human responses to actual or potential health problems. The New York State Nurse Practice Act and A.N.A. Code for Nurses with Interpretive Statements guide the practice of the Registered Professional Nurse. The primary responsibilities of the Registered Professional Nurse as leader of the Patient Care Team is coordination of patient care through the continuum, education, and advocacy.

ESSENTIAL DUTIES AND RESPONSIBILITIES include the following. Other duties may be assigned.

— Performs an ongoing and systematic assessment, focusing on physiologic, psychologic, and cognitive status.
— Develops a goal-directed plan of care which is standards based. Involves patient and/or significant other (S.O.) and health care team members in patient care planning.
— Implements care through utilization and adherence to established standards which define the structure, process, and desired patient outcomes of the nursing process.
— Evaluates effectiveness of care in progressing patients toward desired outcomes. Revises plan of care based on evaluation of outcomes.
— Demonstrates competency in knowledge base, skill level, and psychomotor skills.
— Documents the nursing process in a timely, accurate, and complete manner, following established guidelines.
— Participates in unit and service quality management activities.
— Demonstrates responsibility and accountability for professional standards and for own professional practice.
— Supports research and its implications for practice.
— Establishes and maintains direct, honest, and open professional relationships with all health care team members, patients, and significant others.
— Seeks guidance and direction for successful performance of self and team, to meet patient care outcomes.

QUALIFICATION REQUIREMENTS: To perform this job successfully, an individual must be able to perform each essential duty satisfactorily. The requirements listed below are representative of the knowledge, skill, and/or ability required. Reasonable accommodations may be made to enable individuals with disabilities to perform the essential functions.

EDUCATION and/or EXPERIENCE: Graduate of an approved program in professional nursing. Must hold current New York State registration or possess a limited permit to practice in the State of New York.

LANGUAGE SKILLS: Ability to read and interpret documents such as safety rules and procedure manuals. Ability to document patient care on established forms. Ability to speak effectively to patients, family members, and other employees of organization.

MATHEMATICAL SKILLS: Ability to add, subtract, multiply, and divide in all units of measure, using whole numbers, common fractions, and decimals. Ability to compute rate, ratio, and percent.

REASONING ABILITY: Ability to identify problems, collect data, establish facts, and draw valid conclusions.

PHYSICAL DEMANDS: While performing the duties of this job, the employee is regularly required to stand; walk; use hands to probe, handle, or feel objects, tools, or controls; reach with hands and arms; and speak or hear. The employee is occasionally required to sit or stoop, kneel, or crouch.

The employee must regularly lift and/or move up to 100 pounds and frequently lift and/or move more than 100 pounds. Specific vision abilities required by this job include close vision, distance vision, peripheral vision, depth perception, and the ability to adjust focus.

WORK ENVIRONMENT: While performing the duties of this job, the employee is regularly exposed to bloodborne pathogens.

The noise level in the work environment is usually moderate.

FIGURE 17-4

Albany medical center hospital patient care services job description for registered professional nurses (excerpt).
(*Source:* Courtesy of Albany Medical Center, Albany NY.)

reimbursement benefits are offered? Note the regular salary surveys done by many nursing journals, for example, *RN, Nursing, AORN,* or found on websites such as http://nursing.advanceweb.com/.

Writing a Thank-You Letter

Within 24 hours after your interview, you should send a thank-you letter to the interviewer. Many people do not take the time to write a personal note, but doing so may set you apart from other potential employees as someone who is professional and sincerely interested in joining the organization. Figure 17-5 illustrates a thank-you letter as a follow-up to an interview. Be sure to call your recruiter as you have indicated in your follow-up letter. Have your résumé in front of you when you call him or her. Be professional and call from a landline that will have enough minutes or, if calling from a cell phone, call from a place with an adequate signal that will allow you to concentrate on any recruiter questions. Do not call when you are driving, cooking, or doing something else. Focus on the recruiter and any questions and respect her or his time.

James Mattern
214 Christie Avenue
Gladstone, OH 43523
(604) 775-3424

April 26, 2012

Ms. Eileen Carter, BSN, RN
Director of Human Resources
Concordia Hospital
200 Jones Drive
Austin, OH 43524

Dear Ms. Carter:

Thank you for the time you spent with me as I interviewed for a position as a registered nurse at Concordia Hospital. I enjoyed meeting the emergency department nurse manager and several of the staff nurses yesterday and was especially impressed with the sense of professionalism among the staff.

I have requested that my transcripts be sent directly to your office, and I will have three of my instructors complete the reference forms you gave me. I look forward to hearing from you soon about my second interview and will contact you in two weeks as directed.

Sincerely,

James Mattern

James Mattern

FIGURE 17-5

Follow-up to interview letter.

© Cengage Learning 2014

ORIENTATION TO YOUR NEW JOB

Many health care organizations divide nursing orientation into general and unit-specific sections. Once hired, new nurses receive a general orientation including information and skills that all nurses new to the facility need, regardless of their eventual unit assignment. Figure 17-6 is a sample schedule for the first week of general orientation at one medical center.

General orientations are usually outcome based, requiring the orientee to demonstrate competency, perhaps by written medication or knowledge tests or skills measurement. Information about the Joint Commission, the hospital accrediting body, core measures, and National Patient Safety Goals is also often given at general orientation.

Unit-based orientation, whether it follows the general orientation or is interspersed throughout, focuses on the specific competencies a new nurse needs to care for the diagnoses and ages of patients typical to the assigned unit. Many organizations have developed unit-specific competency tools that list those skills orientees need to demonstrate. These lists provide a useful road map with which to plan a learner-specific orientation. Figure 17-7 is an excerpt from an emergency department's unit-based orientation tool. It is also useful to identify your personal learning needs and set your own learning goals to prepare yourself to deliver quality patient care and to meet your responsibilities in a professional style. See Table 17-10.

Preceptors

Preceptors can play a key role in introducing the new nurse to coworkers and other members of the health team. The orientee needs to be introduced to the specific functions and roles of those people who interact daily with the nurses on the unit. This helps the new nurse identify relationships within the unit and between the unit and the larger health care organization.

A good preceptor is clinically experienced, enjoys teaching, and is committed to the role. If you find it difficult to work with your assigned preceptor, make this known early in the orientation process. The nursing manager or educator should be notified and the situation discussed and resolved. Good preceptors are familiar with the organization's policies and procedures, are willing to share knowledge with their orientees, and model behaviors for their orientees.

Reality Shock

In 1974, Kramer described "reality shock" and discussed the difficulties some new graduates have in adjusting to the work environment. Kramer identified a conflict between new graduates' expectations and the reality of their first nursing position. A skilled preceptor can assist new nurses through this transition by offering them opportunities to validate their impressions. The support of other new nurses in a similar situation, such as those participating in the same core orientation, is particularly helpful. Note that all nurses may experience reality shock throughout their career whenever they enter a new career area (Dyess & Sherman, 2009).

Mentors

Developing a mentoring relationship with a more experienced, successful nurse is another strategy for professional growth and help in setting long-term goals. A mentor coaches a novice nurse and helps the novice develop skills and career direction. A mentor may introduce the new nurse to professional networking opportunities and assist in workplace problems. To find a mentor, a new nurse needs to communicate a willingness to learn and grow. A newer nurse usually needs to seek out a prospective mentor rather than wait to be approached by one. An ideal mentor is an experienced nurse who is willing to support and counsel other nurses when asked. This may lead to a formal structured relationship or a more informal role-modeling association.

PERFORMANCE FEEDBACK

Everyone needs feedback about his or her performance, particularly when in a new position. Some preceptors and managers recognize new employees for their progress, but in many cases, the new nurse needs to solicit their feedback. A concrete mechanism to measure one's own performance is through the objective learning materials, job descriptions, and competency-based orientation tools provided by nurse educators. New nurses must successfully pass the written and technical parts of orientation. While in orientation, and at least annually thereafter, new graduates should meet at regular intervals with their preceptor and manager to review progress.

RN Orientation Template
Week One

Monday **Perdiems/Weekend Staff attend** **May 21**	**Tuesday** **Perdiems/Weekend attend** **May 22** **0745 meet in main lobby**	**Wednesday** **Perdiems/Weekend attend** **May 23**	**Thursday** **Perdiems/Weekend attend** **May 24**	**Friday** **May 25**
Human Resource/ Safety Education ***Remember to sign in on your unit if you want to get paid for the days you attend orientation.**	8:00–11:30 Intro/Tour Nursing at AMC Education Opportunities 11:30–12:00 Tina Raggio-Project Learn 12:00–1:00 Lunch 1:00–2:00 Delegation/Assigning *Donna Harat* 2:00–4:30 Modules on Patient Safety and Quality Improvement *some orientees may need to attend the SMS Computer class in the P building from 11:30–2:30-check with Education**	08:00–11:00 Electronic Documentation Standards of Care, protocols, I/O, graphic, Clinical Pathways Unit Day Prep *(ED exempt: modules)* 11:00–11:30 Restraints 11:30–12:00 Back Video Nurse Scheduling 12:00–1:00 Lunch 1:00–4:30 Skills Lab Afternoon Emergency Care and Mock Code (ACLS or PALS exempt and does not apply to NICU), IV/ Phlebotomy Skills, Accucheck, PCA Pump	08:00–09:30 Modules on Patient Safety and Quality Improvement 09:30–11:00 Epidemiology *Carolyn Scott* 11:00–11:30 Lunch 11:30–2:30 SMS Computer Class 3:00–4:00 Math Calculation Class (**optional-check with Educator**) 4:00–4:30 Planning for next week/ core orientation/orientee assessment forms	07:30–10:30 SMS Computer/ P Building-If needed 10:30–12:00 Independent Activities on Unit of Hire or Modules 12:00–1:00 Meet with Director Main 4 Office Lunch Provided 1:00–2:00 Pastoral Care Room U477 2:00–4:00 Modules on Patient Safety and Quality Improvement

Required Modules:
Age Specific ☐ **IV Therapy** ☐ **Blood and Blood Products** ☐ **RN Medication** ☐ **Patient Rights** ☐
Peds or Adult Emergency Care ☐ **Latex Allergy** ☐ **Patient Classification** ☐
Order Transcription (not for ED, PACU) ☐ **Pain Management** ☐ **Documentation** ☐ **CPR: (see handout)**

Dept of Education- #262–3705

FIGURE 17-6

Registered professional nurse general orientation schedule template—week one.
(*Source:* Courtesy of Albany Medical Center, Albany, NY.)

At each of these sessions, it is important for the new nurse to solicit feedback. Ask, "How do you think I'm doing? Am I at the level you would expect? What should I focus on next?" Answers to questions such as these allow the orientee to measure progress and set goals for the future.

A sample performance goals outline might look like the following:

By the next scheduled performance assessment, nurse Joanne Johnson will do the following:

- Successfully complete the advanced pediatric assessment course
- Assume the primary nurse role for patients with an anticipated length of stay greater than three days
- Become an active participant on a unit-based or hospital-wide interprofessional team committee
- Attend a pediatric nursing conference

TABLE 17-10
Developing a Professional Style

1. Assess your current education and experience.
2. As you start your new nursing role, review the following on your unit:
   - Most common medical diagnoses
   - Most common nursing diagnoses
   - Most common medications and IV solutions
   - Most common diagnostic tests
   - Most common laboratory tests
   - Most common nursing and medical interventions and treatments
3. Set goals for additional education and experience that you may need, both now and for the future.
4. Review your own job description and the roles and job descriptions of nursing and other health care and interprofessional team staff you work with.
5. Identify the names and contact information of all nursing and other interprofessional team staff you work with.
6. Discuss delegation with your preceptor, and observe how the preceptor delegates to others.
7. Observe the impact of delegation on both the delegate and the person delegated to.
8. Remember the golden rule: do unto others as you would want them to do unto you.
9. Recognize that, under the law, the RN holds the responsibility and accountability for nursing care.
10. Practice assertiveness and work at being direct, open, and honest in your new role.
11. Exercise your power with kindness to all.
12. Hold others accountable for their responsibilities as spelled out in their job descriptions.
13. Be open to performance improvement feedback about your personal delegation style.
14. Build rapport and modify your communication approach to fit the needs of patients, staff, the interprofessional team, and yourself.
15. Take action to ensure your patients receive high-quality, safe, evidence-based patient-centered care.
16. Monitor patient satisfaction and patient outcomes.

© Cengage Learning 2014

Name: Preceptor: Unit/Dept.: Emergency Dept: Date:			
At the completion of orientation, the RN will perform technical nursing skills specific to the age and characteristics of the patients served, consistent with the Standards of Nursing Practice.			
Self-Evaluation Scale 1 2 3	RN Technical Skill Checklist	Method of Validation/ Code	Date Met/ Initials
	1. Cardiovascular A. Initiate IV therapy 1. Adult, non-trauma 2. Trauma patient 3. Pediatric 4. Newborn 5. Phlebotomy percutaneous approach B. Blood sampling: 1. Arterial line 2. Blood sampling: port-a-cath 3. Triple lumen/trauma cath/central line C. Central venous line management: securing/dressing/caps/tubing 1. Trauma catheter/triple lumen 2. Implanted device external access (i.e., Hickman) 3. PICC line 4. Port-a-cath D. Infusion pumps 1. IV pumps 2. Syringe pumps 3. Programmable pediatric pump 4. Patient-controlled analgesia E. Spacelab bedside and central monitors 1. Cardiac rhythm interpretation F. Defibrillator operation 1. Zoll 2. Physiocontrol 10 and 9 G. External transcutaneous pacer–Zoll H. Transvenous pacer pack: Emergent I. Transvenous pacer pack: Urgent 1. Pulse generator 2. Ushkow's lead J. Blood products administration K. Level I blood warmer and rapid infuser L. Spun Hct M. Utilization of doppler for vascular assessment 2. Gastrointestinal		

FIGURE 17-7

Emergency department competency-based orientation tool sample page (excerpt).

(*Source:* Courtesy of Albany Medical Center, Albany, NY.)

360-Degree Performance Feedback

Some health care organizations have moved to a performance evaluation program known as **360-degree performance feedback**. In the 360-degree performance feedback system, an individual is assessed by a variety of people in order to provide a broader perspective about his or her performance. For example, a nurse may complete a self-assessment and submit a portfolio that documents competency, critical thinking, values, beliefs, and skills (O'Malley, 2008). The portfolio may include elements of nursing orientation, nursing practice, leadership, teamwork, scholarly activity, documentation, and committee work. The portfolio also documents peer reviews, evaluation by the nurse's immediate supervisor, and patient interviews.

Corrective Action Programs

Sometimes, performance evaluation indicates the need for significant improvement. Most health care organizations have a prescribed corrective action program. One of the first steps in helping employees improve their performance is identifying whether poor performance is developmental or related to a failure to follow policies or procedures. For example, a nurse may be having difficulty completing assignments in an appropriate time frame. The manager needs to coach the nurse, assisting with whatever support will help him or her improve. Another category of corrective action is disciplinary corrective action. Most organizations have a series of progressive steps for corrective action in cases in which employee performance does not improve. For example, a manager may begin by providing a verbal warning to an employee whose attendance is minimally acceptable. If the nurse's attendance problem continues, he or she may receive a written warning. Without improvement, this could proceed to a suspension, final warning, and eventually termination. In a union environment, the employee may have the right to union representation after a verbal reprimand.

Nurses who receive a verbal warning from their manager should immediately demonstrate a commitment to quality patient care and plan for improvement in order to avoid any progression toward corrective action. It is useful, although not always easy, to avoid taking the corrective action personally and to look on the feedback as an opportunity for improvement.

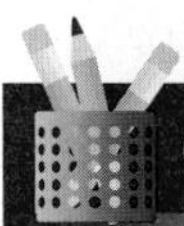

CASE STUDY 17-1

Maria Diaz is a senior nursing student working as a patient care assistant on an oncology floor in a small community hospital. Maria is well liked by the staff of the floor and is offered a full-time registered nurse position upon graduation. While Maria is flattered and relieved that she has an offer, she feels that she should at least interview at another hospital, including a nearby teaching hospital, for comparison.

How would Maria begin her job search at other hospitals? What are the key elements to securing an interview at other hospitals? Once Maria has an interview, what type of questions should she be prepared to answer from the interviewer?

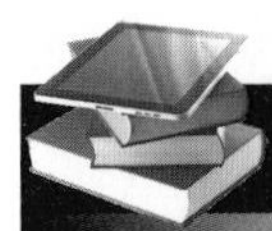

EVIDENCE FROM THE **LITERATURE**

Citation: Heacock, S. (2008). Inspiring the inspirational: Words of hope from nurses to nurses. Retrieved January 3, 2012, from http://www.amazon.com/Inspiring-Inspirational-Words-Hope-Nurses/dp/1438922337

Discussion: The author identifies these elements for a successful career:

RISE AND SHINE: Whether you work 7A–7P, 7P–7A, or any shift in between, arrive at work good to go and in good spirits. There is nothing worse than saying, "Good morning" to a coworker only to be answered with, "What's good about it?" It does not bode well for the positive spirits of those around you for the rest of the day! Shine to your patients, peers, and supervisors every day!

MEASURE TWICE, CUT ONCE: Safety is paramount in nursing. Regardless of how busy or how stressed you feel, you must pay attention to detail to avoid sentinel events or near misses. It is not only the safety of your patients on the line, but your professional reputation as well.

DON'T PUT OFF UNTIL TOMORROW WHAT YOU CAN DO TODAY: Make the best use of your time while at work. Procrastinating and not optimizing your workload are not only unfair to your patients, but affect your peers as well. How many times have you come on shift to find many things were left undone that should have been accomplished? This one goes *hand in hand* with the next one!

DO UNTO OTHERS: I found the true meaning of this statement when I first began working in a pediatric emergency room. I wanted to ensure each patient was treated like he or she were my own child. At the same time, I was constantly cognizant of parental emotions and needs. This philosophy works well with peers too. If your coworker is really busy and you have a slow moment, help him or her out. It will be remembered the next time you need someone to pitch in.

WHEN IN ROME: It is imperative in nursing to be a team player. Those around you rely on your professional standards and behavior. And—there really are reasons for those work site rules and policies! Remember: *There is no "I" in TEAM.*

EVERY ROSE HAS ITS THORN AND STUFF HAPPENS: There is no utopian job, optimum situation, or perfect day. A nurse must take the negatives in stride and focus on the positives. Dwelling on the negatives creates anxiety and makes everything in your day seem worse than it really is! So: *Go with the flow!*

DON'T BITE THE HAND THAT FEEDS YOU AND DON'T BURN YOUR BRIDGES: If you are frustrated with a management decision or your supervisor, *grin and bear it!* Talking about management personnel behind their backs or sabotaging their authority will only *get you in hot water*. Remember, these are the people who create work schedules, complete performance appraisals, and make recommendations for promotions. Also keep in mind that if you ever leave your current position, they control your destiny when new potential employers call!

TURN OVER A NEW LEAF IF YOU ARE BARKING UP THE WRONG TREE: It is okay if you decide your current job is either not for you or you find yourself in need of a new professional challenge. You will not be productive and effective if you are not happy. Find another tree or a new leaf! And never forget that *every cloud has a silver lining* and you need to *take time to smell the roses*.

Implications for Practice: The advice and directives from the author serve as a guideline for most any type of nursing specialty, in any environment. Professional socialization takes time to become a daily "norm" in the lives of nurses.

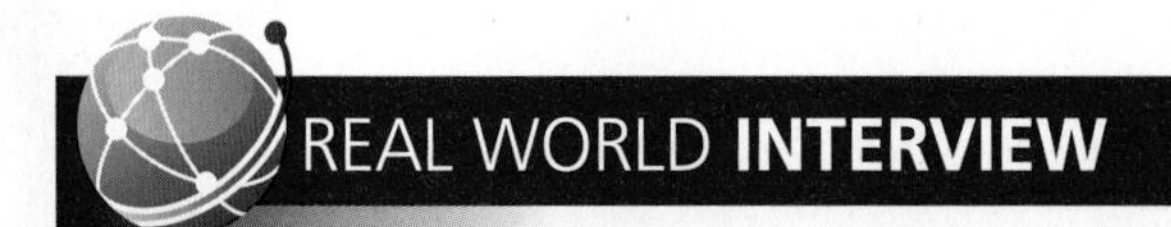

REAL WORLD INTERVIEW

Here are a few lessons I learned as a new graduate:

1. You will manage to get every single type of body fluid on you at one time or another (blood, trach gunk, fistula juice, stomach residual, stool, urine). Bring a pair of backup scrubs to work.
2. You learn from your mistakes. I was taking care of a patient on an insulin drip during the night shift. She was up all night long and her daughter didn't think too highly of the care she was getting. When the patient and her daughter finally fell asleep, I skipped her 3 A.M. Accucheck. Her 4 A.M. Accucheck was 27. Needless to say, I have never skipped an Accucheck since.
3. If a preceptor shows you something, don't say that he or she is doing it wrong and then pull out a policy book. Your preceptor will hate you for life.
4. Never pass up an opportunity to learn something, even if you think you have seen it before. Maybe someone will teach you a new and better way to do it.
5. You will think you are ready for your first really sick patient, but you are not. The senior staff will help you through it. I still replay my first really sick patient in my head and think back to all the things I wish I had done differently. Luckily, no one else dwells on it. I am my worst critic!
6. Find a person besides your preceptor whom you admire, maybe for their nursing skill, their personality, or their way of making everything look easy. Ask if he or she will mentor you. It doesn't need to be a super-serious conversation. I made mine a joke and asked a nurse if she would be my Nighttime Sensei. She accepted and to this day, she has my back when things get crazy.
7. Always do the little things. I was a patient care tech before I was a nurse. I always make sure my rooms are stocked, everything is put away, my patient is clean, the patient's meds are in the drawer, and so forth. Little things like this can really help out your next coworker. There is nothing worse than walking into a patient's room and it looks like a bomb went off.
8. Always help out your coworkers. I work in an ICU, and there is a real sense of teamwork. As a new graduate, I always felt like I never had enough time to do my work, but I always made time to help the other nurses turn their patients, do a bath, move them to a chair, and so on. That stuff doesn't take that long and your coworkers really appreciate it. Plus, next time you need help with something, easy or not, they will be there for you.
9. I think my first month off of orientation, I cried in the shower at least once a week. Some of it was about the patients I took care of; some was about working with not nice people; some of it was just because I needed to cry. I always tried to keep my emotions out of my workplace. Some people are very emotional at work, and it makes others uncomfortable. I am not saying that you can never cry at work or with a patient's family, but if you are crying during every shift, your coworkers will start to think that you can't handle your job.
10. I live by the mottos "never show fear" and "do it right." Always walk into the patient's room with confidence. If you are doing something for the first time, run through it with someone experienced before going into the patient's room. You are taking care of someone's mom, dad, or child, and they are trusting you with their lives. Don't give them a reason to lose that trust.

ERIN MAHONEY, BSN, RN
Loyola University Hospital
Maywood, Illinois

KEY CONCEPTS

- The NCLEX-RN examination tests safe, effective care environment; physiologic integrity; psychosocial integrity; and health promotion and maintenance.
- The NCLEX-RN contains a variety of formats for exam items.
- Multiple factors are associated with NCLEX-RN performance as identified in Table 17-2.
- It is useful to have a plan to review any NCLEX-RN weaknesses.
- Successful NCLEX-RN candidates often practice over 3,000 test questions in preparation for the exam.
- Organizational orientation is both general and unit based. Orientation is a time for developing strong relationships with preceptors and members of other disciplines, as well as for mastering competencies needed for safe patient care.
- Nurses receive performance feedback both informally and as part of periodic evaluations. This input is valuable in developing personal goals.
- Newspapers, electronic media, the Internet, and job fairs are all possible avenues for job opportunities.
- An effective résumé will (1) get the employer's interest; (2) identify critical areas such as education, work experience, and special qualifications; (3) be tailored to the employer's needs; (4) create a favorable first impression about you and your abilities; (5) communicate that you are someone who is a good fit for the position; and (6) be visually appealing.
- When preparing for an interview, practice answering potential interview questions with a colleague, friend, or family member before the actual interview so that you have practiced answers to difficult questions.

KEY TERMS

résumé

360-degree performance feedback

REVIEW QUESTIONS

1. A senior nursing student is preparing for the NCLEX-RN exam. The student realizes a variety of formats for questions will be used that include which of the following? Select all that apply.
   A. Fill-in-the-blank calculation
   B. Multiple responses
   C. Case study scenarios
   D. Ordered response
   E. Hot spots
   F. Matching

2. The nursing student is using the ARKO acronym as a strategy for preparing for the NCLEX-RN. The NCLEX-RN question states: "How would the nurse evaluate if the drug enoxaparin (Lovenox) is effective for the postoperative patient?" Using the second step (R), choose the best answer based on the information provided.
   A. What are the adverse effects of the drug?
   B. How long does it take for the drug to become effective?
   C. What is the intended action of the drug?
   D. How will the nurse administer this drug safely?

3. A nurse is working in a long-term care facility and has an 85-year-old patient with dehydration secondary to diarrhea. The health care provider has ordered to infuse potassium chloride 10 mEq over one hour. Prior to implementation, the nurse's plan should include which of the following?
   A. Validating that the patient has adequate urine output
   B. Obtaining an accurate height and weight
   C. Arranging for a central line IV catheter placement
   D. Assessing possible causes for the diarrhea

4. A nursing student asks an RN preceptor for suggestions to deal with test-taking anxiety prior to the NCLEX-RN exam. The RN explains that the literature supports which of the following actions as a recommendation to deal with test-taking anxiety?
   A. Avoidance of caffeine and concentrated sweets for a month prior to the exam
   B. Walking up to five miles a day in an area with attractive landscape
   C. Keeping well rested with a full night's sleep and a brief afternoon nap
   D. Using guided imagery to create a relaxing visual scene on which to concentrate

5. Nurse residency programs offered by select hospitals across the nation have afforded new graduates which of the following outcomes? Select all that apply.
   A. Better salary/benefit package
   B. Ability to organize and prioritize their work
   C. Increased comfort in communicating with the health care team
   D. Ability to advance into management positions quickly
   E. Ability to provide clinical leadership on the assigned unit
   F. Decreased measurable stress scores

6. A nurse educator is reviewing test-taking strategies in preparation for NCLEX-RN. The nurse educator shares with the class the importance of focusing on setting priorities when meeting patient needs. Put the following items in order of priority from first to last.
   A. A patient requests pain medication
   B. A patient has become confused
   C. A patient with a tracheostomy needs to be suctioned
   D. A patient in shock needs intravenous access for fluid administration

7. A nurse is sending an electronic résumé for a desired position at a local health care clinic. In preparing the electronic résumé, the nurse knows an appropriate step in electronic résumé preparation is which of the following?
   A. Placing the Social Security number in the subject line of the e-mail to increase recognition
   B. Using key nouns associated with the particular job opening in the subject line of the e-mail
   C. Listing the nurse's accomplishments in a three-column format on the résumé
   D. Preparing the entire résumé in a bold font that transmits more clearly electronically

8. A nurse has read a number of articles on interviewing skills and typical topics that a prospective employer might ask during the interview period. The nurse would anticipate which of the following questions in the interview?
   A. "I see on your résumé that you live in a new estate development; do you own the home?"
   B. "Can you share any chronic illnesses you currently have or were treated for in the past?"
   C. "Tell me about the most difficult patient assignment you had while a student in nursing school."
   D. "I know a young man about your age with the same surname; is he your husband?"

9. A graduate-level nursing student is conducting a study on corrective action programs used for nurses working in hospitals. Which issue would most likely require corrective action?

A. Complaints from patients that a nurse has a speech accent which is difficult to understand
B. Complaints from a physician that a nurse who is obese is not setting a good example for patient health behaviors
C. Complaints from colleagues that a nurse arrives late for second-shift handoff report on a continuous basis
D. Complaints from the nurse to the supervisor regarding his/her work schedule being unfair

10. A group of nursing students is discussing the details of the NCLEX-RN. Which of the following is a true statement made in regard to the NCLEX-RN examination?

A. "We can expect to have 100 items on the exam."
B. "This is a computer-adaptive test."
C. "The exam is given at the school of nursing where applicants attended."
D. "The exam measures the highest level of competency of recent graduates."

REVIEW ACTIVITIES

1. Set up a group to study for the NCLEX with several of your friends. Have each member of the group buy an NCLEX review book from a different publisher. Practice answering questions separately for one to two hours daily. Do not mark your answers in the review book. Share your study schedule and your review books with each other to encourage each other and increase your exposure to various authors' test questions.
2. You are graduating in two months from a nursing program. Develop a résumé using the format in this chapter.
3. You are a new nurse who has been asked to interview for a position on the orthopedic floor. Develop a cover letter expressing interest in the position. Make a list of possible interview questions.

EXPLORING THE WEB

- There are many websites specific to nursing employment opportunities. Try some of these:
  http://www.nursingjobs.org
  http://www.healthecareers.com
  http://www.nurse.com
  http://www.discovernursing.com
  http://www.studentdoc.com/nursing-job-site.html
  http://www.healthcareerweb.com
- Look up several of these nursing sites:
  Association of Pediatric Oncology Nurses: *http://www.apon.org*
  Association of Rehabilitation Nurses: *http://www.rehabnurse.org*
  Association of Women's Health, Obstetric and Neonatal Nurses: *http://www.awhonn.org*
  Trauma Nursing: *http://www.trauma.com*
- Check this site for job opportunities: *http://healthcare.monster.com*
- Check this site:
  National Student Nurses' Association: *http://www.nsna.org*
- Go to: *http://www.learningext.com*

Note: NCSBN's Review for the NCLEX is offered through this NCSBN learning extension. This self-paced, online review features NCLEX-style questions, interactive exercises, topic-specific course exams, and a diagnostic pretest that can help you develop a personal study plan. Visit this site every Monday to see its new NCLEX-RN test-question samples.

- Visit: *http://www.nursecredentialing.org*
  Click on "find a facility."
- Check this guide to education in nursing: *http://www.allnursingschools.com*

REFERENCES

American Hospital Association (AHA). (2011). Fast facts on U.S. hospitals. Retrieved from http://www.aha.org/research/rc/stat-studies/fast-facts.shtml

American Nurses Credentialing Center (ANCC). (2011). Retrieved from http://www.nursecredentialing.org/Magnet/FindaMagnetFacility.aspx

Becze, E. (2008). Format your résumé for electronic viewing. *Oncology Nursing Society Connect, 23*(5), 30. Retrieved from http://www.nxtbook.com/nxtbooks/ons/connect_200805/index.php?startid=30

Centers for Disease Control and Prevention (CDC). (2012). Immunization schedules. Retrieved October 8, 2012, from http://www.cdc.gov/vaccines/schedules/hcp/index.html

Centers for Disease Control and Prevention. (2012). Immunization Schedules for Infants and Children. Retrieved November 26, 2012 from, http://www.cdc.gov/vaccines/schedules/easy-to-read/child.html

Doyle, A. (2011a). Illegal interview questions employers should not ask. About.com Guide. Retrieved from http://jobsearch .about.com/od/interviewsnetworking/a/illegalinterv.htm

Doyle, A. (2011b). Nurse interview questions. About.com Guide. Retrieved from http://jobsearch.about.com/od/interviewquestionsanswers/a/nurse-interview-questions.htm

Dyess, S. M., & Sherman, R. O. (2009).The first year of practice: New graduate nurses' transition and learning needs. *Journal of Continuing Education in Nursing, 40*(9), 403–410.

Emery, C. M. (2011). Six interview tips to win the job. *Nursing Link.* Retrieved October 20, 2011, from http://nursinglink.monster.com/benefits/articles/5143-6-interview-tips-to-win-the-job

Gaddis, S. (2009). Ten tips for perfecting a nursing interview. *Tar Heel Nurse, 71*(2), 6–7.

Goode, C. J., Lynn, M. R., Krsek, C., Bednash, G. D., & Jannetti, A. J. (2009) *Nursing Economic$, 27*(3), 142–148.

Heacock, S. (2008). Inspiring the inspirational: Words of hope from nurses to nurses. Retrieved January 3, 2012, from http://www.amazon.com/Inspiring-Inspirational-Words-Hope-Nurses/dp/1438922337

Holden, J. (2006). How can we improve the nursing work environment? *The American Journal of Maternal/Child Nursing, 31*(1), 34–38.

Idris, N. (2011). NCLEX study: Does the NCLEX RN test anxiety monster stalk you? Ezine articles. Retrieved October 20, 2012, from http://ezinearticles.com/?NCLEX-Study:-Does-the-NCLEX-RN-Test-Anxiety-Monster-Stalk-You?&id=6446541

Insider's guide to beating test anxiety. (2010). New York, NY: Bedford-St. Martin's Publishing.

Kelly, P., & Hernandez, G. (2012). Medication Study Guide Starter. Unpublished manuscript.

Kramer, M. (1974). *Reality shock: Why nurses leave nursing.* St. Louis, MO: Mosby.

McGahee, T. W., Gramling, L., & Reid, T. F. (2010). NCLEX-RN® success: Are there predictors? Southern Online Journal of Nursing Research, 10(4). Retrieved December 31, 2010, from http://snrs.org/publications/SOJNR_articles2/Vol10Num04Art13.html

NCLEX-RN® Examination Test Plan for the National Council Licensure Examination for Registered Nurses NCLEX-RN® TEST PLAN. Effective April 2013. Retrieved November 26, 2012, from https://www.ncsbn.org/2013_NCLEX_RN_Test_Plan.pdf

Olmstead, J. (2007, March). Predict future success with structured interviews. *Nursing Management, 38*(3), 52–53.

O'Malley, P. A. (2008, June). Profile of a professional. *Nursing Management, 39*(6), 24–27.

Pescar, S. C. (2009). *Conquering test anxiety.* New York, NY: Grand Central Publishing.

Polifko-Harris, K. (2012). Career Planning. In P. Kelly. (Ed.). *Nursing Leadership and Management* (3rd ed.). Clifton Park, NY: Delmar Cengage Learning.

Schultz, C.M. (2010). Test taking strategies, including NCLEX, GRE, and Certification exams. In Polifko, K.A. (2010). The practice environment of nursing. Delmar Cengage Learning. Clifton Park, NY.

U.S. News & World Report. (2011). 100 best hospitals of America list. Retrieved October 30, 2012, from *http://*www.usnews.com

Winfrey, O. (2012). Search Quotes ©.*Luck is a matter of preparation meeting opportunity*. Retrieved November 26, 2012, from http://www.searchquotes.com/quotation/Luck_is_a_matter_of_preparation_meeting_opportunity./24088/

SUGGESTED READINGS

Affordable Care Act, 2010. Retrieved November 2, 2012, from http://www.healthcare.gov/law/full/index.html

Alameida, M. D., Prive, A., Davis, H. C., Landry, L., Renwanz-Boyle, A., & Dunham, M. (2011). Predicting NCLEX-RN success in a diverse student population. *Journal of Nursing Education, 50*(5), 261–267.

Bonis, S., Taft, L., & Wendler, M. C. (2010). Strategies to promote success on the NCLEX-RN: An evidence-based approach using the ACE Star Model of Knowledge Transformation. *Nursing Education Perspectives, 28*(2), 82–87.

Bruce, C. (2010). Helpful tips on starting a nursing career. The Black Collegian Online. Retrieved from http://www.black-collegian.com/career/industry-reports/helpfultips2001-1st.shtml

Carrick, J. A. (2011). Student achievement and NCLEX-RN success: Problems that persist. *Nursing Education Perspectives, 32*(2), 78–83.

Davenport, N. C. (2007). A comprehensive approach to NCLEX-RN success. *Nursing Education Perspectives, 28*(1), 30–33.

Drenkard, K. (2011). Magnet momentum: Creating a culture of safety. *Nurse Leader, 9*(4), 28-31.

Dudas, K. (2011). Strategies to improve NCLEX® style testing in students who speak English as an additional language. *Journal of Cultural Competence in Nursing & Healthcare, 1*(2), 14–23.

Dumpel, H. (2010). Hospital magnet status: Impact on RN autonomy and patient advocacy. *National Nurse, 106*(3), 22–27.

Future of Nursing Campaign for Action. Retrieved December 26, 2011, from http://thefutureofnursing.org/content/regional-action-coalitions

Garrosa, E., Moreno-Jiménez, B., Rodríguez-Muñoz, A., & Rodríguez-Carvajal, R. (2011). Role stress and personal resources in nursing: A cross-sectional study of burnout and engagement. *International Journal of Nursing Studies, 48*(4), 479–489.

Gordon, S., & Nelson, S. (2006). *Moving beyond the virtue script in nursing in the complexities of care.* Ithaca, NY: ILR Press.

Günüşen, N. P., & Üstün, B. (2010). An RCT of coping and support groups to reduce burnout among nurses. *International Nursing Review, 57*(4), 485–492.

Hader, R. (2011). Education matters. *Nursing Management, 42*(7), 22–27.

Herrman, J. W., & Johnson, A. N. (2009). From beta-blockers to boot camp: Preparing students for the NCLEX-RN. *Nursing Education Perspectives,* (6), 384–388.

Hess, R., DesRoches, C., Donelan, K., Norman, L., & Buerhaus, P. I. (2011). Perceptions of nurses in magnet hospitals, nonmagnet hospitals, and hospitals pursuing magnet status. *Journal of Nursing Administration, 41*(7/8), 315–323.

Ilhan, M. N., Durukan, E., Taner, E., Maral, I., & Bumin, M. A. (2008). Burnout and its correlates among nursing staff: Questionnaire survey. *Journal of Advanced Nursing, 61*(1), 100–106.

Kelly, L. A., McHugh, M. D., Aiken, L. H. (2011). Nurse outcomes in Magnet® and non-Magnet hospitals. *The Journal of Nursing Administration, 41*(10), 428–433.

Lee, J. S., & Akhtar, S. (2011). Effects of the workplace social context and job content on nurse burnout. *Human Resource Management, 50*(2), 227–245.

Leiter, M. P., & Maslach, C. (2009). Nurse turnover: The mediating role of burnout. *Journal of Nursing Management, 17*(3), 331–339.

Manning, L. (2008). Chapter 27: Preparing students for the NCLEX-RN. In B. K. Penn (Ed.), *Mastering the teaching role* (pp. 339–358). Philadelphia, PA: F. A. Davis Company.

Pabst, M. K., Strom, J., & Reiss, P. J. (2010). Use of focus groups to elicit student perception of NCLEX-RN preparation. *Journal of Nursing Education, 49*(9), 534–537.

Pagana, K. D. (2009). 7 tips to improve your professional etiquette. *Nursing 2009, 39*(11), 34–37.

Poorman, S. G., Mastorovich, M. L., Molcan, K. L., & Webb, C. A. (2009). Decreasing performance and test anxiety in practicing nurses. *Journal for Nurses in Staff Development, 25*(1), 13–22.
Romeo, E. M. (2010). Quantitative research on critical thinking and predicting nursing students' NCLEX-RN performance. *Journal of Nursing Education, 49*(7), 378–386.
Tolan, T. (2011). Put your best foot forward: Tips for making sure that your interview produces the best outcome. *Healthcare Informatics, 28*(5), 48.
Uyehara, J., Magnussen, L., Itano, J., & Zhang, S. (2007). Facilitating program and NCLEX-RN success in a generic BSN program. *Nursing Forum, 42*(1), 31–38.

CHAPTER 18

Career Planning and Achieving Balance

TANYA L. TOTH, RN, MSN, MBA, HCM, CNOR, CRNFA;
EDNA HARDNER MATTSON, RN, BN, BA (CSA), MDE; AND
KARIN POLIFKO-HARRIS, RN, PHD, CNAA

To Nurse
To Care
To Solace
To Touch
To Feel
To Hurt
To Need
To Heal others,
As well as ourselves.

—CAROL BATTAGLIA, 1996

OBJECTIVES

Upon completion of this chapter, the reader should be able to:

1. Identify strategies for professional growth.
2. Discuss certification and clinical ladders.
3. Define health.
4. Identify the six concepts of health, namely, physical, intellectual, emotional, professional, social, and spiritual health.
5. Describe selected strategies to maintain physical, intellectual, emotional

You have just started in your new nursing position. You are excited and want to do a good job, as well as plan for the future. You want to continue to grow professionally and yet have a life outside nursing also. You are thinking about many questions. Where do you see yourself one, five, or ten years from now? What opportunities exist for certification and additional education? How can you ensure some balance and less stress in your life both inside and outside nursing?

At the turn of the 21st century, the nursing demand far exceeded the supply of registered professional nurses. As of 2010, the shortage in registered nurses is projected to grow to an estimated 260,000 FTEs by the year 2025, twice as high as any U.S. nursing shortage since the 1960s (AACN, 2012).

Statistical data from 2008 showed that the average age of nurses was 46 years; the average age at graduation for recent RN graduates was 30.8 years; and the number of RNs who were advanced-practice nurses was 250,527. In 2009, the National League for Nursing (NLN) released statistics for enrollment numbers to entry-level RN programs. Enrollment numbers continue to steadily increase from year to year with 315,524 enrollments in 2008; however, this is only a 0.3 percent increase as compared to increases of nearly 20 percent in previous years. According to AACN (2012) in 2010, U.S. nursing schools turned away 67,563 qualified applicants from baccalaureate and graduate nursing programs, and almost 40 percent of all applicants to basic RN programs in 2008–2009. The primary basis for rejection is an insufficient number of faculty.

An issue confronting nursing has been identifying what the appropriate entry-level educational degree should be, and what a nurse really is because of the many levels of educational preparation. In December 1965, the American Nurses Association (ANA) House of Delegates (HOD) adopted a motion that the ANA continue to work toward baccalaureate education as the educational foundation for professional nursing practice. By 1985, the ANA HOD agreed to urge state nursing associations to establish the BS degree with a major in nursing as the minimum educational requirement for licensure and to retain the title of registered nurse (RN) (ANA, 2000). To date, there is still a variety of paths an individual can take to become an RN. These include a two-year associate degree, a three-year diploma, and a four-year baccalaureate degree.

A major advancement within nursing has been the emergence of several areas of advanced nursing practice, namely, the certified registered nurse anesthetist (CRNA), the clinical nurse specialist (CNS), the nurse practitioner (NP), and the certified nurse midwife (CNM). The profession has also significantly upgraded its educational, clinical, research, and managerial focus. This chapter will examine career planning and maintaining balance in your nursing and non-nursing life. The concept of health, the types of health including physical, intellectual, emotional, professional, social, and spiritual health, as well as strategies to maintain health will be discussed.

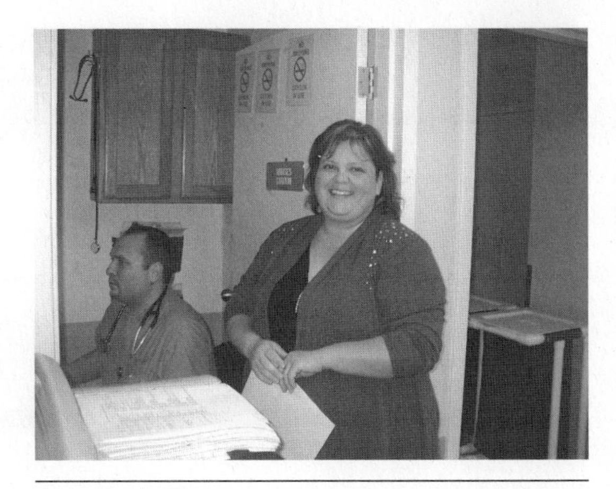

© Cengage Learning 2014

CAREER PLANNING

Career planning is an ongoing process that involves personal and professional self-assessment, setting goals, and regular self-evaluation. Establishing goals creates a written plan for reasonable and measurable, long-term and short-term objectives. Goals should support growth and achievement. Following the SMART model for establishing goals allows you to track your progress (University of Toledo, 2011).

Determining your goals using a common SMART acronym for goal setting is useful. SMART stands for **S**pecific, **M**easurable, **A**chievable, **R**ealistic, and **T**imely goal setting. Being SMART will help you describe specifically what you want to accomplish with your strategic planning for your career. For example, when you are planning your career, you may want to work in a specialty patient care unit after graduation. Your SMART career-planning goals may be as found in Table 18-1. You may want to also

TABLE 18-1
Example of "SMART" Career Planning Goals

Specific	Employment as an RN in an emergency department (ED)
Measurable	Function independently full time
Achievable	Employment at hospital that allows recently graduated RNs to work in ED
Realistic	Presence of other new graduates who were able to achieve goal
Timely	Achieve goal within two years

© Cengage Learning 2014

include goals for continuing your education. Visit www.allnursingschools.com and search for listings of bachelor's, master's, nurse practitioner, and doctoral nursing programs within your geographic location. Career planners suggest setting short-term goals for one to three years, intermediate goals for three to five years, and long-term goals for six to twenty years.

Certification

Certification in nursing represents an example of professional credentialing and is a voluntary process undertaken by practicing nurses. It is a marker of the knowledge and experience of a professional RN and is more than just a symbolic title. The American Board of Nursing Specialists (ABNS) (2009) defines the certification process as the formal recognition of the specialized knowledge, skills, and experience demonstrated by the achievement of standards identified by a nursing specialty to promote health outcomes. Basic eligibility requirements for specialty nursing certification are available at www.nursecredentialing.org.

Professional certification, through a wide variety of organizations, is also monitored by the ABNS and includes the clinical component of nursing (acute care, long-term care and hospice, advanced practice, and outpatient care settings) as well as nursing administration. Certifications for nurses are available in a variety of specialties, including traditional patient care roles, administrative roles, educational roles, and nontraditional nursing roles (Thomas, Benbow, & Ayars, 2010). Several of the larger certifying organizations include the ANA; American Association of Nurse Anesthetists (AANA); National Association of Pediatric Nurse Associates and Practitioners (NAPNAP); Association of Women's Health, Obstetric and Neonatal Nurses (AWHONN); and the Association of Critical-Care Nurses (ACCN).

Competence

Professional growth and practice require competent staff. Professional nursing **competency** is the application of knowledge, and the interpersonal, decision-making, and psychomotor skills expected for the practice role within the context of public health, safety, and welfare. (National Council of State Boards of Nursing, 2011). Competency of professional staff can be ensured through credentialing processes developed either at an agency or through certification by a national nursing organization. See Table 18-2.

Clinical Ladder

A clinical or career ladder may be in place in an agency. A clinical ladder program offers nurses the opportunity to develop their careers, continue their education, and increase their salaries without losing focus on care at the bedside. Although the criteria may vary, most programs have three or four distinct levels. **Clinical ladders** offer the nurse recognition of achievement in clinical practice and provide a means for professional advancement that is separate from progression through other channels, such as education or administration, that have been traditional paths for next steps in career movement within nursing (Burket et al., 2010). For example, to be promoted

TABLE 18-2
Certifications Available from American Nurses Association

Advanced Practice	BS in Nursing or Higher Degree
Nurse Practitioners	◆ Cardiac/Vascular Nurse
◆ Acute Care	◆ Gerontological Nurse
◆ Adult	◆ Informatics Nurse
◆ Adult Psychiatric/Mental Health	◆ Medical-Surgical Nurse
◆ Advanced Diabetes Management	◆ Nursing Administration
◆ Family	◆ Nursing Professional Development
◆ Family Psychiatric/Mental Health	◆ Pediatric Nurse
◆ Gerontological	◆ Perinatal Nurse
◆ Pediatric	◆ Psychiatric/Mental Health Nurse
Clinical Nurse Specialists	◆ Public/Community Health Nurse
◆ Advanced Diabetes Management	**Associate Degree or Diploma in Nursing**
◆ Adult Health (*formerly known as Medical-Surgical*)	◆ Cardiac/Vascular Nurse
◆ Adult Psychiatric/Mental Health	◆ Gerontological Nurse
◆ Child/Adolescent Psychiatric/ Mental Health	◆ Medical-Surgical Nurse
◆ Gerontological	◆ Pediatric Nurse
◆ Pediatric	◆ Perinatal Nurse
◆ Public/Community Health	◆ Psychiatric Mental Health Nurse
Other Advanced-Level Exams	**Diploma, Associate, Baccalaureate or higher degree in Nursing**
◆ Advanced Diabetes Management—Dietician	◆ Ambulatory Care Nurse
◆ Advanced Diabetes Management—Pharmacist	◆ Nursing Case Management
◆ Nursing Administration, Advanced	◆ Pain Management

Source: American Nurses Association (ANA). (2012). ANA handle with care campaign. Retrieved from http://www.nursingworld.org/rnnoharm.

from a new Graduate Level I to a Level II RN, the nurse may be required to complete a specialty course such as Advanced Cardiac Life Support (ACLS) or EKG Interpretation, join a unit- or hospital-based committee, and finish the preceptor course. A clinical ladder program recognizes and rewards nursing's contribution to quality care and highlights evidence-based practices that positively influence patient outcomes (Burket et al., 2010).

The Colorado Differentiated Practice Model (Figure 18-1) builds on the work of Benner (1984) regarding career ladder stages. Stage I is characterized as the entry/learning stage. Stage II is characterized by the individual who competently demonstrates acceptable performance adapting to time and resource constraints. Stage III is characterized by the individual who is proficient. And Stage IV is characterized by the individual who is an expert. The stages in this model are

Colorado Differentiated Practice Model

The Colorado Differentiated Practice Model for Nursing has a separate clinical ladder for the six preparatory backgrounds depicted on the conceptual model (Diagram 1). The framework for each educational ladder has four weighted components as follows:

- Competency Statements 60%
- Skills 10%
- Institutional Goals 15%
- Professional Activities 15%

Conceptual model

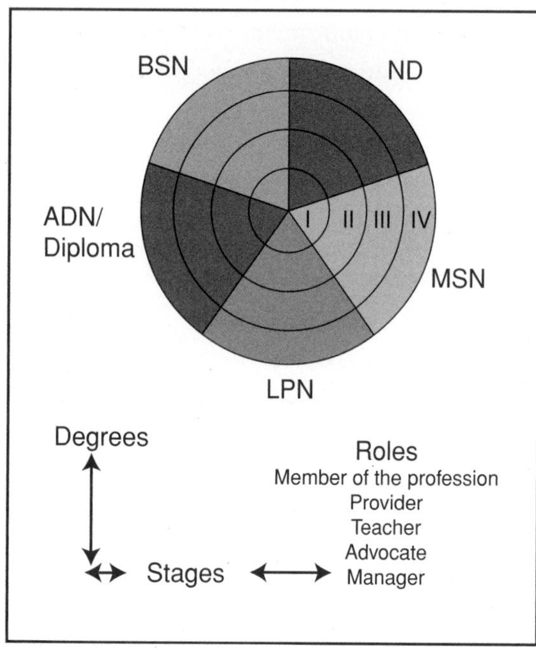

Diagram 1

Sample ladder

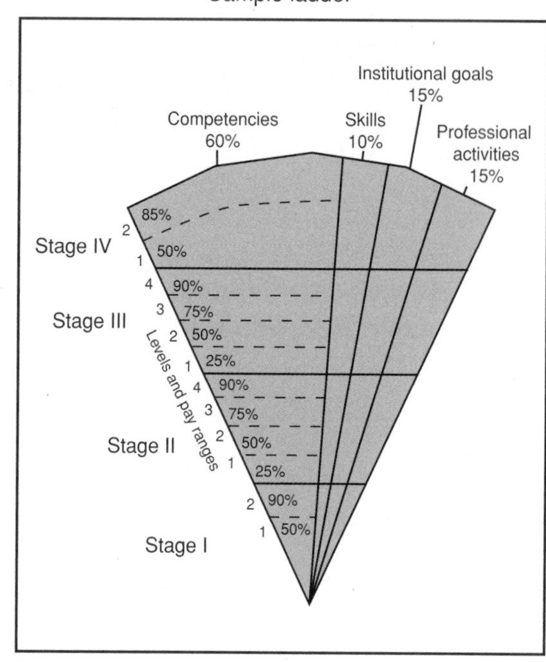

Diagram 2

FIGURE 18-1

Colorado differentiated practice model

(*Source:* Courtesy Marie E. Miller, Colorado Nursing Task Force, 2001.)

specifically defined by behaviors that are consistently exhibited or practiced over a defined period of time.

The Colorado Differentiated Practice Model for Nursing has a separate clinical ladder for the six preparatory backgrounds depicted on the conceptual model (Diagram 1). The framework for each educational ladder has four weighted components as follows:

- Competency Statements 60%
- Skills 10%
- Institutional Goals 15%
- Professional Activities 15%

HEALTHY LIVING—ACHIEVING BALANCE

Nursing is a caring profession. Nurses spend their days helping others, many times at the expense of themselves. But, if there is nothing left for nurses, they will not be able to maintain the strength to care for their patients. Florence Nightingale described health as "being well and using every power the individual possesses to the fullest extent" (Nightingale, 1969 [1860], p. 334). The World Health Organization

(2010) describes **health** as a "state of complete physical, social, and mental well-being, and not merely the absence of disease or infirmity. Health is a resource for everyday life, not the object of living." p. 100.

Goals for Healthy People 2020

In January 2000, more than 1,500 individuals, health professionals, and organizations convened in Washington, D.C. to discuss goals for health promotion and disease prevention for the U.S. population (U.S. Department of Health and Human Services, 2001). Since that time, *Healthy People* has continued to establish benchmarks to develop a society in which all people live long and healthy lives (www.healtypeople.gov). For the next decade *Healthy People* has taken the 10 leading health indicators to

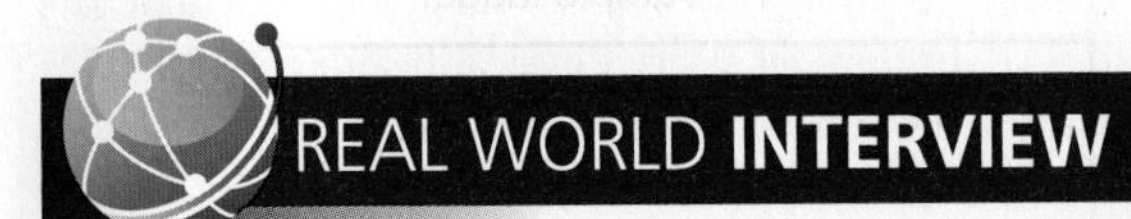

There are five levels of our clinical ladder, which is similar to Benner's novice-to-expert model. The novice RNs are new graduate RNs in orientation. The experts are the clinical specialists. A lot of them have also become nurse practitioners so that the organization can receive some reimbursement for their patient care services. This is a good thing because otherwise I'm afraid we wouldn't have these expert nurses anymore. They are the true mentors for nursing staff, especially when you are working with a very complex or difficult patient situation.

Staff nurses also mentor each other. During orientation, your preceptor guides you along the path from RN I to RN II. When you decide you'd like to advance to RN III, you can choose another mentor. RN IIIs provide much more clinical leadership for staff and for the overall unit. I decided I was ready to be promoted to that level when other staff members consistently were coming to me for clinical guidance and with patient care questions. Now, as an RN III, I am the chairperson of our unit-credentialing committee, which is part of the quality council of our shared-governance model.

Our clinical ladder uses a portfolio as the main tool to evaluate the nurse's readiness to advance. When you are an RN I in orientation, you are first introduced to the idea of a portfolio and how to put it together. It is difficult at first, as people do not know what is expected. However, after that first time when you are promoted from an RN I to an RN II, it becomes easier. You just build on what is already in the portfolio.

A portfolio should include the following:

Licenses
Your résumé
Letters of reference
Evaluations
Clinical documentation of patient care
Validations for competencies related to technical skills (medication administration, IV therapy)
Examples of participation in development of the team plan of care
Exemplars
CEU certificates
Presentations
Publications

The portfolio tells the story of your practice. When a group of people are ready for promotion, the members of the credentialing committee meet. We review the portfolios and make recommendations related to advancement. The nurse manager is a member of this committee. She always reviews the portfolio and gives us her feedback even if she is unable to attend the credentialing meeting. I enjoy reading the exemplars the most. Exemplars are mini stories that paint the pictures of each nurse's practice, and they are all so different.

STACEY CONLEY, RN, BS
Staff Nurse
Cooperstown, New York

a renewed focus on identifying, measuring, tracking, and reducing health disparities through a determinants of health approach. The determinants of health are defined through the range of personal, social, economic, and environmental factors that influence one's overall health status (Healthy People, 2020).

AREAS OF HEALTH

Health is a complex and dynamic state of being. It is a positive concept that emphasizes social and personal resources as well as a person's physical potential. Healthy persons must take into account the implications of their activities in relation to their collective health and well-being. When one area of life is affected, other areas of health are also affected. There is overlap among the areas, but for purposes of discussion in this chapter, health has been divided into the following six elements: physical health, intellectual health, emotional health, professional health, social health, and spiritual health. The tool in Table 18-3 will assist you in identifying your health trends in each of the six areas of health.

Physical Health

Physical health, the first element of health, encompasses nutrition as well as exercise, coupled with a balanced amount of sleep. Physical health also includes health-promotion and disease-prevention behaviors such as avoiding smoking, maintaining a healthy body mass index with healthy nutrition and exercise, and having annual Pap smears and other screening procedures that detect health problems early. Review the 2010 Dietary Guidelines for Americans at www.dietaryguidelines.gov and the physical activity guidelines at www.cdc.gov to make sure you are following the latest guidelines.

TABLE 18-3
Health Assessment Tool

Physical Health	**Yes**	**No**
1. I exercise at least 30 minutes daily.		
2. My BMI meets the optimal health guidelines.		
3. I sleep eight hours a night.		
4. My immunizations are up-to-date.		
5. I avoid risky behaviors, e.g., smoking, drugs, tanning booths, unprotected sex.		
6. I have regular health screenings, dental cleanings, Pap tests, mammograms, and do monthly testicular or breast self-examinations.		
Intellectual Health		
7. I plan to purchase a home soon.		
8. I read at least one book a month and practice critical thinking.		
9. I have a 401K or 403b savings plan for retirement.		
10. I know how much money I have invested in Social Security.		
11. I have invested in diversified mutual stock and bond funds.		
12. I save 10% of my income for the future.		
13. I have a hobby I enjoy.		

(Continues)

TABLE 18-3 (Continued)

Emotional Health

14. I have developed strategies to deal with my own anger.
15. I have developed strategies to deal with the anger of others.
16. I work well with others.
17. I practice stress management techniques.
18. I try to be empathetic and sense what others are feeling.
19. I try to find a reason to laugh daily.
20. I avoid thought distortions.

Professional Health

21. I have professional goals including certification and additional nursing education.
22. I have a mentor.
23. I have attended at least three workshops in the past year.
24. I subscribe to three nursing journals.
25. I belong to at least one professional organization.
26. I use appropriate personal protective equipment.
27. I never recap a needle.
28. I follow safe patient-handling policies when moving patients.
29. I follow standards of care when handling gaseous waste, disinfectants, and chemotherapy.
30. I follow standards of care in dealing with lasers, radiation equipment, and environmental hazards.
31. I avoid workplace violence.

Social Health

32. I go out with my friends at least once a week.
33. I see my family regularly.
34. I have at least one friend I can confide in.
35. I have a wide diversity of professional, family, neighborhood, and church friends.
36. Not all my friends are nurses.
37. I do volunteer work.

Spiritual Health

38. I pray or meditate every day.
39. I believe in a higher power.
40. I attend meetings at a place of worship regularly.
41. I read spiritual books or spend time in quiet meditation daily.
42. I maintain a daily journal.
43. I seek help from professional counselors as needed.

© Cengage Learning 2014

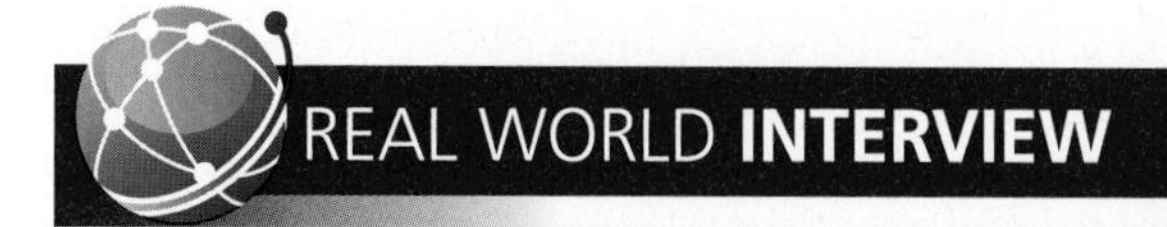

As NPs face the new millennium, it is advisable to listen to the wisdom of the famous author on China, Pearl Buck, who said, "To understand today, you have to search yesterday." Further, to envision the future, think "outside the box" creatively, constructively, and globally. Unfortunately, most people hate change; so do professionals. By their very nature, professionals can become myopic, territorial, and conservative. Some that are so resistant to change become arrogant, self-important, and greedy. Nursing must face the future differently. Tomorrow's practitioners will face globalization, not only of economics but of every field of human endeavor. Demographics, technological advances, transportation, and communication will expand beyond imagination and at lightning speed. Health information will no longer belong exclusively to the health professions. The Internet will see to that. The challenge for NPs is to be proactive rather than reactive in creating a social, cultural, political, and physical environment in which to successfully live, work, and thrive as a responsible member of the new society and as an advocate for our patients and their families. So, thoroughly examine the past, keep the enduring human values of caring, compassion, and courage in nursing, listen to your best teachers—the patients—and create your own future accordingly.

LORETTA FORD, EDD, RN
FAAN Founder, Nurse Practitioner Program
Rochester, New York

Body Mass Index Calculation

You can assess your body weight in relation to your height by calculating your body mass index (BMI). You can calculate this at www.nhlbisupport.com/bmi/bmicalc.htm. The National Institutes of Health (2012) has established the following guidelines for interpretation of the BMI:

- 30 and above is obese
- 25 to 29.9 is overweight
- 18.5 to 24.9 is optimal health
- Below 18.5 is considered underweight

Sleep

Sleep is another component of physical health. It is not uncommon for nurses to sleep less than eight hours per night. Nurses who work nights may find it especially difficult to sleep for an uninterrupted block of time. Nurses who are constantly changing shifts are more susceptible to sleep deprivation. It is estimated that it can take from four to six weeks to change sleeping patterns. In spite of this, nurses may work various shifts within a week. Clockwise or forward shift rotation (i.e., days, evenings, and nights) has been suggested to improve sleep (Berger & Hobbs, 2006).

Studies have shown that individuals who lack sleep are more irritable, have difficulty completing tasks, concentrating, and making decisions, and are unsafe in their actions (www.sleepfoundation.org). Nurses often consider fatigue a normal part of the job, and often do not perceive the connection between working excessive hours and impaired health. Working without adequate sleep between shifts can lead to negative chronic health effects including cardiovascular disease, metabolic syndrome, diabetes, obesity, decreased immune function, and an increased risk of cancer. In respect to job performance and safety to patients, sleep deprivation has been documented as increasing the risk of medical errors (Institute of Medicine [IOM], 2006). Patient safety is the utmost concern.

The drive home after work for a nurse can be dangerous. For each extra shift worked during one month, there is a 9.1 percent increased risk of a motor vehicle accident during the commute home from work. Nurses working nights and rotating shifts rarely obtain optimal amounts of sleep. Nurses who rotate to evenings or nights are almost twice as likely to nod off while driving home. A period of wakefulness over 24 hours can produce performance decrements equivalent to a blood alcohol concentration of 0.01 percent, as well as impaired speed and accuracy, hand-eye coordination, decision making, and memory (Rogers, 2008).

How do you know if you are sleep deprived? Assess your sleepiness index by answering eight simple questions using the Epworth Sleepiness Scale at the following website: http://www.healthcommunities.com/sleep-disorders/epworth-sleepiness-scale-tool.shtml. Test your knowledge regarding sleep deprivation with additional educational resources available at the National Sleep Foundation website: www.sleepfoundation.org; click on Sleep Facts and Information.

Intellectual Health

Intellectual health is the second element of health and encompasses those activities that maintain intellectual curiosity. Intellectually healthy people are able to think critically and make sound decisions. They read, have hobbies, learn from experience, and are flexible and remain open to new ideas. For purposes of this chapter, the term "intellectual health" also includes doing personal financial planning.

Personal Financial Planning

The first step in personal financial planning is to identify your annual salary. In 2009, the average salary for all categories of registered nurses was $66,530. The

CRITICAL THINKING 18-1

Consider the leading health indicators of *Healthy People 2020* at www.healthypeople.gov. How is your personal behavior related to each of the indicators? How can you do better? How can you help your family, friends, and community do better? Keep a diary for one week on how you are doing on five or more of the indicators. The *Healthy People 2020* indicators not on the chart are substance abuse, injury and violence, environmental quality, immunization, and access to health care. See Figure 18-2 for a sample diary. At the end of the week, assess to see how well you have taken care of yourself. Is this a typical week? Do you need to make any changes? Were there any surprises? You can also record for several weeks and compare the outcomes.

	Physical Activity	Overweight and Obesity	Tobacco Use	Responsible Sexual Behavior	Mental Health	Other
Monday						
Tuesday						
Wednesday						
Thursday						
Friday						
Saturday						
Sunday						

FIGURE 18-2

Healthy People 2020 Diary

(*Source: Healthy People 2020* document. Retrieved October 20, 2012, from www.healthypeople.gov/LHI/lhiwhat.htm)

top 10 percent earned over $93,000, while the lowest 10 percent earned less than $44,000 (U.S. Bureau of Labor Statistics, 2009).

Next, begin to think about the percentage of your salary you want to save; most experts recommend 10 to 15 percent. There is no better time than now to invest in your future. Now is the time to begin saving for such things as a home, your children's education, and even retirement, no matter what your age. Note that a nurse who is making $50,000 annually will make $1,800,000 in a 30-year working career. If this nurse invests $200 per month at 12 percent interest for the 30 years, the nurse will have more than $1,000,000 in a retirement account at age 65 (Koren & Christie-McAuliffe, 2012).

Savings for retirement are three-pronged: (1) Social Security funds, (2) employee retirement funds, and (3) additional personal savings. You should annually check the accuracy of your Social Security account by reviewing the information sent to you by the Social Security Administration, available at *www.ssa.gov.*

Employee Retirement Funds: The most common retirement funds are the 401K or 403b plans. The only difference between the two is that the 403b is a plan offered by a nonprofit organization and the 401K is offered by a for-profit organization. Otherwise, the two plans are exactly alike. For purposes of this discussion, the term "401K" will be used.

Often, both the employee and most employers contribute retirement money to a **401K**. This is a great way to save because some health care institutions may match the funds that you contribute. Once your money is put into the fund, it is tax sheltered, meaning you do not pay any taxes on the amount contributed until it is withdrawn. For example, if you earn $58,000 per year and contribute $5,800 to the 401K, you will be taxed on only $52,200 of income. If the money is withdrawn before you reach the age of 59½, you will pay a 10 percent federal penalty. This is an incentive to keep the money in the account until retirement; the plan should be considered a long-term investment.

Once the money is in the fund, you must decide how the company administering the plan will invest it for you. You have two basic choices: bond mutual funds and stock mutual funds. Each of these investment opportunities has risks and benefits. Many financial advisors recommend diversifying and including a mix of these funds in your planning depending on your age. Several reliable information sources rank mutual funds for quality. These include the annual ratings by Consumer Reports and the Morningstar ratings available through the Internet. (See Exploring the Web at the end of this chapter.)

Individual Retirement Account (IRA): Another type of retirement fund is the individual retirement account (IRA). This account is an option for anyone with sufficient employment income. Contributions cannot exceed $5,500 per year. This fund may or may not be tax deductible, depending on what other retirement accounts you hold and which type of IRA you open. There are two kinds of IRAs: the traditional IRA and the Roth. The **Roth IRA** was first introduced in 1998. A Roth IRA is taxed prior to the investment but grows tax-free and there is no penalty for early withdrawal.

Personal Savings and Real Estate: After investing in retirement funds, you also have a few more options for investment. You can open a **money market account**, a short-term investment that is highly liquid and very safe, a checking account, and/or a savings account.

You also have the option to invest in stock or bond mutual funds or individual stocks or bonds outside of your retirement account. You can start your research by reviewing Valueline at your local library (see Exploring the Web at the end of this chapter). The key to successful investment is to diversify, meaning to spread your money around in many different types of investment options, stocks, bonds, mutual funds, and so on.

Owning your own home is a smart investment. When purchasing a home, obtain as much information as possible. Research properties in the area you want to buy. Once you have selected a home that you are interested in, hire your own home inspector to take a look at the property. Investigate the school system, tax base, typical list price, and average time of homes on the market. Drive by and examine the neighborhood. Is this where you would want to live? Next, plan how to finance the property. Work with a real estate agent.

How to Educate Yourself: There are many ways to learn more about investments. Brokerage firms offer classes periodically. Try taking a course on personal finance at a local college. You can also go to the Internet (see Exploring the Web at the end of this chapter).

Another option is to hire a financial planner, but that can become expensive. Check their fees first and educate yourself by reading financial books. Suze Orman (2010) is an author who many find easy to understand and very relevant. Subscriptions to *Money, Barron's,* and *Kiplinger Magazine* can also be educational. Complete your net worth yearly. Knowing your net worth allows you to understand your economic position as it relates to the value of your assets versus your financial liabilities. This can be done by making a list of all your financial assets and deficits. See Table 18-4. Your goal is to see an increase in your assets when you complete this document each year.

Emotional Health

Emotional health is the third element of health. Being emotionally healthy also involves maintaining control of your thoughts and feelings. People with good emotional health are resilient in the face of challenges, find ways to express their creativity, and understand the importance of social connections and having a positive attitude (Emotional Health Center, 2011) Note the discussion of Emotional Intelligence in Chapter 1.

Anger

Anger is a universal, strong feeling of displeasure that is often precipitated by a situation that frustrates or prevents a person from attaining a goal or getting what is wanted from life. Anger is a common emotion that we all may feel at one time or another. As a matter of fact, anger is pervasive in our society today. There is road rage, airplane rage, outraged customers, and rage at sporting events. The causes for the anger are numerous. Some of the anger may be due to: rapid changes in society related to high technology; a lack of privacy, because we are accessible to work at all hours through cell phones, and other electronic devices; a sense of entitlement; a lack of family connection; and overcrowding. There seems to be a spillover of anger into the nursing profession. Many sources for this anger are evident when one considers the increasing complexity of patient care. Add to this economic problems,

TABLE 18-4
Net Worth—Year 1 and 2

Year I Assets		Deficits	
Car	$5,000	School Loan	$2,000
Assets − Deficits = Net Worth		Car Loan	$2,000
$5,000 − $4,000 = $1,000 Net Worth − Year 1			$4,000
Year II Assets		**Deficits**	
Home	$75,000	Home Mortgage	$59,000
Car	$5,000	School Loan	$1,500
Savings	$500	Credit Cards	$200
	$80,500	Car Loan	$1,500
			$62,200
$80,500 − $62,200 = $18,300 Net Worth − Year 2			

© Cengage Learning 2014

staffing shortages, high turnover of experienced staff, and demeaning treatment by other health care staff, and one begins to see some of the causes of anger (Koren & Christie-McAuliffe, 2012).

Ways to Cope with Anger: An effective way of coping with anger is to prevent its development. Teaching resilience as part of nursing education is one approach to this goal. Resilience is the ability to cope with and adapt to adversity, which is a desired quality to have in the stress-filled environment of health care (McAllister & McKinnon, 2009). Evidence is growing that the skill of resilience can be learned.

Sometimes anger and frustration are caused by sensory overload or overcommitment. It is important to have time for yourself. If nurses are to be effective caregivers, they first must care for themselves. Saying no, be it to a supervisor, friend, or family member, may at times be necessary. Learn to say no.

Humor and Stress Management

Laughter is the best medicine (Figure 18-3). Laughter has many benefits such as helping to boost the immune system, promoting relaxation, and decreasing blood pressure, heart rate, and respiratory rate (Mayo Clinic Staff, 2010). But best of all, laughter is contagious and it is free. The ability to laugh, play, and have fun with others not only makes life more enjoyable—it also helps you solve problems, connect with others, and be more creative (Table 18-5). People who incorporate

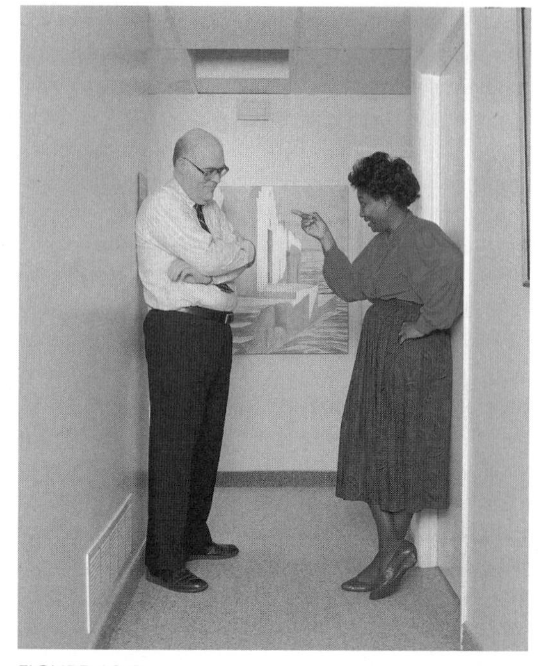

FIGURE 18-3
Laughter Is an Effective Stress Reliever
© Cengage Learning 2014

TABLE 18-5
Stress Management Techniques

Meditate.	Do relaxation exercises.	Be polite to all.
Think peaceful thoughts.	Do something different for lunch.	Take a walk.
See things as others might.	Give yourself a pat on the back.	Read.
Forgive your mistakes.	Join a support group.	Join a club.
Do not procrastinate.	Talk about your worries.	Sing a song.
Set realistic goals.	Be affectionate.	Forgive and forget.
Do a good deed.	View problems as a challenge.	Listen to music.
Vary your routine.	Get/give a massage.	Take a hot bath.
Appreciate what you have.	Say a prayer.	Call an old friend.
Focus on the positive.	Expect to be successful.	Let go of the need to be perfect.

© Cengage Learning 2014

humor and play into their daily lives find that it renews them and all of their relationships (Smith, Kemp, & Segal, 2010).

Avoiding Thought Distortions

Research on thinking processes has shown that people sometimes make mistakes in the way they perceive information and think about the world around them. When people are depressed, their automatic thoughts are loaded with distorted thinking. If one can recognize this distorted thinking (Table 18-6), one can begin to turn his or her life in a more positive direction.

Professional Health

Professional health is the fourth element of health. Persons are professionally healthy when they are satisfied with their career choices and think that there is continual opportunity for growth. The professionally healthy individual is goal directed and seeks every opportunity to obtain knowledge and new learning experiences. This may include going back to school for more education, becoming certified in his or her clinical practice area, and avoiding occupational hazards.

Occupational Hazards Common Among Nurses

An important aspect of professional health is avoidance of occupational hazards. The U.S. Bureau of Labor Statistics (2010) reports that health care and social assistance workers rank second highest in percentage of nonfatal workplace injuries.

The survey reports the number of new, work-related illness cases that are recognized, diagnosed, and reported during the year. Some conditions (e.g., long-term latent illnesses caused by exposure to carcinogens) often are difficult to relate to the workplace and are not adequately recognized and reported. The overwhelming majority of the reported new illnesses are easier to

TABLE 18-6
Thought Distortions

Thought distortion	Example
All-or-nothing thinking: seeing things only in absolutes	"Either you like my proposal and we follow it or you don't."
Overgeneralization: interpreting every small setback as a never-ending pattern of defeat	"As I wasn't given the lead on this project, I'll never lead another one."
Dwelling on negatives: ignoring multiple positive experiences	"I made a mistake. I'm not good enough to be a nurse."
Jumping to conclusions: assuming that others are reacting negatively without definite evidence	"I don't know why I study. Everyone thinks I'm going to fail the NCLEX anyway."
Fortune telling: thinking things will turn out badly without proper evidence	"If I don't get this promotion, I'll be stuck at this level forever."
Emotional reasoning: assuming that your current negative emotions undoubtedly demonstrate the way things really are	"I am scared to go in front of the board, so therefore it must be a scary situation."
Obligations: living life around a succession of too many "shoulds," "shouldn'ts," "musts," "oughts," and "have-tos"	"I must/should never show any weaknesses to my colleagues."

Source: Compiled from Good, D., Yeganeh, B., & Yeganeh, R. (2010). Cognitive Behavioral Executive Coaching. *OD Practitioner, 42*(3), 18–23.

directly relate to workplace activity (e.g., contact dermatitis, carpal tunnel syndrome, or back injuries).

The cumulative weight lifted by a nurse providing direct patient care in a typical eight-hour workday is estimated to be 1.8 tons. Unfortunately, nurses accept back pain as part of their job, with 52 to 63 percent of nurses reporting musculoskeletal pain that lasts for more than 14 days; in 67 percent of cases, pain was a problem for at least six months (Nelson et al., 2007).

The newest approach to this serious occupational problem has been the use of safe patient-handling policies—at the facility level, state level, or national level. In 2009, ANA established ANA's Handle with Care Recognition Campaign™ to recognize health care facilities that have had a safe patient-handling program in place for at least three years and meet high standards for program evaluation, monitoring, planning, policy, and training.

There are numerous suggestions for safeguarding against various hazards in the workplace. Occupational hazards can be divided into four major categories: (1) infectious agents, (2) environmental agents, (3) physical agents, and (4) chemical agents. See Exploring the Web at the end of this chapter and Table 18-7.

INFECTIOUS AGENTS: Infectious agents can be transferred through direct contact with an infected patient or through exposure to infected body fluids. The major infectious agents for health care workers are

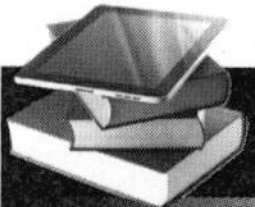

EVIDENCE FROM THE **LITERATURE**

Citation: Waters, T. R. (2007, August). When is it safe to manually lift a patient? *American Journal of Nursing, 107*(8), 53–59.

Discussion: According to the U.S. Bureau of Labor Statistics, in 2005, nursing ranked eighth among occupations reporting work-related musculoskeletal disorders involving days away from work, with more than 9,000 cases of such disorders and a median of seven missed days of work per injury. Nurses' aides, orderlies, and attendants ranked second, behind laborers and freight, stock, and material movers.

Musculoskeletal disorders are often caused by the cumulative effect of repeated patient-handling tasks and high-risk tasks such as lifting, transferring, and repositioning patients. Extensive laboratory-based research has documented high levels of biomechanical stress on caregivers' spines, shoulders, hands, and wrists from patient lifting and repositioning.

Many of these injuries are preventable. A strong body of research has demonstrated that mechanical lifting equipment, as part of a program promoting safe patient handling and movement, can significantly reduce musculoskeletal injuries among health care workers.

Note that for most patient-lifting tasks, the maximum recommended weight limit is 35 pounds—but even less when the task is performed under less than ideal circumstances, such as lifting with extended arms, lifting when near the floor, lifting when sitting or kneeling, lifting with the trunk twisted or the load off to the side of the body, lifting with one hand or in a restricted space, or lifting during a shift lasting longer than eight hours.

In 2003, the American Nurses Association launched its Handle with Care campaign, "a profession-wide effort to prevent back and other musculoskeletal injuries." See www.nursingworld.org/handlewithcare. The ANA also released a position statement, Elimination of Manual Patient Handling to Prevent Work-Related Musculoskeletal Disorders. See www.nursingworld.org. Search for "manual patient handling."

Implications for Practice: Nurses should work to avoid back injuries by following these guidelines. Check the websites for patient-handling information.

TABLE 18-7
Safeguards for Occupational Hazards

Infectious Agents

- Do not recap needles.
- Use needle-free intravascular access devices.
- Place needle disposal containers near point of use of needles.
- Use personal protective equipment.
- Report all needlestick injuries immediately.
- Wash hands before and after each patient contact.

Physical Agents

- Follow standards of care for dealing with radiation/laser equipment.
- Assess work area for amount of noise.
- Eliminate excessive noise in the workplace.
- Implement good body mechanics. Get equipment and help to lift heavy patients.
- Follow ergonomic safety guidelines from OSHA (Department of Government Affairs, 2006b).

Environmental Agents

- Develop a zero tolerance, no abuse policy to protect nurses and all staff.
- Develop a violence reduction plan to protect staff.
- Rotate shifts clockwise—day to evening to night (Rogers, 1997).
- Assess for dangerous chemicals, mold, and fungus in your workplace.
- Review OSHA standards at your facility for environmental agents.
- Develop an agency/facility plan to work with victims of terrorism.
- Maintain air quality; avoid fumes from glutaraldehyde, ethylene oxide, and laser plume smoke.

Chemical Agents

- Utilize effective ventilation systems.
- Develop standards of care for handling gaseous waste, chemotherapy, disinfectants, and anesthetics.
- Protect pregnant nurses from handling chemotherapy during the first trimester.
- Use appropriate nonlatex barrier protections.
- Develop policies and procedures to ensure safety from latex allergies.

© Cengage Learning 2014

HIV, herpes, tuberculosis, and hepatitis. A recent survey of 58 hospitals found that 44 percent of the needlestick injuries were sustained by nurses, compared to 15 percent by medical practitioners (IHCWSC, 2006). Nurses have the largest amount of direct patient contact and are at the greatest risk for exposure to blood-borne pathogens. The chance of a seroconversion, which occurs when a serological test for antibodies changes from a negative reading to a positive reading, varies according to the disease exposure. The estimated risk for infection for HIV after needle exposure is from 0.2 to 0.5 percent. The risk for developing serological evidence of hepatitis B infection is 37 to 62 percent, whereas hepatitis C carries an estimated risk of 1.8 percent (Bahadori & Sadigh, 2010).

Although the majority of infectious agents are transmitted through blood, the herpes simplex virus can be transmitted by direct contact with an infected lesion. Hepatitis A is transmitted primarily via diarrhea as a result of poor hygienic practices among health care workers. The overall incidence of tuberculosis (TB) is gradually increasing, and there are certain regional differences. In 2010, a total of 11,181 TB cases were reported in the United States, equivalent to 3.6 cases per 100,000 population. TB rates in reporting areas ranged from 0.6 (Maine) to 8.8 (Hawaii) cases per 100,000 population (CDC, 2011).

ENVIRONMENTAL AGENTS: Another group of occupational hazards is environmental agents. These include all the agents within the hospital that may lead to injury. The most prevalent include violence, shift work, air quality, mold and fungus, and bioterrorism. Nurses are at risk for workplace violence. Employment in a health care facility is considered one of the most dangerous jobs in the United States. In a recent study, nearly half a million nurses per year reported being victims of some type of violence in the workplace (Department of Government Affairs, 2006a).

Poor air quality in the workplace is yet another environmental risk that may lead to symptoms such as shortness of breath, eye and nose irritation, headaches, contact dermatitis, joint pain, memory problems, and reproductive difficulties. Glutaraldehyde, a chemical used to disinfect many commonly used instruments, can emit a hazardous gas. Ethylene oxide, a chemical commonly used to sterilize surgical equipment, has been reported to have carcinogenic effects. Lasers used in operating rooms can emit hazardous gaseous material in the form of either laser plume or chemical by-products of laser smoke. Laser treatment carries the risk of eye and skin injury if the instruments are not handled properly. Nurses should be educated and aware of the risks of inhalation of smoke plume and develop policies and procedures to protect themselves and patients alike from the harmful effects of surgical smoke (Ulmer, 2008). Air quality can also be influenced by mold and fungus, which are often found in carpeting and in ceiling tiles. The presence of mold and fungus can lead to asthma and other respiratory problems. Most hospitals have some type of bioterrorist alert plan. Nurses play an active role in dealing with any type of bioterrorist disaster.

PHYSICAL AGENTS: Physical agents are another occupational hazard and include radiation, noise, and lifting patients. Radiation exposure is common among health care workers. Radiation is used for both diagnostic and treatment interventions. Persons exposed to excessive amounts of radiation are at risk for cancer. Nurses can protect themselves from the effects of radiation by following agency guidelines and wearing a dosimeter that measures the amount of radiation exposure. Pregnant nurses working with radiation should declare their pregnancy to their employer as soon as possible (Duke University, 2009). Noise is another physical hazard that can lead to hearing loss. Excessive noise that occurs over a long period of time can also lead to irritability and inability to concentrate. High levels of noise are deleterious for both nurses and patients. Special care units are especially noisy with alarms, ventilators, suction equipment, monitors, call lights, and so on.

CHEMICAL AGENTS: Another occupational hazard is chemical agents such as anesthetic agents, antineoplastic drugs, disinfectants, latex gloves, hazardous drugs, and drug and alcohol abuse (Ulmer, 2008). Operating room nurses face many hazards on a daily basis and must take care to identify potential hazards and establish safe practices.

Latex glove exposure is another type of chemical concern for nurses. Nurses and other health care personnel who are frequently exposed to latex can become sensitive to latex proteins. It is estimated that 8 to12 percent of health care workers are latex sensitive with reactions ranging from irritant contact dermatitis and allergic contact sensitivity, to immediate, possibly life-threatening sensitivity (OSHA, 2011). Yet another concern for nurses is the potential for personal misuse of drugs and/or alcohol. Registered nurses have a 50 percent higher rate of substance abuse than the general public, and one in seven nurses remains at risk for addiction (Epstein, Burns, & Conlon, 2010). To reduce the risk of substance abuse among nurses, the primary focus should begin in educating nursing students on the risks of, symptoms of, and resources for drug abuse (Epstein et al., 2010).

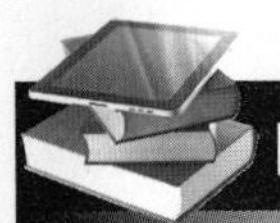

EVIDENCE FROM THE **LITERATURE**

Citation: Franche, R., Murray, E., Ostry, A., Ratner, P., Wagner, S., & Harder, H. (2010). Work disability prevention in rural health care workers. *Rural and Remote Health, 10*(4), 1502.

Discussion: Health care workers appear to be particularly vulnerable to occupational injury and prolonged work-absence duration. In the United States in 2005, the health care sector accounted for the second largest number of nonfatal injuries and illnesses among all sectors, representing over 30 percent of all workplace injuries and illnesses involving time lost from work. Similarly, in British Columbia, Canada, health care is responsible for the second largest proportion of lost work days due to occupational injury or illness, behind construction workers. In Australia, the incidence of serious occupational injury claims is greater in health and community services than in any other industry. Workers in rural areas face three unique challenges that may make them vulnerable to higher rates of poor work-disability outcomes. First, rural residents are less healthy compared with urban residents in Australia, Canada, New Zealand, and many other developed countries. They have overall poorer health, lower life expectancy, and higher infant mortality. Rates of disability, violence, accidents, and poisoning are greater in rural areas than in urban areas. The health of residents in rural communities in Canada has been shown to decrease as the distance to an urban center increases. Second, rural health care systems differ from urban systems in that they are more poorly resourced. In Canada, although the per capita distribution of primary physicians may be relatively equal in rural and urban areas, the availability of specialist care is drastically reduced in rural areas. Distance from and access to primary care services are additional major challenges. Third, rural health care workers are socio-demographically different from urban health care workers. The profile of the health care worker in rural areas emerges as one of an older worker facing extremely high work demands including long hours and high on-call demands, who is expected to be a multispecialist with little educational or professional support, in a context of staffing shortage, and who responds to a patient population that presents with complex health and social needs. Workplace violence, lack of replacement staff, and challenges unique to rural contexts including hazardous roads, harsh climates, long distances, and isolation, are key risk factors for poor disability outcomes in rural health care workers.

Implications for Practice: This literature review suggests two promising future avenues to improve the work disability outcomes of rural health care workers:

1. Health care and workers' compensation policies and processes should be tailored to the unique needs of workers in rural areas, taking into account access to health care challenges.
2. More research is needed about rural-urban differences in work-absence duration and about the relationship between risk factors for occupational injury and work disability-prevention outcomes.

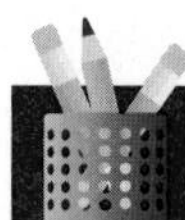

CASE STUDY 18-1

You are a nurse admitting Mrs. Zakima, an 84-year-old female. You received the following report from the emergency department. Her vital signs are BP 140/70, RR 30, HR 80. The patient has bilateral rales, 2+ pitting pedal edema, weighs 350 pounds, and is 5′ 5″ tall. Mrs. Zakima is a transfer from a nursing home. She is being admitted for symptoms related to congestive heart failure. She has a past history of hypertension, diabetes, rheumatoid arthritis, dementia, and MRSA. Mrs. Zakima is being admitted to your unit. In preparing the room that she will be admitted to, what do you need to keep in mind with regard to noise, safety, and universal precautions?

What safety precautions would you put in place to protect yourself, that is, ergonomics, universal precautions, and so forth?

After reviewing her chart, you find she is taking the following medications: methotrexate, zestril, toprol, and lasix. What other precautions should you take with this patient?

Social Health

Social health is another significant element of health. Social health forms the last of the three fundamental and vital forms of health for a person. Social health often deals with how people relate to each other, and how an individual is able to socialize with other people and form relationships, including friendships. Social health has become of increasing importance within the greater overall concept of human health and well-being (Wiesen, 2011).

Impact of Social Relationships

Social support is a communication behavior that plays an important part in physical and mental health maintenance. There is compelling evidence that social support from other people and connectedness with them has a powerful impact on health outcomes and mortality (Segrin & Passalacqua, 2010). If these interactions are frequent, that only adds to good health. In other words, the more you see your friends, the healthier you become. The variety of those relationships may also keep you healthy. The greater the diversity of the relationships, such as professional, family, neighborhood, or church relationships, the more likely you are to remain healthy.

Spiritual Health

Spiritual health is the last area of health. Spirituality is an elusive term that is difficult to define. It can be viewed as the essence of being, that which gives meaning and direction in life, or a feeling of connection with something greater than oneself. Spirituality may be a feeling of well-being in relation to God, or a feeling of purpose and satisfaction in life (Pedrão & Beresin, 2010). Koenig (2007) has extensively researched spirituality, religion, and health. His findings lend some scientific support to the positive effects of prayer and religious involvement.

Dossey and Keegan (2009) describe how nurses can gain insight into their own spirituality by exploring ways to nurture themselves through ritual, rest, play, and expressions of creativity. Nurses function in a fast-paced and stressful environment, which often leads to job dissatisfaction, burnout, and potentially suboptimal patient care. Nurses need to find ways to nurture themselves emotionally and spiritually. Nurturing relationships with a spouse or significant other, children, friends, and other family is a vital part of self-care. For some, engagement in the larger community can enhance well-being. Engaging in self-reflection, including sharing our stories and struggles with partners or friends, can legitimize our challenges and help us gather the strength to persevere or change. A number of studies describe the overall benefit of regular prayer, meditation, and reflective journaling (Chittenden & Ritchie, 2011).

KEY CONCEPTS

- Clinical ladders can guide nursing development.
- There are numerous types of advanced-practice nurses (APNs) within both the hospital and community settings. Some examples of these roles include the CNS, NP, and CRNA.
- To provide quality patient care, nurses need to first take care of themselves and maintain a healthy lifestyle.
- Health is not just the absence of disease; it is the state of complete balance of six elements of health, namely, physical, intellectual, emotional, professional, social, and spiritual health.
- Nurses' physical health encompasses good nutrition, proper exercise, and adequate sleep.
- An important piece of intellectual health is adequate financial planning. Now is the time to begin saving.
- To stay healthy, you must make a conscious decision to maintain each of the six elements of health.
- Establishing short-term, intermediate, and long-term goals will shape your career.

KEY TERMS

401K
anger
certification
clinical ladders
competency
emotional health
health
intellectual health
money market account
physical health
professional health
Roth IRA
social health
spiritual health

REVIEW QUESTIONS

1. Competency of professional nursing staff is identified by which of the following?
   A. Application of knowledge, skill, and decision making
   B. Graduation from an accredited nursing program
   C. Meeting required continuing-education requirements
   D. Promotion through a clinical ladder

2. Establishing professional goals is an example of which of the following?
   A. Aggression
   B. *Healthy People 2020* indicators
   C. Physical health
   D. Professional health

3. You have just seen a CNA wearing a gown, gloves, and mask entering the room of a patient who has recently tested positive for hepatitis B. You can demonstrate to the CNA your understanding of exposure risks by which of the following?
   A. Accompanying the CNA into the room wearing the same protective gear
   B. Explaining to the CNA that she need utilize only universal precautions
   C. Reviewing the infection control manual
   D. Waiting for the CNA to exit and observe the handwashing technique

4. Which of the following is an example of a physical agent that poses occupational hazards to nurses?
   A. Increased incidence of tuberculosis
   B. Latex glove exposure
   C. Manually lifting patients
   D. Workplace violence

5. Social support has been documented in the literature as being essential to health for which of the following reasons?
   A. Assists in weight reduction
   B. Encourages people to attend church
   C. Gives meaning to relationships
   D. Provides an opportunity to interact with others

6. Sleep deprivation has been shown by researchers to result in which of the following?
   A. Decrease in the amount of staff needed to work
   B. Increase in the quality of life of staff
   C. Increase in the risk of injury through medical errors
   D. Increase in the salaries of those who work long hours

7. Examples of activities promoting intellectual health include which of the following? Select all that apply.
   A. Becoming a member of an organization
   B. Drinking coffee
   C. Engaging in a hobby
   D. Reading books
   E. Getting five hours of sleep a night
   F. Snacking

8. Saving for retirement typically includes which of the following? Select all that apply.
   A. Individual retirement accounts
   B. Personal savings accounts
   C. The net worth of your assets
   D. Social Security funds
   E. Gifts from relatives
   F. Percentage of children's earnings

9. An irrational response or emotional response to stress can be defined as which of the following?
   A. Anger
   B. Assertiveness
   C. Disappointment
   D. Laughter

10. Which of the following is the highest risk activity causing nonfatal work-related injuries?
   A. Failure to wear protective gear
   B. Manually lifting patients
   C. Recapping needles
   D. Wearing latex gloves

REVIEW ACTIVITIES

1. Your best friend is getting married next month, and you are the maid of honor. You have already purchased a nonrefundable airline ticket to attend the bridal shower. You work in a very small intensive care unit. You have been working 10- and 12-hour shifts and are near exhaustion. Your head nurse calls you two days before you are to leave for the shower and asks you to work the weekend. One of the staff has been involved in a serious car accident, and there is no one else to work. What would you do?
2. You were recently hired on a nursing unit. What equipment and supplies do you need to protect yourself from occupational hazards?

3. Finally, you have graduated and moved to the city of your choice and are working at the health care facility of your choice. You are starting to apply all the knowledge and skills that you gained at school. You are around all types of nursing mentors and role models and are witnessing first-hand the activities of new and experienced staff nurses, as well as those of advanced practice nurses. Develop some SMART goals regarding where you will be one, three, five, or ten years from now.

EXPLORING THE WEB

- Calculate your BMI and determine your life expectancy and health risks at:
  http://www.healthstatus.com
- Try one of the following sites to retrieve information on dietary supplements, nutrition, and alternative medicine:
  http://www.mypyramid.gov
  http://www.nutritionsite.com
- Retirement Information Sites:
  Charles Schwab:
  http://www.schwab.com
  Click on Retirement Planning.
  Social Security:
  http://www.ssa.gov
  Fidelity Investments:
  http://www.fidelity.com
  Click on Retirement Center; then follow the different retirement options.
  Vanguard:
  http://www.vanguard.com
  Click on Personal Investors; then click on the Planning & Advice tab.
  Valueline:
  http://www.valueline.com
  Click on What's New? Retirement Planners.
  Morningstar:
  http://www.morningstar.com
  Click on Retirement.
- Resources for Violence Prevention:
  The ANA's Workplace Violence: Can You Close the Door? Call (800) 274–4ANA:
  http://www.nursingworld.org
  Guidelines for Preventing Workplace Violence for Healthcare and Social Service Workers.
  U.S. Department of Labor, OSHA 3148–1996, available online:
  http://www.osha-slc.gov
- Resources for Needlesticks:
  Safer Needle Devices: Protecting Health Care Workers:
  http://www.osha-slc.gov
  American Nurses Association:
  http://www.nursingworld.org

Centers for Disease Control and Prevention:
http://www.cdc.gov

- Resources for Latex Allergy:
  ANA's position paper on Latex Allergy:
  http://www.nursingworld.org
  or call (800) 274–4ANA
  OSHA:
  http://ww.osha-slc.gov
- Resource for Back Strain:
  Occupational Safety and Health Administration's ergonomics information:
  http://www.osha-slc.gov
  or call (202) 693–1999
- General Interest and Nursing Issues:
  Centers for Disease Control:
  http://www.cdc.gov
  National Institutes of Health:
  http://www.nih.gov
  National League for Nursing:
  http://www.nln.org
  ANA certification listing:
  http://www.nursingworld.org
  Center for Nursing:
  http://www.nursingcenter.com
  National Council of State Boards of Nursing:
  http://www.ncsbn.org
  General nursing interest site:
  http://www.allnurses.com
  Health care information:
  http://www.medscape.com
  http://www.docguide.com
- Specialty Issues:
  American Association of Nurse Anesthetists:
  http://www.aana.com
  Flight nursing:
  http://www.flightweb.com
  Small Business Administration:
  http://www.sbaonline.sba.gov
  Service Corps of Retired Executives:
  http://www.score.org
  Traveling nurses:
  http://www.springnet.com
  http://www.healthcareers-online.com

REFERENCES

American Association of Colleges of Nursing (AACN). (2012). Nursing shortage. Retrieved October 16, 2012, from http://www.aacn.nche.edu/media-relations/fact-sheets/nursing-shortage

American Board of Nursing Specialties (ABNS). (2009). A position statement on the value of specialty nursing certification. Retrieved August 9, 2011, from http://www.nursingcertification.org/about.html

American Nurses Association (ANA). (2000). Press release. Retrieved February 25, 2000, from http://www.ana.org

American Nurses Association (ANA). (2012). ANA handle with care campaign. Retrieved from http://www.nursingworld.org/rnnoharm

Bahadori, M. M., & Sadigh, G. G. (2010). Occupational exposure to blood and body fluids. *International Journal of Occupational & Environmental Medicine, 1*(1), 1–10.

Battaglia, C. (1996). *Murmurs.* Long Branch, NJ: Vista Publishing, p. 33.

Benner, P. (1984). *From novice to expert.* Menlo Park, CA: Addison-Wesley.

Berger, A. M., & Hobbs, B. B. (2006). Impact of shift work on the health and safety of nurses and patients. *Clinical Journal of Oncology Nursing, 10*(4), 465–471. doi:10.1188/06.CJON.465-471

Burket, T., Felmlee, M., Greider, P., Hippensteel, D., Rohrer, E., & Shay, M. (2010). Clinical ladder program evolution: Journey from novice to expert to enhancing outcomes. *Journal of Continuing Education in Nursing, 41*(8), 369–374. doi:10.3928/00220124-20100503-07

Centers for Disease Control and Prevention (CDC). (2011). Trends in tuberculosis—United States, 2010. *Morbidity and Mortality Weekly Report, 60*(11), 333–337.

Chittenden, E. H., & Ritchie, C. S. (2011). Work-Life balancing: Challenges and strategies. *Journal of Palliative Medicine, 14*(7), 870–874. doi:10.1089/jpm.2011.0095

Department of Government Affairs. (2006a). Health care worker safety. Retrieved January 30, 2006, from www.anapoliticalpower.org

Department of Government Affairs. (2006b). Safe patient handling and the OSHA ergonomics standard. Retrieved January 30, 2006, from http://www.anapoliticalpower.org

Dossey, B. M., & Keegan, L. (2009). *Holistic nursing: a handbook for practice* (5th ed.). Sudbury, MA: Jones and Bartlett Publishers.

Duke University Medical Center. (2009). Radiation safety considerations for nurses at Duke. Retrieved October 20, 2012, from http://www.safety.duke.edu/RadSafety/nurses/default.asp

Emotional Health Center. (2011). Retrieved october 20, 2012, from http://www.everydayhealth.com/emotional-health/index.aspx

Epstein, P. M., Burns, C., & Conlon, H. (2010). Substance abuse among registered nurses. *AAOHN Journal, 58*(12), 513–516. doi:10.3928/08910162-20101116-03

Franche, R., Murray, E., Ostry, A., Ratner, P., Wagner, S., & Harder, H. (2010). Work disability prevention in rural health care workers. *Rural and Remote Health, 10*(4), 1502.

Good, D., Yeganeh, B., & Yeganeh, R. (2010). Cognitive behavioral executive coaching. *Organizational Development Practitioner, 42*(3), 18–23.

Healthy People 2020 document. Retrieved October 20, 2012, from http://www.healthypeople.gov/LHI/lhiwhat.htm

Institute of Medicine. (2006). Sleep disorders and sleep deprivation: An unmet public health problem. H. R. Colten & B. M. Alteveogt (Eds.). Washington, DC: National Academies Press.

International Health Care Worker Safety Center (IHCWSC). (2006). Uniform needlestick and sharp injury report 58 hospitals, 2001. University of Virginia. Retrieved January 28, 2006, from http://www.healthsystem.virginia.edu/internet/epinet/soi01.cfm

Koenig, H. G. (2007). *Spirituality in patient care: Why, how, when, and what.* West Conshohocken, PA: Templeton Foundation Press.

Koren, M. E., & Christie-McAuliffe, C. (2012). Healthy living: Balancing personal and professional needs. In P. Kelly (Ed.), *Nursing leadership and management,* (3rd ed.). Clifton Park, NY: Delmar Cengage Learning.

Mayo Clinic Staff (Eds.). (2010, July 23). Stress relief from laughter: Yes, no joke. Mayo Foundation for Medical Education and Research. Retrieved October 20, 2012, from http://www. MayoClinic.com

McAllister, M., & McKinnon, J. (2009). The importance of teaching and learning resilience in the health disciplines: A critical review of the literature. *Nurse Educator Today, 29*(4), 371–379.

National Council of State Boards of Nursing (NCSBN). (2011). *Meeting the ongoing challenge of continued competency.* Retrieved September 9, 2011, from https://www.ncsbn.org/2900.htm

National Institutes of Health (NIH). (2012). Assessing your weight and health risk. Retrieved October 20, 2012, from http://www.nhlbi.nih.gov/health/public/heart/obesity/ lose_wt/risk.htm

National League for Nursing (NLN). (2010). NLN annual nursing data. Retrieved from http://www.nln.org

Nelson, A. L., Collins, J., Knibbe, H., Cookson, K., de Castro, A. B., Whipple, K. L. (2007, March). Safer patient handling. *Nursing Management,* 26–31.

Nightingale, F. (1969). *Notes on nursing*. New York, NY: Dover. (Original work published 1860.).

Occupational Safety and Health Administration (OSHA). (2011). Latex allergy. Retrieved October 10, 2011, from http://www.osha.gov/SLTC/latexallergy/index.html

Orman, S. (2010). Suze Orman's action plan: New rules for new times. New York, NY: Spiegel and Grau. Random House, Inc.

Pedrão, B., & Beresin, R. (2010). Nursing and spirituality. *Einstein, 8*(1), 86–91.

Rogers, A. (2008). The effects of fatigue and sleepiness on nurse performance and patient safety. In R. G. Hughes (Ed.). (2008). *Patient safety and quality: An evidence-based handbook for nurses* (Chapter 40). AHRQ Publication No. 08-0043, April 2008. Rockville, MD: Agency for Healthcare Research and Quality. Retrieved October 20, 2012, from http://www.ahrq.gov/qual/nurseshdbk

Rogers, B. (1997). Health hazards in nursing and health care: An overview. *American Journal of Infection Control, 25*(3), 248–261.

Segrin, C., & Passalacqua, S. (2010). Functions of loneliness, social support, health behaviors, and stress in association with poor health. *Health Communication, 25*(4), 312–322. doi:10.1080/10410231003773334

Smith, M., Kemp, G., & Segal, J. (2010). Laughter is the best medicine. Retrieved October 20, 2012, from http://www.helpguide .org/life/humor_laughter

Thomas, M., Benbow, D., & Ayars, V. (2010). Continued competency and board regulation: One state expands options. *Journal of Continuing Education in Nursing, 41*(11), 524–528. doi:10.3928/00220124-20100701-04

Ulmer, B. (2008). The hazards of surgical smoke. *AORN Journal, 87*(4), 721–738.

University of Toledo. (2011). SMART goal setting. Retrieved August 10, 2011, from http://www.utoledo .edu/call/CLP/PDFs/smartgoals.htm

U.S. Bureau of Labor Statistics. (2009). Occupational employment and wages, May 2009, 29-1111 registered nurses. Retrieved October 20, 2012, from http://www.bls.gov/oes/current/oes291111.htm

U.S. Bureau of Labor Statistics. (2010). Injuries and illnesses. Retrieved October 20, 2012, from www.bls.gov/iif

U.S. Department of Health and Human Services. (2001). Healthy people 2010: Goals. Retrieved January 2, 2002, from http://www.healthypeople.gov

Waters, T. R. (2007, August). When is it safe to manually lift a patient? *American Journal of Nursing, 107*(8), 53–59.

Wiesen, G. (2011). What is social health? Retrieved October 20, 2012, from http://www.wisegeek.com/what-is-social-health.htm

World Health Organization (WHO). (1946). Preamble to the constitution of the world health organization. Retrieved from http:www.who.int/about/definition/en/print.html

SUGGESTED READINGS

American Nurses Association. (2006). Preventing back injuries: Safe patient handling and movement. Retrieved from http://www.nursingworld.org.

Carta, A., Parmigiani, F., Roversi, A., Rossato, R., Milinic, C., Parrinello, G., & Porru, S. (2010). Training in safer and healthier patient-handling techniques. *British Journal of Nursing (BJN), 19*(9), 576–582.

Centers for Disease Control and Prevention (CDC). (2006). Guidelines for preventing the transmission of Mycobacterium tuberculosis in health care settings. Retrieved January 20, 2006, from http://www.cdc.gov

Certification is an important part of nurse education, career growth. (2010). *American Nurse, 42*(2), 6.

Donner, G., & Wheeler, M. (2011).When it's time to expand your circle. *Canadian Nurse, 107*(7), 38.

Edlin, G., & Golanty, E. (2010). Health & wellness. Retrieved October 20, 2012, from http://health.jbpub.com/hwonline/10e/self_assessments.cfm?chapter=7&step=2

Ersoy-Kart, M. (2009). Relations among social support, burnout, and experiences of anger: An investigation among emergency nurses. *Nursing Forum, 44*(3), 165–174. doi:10.1111/j.1744-6198.2009.00139.x

Hawkins, R., & Nezat, G. (2009). Doctoral education: Which degree to pursue? *American Association of Nurse Anesthetists Journal, 77*(2), 92–96.

Hunt, L. (2005). Sit-down comedy. Meet Ivy Push, nursing's funny girl. *American Journal of Nursing, 105*(7), 110–111.

Institute of Medicine (IOM). (2006). *Keeping patients safe: Transforming the work environment of nurses.* Retrieved August 21, 2006, from http://www.iom.edu/Default.aspx?id=16173

Laughing it off. (2008). Retrieved October 20, 2012, from http://www.asrn.org/journal-nursing-today/358-laughing-it-off.html

National Institutes of Health (NIH). Body mass index calculator. Retrieved January 2, 2012, from http://www.nhlbisupport.com/bmi

Nurses earn more with specialty certification. (2011). *AACN Bold Voices, 3*(9), 5.

Occupational Safety and Health Administration (OSHA). (2003). Guidelines for nursing homes: Ergonomics for the prevention of musculoskeletal disorders. Retrieved October 20, 2012, from http://www.osha.gov/ergonomics

Paniagua, H. (2010). Reviewing the concept of advanced nurse practice. *Practice Nursing, 21*(7), 371–375.

Patient care ergonomics resource guide: Safe patient handling and movement, VA Hospital, Tampa, FL, and Department of Defense, 2001. Revised June 28, 2010. Retrieved October 20, 2012, from http://www.visn8.med.va.gov/patientsafetycenter/safePTHandling

Raines, C., & Taglaireni, M. (2008). Career pathways in nursing: Entry points and academic progression. *Online Journal of Issues in Nursing, 13*(3).

Sabo, B. (2011). Reflecting on the concept of compassion fatigue. *The Online Journal of Issues in Nursing, 16*(1). doi: 10.3912/OJIN.Vol16No01Man01

Seaward, B. L. (2009). *Managing stress: Principles and strategies for health and well-being.* Burlington, MA: Jones & Bartlett Learning.

GLOSSARY

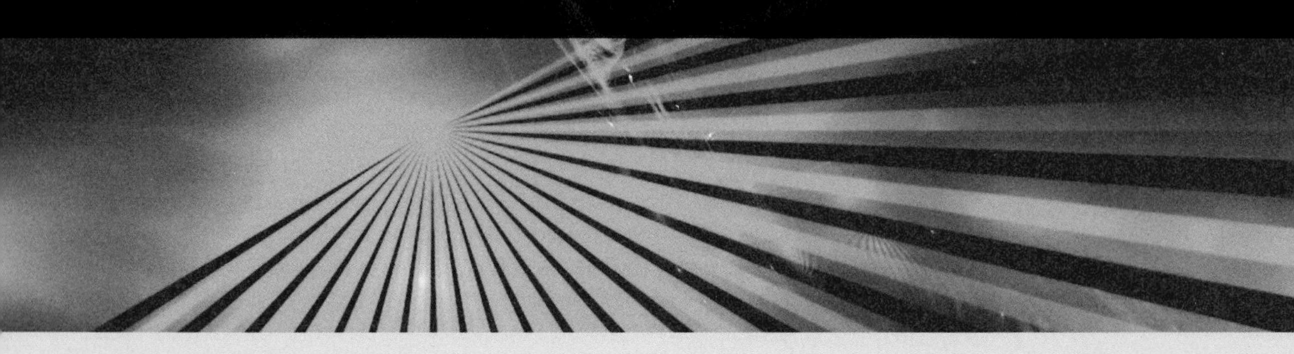

360-degree performance feedback A performance evaluation feedback system in which an individual is assessed by a variety of people in order to provide a broader perspective about his or her performance.

401K A retirement savings account that both employee and for-profit employer contribute to.

A

accountability Being responsible and answerable for the actions or inactions of self (or others in the context of delegation).

accounting An activity that managers engage in to record and report financial transactions and data.

activity log A time management technique to assist in determining how both personal and professional time is used by periodically recording activities.

administrative law A body of law created by administrative agencies in the form of rules, regulations, orders, and decisions that protect the rights of citizens.

anger A universal, strong feeling of displeasure that is often precipitated by a situation that frustrates or prevents a person from attaining a goal or getting what is wanted from life.

assault The offer to touch or the threat of touching another in an offensive manner without that person's permission.

assignment The distribution of work that each staff member is to accomplish during a given period.

authority The right or ability to delegate or direct the actions of others.

autocratic leadership A centralized decision-making style in which the leader makes decisions and uses power to command and control others.

autonomy An individual's right to self-determination and individual liberty.

B

balanced scorecards Balanced scorecards are used to monitor and report customer perspectives; financial perspectives; internal processes and human resources; and learning and growth for strategic management and as a way to examine performance throughout the organization.

battery The touching of another person without that person's consent.

benchmarking A continuous process of measuring products, services, and practices against the toughest competitors or those customers recognized as industry leaders.

beneficence The duty to do good to others and to maintain a balance between benefits and harms.

budget A plan that provides formal quantitative expression for acquiring and distributing funds over the ensuing time period (generally one year).

C

capital budget Accounts for the purchase of major new or replacement equipment.

case management A strategy to improve patient care and reduce hospital costs through coordination of care.

certification A process by which a nongovernmental agency or association asserts that an individual licensed to practice a profession has met certain predetermined standards specified by that profession for practice.

change Making something different from what it was.

change agent One who is responsible for implementation of a change project.

civil law That body of law that governs how individuals relate to each other in everyday matters.

clinical ladders A promotional model that acknowledges that staff members have varying skill sets based on their education and experience, and may be rewarded differently and may carry differing responsibilities.

clinical pathways A care management tool that outlines the expected clinical course and outcomes for a specific patient type.

coercive power Power that comes with the ability to punish others to influence them to change their behavior.

collective bargaining A group working with management to achieve what the group desires.

common law The body of law that develops from precedents set by judicial decisions that, over time, have the force of law, as distinguished from legislative enactments.

communication Communication is an interactive process that occurs when a person (the sender) sends a verbal or nonverbal message to another person (the receiver) and receives feedback.

compassion A deep awareness of the suffering of another along with the desire to relieve it.

competence The ability of a person to act with and integrate the knowledge, skills, values, attitudes, abilities, and professional judgment that underpin effective, quality service; it is required to practice safely and ethically in a designated role and setting.

competency The application of current knowledge and the interpersonal, decision-making and psychomotor skills expected to provide safe and effective care.

confidentiality Keeping information private and undisclosed.

conflict A disagreement about something of importance to each person involved.

connection power A strength that comes from the extent to which persons are connected with others having power.

consensus A situation in which all group members agree to live with and support a decision, regardless of whether they totally agree.

consideration The dimension of consideration involves activities that focus on the employee and emphasize relating and getting along with people.

constitution A set of basic laws that specifies the powers of the various segments of a government and how these segments relate to each other.

construction budget A budget that is developed when renovations or new structures are planned.

contingency theory A leadership theory that acknowledges that other factors in the environment influence outcomes as much as leadership style and that leader effectiveness is contingent upon or depends upon something in addition to the leader's behavior.

contract law Rules that regulate certain transactions between individuals and/or legal entities such as businesses.

co-payments A fixed health care fee paid by the patient to the health care provider at the time of service; this amount is paid in addition to the money the health care provider will receive from the insurance company.

core measures A grouping of Joint Commission–required quality measures established using evidence-based practice that reflect the quality of care delivery to a patient population.

cost centers A nursing or hospital unit, department, or section commonly used for organizational purposes to track financial data.

cost shifting The practice of cost shifting, whereby health care providers raise prices for the privately insured to offset the lower health care payments from both Medicare and Medicaid as well as the often nonpayment of health care premiums from the uninsured, continues to raise the cost of health care.

criminal law A branch of law that focuses on the actions of individuals that can intentionally do harm to others.

critical thinking Actively thinking about your thinking while you are thinking in order to provide deeper insight about what you are thinking about.

culturally competent care Care that intgrates knowledge, skills and attitudes that enhance cross-cultural communication and appropriate interactions.

culture Patterns of thought and action contributing to a group's social and physical survival.

culture of safety The culture that is the result of shared values and behaviors that demonstrate communications based on mutual trust, agreement on the importance of safety, and confidence in the ability to prevent errors through the use of known safety practices.

culture shock The reaction when the values and beliefs upheld by a person's new culture are radically different from those of the person's native culture.

customers Everyone internal or external to the organization who receives the product or service of the workers.

D

dashboard A documentation tool providing a snapshot image of pertinent quality information and activity reflecting a point in time.

decision making Considering and selectiong interventions from many possibilities to achieve a desired outcome.

deductibles A predetermined out-of-pocket fee paid by a patient for health care services before reimbursement through health insurance begins to be paid.

defamation An intentionally false communication either published or publicly spoken.

delegation The transfer of responsibility for the performance of a task from one individual to another while retaining accountability for the outcome.

democratic leadership A style in which participation is encouraged and authority is delegated to others.

diagnostic-related groups (DRGs) A federal government–established payment system for hospitals based on diagnosis.

direct care The time spent providing hands-on care to patients.

direct expenses Direct expenses are those expenses directly associated with the patient, such as medical and surgical supplies, wages, and drugs.

disaster An incident where human suffering and needs cannot be managed or alleviated by the victims without assistance and that requires extraordinary efforts beyond those needed for everyday emergencies.

discernment The possession of acuteness of judgment.

E

economics Economics is the study of how scarce resources are allocated among possible uses in order to make appropriate choices among the increasingly scarce resources.

emotional health The healthy expression of emotions or feelings about an event.

emotional intelligence Emotional intelligence is a component of leadership and refers to the capacity for recognizing your own feelings and those of others, for motivating yourself, and for managing emotions well in yourself and in your relationships.

employee-centered leadership A style with a focus on the human needs of subordinates.

ethical dilemma A conflict between two or more ethical principles for which there is no obviously correct decision.

ethics The branch of philosophy that concerns the distinction between right from wrong on the basis of a body of knowledge, not just on the basis of opinions.

evidence-based practice (EBP) A problem-solving approach to clinical decision making that integrates the best available scientific evidence with the best available experiential (patient and practitioner) evidence.

expert power power derivied from the knowledge and skills nurses possess. The more proficient and knowledgable a nurse is, the more they are percieved as an expert.

F

false imprisonment Imprisonment that occurs when people are incorrectly led to believe they cannot leave a place.

fee for service Payment of a fee for delivery of a health care service.

fidelity The principle of keeping a promise; the duty to keep one's promise or word.

fixed costs Fixed costs are those expenses that are constant and are not related to productivity or volume.

focus groups A small group of individuals selected because of a common characteristic who meet in a group and respond to questions about a topic in which they have interest or expertise.

formal leadership A leadership role in which a person is in a position of authority or in a sanctioned role within an organization that connotes influence.

full-time equivalent The measure of the work-time commitment of a full-time employee.

functional nursing A care delivery model that divides nursing work into functional roles that are then assigned to individual team members.

G

generation A group that shares birth years, age, location, and significant life events.

goal A specific aim or target that a unit wishes to attain within a specified time span.

Good Samaritan laws The laws that have been enacted to protect the health care professional from legal liability for actions rendered in an emergency when the professional is giving service without pay.

grapevine The grapevine is an informal avenue in which rumors circulate.

gross domestic product (GDP) The economic measure of a country's national income and output within a year that reflects the market value of goods and services produced within the country within that year.

group process The stages that a group progresses through as it matures, consisting of the following: forming, storming, norming, performing, and adjourning.

H

health A state of complete physical, social, and mental well-being, and not merely the absence of disease or infirmity.

health care disparities The persistent inequalities between the health outcomes of people in one group versus another group, due to such variables as gender, sexuality, age, ethnicity, socioeconomic group, lifestyle, and/or health care access.

high reliability organization High reliability organizations create a culture and work processes that radically reduce system failures and effectively respond when failures do occur, thus helping to achieve safety, quality, and efficiency goals.

I

indirect care The activities that support patient care but are not done directly to the patient.

indirect expenses Indirect expenses are expenses for items such as utilities—gas, electric, and phones—that are not directly related to patient care but are necessary to support care.

informal leadership An informal leader is an individual who demonstrates leadership outside the scope of a formal leadership role, such as a member of a group rather than the head or leader of the group.

information power The power persons have who influence others through the knowledge they provide to the group.

initiating structure Initiating structure involves an emphasis on the work to be done, a focus on the task and production.

innovation The process of creating new services or products.

inpatient unit A hospital unit that provides care to patients in a hospital 24 hours a day, 7 days a week.

integrity The firm adherence to a code of conduct or an ethical value.

intellectual health The element of health that encompasses those activities that maintain intellectual curiosity.

intuitive thinking A "gut" feeling regarding a situation based on prior experiences.

J

job-centered leaders Job-centered leaders are seen as less effective because of their focus on schedules, cost, and efficiency, resulting in a lack of attention to developing work groups and high performance goals.

justice The principle of fairness that is served when an individual is given that which he or she is due, owed, deserves, or can legitimately claim.

K

knowledge workers Workers who are involved in serving others through their special knowledge.

L

laissez-faire leadership A passive and permissive leadership style in which the leader defers decision making.

leader-member relations Leader-member relations are the feelings and attitudes of followers regarding acceptance, trust, and credibility of the leader.

leadership A process of influence whereby the leader influences others toward goal achievement.

learning organization theory A theory based on five learning disciplines (personal mastery, mental models, shared vision, team learning, and systems thinking) that demonstrate responsiveness and flexibility.

legitimate power The power derived from the position a person holds in a group; it indicates the person's degree of authority.

living will A document voluntarily signed by patients that specifies the type of care they desire if and when they are in a terminal state and cannot sign a consent form or convey this information verbally.

length of stay (LOS) The average number of days a patient is hospitalized from day of admission to day of discharge.

M

magnet hospital A health care organization that has met the rigorous nursing excellence requirements of the American Nurses Credentialing Center (ANCC), a division of the American Nurses Association (ANA).

malpractice A professional's wrongful conduct in discharge of professional duties or failure to meet standards of care for the profession, which results in harm to an individual entrusted to the professional's care.

management The process of planning, organizing, coordinating, and controlling resources and staff to achieve organizational goals.

margin Not for-profit organizations desiring a purer image than the term "profit" engenders refer to their profit as a contribution to margin, with the rule of thumb being to secure 4 to 5 percent of the total budget as profit or margin.

marginalization The separation of some cultural groups away from the mainstream.

medical preparedness The ability of the health care system to prevent, protect against, quickly respond to, and recover from health emergencies, particularly those whose scale, timing, or unpredictability threaten to overwhelm routine capabilities.

mission statement A formal expression of the purpose or reason for existence of an organization.

modular nursing A care delivery model that divides a geographical space into modules of patients, with each module having a team led by an RN to care for its patients.

money market account A type of bank checking account, though it often requires a larger minimum amount of money to open and often has a higher interest rate.

moral courage Acting when unsafe, illegal, or unethical practice occurs, even if the action is unpopular, or call for one to stand alone, in order to defend patients and maintain ethical standards of care.

morality Behavior in accordance with custom or tradition; usually reflects personal or religious beliefs.

motivation Whatever influences one's choices and creates direction, intensity, and persistence in one's behavior.

N

negligence Failure to provide the care a reasonable person would ordinarily provide in a similar situation.

never events Preventable, serious events that should never occur in a hospital; they include items such as patient incidence of pressure ulcers, surgery on the wrong leg, etc.

nonmaleficence The principle of doing no harm.

nonproductive hours Paid time not devoted to patient care; it includes benefit time such as vacation, sick time, and education time.

nursing care delivery model A method to organize the work of caring for patients.

nursing hours per patient day (NHPPD) The amount of nursing care required per patient in a 24 hour period based on standards such as past unit needs or national benchmarks.

nursing informatics The integration of nursing, its information, and information management with information-processing and communication technology to support the health of people worldwide.

nursing-sensitive indicators Nursing sensitive indicators reflect the structure, process and outcomes of nursing care. The structure of nursing care is indicated by the supply of nursing staff, the skill level of the nursing staff, and the education/certification of nursing staff. Process indicators measure aspects of nursing care such as assessment, intervention, and RN job satisfaction. Patient outcomes that are determined to be nursing sensitive are those that improve if there is a greater quantity or quality of nursing care (e.g., pressure ulcers, falls, and intravenous infiltrations). (American Nurses Association, 2012).

O

operational budget Accounts for the income and expenses associated with day-to-day activity within a department or organization.

organizational power The power acquired and exercised through formal and informal roles in the workplace and the health care system.

outcome The outcome component of health care refers to the results of good care delivery achieved by using quality structures and quality processes and includes the achievement of outcomes such as patient satisfaction, good health and functional ability, and the absence of health care-acquired infections and morbidity.

P

Pareto Principle The principle developed by Pareto, a 19th-century economist, that states that 20% of focused effort results in 80% of results, or conversely, that 80% of unfocused effort results in 20% of results.

patient acuity The measure of nursing workload that is generated for each patient based on the patient's needs.

patient-centered care A patient care delivery model in which care and services are brought to the patient.

patient classification system (PCS) A system for identifying different patients based on their acuity, functional ability, or resource needs.

patient-focused care A model of differentiated nursing practice that emphasizes quality, cost, and value.

personal power The power an individual acquires and exercises through informal and formal roles in the family and community.

philosophy A statement of beliefs based on core values; rational investigations of the truth and principles of knowledge, reality, and human conduct.

physical health Encompasses nutrition, exercise, a balanced amount of rest, health preventive measures, and health-screening behaviors to detect problems early.

politics The process by which people use a variety of methods to achieve their goals.

population-based health care practice Population-based health care practice is the development, provision, and evaluation of inter-professional health care services to population groups experiencing increased health risks or disparities.

position power Position power is the degree of formal authority and influence associated with the leader.

power The ability to create, get, and use resources to achieve one's goals.

power of attorney A legal document executed by an individual (principal) granting another person (agent) the right to perform certain activities in the principal's name.

pre-authorization An approval obtained from the insurance company before care or treatment such as hospitalization or diagnostic testing is initiated if such services are to be reimbursed by the patient's health insurance plan.

primary nursing A care delivery model that clearly delineates the responsibility and accountability of the RN and reinforces the RN as the primary provider of nursing care to patients.

problem solving An active a process that starts with a problem and ends with a solution.

process The process component of health care includes the quality activities, procedures, tasks, communications, and processes performed within the health care structures, such as hospital admissions, surgical.

productive hours The hours worked by staff and available for patient care.

professional health A satisfaction with personal career choices and continued opportunities for growth.

professional power The power acquired and exercised through a formal role in a profession.

profit The measurement of the relationship of income to expenses and results when income is higher than expenses.

public health preparedness Public health preparedness is the ability of the public health system, community, and individuals to prevent, protect against, quickly respond to, and recover from health emergencies, particularly those in which scale, timing, or unpredictability threaten to overwhelm routine capabilities.

public law A general classification of law, consisting usually of constitutional, administrative, and criminal law; public law defines a citizen's relationship to the government.

Q

quality Quality is defined by the Institute of Medicine (1990) as "the degree to which health services for individuals and populations increase the likelihood of health outcomes and are consistent with current professional knowledge".

quality improvement A management philosophy to improve the organizational structure and the level of performance of key processes in the organization to achieve high-quality outcomes.

R

race A geographical or global segment of a human population as distinguished by genetic traits and physical characteristics.

referent power The power derived from how much others respect and like any individual, group, or organization.

reflective thinking Observing or thnking back about a task or decision made in a sitution to help in future tasks or decisions.

respect for others The acknowledgment of the right of people to make their own decisions.

responsibility The obligation to accomplish a task or duty.

résumé A brief summary of a person's background, training, and experience, as well as their qualifications for a position.

revenue Revenue is income generated through a variety of means, including billable patient services, investments, and donations to the organization.

reward power The power to reward others.

Roth IRA An individual retirement account that allows one to set aside after-tax income up to a specified amount each year.

S

self-scheduling The process in which unit staff take leadership in creating and monitoring the work schedule while working within defined guidelines.

shared governance An organizational framework grounded in a philosophy of decentralized leadership that fosters autonomous decision making and professional nursing practice.

skill mix The percentage of RN staff to other direct care staff, LPNs, and NAP.

social health The ability to relate to and interact with others.

sources of power A combination of conscious and unconscious factors that allow an individual to influence others to do as the individual wants.

spiritual distress A condition in which an individual has an impaired ability to integrate meaning and purpose in life through the individual's connectedness with self, others, art, music, literature, nature, or a power greater than self.

spiritual health The human capacity to find strength from within; results from a connection with a higher being or power.

staffing pattern A plan that articulates how many and what kind of staff are needed by shift and day to staff a unit or department.

stakeholder assessment A systematic consideration of all potential stakeholders' needs to assure that these are considered for incorporation into the planning phase of a program, project, or quality initiative.

structure The structure component of health care includes resources or structures needed to deliver quality health care, for example, human and physical resources, such as nurses and nursing and medical practitioners; hospital buildings; medical records; and pharmaceuticals.

substitutes for leadership Substitutes for leadership are variables that may influence followers to the same extent as the leader's behavior.

supervision The provision of guidance or direction, oversight, evaluation, and follow-up by the person in charge for the accomplishment of a delegated task by assistive personnel.

T

task structure Task structure refers to the degree to which work is defined, with specific procedures, explicit directions, and goals.

team nursing A care delivery model that assigns staff to teams that are then responsible for a group of patients.

time management A set of related, common-sense skills that help a person use time in the most effective and productive way possible.

tort A civil wrong for which a remedy may be obtained.

total patient care A care delivery model in which nurses are responsible for the total nursing care for their patient assignment for the shift they are working.

transactional leader The traditional manager, concerned with day-to-day operations, is called the transactional leader.

trustworthiness The quality existing in a person when trust is well founded or deserving.

U

units of service A measure of patient encounters to help in determining nursing workload.

universal health care (UHC) A government-sponsored system that ensures health care coverage for all eligible residents of a nation regardless of income level or employment status.

V

values Personal belief about the truth of ideals, standards, principles, objects, and behaviors that gives meaning and direction to life.

values clarification The process of analyzing one's own values to better understand what is truly important.

variable costs Variable costs fluctuate depending upon the volume or census and types of care required.

variance The difference between what was budgeted and the actual cost.

veracity The obligation to tell the truth.

W

workplace advocacy Activities that persons undertake to address problems in their everyday workplace setting.

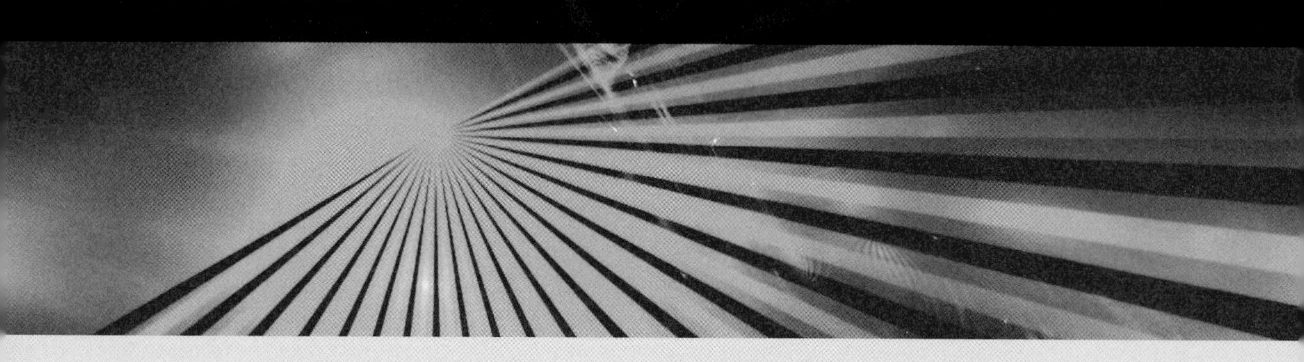

INDEX

D

E

O

P

Q

R

U

V